Contemporary Nursing

Issues, Trends, & Management

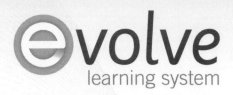
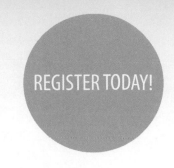

Edition
5

Contemporary Nursing

Issues, Trends, & Management

Barbara Cherry, DNSc, MBA, RN, NEA-BC
Department Chair for Leadership Studies and Associate Professor
Texas Tech University Health Sciences Center
School of Nursing
Lubbock, Texas

Susan R. Jacob, PhD, MSN, RN
Executive Associate Dean and Professor
The University of Tennessee Health Science Center
College of Nursing
Memphis, Tennessee

ELSEVIER
MOSBY

ELSEVIER
MOSBY

3251 Riverport Lane
St. Louis, Missouri 63043

CONTEMPORARY NURSING: ISSUES, TRENDS, AND MANAGEMENT, ed 5   9780323069533
Copyright 2011 by Mosby, Inc., an affiliate of Elsevier Inc.

Notice

Knowledge and best practice in this field are constantly changing. As new research and experience broaden our understanding, changes in research methods, professional practices, or medical treatment may become necessary.

Practitioners and researchers must always rely on their own experience and knowledge in evaluating and using any information, methods, compounds, or experiments described herein. In using such information or methods they should be mindful of their own safety and the safety of others, including parties for whom they have a professional responsibility.

With respect to any drug or pharmaceutical products identified, readers are advised to check the most current information provided (i) on procedures featured or (ii) by the manufacturer of each product to be administered, to verify the recommended dose or formula, the method and duration of administration, and contraindications. It is the responsibility of practitioners, relying on their own experience and knowledge of their patients, to make diagnoses, to determine dosages and the best treatment for each individual patient, and to take all appropriate safety precautions.

To the fullest extent of the law, neither the Publisher nor the authors, contributors, or editors assume any liability for any injury and/or damage to persons or property as a matter of product liability, negligence or otherwise, or from any use or operation of any methods, products, instructions, or ideas contained in the material herein.

Previous editions copyrighted 2008, 2005, 2002, 1999

Library of Congress Cataloging-in-Publication Data
Contemporary nursing : issues, trends, and management / [edited by]
Barbara Cherry, Susan R. Jacob. -- Ed. 5.
  p. ; cm.
  Includes bibliographical references.
  ISBN 978-0-323-06953-3 (pbk. : alk. paper) 1. Nursing. I. Cherry,
Barbara, MSN. II. Jacob, Susan R.
  [DNLM: 1. Nursing--United States. 2. Nursing Care--United States.
WY 100 AA1 C761 2011]
  RT41.C564 2011
  610.73--dc22

2010022009

Executive Editor: Darlene Como
Acquisitions Editor: Maureen Iannuzzi
Senior Developmental Editor: Robin Levin Richman
Publishing Services Manager: Jeff Patterson
Project Manager: Jeanne Genz
Design Direction: Andrea Lutes

Printed in the United States

Last digit is the print number: 9   8   7   6   5   4   3   2   1

To all the student nurses whose curiosity and enthusiasm for nursing created the inspiration to develop this text and to all practicing nurses who face serious challenges but reap great rewards for providing high-quality patient care

Being a Nurse Means . . .

You will never be bored,
You will always be frustrated,
You will be surrounded by challenges,
So much to do and so little time.
You will carry immense responsibility
And very little authority.
You will step into peoples lives,
And you will make a difference.
Some will bless you.
Some will curse you.
You will see people at their worst,
And at their best.
You will never cease to be amazed at peoples capacity
For love, courage, and endurance.
You will see life begin
and end.
You will experience resounding triumphs
And devastating failures.
You will cry a lot.
You will laugh a lot.
You will know what it is to be human
And to be humane.

Melodie Chenevert, RN

Contributors

L. Antoinette (Toni) Bargagliotti, DNSc, RN, ANEF
Professor
Loewenberg School of Nursing
University of Memphis
Memphis, Tennessee

Virginia Trotter Betts, MSN, JD, RN, FAAN
Commissioner of Tennessee Department of Mental Health and Developmental Disabilities
Tennessee Department of Mental Health
Nashville, Tennessee

Barbara Cherry, DNSc, MBA, RN, NEA-BC
Department Chair for Leadership Studies and Associate Professor
Texas Tech University Health Sciences Center
School of Nursing
Lubbock, Texas

Genevieve Conlin, MS, MBA, MEd, RN, NEA-BC
Patient Access Team Leader
Partners Health System, Inc.
Charlestown, Massachusetts

Charlotte Eliopoulos, PhD, RN, MPH, ND
Author, Speaker, Specialist: Holistic Long-Term and Gerontologic Care
Health Education Network
Glen Arm, Maryland

Debra D. Hatmaker, PhD, RN-BC, SANE-A
Chief Programs Officer
Georgia Nurses Association
Southern Performance Assessment Center
Atlanta, Georgia

Rodney (Rod) W. Hicks, PhD, RN, FNP-BC, FAANP, FAAN
Lubbock, Texas

Susan R. Jacob, PhD, MSN, RN
Executive Associate Dean and Professor
The University of Tennessee Health Science Center
College of Nursing
Memphis, Tennessee

Marylane Wade Koch, MSN, RN, CNAA, CPHQ
Adjunct Faculty
Loewenberg School of Nursing
The University of Memphis
Memphis, Tennessee

Robert W. Koch, DNS, RN
Associate Dean—Graduate Studies
Loewenberg School of Nursing
The University of Memphis
Memphis, Tennessee

Carrie B. Lenburg, EdD, RN, FAAN, ANEF
President and Consultant
Creative Learning and Assessment Systems, Inc.
Roan Mountain, Tennessee

Laura R. Mahlmeister, PhD, RN
President, Mahlmeister and Associates
Belmont, California
Clinical Professor of Nursing
University of California, San Francisco
Staff Nurse, Birth Center
San Francisco General Hospital
San Francisco, California

Linda D. Norman, DSN, RN, FAAN
Professor of Nursing
Senior Associate Dean
School of Nursing
Vanderbilt University
Nashville, Tennessee

Tommie L. Norris, DNS, RN
Director Professional Entry Program and Associate
    Professor
College of Nursing
The University of Tennessee Health Science Center
Memphis, Tennessee

Patricia Reid Ponte, DNSc, RN, FAAN, NEA-BC
Senior Vice President for Patient Care Services
Chief of Nursing
Dana-Farber Cancer Institute
Director, Oncology Nursing & Clinical Services
Brigham and Women's Hospital
Boston, Massachusetts

Carolyn Roe, MSM, BSN
Permanent Solutions Labor Consultants
Riverview, Michigan

Cynthia K. Russell, PhD, APN
Professor, Acute and Chronic Care Department
Assistant Vice Chancellor, Faculty Administration
The University of Tennessee Health Science Center
College of Nursing
Memphis, Tennessee

Anna Marie Sallee, PhD, MSN, RN, CCRN
Assistant Professor
College of Nursing
Prairie View A & M University
Houston, Texas

Carla D. Sanderson, PhD, RN
Provost and Professor of Nursing
Union University
Jackson, Tennessee

Gwen Sherwood, PhD, RN, FAAN
Professor and Associate Dean
University of North Carolina at Chapel Hill School of
    Nursing
Chapel Hill, North Carolina

Margaret Elizabeth Strong, MSN, RN, CNA
Nurse Consultant
Memphis, Tennessee

Jill J. Webb, PhD, MSN, RN, CS
Professor
School of Nursing
Union University
Jackson, Tennessee

Elizabeth E. Weiner, PhD, RN, BC, FAAN
Senior Associate Dean for Informatics
School of Nursing
Vanderbilt University
Nashville, Tennessee

Kathleen M. Werner, MS, BSN, RN
Clinical Nurse Educator
Meriter Hospital
Madison, Wisconsin

Reviewers

Michael D. Aldridge, MSN, RN, CCRN, CNS
Clinical Instructor in Nursing
The University of Texas
School of Nursing
Austin, Texas

Marylee Bressie, MSN, RN, CCRN, CCNS, CEN
Instructor
Division of Nursing
Spring Hill College
Mobile, Alabama
PRN Critical Care Clinical Nurse Specialist
Providence Hospital
Mobile, Alabama

Sherri Denise Caldwell, RN, BSN, CEN
Chesapeake Regional Medical Center
Chesapeake, Virginia

Karen Clark, PhD, MSN, BSN, AD, CCRN
School of Nursing Baltimore
University of Maryland
Baltimore, Maryland

Margaret M. Dean, RN, CS-BC, GNP-BC, MSN
Instructor
Graduate Program
School of Nursing
Texas Tech University Health Sciences Center
Lubbock, Texas

Maurice H. Espinoza, RN, CNS, BSN, MSN, CCRN
University of California Irvine Medical Center
Orange, California

Joellen W. Hawkins, RN, PhD, WHNP-BC, FAAN, FAANP
Professor Emeritus
William F. Connell School of Nursing
Boston College
Chestnut Hill, Massachusetts

Patricia Hindin, PhD, CNM
Assistant Professor
School of Nursing
University of Medicine and Dentistry of New Jersey
Newark, New Jersey

Barbara Ann Konopka, RN, MSN, CCRN, CEN, CNE
Instructor
School of Nursing
Pennsylvania State University
Worthington Scranton
Dunmore, Pennsylvania

Mary Beth Flynn Makic, RN, PhD, CNS, CCNS, CCRN
Research Nurse Scientist, Critical Care
University of Colorado Hospital
Aurora, Colorado
Assistant Professor, Adjoint
College of Nursing
University of Colorado
Aurora, Colorado

Ruby J. Martinez, RN, PhD, PMHCNS-BC
Associate Professor Emeritus
College of Nursing
University of Colorado
Denver, Colorado

Arlene H. Morris, RN, MSN, EdD, CNE
Distinguished Teaching Associate Professor of
    Nursing
Auburn University
Montgomery, Alabama

Cherie R. Rebar, MSN, MBA, RN, FNP, PhD
Kettering College of Medical Arts
Kettering, Ohio

Mary Beth Reid, PhD, RN, CNS, CCRN, CEN
Kindred Healthcare
Arlington, Texas

Cheryl Christine Rodgers, PhD, CPNP, CPON
Pediatric Nurse Practitioner
Texas Childrens Cancer Center and Hematology
    Service
Houston, Texas
Clinical Instructor
Baylor College of Medicine
Houston, Texas

Mitchell J. Seal, EdD, MEd-IT, BSN, AS, RNBC
Lieutenant Commander
Nurse Corps
U.S. Navy
Naval School of Health Sciences
San Diego, California
Cerro Coso College
Ridgecrest, California

Susan Seiboldt, MSN, RN, CNE
Assistant Nursing Professor
Allied Health Department
Carl Sandburg College
Galesburg, Illinois

Joyce A. Shanty, MS, RN
Assistant Professor
Indiana University of Pennsylvania
Indiana, Pennsylvania

Sandra L. Siedlecki, PhD, RN, CNS
Assistant Professor
Ursuline College
Pepper Pike Ohio
Senior Nurse Researcher
Cleveland Clinic
Cleveland, Ohio

Erma Jean Smith-King, RN, MPH, MBA
Clinical Instructor
Department of Nursing
North Carolina Central University
Durham, North Carolina

Linda H. Snell, DNS, RN, WHNP-C
The College at Brockport
Brockport, New York

**Sharon Wallace Stark, PhD, RN, ANP-BC, GNP-
    BC, CFN**
Monmouth University
West Long Branch, New Jersey

M. Terese Verklan, PhD, CCNS, RNC
School of Nursing
University of Texas Health Science Center at Houston
Houston, Texas

Gerry Walker, DHeD, MSN, RN
Park University
Parkville, Missouri

Mary A. Wcisel, RN, MSN
Associate Professor of Nursing
Saint Marys College
Notre Dame, Indiana

**Barbara Weintraub, RN, MSN, MPH, APN, CEN,
    FAEN**
Director
Adult and Pediatric Emergency and Trauma Services
Northwest Community Hospital
Arlington Heights, Illinois

Susan A. Weitzel, RN, MN
New Mexico State University
Alamogordo, New Mexico

Preface

At no other time in the history of modern nursing have nurses been presented with such tremendous opportunities to improve health care and advance the nursing profession. By understanding and providing leadership to address the very serious issues currently facing the U.S. health care system, nurses can advance health care delivery to promote the health and well-being of each individual in our society. These important issues include patient safety and quality care, health care reform and the uninsured population, the nursing shortage, advancing technology, changing legal and ethical concerns, evolving nursing education trends, rising health care costs, and working within a multicultural society.

WHO WILL BENEFIT FROM THIS BOOK?

The fifth edition of *Contemporary Nursing: Issues, Trends, & Management* is an excellent resource to help nursing students and practicing nurses understand these very complex issues and implement strategies from the direct patient care level to the national legislative arena that can significantly improve patient care, the health care system, and the nursing profession. The American Association of Colleges of Nursing (AACN) (2008) *Essentials of Baccalaureate Education* is reflected throughout this text. A valuable and useful table that maps the *BSN Essentials* to the chapter content is located on page xvii.

ORGANIZATION
Unit One: The Development of Nursing

The book opens with a presentation about the exciting evolution of nursing, its very visible public image, and its core foundations, which include nursing education, licensure and certification, nursing theory, and nursing research and evidence-based practice. These opening chapters provide the reader with a solid background for understanding and studying current and future trends.

Unit Two: Current Issues in Health Care

This unit provides a comprehensive overview of the most current trends and issues occurring today in nursing and health care, including health care financing and economics, legal and ethical issues, cultural and social issues, complementary and alternative healing, workplace issues and the nursing shortage, collective bargaining and unions, technology in the clinical setting, and emergency preparedness. Students, faculty, and veteran nurses will be challenged to critically examine each of these significant issues that are shaping the practice of professional nursing and the health care delivery system.

Unit Three: Leadership and Management in Nursing

This unit offers a foundation of knowledge in nursing leadership and management, with a focus on the basic skills that are necessary for nurses to function effectively in the professional nursing role. Chapters examine leadership and management theory and roles, budgeting basics, effective communication, delegation and supervision, staffing and nursing care delivery models, quality improvement and patient safety, quality and safety education in nursing, and health policy and politics. The updated content in this unit provides the most current information available related to nursing leadership and management and will serve as both a valuable educational tool for students and a very useful resource for practicing nurses.

Unit Four: Career Management

The final unit prepares the student to embark on a career in nursing. Making the transition from student to professional, managing time, understanding career opportunities, finding a good match between the nurse and the employer, and passing the NCLEX-RN examination are all presented with practical, useful advice that will serve as an excellent resource for both students and novice nurses as they build their careers in professional nursing.

LEARNING AIDS

Each chapter in the fifth edition contains the same features that made the previous editions so successful:

◆ Real-life **Vignettes** and **Questions to Consider** at the beginning of each chapter, which pique the readers interest in the chapter content and stimulate critical thinking
◆ **Key Terms** that contain clear and concise definitions of terms that are critical to enhance readers understanding of the topics and expand their vocabulary related to health care issues
◆ Integrated **Learning Outcomes** that provide instructors and students with a clear understanding of what behaviors can be expected after a study of the chapter is completed
◆ **Chapter Overview** is an overall perspective and guidelines to the chapter content
◆ **Case Studies,** included as appropriate, apply theory to clinical practice
◆ **Summary** at the end of each chapter provides a wrap-up and helps students focus on points to remember
◆ **References** related to chapter content help students explore further the issues that were covered
◆ **Helpful Websites and Online Resources** that are particularly relevant for further exploration of the topic are included at the back of selected chapters

NEW TO THIS EDITION

Every chapter in the fifth edition has been updated to include the most current and relevant information available. The following are new to this edition:

◆ **Two new chapters** reflect todays important focus on patient safety and quality improvement and the nurses work environment: Chapter 13: *Collective Bargaining and Unions in Todays Workplace* and Chapter 22: *Quality and Safety Education in Nursing.*
◆ **New Case Studies** for each chapter illustrate application to real-life scenarios
◆ **New and expanded content** on:
  ◆ Nursing shortage
  ◆ New technologies in health care, including point-of-care technology and information literacy

- Disaster planning for mass casualty events
- Collective bargaining and unions
- Patient safety and improving the quality of health care and nurses work environments
- Most current legal issues facing nurses
- 2010 NCLEX-RN Examination Test Plan

ANCILLARIES

The student and instructor resources for the fifth edition have been expanded to provide numerous activities to engage the students in active learning, both within and outside the classroom.

Student Resources

At the beginning and end of every chapter students are referred to the dedicated **Evolve website** for the book, http://evolve.elsevier.com/Cherry, where they can find additional online resources that provide them with the opportunity to become actively engaged in the learning process:

- **Student Learning Activities** cover the major content in the chapter with fill-in-the-blank, short answer, complete-the-chart, true-false exercises, and crossword puzzles.
- **Case Studies** bring the content alive with answers to help instructors facilitate discussion about the cases.
- **Critical Thinking Questions** and **Answer Scenarios** allow students to apply critical analysis to what theyve learned and to develop problem-solving skills.
- **Resumé Builder** offers templates and samples of resumés and cover letters.

Instructor Resources

On the same dedicated website, instructors will have access to all of the Student Resources as well as the following resources that are designed to engage the student in active learning within the classroom and provide instructors with excellent in-class and online teaching-learning activities:

- **PowerPoint** slides and **Audience Response** questions giving rationale and level of difficulty for each chapter
- **Test Bank** with NCLEX-RN-exam alternative-format questions and rationales and level of difficulty based on Blooms Taxonomy
- **Suggested Annotated Outlines** for lectures and discussion
- **Interactive Teaching-Learning Activities** for small-group problem solving and extra credit assignments
- **Questions** to guide in-class or online discussion
  All instructor resources are password-protected, so please contact your local sales representative for further details.

About the Authors

Barbara Cherry, DNSc, MBA, RN, NEA-BC, received her diploma in nursing from Methodist Hospital School of Nursing in 1973, her BSN from West Texas A&M University in 1980, her MBA from Texas Tech University in 1995, her MSN from Texas Tech University Health Sciences Center in 1997, and a Doctor of Nursing Science from the University of Tennessee Health Science Center in 2006. Dr. Cherrys clinical background is in critical care, medical-surgical, and nephrology nursing, and her research is focused on the long-term care nursing workforce and technology. She has more than 20 years clinical and nursing management experience and is currently Associate Professor and Department Chair for Leadership Studies at Texas Tech University Health Sciences Center School of Nursing in Lubbock, Texas.

Susan R. Jacob, PhD, MSN, RN, received her BSN from West Virginia University in 1970, her MSN from San Jose State University in 1975, and her PhD from the University of Tennessee, Memphis in 1993. Her extensive experience as a clinician, educator, and researcher has been focused in the community health arena, specifically home health and hospice. She has been an educator for more than 25 years and has taught at both the undergraduate and graduate levels. Dr. Jacobs research has addressed the bereavement experience of older adults and enhanced models of home health care delivery. Dr. Jacob is Executive Associate Dean and Professor in the College of Nursing at The University of Tennessee Health Science Center, Memphis, Tennessee.

Acknowledgments

Our contributors deserve our most sincere thanks for their high-quality timely work that demonstrates genuine expertise and professionalism. Their contributions have made this book a truly first-rate text that will be invaluable to nursing students and faculty and will serve as an outstanding resource for practicing nurses. We extend a special thanks to our reviewers who gave us helpful suggestions and insights as we developed the fifth edition.

We would like to express our grateful appreciation to the Elsevier staff—Maureen Iannuzzi, Acquisitions Editor, and Robin Levin Richman, Senior Developmental Editor—for their very capable and professional support, guidance, and calm reassurance.

Our deepest appreciation goes to the most important people in our lives—our husbands, Mike and Dick, our families, and our friends. Their enduring support and extreme patience have allowed us to accomplish what sometimes seemed to be the impossible.

How this Text Reflects the Essentials of Baccalaureate Education for Professional Nursing Practice

2008 BSN ESSENTIAL I: LIBERAL EDUCATION FOR BACCALAUREATE GENERALIST NURSING PRACTICE

Chapter 3: *The Influence of Contemporary Trends and Issues on Nursing Education*	• Integrate knowledge of 10 current trends and issues in society and health care into a more holistic perception of their influence on nursing, nursing education, students, faculty, and practitioners. • Integrate knowledge of current trends and issues into a personal contemporary philosophy of ongoing professional development and practice. • Differentiate among various types of conventional, mobility, and new nursing education programs and the issues associated with them. • Access and evaluate pertinent current information resources related to evolving trends and issues as a component of ongoing professional development.
Chapter 9: *Ethical and Bioethical Issues in Nursing and Health Care*	• Integrate basic concepts of human values that are essential for ethical decision making. • Analyze selected ethical theories and principles as a basis for ethical decision making. • Analyze the relationship between ethics and morality in relation to nursing practice. • Use an ethical decision-making model framework for resolving ethical problems in health care. • Apply the ethical decision-making process to specific ethical issues encountered in clinical practice.
Chapter 10: *Cultural Competency and Social Issues in Nursing and Health Care*	• Integrate knowledge of demographic and sociocultural variations into culturally competent professional nursing care. • Provide culturally competent care that incorporates variations in biologic characteristics, social organization, environmental control, communications, and other phenomena. • Critique education, practice, and research issues that influence culturally competent care. • Incorporate respect for differences in the beliefs and values of others as a critical component of nursing practice.

2008 BSN ESSENTIAL II: BASIC ORGANIZATIONAL AND SYSTEMS LEADERSHIP FOR QUALITY CARE AND PATIENT SAFETY

Chapter 12:
*Workforce Advocacy
and the Nursing
Shortage*

- Describe workforce advocacy as a means of improving the quality of health care delivery.
- Identify issues that are affecting the practice of professional nursing in the health care workplace.
- Identify available resources to assist in improving the workplace environment.
- Define the role of nurses in advocating for safe and effective workplace environments.
- Describe internal and external workplace strategies that support efficient and effective quality patient care.
- Identify unique opportunities within the organization to improve the work environment for nurses.

Chapter 13:
*Collective
Bargaining and
Unions in Todays
Workplace*

- Use terms associated with collective bargaining correctly in written and oral communications.
- Examine key events in the historical development of collective bargaining and unions.
- Recognize questionable labor or management practices in the workplace.
- Analyze collective bargaining as a method for achieving power sharing in the workplace.
- Evaluate current conflicts and controversies associated with collective bargaining by professional nurses.

Chapter 15:
*Emergency
Preparedness and
Response for Todays
World*

- Describe the interaction between local, state, and federal emergency response systems.
- Examine the roles of public and private agencies in preparing for and responding to a mass casualty event.
- Compare and contrast chemical, biologic, radiologic, nuclear, and explosive agents and treatment protocols.
- Access resources related to disaster preparedness on the Internet.
- Communicate effectively (using correct emergency preparedness terminology) with regard to a mass casualty incident.

Chapter 16: *Nursing
Leadership and
Management*

- Relate leadership and management theory to nursing leadership and management activities.
- Differentiate among the five functions of management and essential activities related to each function.
- Integrate principles of patient-centered care and customer service in professional nursing practice.
- Implement effective team-building skills as an essential component of nursing practice.
- Implement the nursing process as a method of problem solving and planning.
- Apply principles and strategies of change theory in the management role.
- Discuss implications of leadership and management challenges of the twenty-first century.

Chapter 20: *Staffing
and Nursing Care
Delivery Models*

- Outline key issues surrounding staffing for a health care organization.
- Evaluate lines of responsibility and accountability associated with various types of nursing care delivery models.
- Analyze the advantages and disadvantages of nursing care delivery models in relation to patient care in various settings.

- Integrate essential components of clinical pathways into patient care planning.
- Differentiate among several nursing care delivery models by evaluating their defining characteristics.
- Explain the purpose and components of nursing case management.
- Summarize criteria to be considered in the development of future models of nursing care delivery.

Chapter 21: *Quality Improvement and Patient Safety*

- Apply principles of quality management to the role of the professional nurse.
- Analyze the basis for the increasing emphasis on health care quality and medical errors.
- Analyze the role of health care regulatory agencies and how they have embodied the principles of quality management.
- Critique key evolutionary facts that led to the development of quality management in health care.
- Discuss the role process improvement can play in ensuring patient safety and improving quality in the health care system.
- Describe the tools and skills necessary for successful quality management activities.
- Discuss the professional nurses role in reducing medical errors and improving health care quality.

Chapter 22: *Quality and Safety Education in Nursing (QSEN)*

- Describe driving forces for quality and safety competency in nursing.
- Define the six core quality competencies integrated into nursing curricula to prepare nurses for working in systems focused on quality.
- Base nursing care delivery on the knowledge, skills, and attitudes defining the six core competencies.
- Evaluate nurses roles in improving health care quality.

2008 BSN ESSENTIAL III: SCHOLARSHIP FOR EVIDENCE-BASED PRACTICE

Chapter 5: *Theories of Nursing Practice*

- Differentiate between a science and a theory.
- Identify the criteria necessary for science.
- Identify the criteria necessary for a theory.
- Explain a nursing theory and a nursing model.
- Discuss two early and two contemporary nursing theorists and their theories.
- Explain the effect of nursing theory on the profession of nursing.

Chapter 6: *Nursing Research and Evidence-Based Practice*

- Summarize major points in the evolution of nursing research in relation to contemporary nursing.
- Evaluate the influence of nursing research on current nursing and health care practices.
- Differentiate among nursing research methods.
- Use established criteria to evaluate the quality of research studies.
- Participate in the research process.
- Use research findings to improve nursing practice.

2008 BSN ESSENTIAL IV: INFORMATION MANAGEMENT AND APPLICATION OF PATIENT CARE TECHNOLOGY

Chapter 14:
*Information
Technology in the
Clinical Setting*

- Describe the role of clinical information systems in patient care.
- Explain the importance of security and confidentiality in the use of various clinical information systems.
- Predict future trends in computing as they relate to health care and nursing practice.
- Conduct Internet searches for relevant health-related information.
- Use established criteria to evaluate the content of health-related sites found on the Internet.

2008 BSN ESSENTIAL V: HEALTH CARE POLICY, FINANCE, AND REGULATORY ENVIRONMENTS

Chapter 4: *Nursing
Licensure and
Certification*

- Explain the development of licensure requirements in the United States.
- Summarize current licensure requirements in the context of historical developments.
- Analyze the various components of a nurse practice act.
- Discuss mutual recognition of nursing practice and identify Nurse Licensure Compact states.
- Describe the development of certification requirements for advanced practice.
- Identify requirements for certification for advanced practice in different specialties.
- Use appropriate resources to obtain current information on licensure and certification.

Chapter 7:
*Paying for Health
Care in America:
Rising Costs and
Challenges*

- Analyze major factors that have influenced health care access and financing since the middle of the twentieth century.
- Analyze the relationship between market issues and health care resource allocation.
- Integrate knowledge of health care resources, access, and financing into managing professional nursing care.
- Critique the relationship between contemporary economic issues and trends and professional nursing practice.

Chapter 8: *Legal
Issues in Nursing
and Health Care*

- Differentiate among the three major categories of law on which nursing practice is established and governed.
- Analyze the relationship between accountability and liability for ones actions in professional nursing practice.
- Outline the essential elements that must be proven if a claim of negligence or malpractice is to be substantiated.
- Distinguish between intentional torts and unintentional torts in relation to nursing practice.
- Incorporate fundamental laws and statutory regulations that establish the patients right to self-determination in the health care setting.

Chapter 17:
*Budgeting Basics for
Nurses*

- Explain the basic terminology of budgeting in the health care industry.
- Contribute to the budget development process for a nursing/clinical department.
- Contribute to the capital budget development process for a nursing/clinical department.
- Explain aspects of monitoring financial performance against an operational budget.
- Understand the overall role of nursing in a health care organizations budget process.

Chapter 19: *Effective Delegation and Supervision*

- Evaluate the effect of changes in the current health care system on nurse staffing patterns and responsibilities.
- Outline six topic areas that the professional nurse should consider when making delegation decisions.
- List nine essential requirements for safe and effective delegation.
- Incorporate principles of delegation and supervision in professional nursing practice to ensure safe and legal patient care.

Chapter 23: *Health Policy and Politics: Get Involved!*

- Differentiate between policy and politics.
- Discuss the roles of the legislative, administrative, and judicial levels of government.
- Differentiate among federal, state, and local governments and their roles in governing and influencing health care and nursing practice.
- Identify three policy issues of significant consequence to nurses and nursing.
- Demonstrate the knowledge to be a responsible, informed, and politically active nurse.
- Use diverse technologic resources to obtain information about current health policy developments and political issues.

Chapter 21: *Quality Improvement and Patient Safety*

- Apply principles of quality management to the role of the professional nurse.
- Analyze the basis for the increasing emphasis on health care quality and medical errors.
- Analyze the role of health care regulatory agencies and how they have embodied the principles of quality management.
- Critique key evolutionary facts that led to the development of quality management in health care.
- Discuss the role process improvement can play in ensuring patient safety and improving quality in the health care system.
- Describe the tools and skills necessary for successful quality management activities.
- Discuss the professional nurses role in reducing medical errors and improving health care quality.

Chapter 28: *NCLEX-RN Examination*

- Explain the purpose of the NCLEX-RN examination.
- Evaluate various methods of preparation for the NCLEX-RN examination.
- Create a personal plan for preparing for the NCLEX-RN examination.
- Analyze the relationship between the nursing process and client needs as they relate to NCLEX-RN examination test items.
- Compare various review courses designed to aid in review for the NCLEX-RN examination.

2008 BSN ESSENTIAL VI: INTERPROFESSIONAL COMMUNICATION AND COLLABORATION FOR IMPROVING PATIENT HEALTH OUTCOMES

Chapter 18: *Effective Communication and Conflict Resolution*

- Outline factors that can influence the communication process.
- Communicate effectively with diverse intergenerational and interdisciplinary team members.
- Apply positive communication techniques in diverse situations.
- Identify negative communication techniques.
- Evaluate conflicting verbal and nonverbal communication cues.
- Examine constructive methods of communicating in conflict situations.
- Respond to inappropriate use of logical fallacies in communication.

Chapter 19: *Effective Delegation and Supervision*	• Evaluate the impact of changes in the current health care system on nurse staffing patterns and responsibilities. • Outline six topic areas that the professional nurse should consider when making delegation decisions. • List nine essential requirements for safe and effective delegation. • Incorporate principles of delegation and supervision in professional nursing practice to ensure safe and legal patient care.
Chapter 22: *Quality and Safety Education in Nursing (QSEN)*	• Describe driving forces for quality and safety competency in nursing. • Define the six core quality competencies integrated into nursing curricula to prepare nurses for working in systems focused on quality. • Base nursing care delivery on the knowledge, skills, and attitudes defining the six core competencies. • Evaluate nurses roles in improving health care quality.
Chapter 24: *Making the Transition from Student to Professional Nurse*	• Compare and contrast the phases of reality shock. • Differentiate between the novice nurse and the expert professional nurse. • Design strategies to ease the transition from novice to professional nurse. • Differentiate between compassion fatigue and burnout. • Make the transition from novice to professional nurse.

2008 BSN ESSENTIAL VII: CLINICAL PREVENTION AND POPULATION HEALTH

Chapter 11: *Complementary and Alternative Healing*	• Describe various complementary and alternative healing processes. • Effectively incorporate pertinent alternative therapies into patient care. • Provide patient education regarding uses, limitations, and precautions associated with alternative healing practices and products.

2008 BSN ESSENTIAL VIII: PROFESSIONALISM AND PROFESSIONAL VALUES

Chapter 1: *The Evolution of Professional Nursing*	• Summarize health practices throughout the course of history. • Analyze the impact of historical, political, social, and economic events on the development of nursing. • Describe the evolution of professional challenges experienced by nurses of diverse ethnic, racial, and educational backgrounds.
Chapter 2: *The Contemporary Image of Professional Nursing*	• Summarize health practices throughout the course of history. • Analyze the impact of historical, political, social, and economic events on the development of nursing. • Describe the evolution of professional challenges experienced by nurses of diverse ethnic, racial, and educational backgrounds.
Chapter 4: *Nursing Licensure and Certification*	• Explain the development of licensure requirements in the United States. • Summarize current licensure requirements in the context of historical developments. • Analyze the various components of a nurse practice act. • Discuss mutual recognition of nursing practice and identify Nurse Licensure Compact states. • Describe the development of certification requirements for advanced practice. • Identify requirements for certification for advanced practice in different specialties. • Use appropriate resources to obtain current information on licensure and certification.

Chapter 25: *Managing Time: The Path to High Self-Performance*	• Describe the unique demands of complex health care environments in todays fast-paced world of high technology and communication transfer and its effects on personal time management. • Explain the relationship between personal performance and time management. • Explain ones time management preferences and style. • Create an action plan to manage procrastination, distraction, and anxiety. • Describe how ones communication styles interact with ones ability to manage time effectively. • Adopt into daily practice a time management strategy plan unique to ones own style to ensure high-level personal performance in work and home life.
Chapter 26: *Contemporary Nursing Roles and Career Opportunities*	• Evaluate the impact of the current health care environment on the future role of nurses. • Analyze the influence of current demographic characteristics of RNs in the United States on contemporary nursing roles. • Differentiate among various innovative nursing practice roles today. • Differentiate between the roles of advanced practice nurses and other RNs in various settings. • Describe the role of the clinical nurse leader (CNL).
Chapter 27: *Job Search: Finding Your Match*	• Use the interview process to evaluate potential employment opportunities. • Prepare an effective résumé and nursing portfolio. • Compare and contrast various professional nursing employment opportunities. • Summarize the employment process.

Data from American Association of Colleges of Nursing, 2008.

Contents

CHAPTER

1

The Evolution of Professional Nursing

Susan R. Jacob, PhD, RN

evolve Additional resources are available online at: http://evolve.elsevier.com/Cherry/

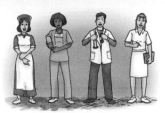

Building on a strong foundation for a bright future.

VIGNETTE

Toba Kamotu is a 17-year-old African-American college freshman who has been treated for depression for the past year at a local mental health center. It has also been reported that she suffered from anorexia and bulimia, in that she was vomiting frequently. Her treatment consisted of Zoloft 100 mg once daily and psychotherapy sessions once each week. Toba also had been complaining of somatic pain for the past 6 months. The pain radiated up her right leg and had a "pins and needles sensation." Her therapist told her that these symptoms sometimes accompany depression and would dissipate as her depression improved. The pain in her leg kept her awake at night and was affecting her ability to study.

Toba's college roommate was a nursing student who insisted that she be seen for her physical complaints. Because Toba had no insurance, she knew that her access to care would be limited. Therefore, she was reluctant to seek health care services. The clinic that she preferred did not take Medicaid or medical assistance patients of any kind. Her roommate asked one of her nursing professors what Toba should do, and the professor referred them to a clinic that provided care to individuals in the community who had limited funds. Toba called immediately but was told that the earliest available appointment would be 2 months later. She made the appointment and placed her name on a waiting list to be seen earlier.

Within 2 weeks Toba awakened vomiting and complaining to her roommate of feeling very hot. She was unable to walk because of excruciating pain in her right leg and was taken to the hospital by ambulance. When she arrived, her temperature was 103° F. A computed tomography (CT) scan was performed that indicated she had a liver mass measuring 10 cm. On biopsy the mass was determined to be malignant. Dr. Tabitha Winthrop, her oncologist, recommended chemotherapy to decrease the size of the mass so that surgery could be performed. It was also speculated that if this therapy worked, she could become a candidate for liver transplant and would be placed on the transplant list. Ms. Kamotu was placed under the care of the palliative care team, an interprofessional group of health professionals that was coordinated by an advanced practice nurse who was nationally certified by the National Board for Certification of Hospice and Palliative Nurses. The palliative care team consisted of a clinical nurse leader, clinical

We thank Shiprah A. Williams-Evans, PhD, APRN, BC for her contribution to this chapter in the 4th edition.

nurse specialist, and a registered nurse (RN), all nationally certified in palliative and hospice nursing; a counselor; medical director; case manager; and a representative from pastoral care. In this case, a child life specialist was also included as part of the team, as a result of the patient's age. Palliative care at this institution was defined as treatment of any patient who was experiencing a life-altering, debilitating, and/or life-threatening illness or injury. Ms. Kamotu was definitely experiencing a condition that would alter her life as an adolescent and might eventually become debilitating and life threatening, depending on the disease process and treatment options.

The palliative care team assists with symptom management and assessment of family dynamics, and provides emotional and spiritual support. The team also assists the patient to set goals to maintain her optimal level of functioning throughout treatment, with consideration of cultural aspects of care, in addition to discharge planning and communication deficits that are prominent in patients who are undergoing life-altering experiences. The ultimate goal is to maintain the highest optimal functioning and provide the highest-quality comprehensive care.

Florence Nightingale and Mary Seacole were trailblazers who began the work of organized nursing. Since their time, nursing has evolved into a profession that is focused on meeting the needs of the people it serves and preparing providers who can meet those needs. This vignette demonstrates just one instance of how a variety of nurse providers can assist in enhancing the quality of care.

■ QUESTIONS TO CONSIDER WHILE READING THIS CHAPTER:

1 What were the challenges faced by nurses historically?

2 How has access to care and managed care affected professional nursing practice?

3 What are the challenges facing nurses in the twenty-first century?

4 What areas of nursing specialization enhance patient care?

KEY TERMS

Clinical nurse leader (CNL) A master's degree–educated RN who assumes accountability for client care outcomes through the assimilation and application of research-based information to design, implement, and evaluate client plans of care. The CNL is a provider and a manager of care at the point of care to individuals and cohorts or populations. The CNL designs, implements, and evaluates client care by coordinating, delegating, and supervising the care provided by the health care team, including licensed nurses, technicians, and other health professionals (AACN Updated White Paper on the Role of the Clinical Nurse Leader, July 2007).

Doctor of nursing practice (DNP) A practice focused doctoral degree in nursing. The degree that is recommended by the American Association of Colleges of Nursing (AACN) for all advanced practice nurses by 2015.

Clinical nurse specialist (CNS) An advanced practice nurse who possesses expertise in a defined area of nursing practice for a selected client population or clinical setting. The CNS functions as an expert clinician, educator, consultant, researcher, and administrator.

Florence Nightingale (1820 to 1910) Considered the founder of organized, professional nursing. She is best known for her contributions to the reforms in the British Army Medical Corps, improved sanitation in India, improved public health in Great Britain, use of statistics to document health outcomes, and the development of organized training for nurses.

Professional nurse A specially trained *professional* that addresses the humanistic and holistic needs of patients, families, and environments and provides responses to patterns and/or needs of patients, families, and communities to actual and potential health problems. The professional nurse has diverse roles, such as health care provider, client advocate, educator, care coordinator, primary care practitioner, and change agent (Katz et al, 2009).

After studying this chapter, the reader will be able to:

1 Summarize health practices throughout the course of history.
2 Analyze the effect of historic, political, social, and economic events on the development of nursing.
3 Describe the evolution of professional challenges experienced by nurses of diverse ethnic, racial, and educational backgrounds.

CHAPTER OVERVIEW

Throughout the pages of recorded history nursing has been integrated into every facet of life. A legacy of human caring was initiated when, according to the book of Exodus, two midwives, Shiphrah and Puah, rescued the baby Moses and hid him to save his life. This legacy of caring has progressed throughout the years, responding to psychologic, social, environmental, and physiologic needs of society. Nurses of the past and present have struggled for recognition as knowledgeable professionals. The evolution of this struggle is reflected in political, cultural, environmental, and economic events that have sculpted our nation and world history (Katz et al, 2009; Snodgrass, 2004).

In the beginning, men were recognized as health healers. Women challenged the status quo and transformed nursing from a mystical phenomenon to a respected profession (Snodgrass, 2004). Florence Nightingale and Mary Seacole played major roles in bringing about changes in nursing. Using the concept of role modeling, these women demonstrated the value of their worth through their work in fighting for the cause of health and healing. During the twentieth century, nurses made tremendous advancements in the areas of education, practice, research, and technology. Nursing as a science progressed through education, clinical practice, development of theory, and rigorous research. Today nurses continue to be challenged to expand their roles and explore new areas of practice and leadership. This chapter provides a brief glimpse of health care practices and nursing care in the prehistoric period and early civilization and then describes the evolution of professional nursing practice. Box 1-1 summarizes some of the important events in the evolution of nursing.

PREHISTORIC PERIOD

Nursing in the prehistoric period was delineated by health practices that were strongly guided by beliefs of magic, religion, and superstition. Individuals who were ill were considered to be cursed by evil spirits and evil gods that entered the human body and caused suffering and death if not cast out. These beliefs dictated the behavior of primitive people, who sought to scare away the evil gods and spirits. Members of tribes participated in rituals, wore masks, and engaged in demonstrative dances to rid the sick of demonic possession of the body. Sacrifices and offerings, sometimes including human sacrifices, were made to rid the body of evil gods, demons, and spirits. Many tribes used special herbs, roots, and vegetables to cast out the "curse" of illness.

EARLY CIVILIZATION
Egypt

Ancient Egyptians are noted for their accomplishments in health care at an early period in civilization. They were the first to use the concept of suture in repairing wounds. They also were the first to be recorded as developing community planning that resulted in a decrease in

BOX **1-1**

Important Events in the Evolution of Nursing

1751 The Pennsylvania Hospital is the first hospital established in America.

1798 The U.S. Marine Hospital Service comes into being by an act of Congress on July 16. It is renamed the U.S. Public Health Service in 1912.

1840 Two African-American women, Mary Williams and Frances Rose, who founded Nursing Sisters of the Holy Cross, are listed as nurses in the City of Baltimore Directory.

1851 Florence Nightingale (1820-1910) attends Kaiserswerth to train as a nurse.

1854 During the Crimean War, Florence Nightingale transforms the image of nursing. Mary Seacole, a black woman from Jamaica, West Indies, nurses during the same time.

1861 The outbreak of the Civil War causes African-American women to volunteer as nurses. Among these women are Harriet Tubman, Sojourner Truth, and Susie King Taylor.

1872 Another school of nursing opens in the United States: the New England Hospital for Women and Children in Boston, Massachusetts.

1873 Linda Richards is responsible for designing a written patient record and physician's order system—the first in a hospital.

1879 Mary Mahoney, the first trained African-American nurse, graduates from the New England Hospital for Women and Children in Boston, Massachusetts.

1882 The American Red Cross is established by Clara Barton.

1886 The Visiting Nurses Association (VNA) is started in Philadelphia; Spelman College, Atlanta, Georgia, establishes the first diploma nursing program for African-Americans.

1893 Lillian Wald and Mary Brewster establish the Henry Street Visiting Nurse Service in New York.

1896 The Nurses' Associated Alumnae of the United States and Canada is established

1898 Namahyoke Curtis, an untrained African-American nurse, is assigned by the War Department as a contract nurse in the Spanish-American War.

1899 The International Council of Nurses (ICN) was founded.

1900 The first issue of the *American Journal of Nursing* is published.

1901 The Army Nurse Corps is established under the Army Reorganization Act.

1902 School of nursing is established in New York City by Linda Rogers.

1903 The first nurse practice acts are passed, and North Carolina is the first state to implement registration of nurses.

1908 The National Association of Colored Graduate Nurses is founded; it is dissolved in 1951.

1909 Ludie Andrews sues the Georgia State Board of Nurse Examiners to secure African-American nurses the right to take the state board examination and become licensed; she wins in 1920.

1911 The American Nurses Association (ANA) is established.

1912 The U.S. Public Health Service and the National League for Nursing (NLN) are established.

1918 Eighteen black nurses are admitted to the Army Nurse Corps after the armistice is signed ending World War I.

1919 *Public Health Nursing* is written by Mary S. Gardner. A public health nursing program is started at the University of Michigan.

1921 The Sheppard-Towner Act is passed providing federal aid for maternal and child health care.

1922 Sigma Theta Tau is founded (becomes the International Honor Society of Nursing in 1985).

1923 The Goldmark Report criticizes the inadequacies of hospital-based nursing schools and recommends increased educational standards.

1924 The U.S. Indian Bureau Nursing Service is founded by Eleanor Gregg.

1925 The Frontier Nursing Service is founded by Mary Breckenridge.

1935 The Social Security Act is passed.

1937 Federal appropriations for cancer, venereal diseases, tuberculosis, and mental health are begun.

1939 World War II begins.

1941 The U.S. Army establishes a quota of 56 African-American nurses for admission to the Army Nurse Corps. The Nurse Training Act is passed.

1943 An amendment to the Nurse Training bill is passed that bars racial bias.

1945 The U.S. Navy drops the color bar and admits four African-American nurses.

BOX **1-1**

Important Events in the Evolution of Nursing—cont'd

1946 Nurses are classified as professionals by the U.S. Civil Service Commission. The Hospital Survey and Construction Act (Hill-Burton) is passed.

1948 The Brown Report discusses the future of nursing

1948 Estelle Osborne is the first African-American nurse elected to the board of the ANA. The ANA votes individual membership to all African-American nurses excluded from any state association.

1949 M. Elizabeth Carnegie is the first African-American nurse to be elected to the board of a state association (Florida).

1950 The Code for Professional Nurses is published by the ANA.

1952 National nursing organizations are reorganized from six to two: ANA and NLN.

1954 The Supreme Court decision *Brown v. Board of Education* asserts that "separate educational facilities are inherently unequal."

1965 The Social Security Amendment includes Medicare and Medicaid.

1971 The National Black Nurses Association is organized.

1973 The ANA forms the American Academy of Nursing.

1974 The American Assembly of Men in Nursing was founded.

1978 Barbara Nichols is the first African-American nurse elected president of the ANA. M. Elizabeth Carnegie, an African-American nurse, is elected president of the American Academy of Nursing.

1979 Brigadier General Hazel Johnson Brown is the first African-American chief of the Army Nurse Corps.

1985 Vernice Ferguson, an African-American nurse, is elected president of Sigma Theta Tau International.

1986 The Association of Black Nursing Faculty is founded by Dr. Sally Tucker Allen.

1990 Congress proclaims March 10 as Harriet Tubman Day in the United States, honoring her as a brave African-American freedom fighter and nurse during the Civil War. The Bloodborne Pathogen Standard is established by OSHA.

1991 *Healthy People 2000* is published.

1993 The National Center for Nursing Research is upgraded to the National Institute of Nursing Research within the National Institutes of Health.

1994 NCLEX-RN®, a computerized nurse-licensing examination, is introduced.

1996 The Commission on Collegiate Nursing Education is established as an agency devoted exclusively to the accreditation of baccalaureate and graduate-degree nursing programs.

1999 Beverly Malone, the second African-American president of the ANA, is named Deputy Assistant Secretary for Health, Department of Health and Human Services, Office of Public Health and Science. The IOM releases its landmark report: *To Err Is Human: Building a Safer Health System.*

2000 M. Elizabeth Carnegie is inducted into the ANA Hall of Fame. The American Nurses Credentialing Center gives its first psychiatric mental health nurse practitioner examination. *Healthy People 2010* is published. AACN reports a faculty vacancy rate of 7.4% among the 220 nursing schools that responded to a survey. According to the AACN, the average age of full-time faculty is more than 50 years old; average age of doctorally prepared professors is 55.9.

2001 Beverly Malone is appointed General Secretary, Royal College of Nursing, London. Health Care Financing Administration (HCFA) becomes Centers for Medicare & Medicaid Services (CMS).

2002 Johnson and Johnson Health Care Systems, Inc. launches The Future of Nursing, a national publicity campaign to address the nursing shortage.

2002 To address the shortage of nurses the Nurse Reinvestment Act is signed into law by President George W. Bush.

2002 Significant funding is obtained for geriatric nursing initiatives.

2003 The American Nurses Foundation launches an "Investment in Nursing" Campaign to deal with the nursing shortage.

2003 IOM report *Keeping Patients Safe: Transforming the Work Environment of Nurses* is released.

2003 AACN White Paper on the Role of the Clinical Nurse Leader.

Continued

BOX **1-1**

Important Events in the Evolution of Nursing—cont'd

2005 CCNE decides that only programs that offer practice doctoral degrees with the Doctor of Nursing Practice (DNP) title will be eligible for CCNE accreditation.

2005 NLN offers and certifies the first national certification for nurse educators; the initials CNE may be placed behind the names of those certified.

2006 AACN approves essentials of doctoral education for advanced nursing practice (DNP) (www.aacn.nche.edu/DNP/pdf/Essentials.pdf).

2007 Commission on Nurse Certification, an autonomous arm of AACN, began certifying clinical nurse leaders (CNLs).

2008 Commission on Collegiate Nursing Education begins accrediting DNP programs.

Sources: AACN, 2003; Carnegie, 1995; Deloughery, 1998; Donahue, 1999; Kalisch and Kalisch, 1995; IOM, 2003.

public health problems. One of the main early public health problems was the spread of disease through contaminated water sources. Specific laws on cleanliness, food use and preservation, drinking, exercise, and sexual relations were developed. Health beliefs of Egyptians determined preventive measures taken and personal health behaviors practiced. These health behaviors were usually carried out to accommodate the gods. Some behaviors were also practiced expressly to appease the spirits of the dead (Kalisch and Kalisch, 2003). The Egyptians developed the calendar and writing, which initiated recorded history. The oldest records date back to the sixteenth century BC in Egypt. A pharmacopoeia that classified more than 700 drugs was written to assist in the care and management of disease (Ellis and Hartley, 2008). As in the case of Shiphrah and Puah, the midwives who saved the baby Moses, nurses were used by kings and other aristocrats to deliver babies and care for the young, older adults, and those who were sick.

Palestine

From 1400 to 1200 BC, the Hebrews migrated from the Arabian Desert and gradually settled in Palestine, where they became an agricultural society. Under the leadership of Moses, the Hebrews developed a system of laws called the Mosaic Code. This code, one of the first organized methods of disease control and prevention, contained public health laws that dictated personal, family, and public hygiene. For instance, laws were written to prohibit the eating of animals that were dead longer than 3 days and to isolate individuals who were thought to have communicable diseases. Hebrew priests took on the role of health inspectors (Ellis and Hartley, 2004).

Greece

From 1500 to 100 BC, Greek philosophers sought to understand man and his relationship with the gods, nature, and other men. They believed that the gods and goddesses of Greek mythology controlled health and illness. Temples built to honor Aesculapius, the god of medicine, were designated to care for the sick. Aesculapius carried a staff that was intertwined with serpents or snakes, representing wisdom and immortality. This staff is believed to be the model of today's medical caduceus. Hippocrates (460 to 362 BC), considered the "Father of Medicine," paved the way in establishing scientific knowledge in medicine. Hippocrates was the first to attribute disease to natural causes rather than supernatural causes and curses of the gods. Hippocrates' teachings also emphasized the patient-centered approach and use of the scientific method for solving problems (Ellis and Hartley, 2004).

India

Dating from 3000 to 1500 BC, the earliest cultures of India were Hindu. The sacred book of Brahmanism (also known as Hinduism), the Vedas, was used to guide health care practices. The Vedas, considered by some to be the oldest written material, emphasized hygiene and prevention of sickness and described major and minor surgeries. The Indian practice of surgery was very well developed. The importance of prenatal care to mother and infant was also well understood. Public hospitals were constructed from 274 to 236 BC and were staffed by male nurses with qualifications and duties similar to those of the twentieth-century practical nurse. In rare instances, older women were allowed to assume a nursing role outside the home (Ellis and Hartley, 2008).

China

The teachings of the Chinese scholar Confucius (551 to 479 BC) had a powerful effect on the customs and practices of the people of ancient China. Confucius taught a moral philosophy that addressed one's obligation to society. Several hundred years after his death, Confucius' philosophy became the basis for Chinese education and government. Central to his teachings were service to the community and the value of the family as a unit.

The early Chinese also placed great value on solving life's problems. Their belief about health and illness was based on the yin and yang philosophy. The yin represented the feminine forces, which were considered negative and passive. The yang represented the masculine forces, which were positive and active. The Chinese believed that an imbalance between these two forces would result in illness, whereas balance between the yin and yang represented good health (Ellis and Hartley, 2008). The ancient Chinese used a variety of treatments believed to promote health and harmony, including acupuncture. Acupuncture involves insertion of hot and cold needles into the skin and underlying tissues to manage or cure conditions (such as pain, stroke, or breathing difficulty) and ultimately to affect the balance of yin and yang. Hydrotherapy, massage, and exercise were used as preventive health measures (Giger and Davidhizar, 2004). The Chinese also used drug therapy to manage disease conditions; they recorded more than 1000 drugs derived from animals, vegetables, and minerals (Walton, Barondess, and Locke, 1994). Many of the drugs used by the Chinese in ancient times, such as ephedrine, continue to be used today (Ellis and Hartley, 2004).

Rome

The Roman Empire (27 BC to 476 AD), a military dictatorship, adapted medical practices from the countries they conquered and the physicians they enslaved. The first military hospital in Europe was established in Rome. The physicians were enslaved and forced to provide details about their medical practice. Both male and female attendants assisted in the care of the sick. Galen was a famous Greek physician who worked in Rome and made important contributions to the practice of medicine by expanding his knowledge in anatomy, physiology, pathology, and medical therapeutics (Walton et al, 1994).

THE MIDDLE AGES

The Middle Ages (476 BC to 1450 AD) followed the demise of the Roman Empire (Walton et al, 1994). Women used herbs and new methods of healing, whereas men continued to use purging, leeching, and mercury. This period also saw the Roman Catholic Church become a central figure in the organization and management of health care. Most of the changes in health care were based on the Christian concepts of charity and the sanctity of human life. Wives of emperors and other women considered noble became nurses. These women devoted themselves to caring for the sick, often carrying a basket of food and medicine as they journeyed from house to house (Bahr and Johnson, 1997). Widows and unmarried women became nuns and deaconesses. Two of these deaconesses, Dorcas and Phoebe, are mentioned in the Bible as outstanding for the care they provided to the sick (Freedman, 1995).

During the Middle Ages, physicians spent most of their time translating medical essays; they actually provided little medical care. Poorly trained barbers, who lacked any formal medical education, performed surgery and medical treatments that were considered "bloody" or "messy." Nurses also provided some medical care, although in most hospitals and monasteries, female nurses who were not midwives were forbidden to witness childbirth, help with gynecologic examinations, or even diaper male infants (Kalisch and Kalisch, 1986). In addition these nurses were not permitted to have contact with male patients, administer enemas, or care for a man with a venereal disease. Female nurse midwives did, however, provide the bulk of obstetric care within the community (Ellis and Hartley, 2008).

During the Crusades, which lasted for almost 200 years (from 1096 to 1291), military nursing orders, known as Templars and Hospitalers, were founded. Monks and Christian knights provided nursing care and defended the hospitals during battle, wearing a suit of armor under their religious habits. The habits were distinguished by the Maltese cross to identify the monks and knights as Christian warriors. The same cross was used years later on a badge designed for the first school of nursing and became a forerunner for the design of nursing pins (Ellis and Hartley, 2004).

THE RENAISSANCE AND THE REFORMATION PERIOD

Following the Middle Ages came the Renaissance and the Reformation, also known as the rebirth of Europe (the fourteenth through the sixteenth centuries AD). Major advancements were made in pharmacology, chemistry, and medical knowledge, including anatomy, physiology, and surgery. During the Renaissance, new emphasis was given to medical education, but nursing education was practically nonexistent.

The Reformation was a religious movement that resulted in a dissention between Roman Catholics and Protestants. During this period, religious facilities that provided health care closed. Women were encouraged toward charitable services, but their main duties included bearing and caring for children in their homes. Furthermore, hospital work was no longer appealing to women of high economic status, and the individuals who worked as nurses in hospitals were often female prisoners, prostitutes, and drunks. Nursing was no longer the respected profession it had once been. This period is referred to as the "Dark Ages" of nursing (Ellis and Hartley, 2008).

During the sixteenth and seventeenth centuries, famine, plague, filth, and horrible crimes ravaged Europe. King Henry VII eliminated the organized monastic relief programs that aided the orphans, poor, and other displaced people. It became common to encounter homeless men, women, and children begging in the streets. Beggars were beaten, branded, and chained to the galleys of boats as punishment for their disgraceful behavior (Ellis and Hartley, 2004).

Out of great concern for social welfare, several nursing groups, such as the Order of the Visitation of St. Mary, St. Vincent de Paul, and the Sisters of Charity, were organized to give time, service, and money to the poor and sick. The Sisters of Charity recruited young women for training in nursing, developed educational programs, and cared for abandoned children.

In 1640 St. Vincent de Paul established the Hospital for the Foundling to care for the many orphaned and abandoned children (Ellis and Hartley, 2008).

THE COLONIAL AMERICAN PERIOD

The first hospital and the first medical school in North America were founded in Mexico—the Hospital of the Immaculate Conception in Mexico City and the medical school at the University of Mexico. During this time in the American colonies, individuals with infectious diseases were isolated in almshouses or "pesthouses" (Ellis and Hartley, 2008). Procedures, such as purgatives and bleeding, were widely used, leading to shortened life expectancy. Plagues, such as yellow fever and smallpox, caused thousands of deaths. Benjamin Franklin, who was outspoken regarding the care of the sick, insisted that a hospital be built in the colonies. He believed that the community should be responsible for the management and treatment of those who were ill. Through his efforts, the first hospital, called the Pennsylvania Hospital, was built in the United States in Philadelphia in 1751 (Ellis and Hartley, 2008).

FLORENCE NIGHTINGALE

Florence Nightingale was born in Florence, Italy, on May 12, 1820. The Nightingale family was wealthy, well traveled, and well educated. Nightingale was a highly intelligent, talented, and attractive woman. From an early age she demonstrated a deep concern for the poor and suffering. At the age of 25 she became interested in training as a nurse. However, her family was strongly opposed to this choice and preferred that she marry and take her place in society (Joel, 2006). In 1851 her parents finally permitted her to pursue training as a nurse. Nightingale attended a 3-month nursing training program at the Institution of Deaconesses at Kaiserswerth, Germany. In 1854 she began training nurses at the Harley Street Nursing Home and served as superintendent of nurses at King's College Hospital in London (Small, 2002).

The outbreak of the Crimean War marked a turning point in Nightingale's career. In October 1854, Sidney Herbert, British Secretary of War and an old friend of the Nightingale family, wrote to Nightingale and asked her to lead a group of nurses to the Crimea to work at one of the military hospitals under government authority and expense. Nightingale accepted his offer and assembled 38 nurses who were sisters and nuns from various Catholic and Anglican orders (Joel, 2006; Small, 2002).

Nightingale and her team were assigned to the Barracks Hospital at Scutari. The Barracks Hospital actually was a dilapidated, barnlike building that had been formerly used as artillery barracks. Thousands of cholera victims and hundreds of battle casualties were taken to Scutari. To get to the hospital from the front lines, the wounded and ill soldiers were put aboard hospital ships to cross the long Black Sea (Small, 2002).

When Nightingale arrived at the Barracks Hospital, she found deplorable conditions. Between 3000 and 4000 sick and wounded men were packed into the hospital, which was originally designed to accommodate 1700 patients. There were no beds, blankets, food, or medicine. Many of the wounded soldiers had been placed on the floor, where lice, maggots, vermin, rodents, and blood covered their bodies. There were no candles or lanterns. All medical care had to be rendered during the light of day (Small, 2002).

Despite the distressing conditions at the Barracks Hospital, the army physicians and surgeons at first refused Nightingale's assistance. However, within a week, faced with scurvy, starvation, dysentery, and the eruption of more fighting, the physicians, in desperation, called her to help. Nightingale immediately purchased medical supplies, food, linen, and hospital equipment, using her own money and that of the Times Relief Fund. Within 10 days she had set up a kitchen for special diets and had rented a house that she converted into a laundry (Gill 2004; Small, 2002). The wives of soldiers were hired to manage and operate the laundry service. She assigned soldiers to make repairs and clean up the building. Just weeks later she initiated social services, reading classes, and even coffeehouses, where soldiers could enjoy music and recreation (Small, 2002).

Nightingale worked long, hard hours to care for these soldiers. She spent up to 20 hours each day caring for wounds, comforting soldiers, assisting in surgery, directing staff, and keeping records. Nightingale introduced principles of asepsis and infection control, a system for transcribing physicians' orders, and a procedure to maintain patient records. By the end of the Crimean War, Nightingale had trained as many as 125 nurses to care for the wounded and ill soldiers (Small, 2002).

Nightingale is credited with using public health principles and statistical methods to advocate for improved health conditions for British soldiers. Through carefully recorded statistics, Nightingale was able to document that the soldiers' death rate decreased from 42% to 2% as a result of health care reforms that emphasized sanitary conditions. Because of her remarkable work in using statistics to demonstrate cause and effect and improve the health of British soldiers, Nightingale is recognized for her contributions to nursing research (Nies and McEwen, 2007).

Nightingale also demonstrated the power of political activism to effect health care reform by writing letters of criticism accompanied by constructive recommendations to British army leaders. Nightingale's ability to overthrow the British army management method that had allowed the deplorable conditions to exist in the army hospitals was considered one of her greatest achievements (Dossey et al, 2005; Gill, 2004; Nies and McEwen, 2007).

In 1855 after visiting the front lines and hospitals in Balaclava, Nightingale contracted "Crimean fever" and was taken to the Castle Hospital. There she received intensive care from the physicians and nurses she trained. She remained in poor condition for several weeks. Soldiers wept when they heard of her illness and near death. She eventually recovered, but the illness had taken a heavy toll on her overall health (Luddy et al, 2004).

In 1860 Nightingale established the first nursing school in England. By 1873 graduates of Nightingale's nurse training program in England migrated to the United States, where they became supervisors in the first of the hospital-based (diploma) nursing schools: Massachusetts General Hospital in Boston, Bellevue Hospital in New York, and the New Haven Hospital in Connecticut.

Florence Nightingale's work, from the Crimean War to the establishment of formal nursing education programs, was a catapult for the reorganization and advancement of professional nursing. Until her death in August 1910, Nightingale demonstrated the powerful effect that well-educated, creative, skilled, and competent individuals have in the provision of health care. She is honored as the founder of professional nursing (Small, 2002). Nightingale had the means to support her work and the stamina to drive forward in her belief concerning health care. Her theory of environmental cleanliness is still applicable today, even though Louis Pasteur's germ theory was not widely known and was very controversial at the time.

MARY SEACOLE

Mary Seacole was a Jamaican nurse who learned the art of caring and healing from her mother. In her native land of Jamaica, British West Indies, she was nicknamed "Doctress" because of her administration of care to the sick in a lodging house in Kingston (Carnegie, 1995). Seacole learned of the Crimean War and wrote to the British government requesting to join

Nightingale's group of nurses. However, she was denied the right to join because she was black. She was confused about this denial because many of the British soldiers had lived in Jamaica, where she had already provided health care to them.

Seacole had previously served as a nurse in Cuba and Panama during the yellow fever and cholera epidemics. She had also conducted forensic studies on an infant who died of cholera in Panama. She felt that her experience would be valuable in treating disease in the Crimean War, and she sailed to England at her own expense. She provided a letter of introduction to Nightingale, which was blocked because Seacole was black, even though she had been trained by British army physicians (Carnegie, 1995).

After several efforts to join Nightingale's group failed, Seacole, who was not a woman of wealth, purchased her own supplies and traveled more than 3000 miles to the Crimea, where she built and opened a lodging house. On the bottom floor of the house was a restaurant, and on the top floor an area was arranged like a hospital to nurse sick soldiers (Carnegie, 1995).

When Seacole finally met Nightingale, the response was still the same: "no vacancies" (Carnegie, 1995). However, being denied enlistment did not deter Seacole; she remained faithful and nursed the sick throughout the Crimean War. Her efforts did not go unnoticed by the English people. Long after the war was over, the British government finally honored Seacole with a medal in recognition of her efforts and the services she provided to the sick and injured soldiers.

NURSING IN THE UNITED STATES
The Civil War Period

During the United States Civil War, or the War Between the States (1861 to 1865), health care conditions in the United States were similar to those encountered by Nightingale and Seacole. Numerous epidemics plagued the country, including syphilis, gonorrhea, malaria, smallpox, and typhoid (Nelson, 2001; Oermann, 1997).

The Civil War was initiated by the attack on Fort Sumter, South Carolina, April 17, 1861. At this time, there were no nurses formally trained to care for the sick. However, thousands of men and women from the South and North volunteered to care for the wounded. Hospitals were set up in the field, and transports were put in place to carry the wounded to the hospitals (Carnegie, 1995).

Secretary of War Simon Cameron appointed a schoolteacher named Dorothea Dix to organize military hospitals and provide medical supplies to the Union Army soldiers. Dix received no official status and no salary for this position.

Women providing nursing care during the Civil War worked under very primitive conditions. Maintaining sanitary conditions was an overwhelming challenge and often not possible. Greater than 6 million patients were admitted to hospitals. There were approximately one-half million surgical cases performed. Unfortunately there were only about 2000 individuals who served as nurses, far less than the number needed to provide adequate care (Fitzpatrick, 1997; Kalisch and Kalisch, 1995). According to records kept at three hospitals, 181 men and women African-American nurses served between July 16, 1863, and June 14, 1864. White nurses were paid $12 per month; African-American nurses received $10 per month (Carnegie, 1995).

Three African-American nurses made particularly important contributions to nursing efforts during the Civil War: Harriet Tubman cared for the sick as a nurse in the Sea Islands off the coast of South Carolina and was later known as the "conductor of the underground railroad." It is also reported that she was the first woman to lead American troops into battle (Carnegie, 1995). Sojourner Truth, known for her abolitionist and nursing efforts, was an advocate of clean and sanitary conditions for patients. She insisted that these conditions were needed for patients to heal. Susie King Taylor, although hired to work in the laundry, served as a nurse because of the growing number of wounded who needed care. Having learned to read and write, which was against the law for African-Americans at the time, she also taught many of her comrades in Company E to read and write (Carnegie, 1995).

Many other volunteer nurses made important contributions during the Civil War: Clara Barton served on the front line during the Civil War and operated a war relief program to provide supplies to the battlefields and hospitals. Barton also set up a postwar service to find missing soldiers and is credited with founding the American Red Cross (Nelson, 2001; Oermann, 1997). Louisa May Alcott, who served as a nurse for 6 weeks until stopped by ill health, authored detailed accounts of the experiences encountered by nurses during the war for a newspaper publication titled *Hospital Sketches* (Kalisch and Kalisch, 1995; 2003).

When the Civil War ended, the number of nurse training schools increased. The war had proven the need for more nurses to be formerly trained. These early nursing programs offered little or no classroom education, and on-the-job training occurred in the hospital wards. The students learned routine patient care duties, worked long hours 6 days a week, and were used as supplemental hospital staff. After graduation most of the nurses practiced as private duty nurses or hospital staff (Lindeman and McAthie, 1990). The first nursing textbook, titled *A Manual of Nursing*, was published in 1876 and was used by the New York Training School for Nurses at Bellevue Hospital (Kalisch and Kalisch, 1995).

During the 1890s, the nationwide establishment of African-American hospitals and nursing schools gained momentum as African-American musicians, educators, and community leaders became alarmed at the high rates of African-American morbidity and mortality. Because of segregation and discrimination, African-Americans had to establish their own health care institutions to provide African-American patients with access to quality health care and to provide African-American men and women with opportunities to enter the nursing profession. In 1886 John D. Rockefeller funded the establishment of the first school of nursing for African-American women at the Atlanta Baptist Seminary—now known as Spelman College (Jones, 2004; Salzman, Smith, and West, 1996).

1900 to World War I

In the 1900s states began to require nurses to become registered before entering practice. By 1910 most states had upgraded education requirements to high school, upgraded training, and required registration before practice (Deloughery, 1998; Donahue, 1999).

Lillian Wald, a pioneer in public health nursing, is best known for the development and establishment of a viable practice for public health nurses in the twentieth century. The main location for this practice was the Henry Street Settlement House, located in the Lower East Side of New York City. Its purpose was to provide well-baby care, health education, disease prevention, and treatment of patients with minor illnesses. Nursing practice based at the Henry Street Settlement House formed the basis of public health nursing for the entire country. Instead of relying on patients visiting the clinic, public health nurses made their way to the various tenements located around Henry Street (Snodgrass, 2004; Stanhope and Lancaster, 2008).

Lillian Wald also developed the first nursing service for occupational health. She believed that prevention of disease among workers would improve productivity and was able to convince the Metropolitan Life Insurance Company that her ideas had merit. As a result, nursing agencies, such as those in place at the Henry Street Settlement House, provided skilled nursing services to employees. Another innovation that emerged from this program was the sliding fee scale, by which patients were billed according to their income or their ability to pay. This innovative nursing service existed for 44 years before it was dissolved by the Metropolitan Life Insurance Company (Stanhope and Lancaster, 2008).

In 1911 Wald chaired a committee formed by members of the Associated Alumnae of Training Schools for Nurses, later to become the American Nurses Association (ANA), and the Society of Superintendents of Training Schools for Nurses, the precursor of the National League for Nursing (NLN). The purpose of the committee was to develop standards for nursing services performed outside of the hospital environment. The committee determined that a new organization was necessary to meet the needs of community health nurses. The result of the committee's recommendation was the formation of the National Organization for Public Health Nursing, whose goals were to establish educational and practice standards for community health nursing (Stanhope and Lancaster, 2008).

The ANA and the NLN are still leading nursing organizations today. The ANA has focused primarily on professional aspects of nursing, and the NLN was the only accrediting body for nursing schools until 1996, when the Commission on Collegiate Nursing Education (CCNE), an autonomous arm of the AACN, was established as an agency devoted exclusively to the accreditation of baccalaureate and graduate degree nursing programs (Stanhope and Lancaster, 2008).

World War I and the 1920s

During the early 1900s the world was rapidly changing and moving toward global conflict. Germany was arming, and the rest of Europe was trying to ignore the threat. "Prosperous" was the word used to describe the U.S. economy. Women were granted the right to vote and were moving into the workforce on a regular basis.

Advancements in medical care and public health were being made. The primary site for medical care moved from the home to the hospital, and surgical and diagnostic techniques were improved. Pneumonia management was the focus of scientific study. Insulin was discovered in 1922, and in 1928 Alexander Fleming discovered the precursor of penicillin, which would eventually be used to successfully treat patients with pneumonia and other infections (Kalisch and Kalisch, 1995) (Box 1-2).

Environmental conditions improved, and the serious epidemics of the previous century became nonexistent. Lillian Wald, in *The House on Henry Street*, linked poor environmental and social conditions to prevalent illnesses and poverty and used this information to lead the fight for better sanitation and housing conditions (Nies and McEwen, 2007).

With the outbreak of World War I in 1914, nurses were desperately needed to care for the soldiers who were injured or who suffered from the many illnesses that were a result of trench warfare (Nies and McEwen, 2007). The war offered nurses a chance to advance into new fields of specialization. For example, nurse anesthetists made their first appearance as part of the surgical teams at the front lines. More than 20,000 U.S.-trained nurses served in WWI (Oermann, 1997).

Because many nurses volunteered to provide services during the war, the community health nursing movement in the United States stalled. However, the American Red Cross, founded by Clara Barton in 1882, assisted in efforts to continue public health nursing. The Red Cross nurses originally focused on the rural communities that were not able to access health care services. As the war continued, however, the Red Cross nurses also moved into urban areas to provide health care services (Chitty and Black, 2007).

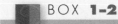

BOX **1-2**

Duties of the Hospital Floor Nurse in 1887

In addition to caring for your 60 patients, each nurse will follow these regulations:
1. Daily sweep and mop the floors of your ward; dust the patient's furniture and windowsill.
2. Maintain an even temperature on your ward by bringing in a scuttle of coal for the day's business.
3. Light is important to observe the patient's condition; therefore, each day fill kerosene lamps, clean chimneys, and trim wicks. Wash the windows once a week.
4. The nurse's notes are important in aiding the physician's work. Make your pens carefully; you may whittle nibs to your individual taste.
5. Each nurse on day duty will report every day at 7 AM and will leave at 8 PM except on Sabbath, on which day you will be off from 12 noon to 2 PM.
6. Graduate nurses in good standing with the director of nurses will be given an evening off each week if you regularly attend church.
7. Each nurse should lay aside from each payday a good sum of her earning for her benefits during her declining years so that she will not become a burden. For example, if you earn $20 a month, you should set aside $10.
8. Any nurse who smokes, uses liquor in any form, gets her hair done at a beauty shop, or frequents dance halls will have given the director of nurses good reason to suspect her worth, intentions, and integrity.
9. The nurse who performs her labors, serves her patients and physicians faithfully and without fault for a period of 5 years will be given an increase by the hospital administration of 5 cents per day, providing there are no hospital debts that are outstanding.

From Lois Turley © 1981-2004. Used by permission. All rights reserved. From CareNurse.com.

During WWI, the U.S. Public Health Service, founded in 1798 to provide health care services to merchant seamen, was charged with the responsibility to provide health services at the military posts located within the United States. A nurse, "loaned" by the National Organization for Public Health Nursing, established nursing services at U.S. military outposts. The responsibilities of the U.S. Public Health Service continued to grow; eventually it was composed of physicians, nurses, and other allied health professionals, who provided indigent care and practiced in community health programs (Stanhope and Lancaster, 2008).

Further changes were in store for nursing during WWI. In 1918 the Vassar Camp School for Nurses was established. Its purpose was to provide an intensive 2-year nurses' training program for college graduates. Graduates of the program were given an army reserve commission and would be activated during times of war to meet increased nursing needs. Sponsored by the American Red Cross and the Council of National Defense, the school graduated 435 nurses. The Vassar Camp School for Nurses was a short-lived enterprise. When peace was declared in 1919, the program was permanently disbanded (Snodgrass, 2004; Stanhope and Lancaster, 2008).

In 1921 the federal government recognized the need to improve the health of women and children and passed the Sheppard-Towner Act, one of the first pieces of federal legislation passed to provide funds to assist in the care of special populations (Oermann, 1997). This funding provided public health nurses with resources to promote the health and well-being of women, infants, and children.

Following these improvements, the Frontier Nursing Service (FNS) was established in 1925 by Mary Breckenridge of Kentucky. Born into a wealthy family, Breckenridge learned the value of providing care to others from her grandmother. Breckenridge began her career in

New York's St. Luke's Hospital School of Nursing. After serving as a nurse during WWI, she returned to Columbia University to learn more about community health nursing. Armed with her new knowledge and a passion to assist disadvantaged women and children, Breckenridge returned to Kentucky and the rural Appalachian Mountains (Oermann, 1997; Stanhope and Lancaster, 2008).

Breckenridge believed that the rural mountain area of Kentucky, cut off from many modern conveniences, was an excellent place to prove the value of community health nursing. She established the FNS in a five-room cabin in Hyden, Kentucky. After overcoming serious obstacles, such as no water supply or sewage disposal, six other nursing outposts were constructed in the rural mountains from 1927 to 1930. The FNS based its hospital in Hyden and eventually attracted physicians and nurses to provide medical, dental, surgical, nursing, and midwifery services to the rural poor. Financial support for the FNS ranged from fees for labor and supplies to funds raised through annual family dues to donations and fundraising efforts. Nurses working for the FNS traveled a 700-square mile area, often on horseback, to provide services to approximately 10,000 patients (Oermann, 1997).

Breckenridge established an important health care service for rural Kentucky communities. Equally important was her documentation of the results of community health nursing in rural communities. Breckenridge followed the advice of a consulting physician and collected mortality data on the communities before nursing services actually were started. The results were startling; mortality was significantly reduced, and the need for the nursing services was clearly documented. Breckenridge proved that even in appalling environmental conditions without heat, electricity, or running water, nursing services could make a substantial positive impact on the health of the community (Stanhope and Lancaster, 2008). The FNS is still in operation today and provides vital service to the rural communities of Kentucky.

The Great Depression (1930 to 1940)

The U.S. economy prospered during WWI and well into the 1920s. However, after the stock market crash in October 1929, economic prosperity quickly dissipated. Millions of men and women became unemployed. Before the depression many people had private-duty nurses. However, during the depression, many nurses found themselves unemployed because most families could no longer afford private-duty nurses.

Franklin D. Roosevelt, elected president of the United States in 1932, faced a country in shambles. He responded with several innovative and necessary interventions and ushered in the first major social legislation that had been enacted in U.S. history. Titled the "New Deal," the legislation had several social components that affected the provision of medical care and other services for indigent people across the country (Karger and Stoesz, 2005).

The piece of legislation that had the greatest effect on health care in the United States was the Social Security Act of 1935, which set the precedent for the passage of the Medicare and Medicaid acts that followed in 1965. The main purposes of the 1935 Social Security Act were to provide (1) a national old-age insurance system, (2) federal grants to states for maternal and child welfare services, (3) vocational rehabilitation services for the handicapped, (4) medical care for crippled children and blind people, (5) a plan to strengthen public health services, and (6) a federal-state unemployment system (Karger and Stoesz, 2005).

The passage of the 1935 Social Security Act provided avenues for nursing care, and nursing jobs were created. With funds from the Social Security Act, public health nursing became the major source of health care for dependent mothers and children, the blind, and crippled children. Nurses found employment as public health nurses for county or state health departments

(Chitty and Black, 2007). Hospital job opportunities also were created for nurses, and the hospital became the usual employment setting for graduate nurses.

World War II (1940 to 1945)

The United States officially entered World War II after the bombing of Pearl Harbor in December 1941. At that time the nursing divisions of all of the military branches had inadequate numbers of nurses. Congress passed legislation to provide needed funds to expand nursing education. A committee of six national nursing organizations, called the National Nursing Council, received a million dollars to accomplish the needed expansion. The U.S. Public Health Service became the administrator of the funds, which further strengthened the tie between the U.S. Public Health Service and nursing (Sarnecky, 2001; Stanhope and Lancaster, 2008).

The war was considered a global conflict, and nursing became an essential part of the military advance. Nurses were required to function under combat conditions and had to adapt nursing care to meet the challenges of different climates, facilities, and supplies. As a result of their service during WWII, nurses finally were recognized as an integral part of the military and attained the ranks of officers in the army and navy. Colonel Julie O. Flikke was the first army nurse to be promoted to colonel in the U.S. Army and served as Superintendent of the Army Nurse Corps from 1937 to 1942 (Deloughery, 1998; Robinson and Perry, 2001).

Post-World War II Period (1945 to 1950)

The period after WWII was a time of prosperity for the average American. The GI Bill enabled returning veterans to complete their interrupted education. The unemployment rate dropped to an all-time low in the United States. In an effort to provide more areas of employment for the returning men, the government mounted a massive campaign to encourage women to return to the more traditional roles of wife and mother. Consequently, numerous women in all professions, including nursing, chose to return to marriage and childrearing rather than continue employment outside the home.

After WWII communism demonstrated its strength more than ever as the Soviet Union began invading and taking over Eastern European countries. With support from China, the North Koreans made a grab for South Korea, resulting in the Korean War. Again, nurses volunteered for the armed services to provide care to patients near the battlefields in Korea. This time they worked in mobile army surgical hospitals, better known as MASH units, where medical and surgical techniques were further refined.

The two decades after WWII saw the emergence of nursing as a true profession. Minimal national standards for nursing education were established by the National Nursing Accrediting Service. In 1945 state boards of nurse examiners in 25 states adopted the state board test pool. By 1950 all state boards were participating in the test pool; they continue to do so today. Nursing continued to improve the quality and quantity of educational programs as the number of nursing baccalaureate programs grew and associate degree programs developed in community or junior colleges (Kalisch and Kalisch, 1995; Robinson and Perry, 2001) (Box 1-3).

The end of WWII and the early 1950s marked the beginning of significant federal intervention in health care. The Nurse Training Act of 1943 was the first instance of federal funding being used to support nurse training. The passage of the Hill-Burton Act, or the Hospital Survey and Construction Act of 1946, marked the largest commitment of federal dollars to health care in the country's history. The purpose of the act was to provide funding to construct hospitals and to assist states in planning for other health care facilities based on the needs of the communities. Nearly 40% of the hospitals constructed in the late 1940s and the early 1950s were built with Hill-Burton funds. The hospital construction boom created by the Hill-Burton Act led to an increased demand for professional nurses to provide care in hospitals (Chitty and Black, 2007).

It was also in the early 1950s that the National Association of Colored Graduate Nurses (NACGN) went out of existence. This was the organization that fought for integration of the African-American nurse into the ANA. From 1916 to 1948, African-American nurses in the South were barred from membership in the ANA because of segregation laws in the Southern states. In the 1940s, the NACGN began to wage an all-out war against discrimination by the Southern constituents of the ANA. The NACGN chose as its central issue the route to membership in ANA. This issue was raised by the NACGN on the floor at every national convention of the ANA, and it evoked strong opposition from the Southern state constituents. Speaking from the floor of the House of Delegates at the 1946 convention in Atlantic City, a white nurse from Georgia referred to African-American nurses as "our darkies." Immediately a motion was passed to strike the reference from the record. However, this comment caused an uproar, and the African-American nurses who were barred from membership in the Southern states started the wheels turning to bypass the states and join ANA directly. This arrangement, known as individual membership, was put into effect in 1948. With the establishment of individual membership, African-American nurses in the South could bypass their states and become members of the ANA. This type of individual membership continued until all barriers had been dropped in the early 1960s (Carnegie, 1995).

Nursing in the 1960s

Federal legislation enacted during the 1960s had a major and lasting effect on nursing and health care. The Community Mental Health Centers Act of 1963 provided funds for the construction of community outpatient mental health centers; opportunities for mental health nursing were expanded when funds to staff these centers were appropriated in 1965 with the passage of the Medicare and Medicaid acts (Boschma, 2003). Medicaid, Title XIX of the Social Security Act, was enacted and replaced all programs previously instituted for medical assistance. The purpose of the Medicaid program, which was jointly sponsored and financed with matching funds from federal and state governments, was to serve as medical insurance for those families, primarily women and children, with an income at or below the federal poverty level. Medicaid quickly became "the largest public assistance program in the nation, covering about 9.7% of the population, including more than 15% of all children," (Baer, D'Antonio, and Rinker, 2002).

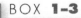

BOX **1-3**

Qualities of Good Nurses During Post–World War II

1. Tidy and loyal to the hospital and its personnel
2. Compliant with the orders of the physicians and directives of nursing management
3. Always busy
4. If census was low, fold laundry, clean shelves, prepare supplies to be sterilized
5. Ability to get work done no matter how many patients assigned

From Martell LK: Maternity care during the post World War II baby boom: the experience of general duty nurses, *West J Nurs Res* 96(3):387-391, 1999.

Health departments employed public health nurses to provide the bulk of the care needed by children and pregnant women in the Medicaid population. Services provided by these nurses included family planning, well-child assessments, immunizations, and prenatal care. A physician assigned as the district health officer supervised the nurses. Without the public health nurses and local health departments, many women and children in the inner city areas and rural communities would have been without access to basic health care.

Another important amendment to the Social Security Act was Title XVIII, or Medicare, passed in 1965. The Medicare program provides hospital insurance, part A, and medical insurance, part B, to all people ages 65 and older who are eligible to receive social security benefits; people with total, permanent disabilities; and people with end-stage renal disease. As a result of Medicare reimbursement, many hospitals began catering to physicians who treated Medicare patients. Medicare patients were attractive to the hospitals because all hospital charges, regardless of amount or appropriateness of services, were reimbursed through the Medicare program (Chitty and Black, 2007).

As a result of Medicare reimbursement, hospital-bed occupancy increased, which led to increased numbers of nurses needed to staff hospitals. Nursing embraced the hospital setting as the usual practice area and moved away from the community as the preferred practice site. Nursing schools also followed the trend by reducing the number of curriculum hours devoted to community health and concentrated their efforts on hospital-based nursing (Stanhope and Lancaster, 2008).

Another outcome of the Medicare legislation was the home health movement. To receive Medicare reimbursement for home health services, patients had to have (1) home-bound status; (2) a need for part-time or intermittent, skilled nursing care; (3) a medically reasonably and necessary need for treatment; and (4) a plan of care authorized by a physician. Home health agencies were established and began to employ increasing numbers of nurses. The number of home health agencies began to grow in the mid-1960s, and as a result of Medicare reimbursement and other influences, including a growing older adult population, advances in medical technology, and public demand for increased access to health care, the home health industry continued unprecedented growth into the 1990s. Home health was one of the first employment settings that provided nurses the opportunity to work weekdays only.

Nursing in the 1970s

The women's movement of the 1970s greatly influenced nursing. Nurses began to focus not only on providing quality care to patients but also on enhancing the economic benefits of the profession. Hospitals were receiving significant reimbursements for patient care; however, nurses' salaries did not reflect an adequate percentage of that reimbursement. Health care costs soared. This increase in health care costs built the framework for mandated changes in reimbursement. Nursing practice and the educational focus remained in the hospital setting.

During this time nurses played a major role in providing health care to communities and were instrumental in developing hospice programs, birthing centers, and daycare centers for older adults (Buhler-Wilkerson, 2001). Although basic educational programs for nurse practitioners expanded during the 1970s and master's-level preparation was developed as the requirement for graduation and practice, certification was also required to practice as a nurse practitioner. Before this time, only certification was required. State nursing practice acts were amended to provide for monitoring and licensing advanced practice nurses. Men also began to increase in numbers in this female-dominated profession (O'Lynn and Tranbarger, 2006).

In 1974 the ANA conducted research in the area of ethnic minorities and submitted a proposal to the National Institute of Mental Health to fund a project to permit minority nurses—African-Americans, Hispanics, Asians, and American Indians—to earn PhDs. Of the graduates of the project, the vast majority serve on faculties of universities and are conducting research on factors in mental health and illness related to ethnicity and cross-cultural conflict, thereby fulfilling their commitment to advance the cause of quality health care for people of all ethnicities.

Despite past laxity, the ANA House of Delegates at its 1972 convention did pass an affirmative action resolution calling for a task force to develop and implement a program to correct inequities. The house also provided for the position of an ombudsman to evaluate involvement of minorities in leadership roles within the organization and to treat complaints by applicants for membership or by members of the association who had been discriminated against because of nationality, race, creed, lifestyle, color, age, or sex. It was also in the 1970s that the ANA elected its first African-American president, Barbara Nichols, who served two terms.

Within the structure of many professional organizations is a unit referred to as an academy, which is composed of a cadre of scholars who deal with issues that concern the profession and take positions in the name of the academy. The American Academy of Nursing (AAN) was created by the ANA board in 1973. An elected group of highly accomplished leaders across all sectors of nursing (education, research, and practice), it uses the credential FAAN (Fellow, American Academy of Nursing). Through the application of visionary leadership, the intent of the AAN is to transform health care policy through nursing knowledge to optimize the well-being of the American people.

At its convention in Atlantic City in 1976, the ANA launched its Hall of Fame to pay tribute to those nurses who had not only paved the way for others to follow but also made outstanding contributions to the profession.

Nursing in the 1980s

The types of patients needing health care changed in the 1980s. Homelessness became a common problem in large cities. Unstable economic developments contributed to an increase in indigent populations (Baer et al, 2002). Acquired immunodeficiency syndrome (AIDS) emerged as a frightening, fatal epidemic.

Runaway health care costs became a national issue in the 1980s. Medicare was still reimbursing for any and all hospital services provided to recipients. From 1966 to 1981, the federal contribution to hospital care rose from 13% to 41% (Baer et al, 2002). In 1983 in an attempt to restrain hospital costs, Congress passed the Diagnosis-Related Group system for reimbursement, better known as the DRG system.

Before 1983 Medicare payments were made to the hospital after the patient received services. Although there were restrictions, the entire bill generally was paid without question. DRGs were implemented to provide prospective payment for hospital services based on the patient's admitting diagnosis and thereby to reduce the overall cost to Medicare. Hospitals now were to be reimbursed one amount based on the patient's diagnosis, not on hospital charges. The system was developed by physicians at the Yale–New Haven Hospital and addressed approximately 468 diagnoses classified according to length of stay and cost of procedures associated with the diagnosis (Nies and McEwen, 2007).

As a result of the DRG reimbursement system, hospitals were forced to increase efficiency and more closely manage hospital services, including the patient's length of stay, laboratory and radiographic testing, and diagnostic procedures. Case management and critical pathways were developed to more efficiently manage patient care, and case management became a new area of specialization for the professional nurse.

Despite the high cost of health care, medicine prospered. Medical care advanced in areas such as organ transplantation, resuscitation and support of premature infants, and critical care techniques. Physician specialization and advances in medical technology flourished. Medical specialties, such as nephrology, cardiology, endocrinology, orthopedics, neurosurgery, cardiovascular surgery, and advanced practices for obstetrics all led to improved health care services and costs in the hospital setting. The advanced technology also led to the development of outpatient surgery units.

Outpatient surgery services blossomed and provided a quick and efficient site for surgery that did not require extended hospital stays. Costs were greatly reduced because of fewer staff members needed for coverage, fewer supplies, and reduced facility costs. Nurses were interested in employment opportunities in outpatient facilities because they afforded a chance to work only during the day with no weekend assignments.

As the concern over increasing health care costs heightened, use of ambulatory services increased and enrollment in health maintenance organizations grew. Advanced nurse practitioners increased in popularity as cost-effective providers of primary and preventive health care. A growing number of nurses moved from the hospital setting into the community to practice in programs, such as hospice and home health. Consumers began to demand bans on unhealthy activities, such as smoking in public. Health education became more important as consumers were encouraged to take responsibility for their own care (Stanhope and Lancaster, 2008). Even the terminology changed; the individual once known as the patient became known as the client or consumer and was afforded respect as a person who purchases a service.

Public health programs struggled to survive as counties and states cut health department budgets. A landmark study conducted by the Institute of Medicine (IOM) in 1988, titled *The Future of Public Health*, indicated a dismal picture for public health. The study determined that public health had moved away from its traditional role and core functions and that no strategy was in place to bring public health back to its original purpose (Stanhope and Lancaster, 2008). Inadequate funding for public health continues to be a problem; however, it is hoped that soon public health will be restored to its original function and purpose.

Nursing enrollments dropped drastically in the late 1980s. This drop in enrollment occurred as the complexity of health care was rapidly increasing and more nurses were assuming expanded roles. As a result of these trends, a serious national shortage of nurses occurred across all settings (Ellis and Hartley, 2004).

Toward the end of the 1980s, the American Medical Association announced its answer to the nursing shortage. It proposed to establish a 9-month program to prepare registered care technologists. This proposal incensed nurses who unified to fight against it. As a result, the proposal was rejected (Schorr and Kennedy, 1999).

Also in the late 1980s several nursing scholars suggested that nursing research be firmly focused on the substantive information required to guide practice, rather than on philosophic and methodologic dilemmas of scientific inquiry. In 1985 the creation of the National Center for Nursing Research at the National Institutes of Health brought with it an increase in federal resources for nursing research and research training (Baer et al, 2002; Hinshaw, 1999).

Nursing in the 1990s

The 1990s began with alarm over the state of the U.S. economy. Government statisticians reported an alarming increase in the national debt complicated by slow economic growth. In the early 1990s, average household incomes were stagnating. More women with families entered the workforce to afford the increasing cost of living. More nurses selected jobs in which they could work more hours in fewer days for more money, sometimes sacrificing the fringe benefits, allowing them to work a second job or earn higher pay through shift differential for working evening and night shifts. Creative shifts, such as the 10-hour day, 4-day work week or the 12-hour day, 3-day work week became commonplace in health care facilities. Just as in the 1980s, the cost of health care continued to increase with the technologic advancements in medical care. Men were considered a minority in nursing, and salaries were thought to be on the increase as a result of male presence in the profession (O'Lynn and Tranbarger, 2006).

There also were growing concerns in the 1990s about the health of the nation, which prompted the *Healthy People 2000* initiative. Many diseases associated with preventable causes characterized mortality in the United States. In 1990 more than 2 million U.S. residents died from diseases, such as heart disease, cancer, cerebral vascular disease, accidents, chronic obstructive pulmonary disease, liver cirrhosis, tuberculosis, and human immunodeficiency virus infection. The inner city became a concern of disparities in these diseases with issues related to access and quality of care (Karels, 2005). Factors contributing to these common diseases state related to lifestyle patterns, behaviors, and habits (modifiable risk factors). More youth were at risk because of behavior such as smoking cigarettes, using abusive drug substances, eating poorly balanced diets, failing to exercise, having sex with multiple partners, and being subjected to acts of violence. *Healthy People 2000: National Health Promotion and Disease Prevention Objectives* was published in 1991 by the U.S. Department of Health and Human Services as a nationwide effort to help states, cities, and communities identify health promotion and disease prevention strategies to address these health risk problems.

The AIDS epidemic radically changed the process for infection control among health care workers in health care institutions across the nation. Recapping needles, wearing latex gloves, and using isolation precautions were issues that triggered much dialogue and debate among health care workers. Health care workers were mandated to use preventive measures in the form of Universal Precautions; all contact with blood and body fluids from all patients was considered potentially infectious.

Exposure to hazardous materials became a major issue of concern for not only health care workers but also the general public. Chemical and radioactive substances that created dangerous exposure and health risks were increasingly used in the workplace. Employers were held legally accountable for informing their employees of the actual or potential hazards and for reducing their exposure risk through training and the use of protective equipment. The hazardous materials issue was especially important in nursing and medicine, particularly with regard to exposure to carcinogenic chemicals used in drug therapy and in environmental infection control.

In 1990 the increasing costs of Medicaid and Medicare triggered political action for health care reform. Findings of a federal commission appointed to evaluate the American health care system included the following (Chitty and Black, 2007):

♦ Fifteen percent of the gross national product was related to health care expenditures (this amounts to approximately $1 trillion annually).

♦ The United States spent more than twice as much as any industrialized nation for health care services.

◆ Americans were living longer, which indicated a growing demand for home health and nursing home care, in addition to increased Medicare expenditures.

It became apparent that if health care spending continued to increase, the U.S. economy would be in danger of collapse. Thus the health care system moved toward managed care in an attempt to control health care expenditures. The managed care movement has had a tremendous effect on nursing.

The focus of managed care was on providing more preventive and primary care, using outpatient and home settings when possible, and limiting expensive hospitalizations. Massive downsizing of hospital nursing staff occurred, with an increased use of unlicensed assistive personnel to provide care in hospitals. There was an increasing demand for community health nurses and advanced practice nurses to provide primary care services. The nurse of the 1990s had to be focused on delivering health care services that (1) encompassed health risk assessment based on family and environmental factors, (2) supported health promotion and disease prevention, and (3) advanced counseling and health education (Jones, 2004).

In June 1993, the National Center for Nursing Research was renamed the National Institute of Nursing Research. Moving nursing research into the National Institutes of Health enhanced the interprofessional possibilities for collaborative investigation. As a result, nursing research grew rapidly during the 1990s. Multiple research programs focused on important health issues, such as health promotion across the life span. Nursing research began to inform health care policy through federal commissions and agency programs (Hinshaw, 1999; Jones, 2004).

In the 1990s, a partnership was forged between mandatory state licensure authorities, which set practice standards at the level of entering associate-degree graduates, and national, nongovernmental bodies that certify graduate-prepared specialists. These national certifying agencies were intensely engaged in improving methods for determining the continual competence of certified nurse practitioners within the swift current of health care change. The consumer's voice in the partnership was heard via collaboration with advocacy organizations and the appointment of more public members to licensing, certifying, and accreditation boards. Voluntary credentialing bodies recognized that if they were to serve effectively, they had to engage in active public information campaigns to inform consumers about their health care choices (Buhler-Wilkerson, 2001).

Nursing in the Twenty-First Century

Professional nurses in the twenty-first century are faced with many challenges within the dynamic state of health care. In addition to the issues of access, cost, quality, safety, and accountability in health care, nurses today are challenged by an aging population, a serious nursing shortage, generational differences in an aging workforce with poor prospects for replacements, high acuity and short staffing, conflict in the workplace, expanding technology, complex consumer health values, and an increasingly intercultural society. Nurses have identified numerous areas of concern, including insufficient staffing, inadequate salaries, effects of stress and overwork, lack of participation in decision making, and dissatisfaction with the quality of their own nursing care.

Changing duties, responsibilities, and conflicts amid nursing shortages and public concern over patient safety and quality of care characterize present-day practice. These changes require professional nurses to have core competency in critical thinking, communication, interprofessional collaboration, assessment, leadership, and technical skills, in addition to knowledge of health promotion and disease prevention, information technology, health systems, and public policy.

According to AACN's report on 2008-2009 Enrollment in Baccalaureate and Graduate Programs in Nursing, U.S. nursing schools turned away 49,948 qualified applicants due to insufficient number of faculty, clinical sites, classroom space, clinical preceptors, and budget constraints. Like the overall nursing workforce, mean age of faculty has increased steadily from 49.7 years in 1993 to 54 in 2008 (AACN, 2009). Public funding to schools of nursing needs to be increased to attract and retain nursing faculty. In support of the nursing profession, the U.S. Congress adopted the Nurse Reinvestment Act to provide funds for nursing education, recruitment, and retention programs. President George W. Bush signed the bill into law in August 2002.

In May 2003 the IOM released recommended partnerships of academic institutions, local and state public health departments, community health agencies, and schools of public health to establish training for medical and nursing school curricula. The future of public health in our nation depends on a competent, well-trained public health workforce. A well-trained workforce is in the best interest of all those concerned with maintaining a healthy society (Institute of Medicine [IOM], 2003).

Nursing is the nation's largest health care profession with more than 2.9 million RNs nationwide. Nurses make up the largest single component of hospital staff, are the primary providers of hospital patient care, and deliver most of the nation's long-term care. According to the U.S. Bureau of Labor Statistics, registered nursing is the occupation with the largest job growth from 2002 to 2012 (Hecker, 2004). Nursing students account for more than half (52%) of all health professions students in the United States. The nursing profession has risen to the challenges of the twenty-first century by uniting efforts to shape health care and the profession. Numerous coalitions have been formed to address the critical nursing shortage; increased political liaisons have influenced health policy; and involvement in evidence-based practice is more prevalent than ever and continues to improve health outcomes for individuals, groups, communities, and the nation (Connelly, 2004).

SUMMARY

Nursing is a dynamic profession that has evolved into a theory, research, and evidence-based practice. From its unorganized and variably defined beginnings, a profession based on the framework of competence, autonomy, determination, and human caring has developed. The challenges and opportunities have paralleled the path of world history and have brought about significant changes in the profession. From the men who opened the path, to the women who brought dignity and respect to their philosophy of caring, to the pioneers who brought unity to the profession plagued by a history of racism, sexism, and sometimes disgrace, nursing has become recognized as critical to the health of the nation. Despite myriad challenges, the practice of nursing has been distinguished and qualified by the intellect, skill, commitment, and contribution of countless sisters, deaconesses, and individuals, such as Seacole, Dix, Barton, Wald, Breckenridge, and Nightingale.

The nursing shortage has forced the nation to focus on a variety of ways to educate and use nurses of the future. Nurses play an important role in determining that future and the future of health care in America. Congress will continue to play a major role in providing funding to alleviate the shortage of faculty, clinical practitioners, and advanced practice nurses. As society changes, so does the role of the nurse. The quality of health care provided to our citizens cannot be compromised. Therefore, nurses must continue to play major roles in future health care initiatives (Connelly, 2004; Jones, 2004).

SUMMARY—cont'd

Through periods of war, socioeconomic change, and health care reform, nurses have played a vital role in initiating change to improve the health care arena. Nurses have provided the integrity to maintain the quality of care in all health care settings. The evolution of the practice from the treatment of disease to health promotion and disease prevention has led the way in determining the type of providers needed to care for patients in the future (Connelly, 2004). This evolution will continue to provide the foundation for the scope of practice, educational curricula, scholarship, and research necessary for nurses to lead and manage the health care environment of the future (Catalano, 2009). Nurses will continue to increase knowledge, manage technology, and maintain ethical standards to provide high-quality, patient-centered, safe care to individuals, families, communities, and populations throughout the world (Box 1-4).

evolve Additional resources are available online at: http://evolve.elsevier.com/Cherry/

BOX **1-4**

Helpful Websites

HISTORICAL NURSING REFERENCES
www.aacn.nche.edu/Publications/issues/96july.
  htm
www.mtsu.edu/~kmiddlet/history/women/
  wh-med.html
www.nursingworld.org/pressrel/2002/ltr0726.
  htm
www4.umdnj.edu/camlbweb/blacknurses.html
www.contemporarynurse.com/vol12_1.htm
www.aahn.org
www.firstaid.about.com/cs/historyofnursing
www.umich.edu/~inden/papers/sindhu.html
www.internurse.com/history

http://womenshistory.about.com/cs/medicine
www.geocities.com/Athens/Forum/6011
http://womenshistory.about.com/cs/
  nursesandnursing
www.nurseweek.com/features/98-7/forensic.
  html
www.aahn.org/resource.html
Women in Medicine
www.med.virginia.edu/hs-library/historical/
  antiqua/stext.htm
Nursing Individuals
www.bu.edu/archives/holdings/historical/nursing.
  html

REFERENCES

American Association of Colleges of Nursing (AACN): *Faculty shortages in baccalaureate and graduate nursing programs: scope of the problem and strategies for expanding the supply*, Washington, DC, June 2005.

American Association of Colleges of Nursing (AACN): *Essentials of doctoral education for advanced nursing practice*. 2006. Available at: www.aacn.nche.edu/DNP/pdf/Essentials.pdf.

American Association of Colleges of Nursing (AACN): 2007 *White paper on the role of the clinical nurse leader*. Retrieved July 21, 2007, from: www.aacn.nche.edu/Publications/*WhitePapers*/Clinicalnurseleader.htm.

American Association of Colleges of Nursing (AACN): *2008-2009 Salaries of instructional and administrative nursing faculty in baccalaureate and graduate programs in nursing*, Washington, DC, 2009.

Baer ED, D'Antonio P, Rinker S: *Enduring issues in American nursing*, New York, 2002, Springer.

Bahr L, Johnson B: *Collier's encyclopedia* (vol 18), New York, 1997, Simon and Schuster.

Boschma G: *The rise of mental health nursing: a history of psychiatric care in Dutch asylums 1890-1920*, University of Chicago Press, Chicago, 2003, Amsterdam University Press in US.

Buhler-Wilkerson K: *No place like home: a history of nursing and home care in the United States*, Baltimore, 2001, Johns Hopkins.

Carnegie ME: *The path we tread: blacks in nursing worldwide: 1854-1994*, ed 3, New York, 1995, National League for Nursing, Jones and Bartlett.

Catalano JT: *Nursing now: today's issues, tomorrow's trends*, ed 4, Philadelphia, 2009, FA Davis.

Chitty KB, Black BP: *Professional nursing: concepts and challenges*, ed 5, St Louis, 2007, Saunders.

Collins H: Mission for the millennium: choke out remains of polio, *Charlotte Observer*, March 14, 1999, pp 1A, 10A.

Connelly CA: Beyond social history: new approaches to understanding the state of and the state in nursing history, *Nurs Hist Rev* 12:5–24, 2004.

D'Antonio P: *Founding friends: families, staff and patients at the Friends Asylum in early nineteenth century Philadelphia*, Bethlehem, PA, 2006, Lehigh University Press.

Deloughery GL: *Issues and trends in nursing*, ed 3, St Louis, 1998, Mosby.

Doheny MD, Cook CB, Stopper MC: *The discipline of nursing: an introduction*, ed 4, Stamford, CT, 1997, Appleton and Lange.

Donahue MP: *Nursing: the finest art—an illustrated history*, St Louis, 1999, Mosby.

Dossey BM et al, editors: *Florence Nightingale today: healing, leadership, global action*, Washington DC, 2005, Nursesbooks.org.

Ellis JR, Hartley CL: *Nursing in today's world: challenges, issues and trends*, ed 8, Philadelphia, 2004, Lippincott.

Ellis JR, Hartley CL: *Nursing in today's world: challenges, issues and trends*, ed 9, Philadelphia, 2008, Wolters Kluwer/Lippincott Williams & Wilkins.

Fitzpatrick MF: The mercy brigade, *Civil War Times* 36(3):34–40, 1997.

Freedman D: *The Anchor bible dictionary*, New York, 1995, Doubleday.

Giger J, Davidhizar R: *Transcultural nursing: assessment and intervention*, ed 4, St Louis, 2004, Mosby.

Gill G: *Nightingales: the extraordinary upbringing and curious life of Miss Florence Nightingale*, New York, 2004, Ballantine Books.

Hecker DE: *Occupational employment projections to 2012*, Washington, DC, 2004, US Department of Labor, Bureau of Labor Statistics.

Hinshaw AS: Nursing research and the explosion of knowledge. In Schorr TM, Kennedy MS, editors: *One hundred years of American nursing*, New York, 1999, Lippincott.

Institute of Medicine (IOM): Who will keep the public healthy? Workshop summary. In Hernandez I, editor: *Committee on Education, Public Health Professionals for the 21st Century*, 2003, The National Academy of Sciences Press.

Joel L: *The nursing experience: trends, challenges and transition*, ed 5, New York, 2006, McGraw-Hill.

Jones ZO: Knowledge systems in conflict: the regulation of African American midwifery, *Nurs Hist Rev* 12:167–184, 2004.

Kalisch P, Kalisch B: *The advance of American nursing*, ed 2, Philadelphia, 1986, JB Lippincott.

Kalisch P, Kalisch B: *The advance of American nursing*, ed 3, Philadelphia, 1995, JB Lippincott.

Kalisch B, Kalisch P: *American nursing: a history*, ed 4, Philadelphia, 2003, Lippincott Williams & Wilkins.

Karels C: *Cooked: an inner city nursing memoir*, ed 2, Hackensack, NJ, 2005, Arcania Press.

Karger HJ, Stoesz D: *American social welfare policy: a pluralist approach*, ed 5, New York, 2005, Allyn and Bacon.

Katz JR, Carter C, Bishop J, Kravits SL, Block J: *Keys to nursing success*, ed 3, Columbus, OH, 2009, Pearson/Prentice-Hall.

Lindeman C, McAthie M: *Nursing trends and issues*, Springhouse, PA, 1990, Springhouse Corporation.

Luddy M, et al, editors: *The Crimean journals of the Sisters of Mercy 1854-1856*, Dublin, Ireland, 2004, Four Courts Press.

Nelson S: *"Say little, do much": nineteenth century religious women and care of the sick*, Philadelphia, 2001, University of Pennsylvania Press.

Nies MA, McEwen M: *Community/public health nursing: promoting the health of populations*, ed 4, Philadelphia, 2007, Saunders.

Oermann MH: *Professional nursing practice*, Stamford, CT, 1997, Prentice-Hall.

O'Lynn CO, Tranbarger R: *Men in nursing: history, challenges, and opportunities*, New York, 2006, Springer.

Robinson TM, Perry PM: *Cadet nurse stories: the call for and response of women during World War II*, Indianapolis, 2001, Center Nursing Press.

Salzman J, Smith D, West C, editors: *Encyclopedia of African-American culture and history*, vol 3, New York, 1996, Macmillan Library Reference USA, Simon and Schuster Macmillan.

Sarnecky M: Nurses at Pearl Harbor: the true story, *Reflect Nurs Leadersh* 27(4):16–21, 2001.

Schorr TM, Kennedy MS: *One hundred years of American nursing*, New York, 1999, Lippincott.

Small H: *Florence Nightingale: avenging angel*, London, 2002, Constable and Robinson.

Snodgrass ME: *Historical encyclopedia of nursing*, Santa Barbara, CA, 2004, Diane Publishing Co.

Stanhope M, Lancaster J: *Community and public health nursing*, ed 7, St Louis, 2008, Mosby.

Walton J, Barondess J, Locke S: *The Oxford medical companion*, New York, 1994, Oxford University Press.

ADDITIONAL RESOURCES

American Association of Colleges of Nursing (AACN). (2008): *The essentials of doctoral education for advanced nursing practice*, www.aacn.nche.edu.

Carnegie ME: Black nurses at the front, *Am J Nurs* 84(10):1250–1252, 1984.

Rosseter R: A new role for nurses: making room for clinical nurse leaders, *Jt Comm Perspect* 9(8):5 7, 2009.

Tornabeni J: The evolution of a revolution in nursing, *J Nurs Admin* 36:3–6, 2006.

The Contemporary Image of Professional Nursing

L. Antoinette (Toni) Bargagliotti, DNSc, RN, ANEF

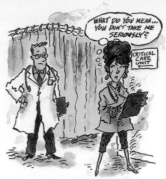

Each nurse forms the image of nursing every day.

Ⓔvolve Additional resources are available online at: http://evolve.elsevier.com/Cherry/

"People are always blaming their circumstances for what they are. I don't believe in circumstances. The people who get on in this world are the people who get up and look for the circumstances they want, and if they can't find them, make them."

GEORGE BERNARD SHAW

VIGNETTE

Mary is a senior nursing student who asks a faculty member, "Why can't we wear different scrubs and jewelry to clinical? Have you seen what nurses wear? I don't know what difference it makes anyway. Patients don't care what we're wearing. They care that we know how to take care of them. You know, 2 months after we graduate, we'll be wearing what everyone else does. Yes, I know we look better than everyone else does. But why?"

■ QUESTIONS TO CONSIDER WHILE READING THIS CHAPTER:

1 How does the image of a nurse differ from that of a physician?

2 How does the nurse's appearance affect the patient's opinion of the quality of care the nurse provides?

KEY TERMS

Art Any branch of creative work, especially painting and drawing, that displays form, beauty, and any unusual perception.
Literature All writings in prose or verse.
Media All the means of communication, such as newspapers, radio, and television.
Stereotype A fixed or conventional conception of a person or group held by a number of people that allows for no individuality.

LEARNING OUTCOMES

After studying this chapter, the reader will be able to:

1 Describe the image of nursing in art, media, and literature over time.

2 Identify nursing actions that convey a negative image of nursing.

3 Suggest strategies that would enhance the image of nursing.

4 Create an individualized plan to promote a positive image of nursing in practice.

CHAPTER OVERVIEW

This chapter describes how the image of nursing has been shaped and suggests strategies that nurses can use to forge a positive public and professional image of their practice. Because nurses have been the subjects of artists, sculptors, and writers for thousands of years, a historic perspective is used to illustrate the contextual background for the evolving image of the profession.

IMAGES OF NURSING

When you imagine a nurse, what mental picture comes to mind? Do you think of *LIFE* magazine's 1942 nurse in a starched white uniform with a cap, the nurses portrayed in Johnson & Johnson's *Campaign for Nursing's Future* (2007), or your colleagues with whom you practiced yesterday? The contemporary image of professional nursing in the United States is an ever-changing kaleidoscope created by the 3.4 million men and women of all ages, races, and religious beliefs who are registered nurses (RNs). Adding to this multifaceted collage are the numerous snapshots of nurses and nursing as portrayed in television commercials, bumper stickers, art, poetry, architecture, postage stamps, television dramas, television series, movies, newspaper comic strips, stained-glass windows, and statues. Second in size to the profession of teaching, nurses have been alternatively described as either saints or sinners, powerless or powerful, admired or ignored, and, most recently, those who dare to care. Their practice has captured the attention of historians, economists, and sociologists who have studied this unusual group of people.

Since Florence Nightingale reduced mortality rates from 42% to 2% in a Crimean hospital constructed over an open sewer, nurses have been reformers who use limited resources to address unlimited "wants" for health care. The request for Nightingale's nursing services in the Crimea was born out of newspaper reports about the devastating health care conditions in the Crimean War. However, the outcome that Nightingale and these nurses achieved changed conditions in the British Army, forged a system of nursing education, and continues to strongly influence the profession.

Although nurses have become concerned with their public image and media portrayal, Kalisch and Kalisch's (1995) extensive work outlining the image of nursing in film and media over time permanently etched the image issue into the professional radar screen.

WHY IMAGE IS IMPORTANT

Publicly, concerns about the image of nursing are most often associated with a deepening national and global concern about the evolving nursing shortage. However, the image of nursing has far more serious effects than the numbers of nurses who are not there. RNs, who are 40% of the entire health professional workforce, are the "glue" that binds the health care of many into a more seamless experience for the patient. Safe patient care demands coordination of the armada of health professionals who use many technologies and many handoffs to provide care to a single person in intensive care and other technology-driven areas. The health care system's failure to recognize the criticality of seamless health care has allowed many medical errors to occur (Wachter, 2004). How nursing is perceived inside and outside of the health care system directly affects how successful nurses will be in coordinating patient care.

From the individual patient perspective, more often than not the requirement for health care comes unexpectedly and without warning. When patients seek health care in a hospital, they are entrusting their life and well-being to the one person who has 24/7 direct responsibility for their care and their environment—the RN. Unlike their personal physician, with whom patients may have had a long-term relationship, the RN, who is coordinating all of their care, is new to them and changes every 8 to 12 hours. It is important that the public trusts and believes in this nurse and the profession the nurse represents.

THE NURSING SHORTAGE

The specter of a growing nursing shortage will continue to loom large as an image-maker for nursing. According to the U.S. Bureau of Labor, the employment rate of RNs has one of the highest growth rates of employment of all occupations. With an employment rate expected to increase by more than 23%, nursing is projected to grow faster than the average of all occupations until 2010 (Bureau of Labor Statistics, 2009). However, by 2020 the United States is projected to need 1,016,900 more RNs than will be available and to have only 64% of the RN workforce required to meet the demand (Biviano et al, 2004).

The unprecedented magnitude of this shortage is a problem because the strategies that have been used in the past to ameliorate nursing shortfalls, such as the migration of foreign nurses, are insufficient to ameliorate this shortage. The numbers of foreign nurse graduates who become licensed for practice in the United States are too small. For example, only 36% ($n = 9211$) of the foreign nurse graduates ($n = 25,607$) who took the Commission on Graduates of Foreign Nursing Schools qualifying examination in 2005 to enable them to take the NCLEX-RN® examination passed the qualifying examination (Commission on Graduates of Foreign Nursing Schools, 2006). Similarly, strategies to entice nurses back into nursing will produce little for a profession that already has 83% of its licensed members in nursing practice (U.S. Department of Health and Human Services, 2006).

To begin to address the nursing shortage, President George W. Bush signed the Nurse Reinvestment Act P.L. 107-205 into law in August 2002. This act was funded at $20 million to provide nursing scholarships, public service announcements promoting nursing as a career, faculty loan cancellation programs, geriatric training grants, and nurse retention and safety enhancement grants.

NURSING IN ART AND LITERATURE

Although the way that nursing has been portrayed in art and literature over time may seem to be unrelated to the contemporary image of nursing, the mental image of contemporary nursing is enmeshed with these earliest images.

Art and literature have been the way in which people describe the human condition and cultural values of their time. In these earliest descriptions of nurses and nursing are found the enduring fundamental and essential tensions that exist within the profession today. Found within art and literature is the eternal question asked by those who know they will one day require nursing care, "Can I trust and entrust my life to this nurse?"

Antiquity Image of Nursing

The earliest literary reference to nursing chronicles the actions of two nurse midwives in approximately 1900 BC in Exodus 1 of the Old Testament, which indicates that the practice of two midwives became the vehicle through which the Israelites, the Jewish race, and the resultant Judeo-Christian heritage survived. From the sixth century until the 1800s, nurses were imaged as either untrained servants, soldiers, women of religious orders, or wealthy people performing acts of Christian charity (Kalisch and Kalisch, 1995; Kampen, 1988). These meager artistic renderings of nurses convey images that continue to be familiar to contemporary nurses.

Victorian Image of Nursing

In 1844 when Nightingale was "called" to become a nurse, Charles Dickens immortalized a different kind of nurse through Sairy Gamp, the nurse for whom nursing was endured because of the lack of other opportunities. For Sairy Gamp, a drunken, physically unkempt, uncaring nurse in *Martin Chuzzlewit*, nursing provided a way to profit from the sick and dying. Reflecting the concern of Victorian England for untrained caregivers, Dickens advised Sairy of the advantages of "a little less liquor, and a little more humanity, and a little less regard for herself, and a little more regard for her patients, and perhaps a trifle of additional honesty" (Dickens, 1910, p. 894).

Fortunately Sairy's literary arrival was followed by Longfellow's portrayal of the heroic Nightingale in *Santa Filomena* (1857). As important as Nightingale was to the improved health care of British soldiers and to the development of modern nursing, the ever-increasing positive images of Nightingale occurred solely because she was able to succinctly demonstrate the aggregate outcomes of nursing practice. To do so, she became one of the earliest users of the emerging body of knowledge called statistics and developed the pie chart that remains in common use. Notably, nursing emerged at a time of turbulent social change and reform in Great Britain.

Early Twentieth-Century Nursing

Toward the end of the Nightingale period at the turn of the century, nurses in war settings vividly capture the attention of artists. The most compelling image is Bellows' 1918 canvas, *Edith Cavell Directing the Escape of Soldiers from Prison Camp* (Donahue, 1985). World War I (WWI) Germany shocked the world with its 1915 firing squad execution of Edith Cavell, founder of the first nursing school in Belgium, who aided soldiers escaping prison camps. The art of heroic nursing expressed in several famous paintings reflected the reality of WWI nurses who were also the recipients of three Distinguished Service Crosses, 23 Distinguished Service Medals, 28 French Croix de Guerres, 69 British Military Medals, and 4 U.S. Navy Crosses (Donahue, 1985). Notably, American nurses who served in WWI were not commissioned in the military services. One in every three nurses served in WWI.

The 1930s Nurse as Angel of Mercy

On a grander scale, Warner Brothers' film *The White Angel* (1936) chronicled the professional life of Florence Nightingale (Jones, 1988). Endorsed by the American Nurses Association (ANA), *The White Angel* clearly portrayed Nightingale's persistence and head-to-head confrontation with medicine. Anticipating that the medical staff would deny her nurses rations, she brought provisions for them. When the medical staff locked her out of the hospital, Nightingale sat outside in the snow until patients and soldiers required physicians to admit these nurses. *The White Angel* conveyed to the public that nursing is a holy vocation, nurses have professional credentials, and their career choice is opposed because women belong at home (Jones, 1988). A subtle inference of the film is that Nightingale was smart enough to overcome the obstacles of medicine.

In 1938 Rich's tall and imposing white limestone statue, the *Spirit of Nursing*, was placed in Arlington National Cemetery to honor military nurses. Similarly, Germany's 1936 stamp commemorated nursing with a larger-than-life nurse compassionately overlooking people (Donahue, 1985).

The 1940s Nurse as Heroine

Considered to be the most positive movie about nursing, *So Proudly We Hail* is the 1942 story of nurses in Bataan and Corregidor. The film, starring Claudette Colbert, portrayed a small group of nurses rerouted to the Philippines after the attack on Pearl Harbor. Soon cut off from supplies and replacements as the Japanese took over the Philippines, these nurses provided care with few supplies and no staff to the thousands of soldiers in the Philippines. When the last nurses were to be evacuated from the occupied islands, a number of nurses voluntarily stayed behind, made the march to Bataan, and were interned as prisoners of war. Norman's *We Band of Angels: the Untold Story of American Nurses Trapped on Bataan by the Japanese* (1999) tells via their diaries and interviews the gritty, difficult, and heroic story of these nurses who served on Bataan.

Nursing was depicted positively on a 1940 Australian stamp as a larger-than-life figure looking over a soldier, a sailor, and an aviator; in Costa Rica's 1945 stamp of Florence Nightingale and Edith Cavell; and in the 1945 commissioning of the *USS Higbee*, a Navy destroyer named in honor of a Navy nurse (Donahue, 1985).

After nursing's glorious contributions to World War II, nurses returned home to find low salaries, long hours, too few staff, and too many patients. However, nursing continued to be glamorized through the Cherry Ames book series, the Sue Barton series, and other romance novels.

Nursing in the Antiestablishment Era of the 1960s

Ken Kesey developed the modern version of Sairy Gamp through the character of Nurse Ratched in *One Flew Over the Cuckoo's Nest* (1962). This best-selling novel later became a play and motion picture (1975) that won six Oscars, including Best Picture. Entrusted with the care of the mentally ill, Nurse Ratched, a military nurse in a starched white uniform, was the ultimate power figure who punished patients to cure their psychosis through conformity to a "system" (Jones, 1988). However, the reality of the turbulent period of the 1960s is that nursing was one of President Johnson's first salvos in the war on poverty. The Nurse Training Act of 1964 was funded at $250 million ($1.63 billion in 2006 dollars) (Federal Reserve Bank of Minneapolis, 2006). Although nurses also dramatically shaped the future of health care through the development of coronary care units, intensive care units, hemodialysis, and Silver and Ford's first nurse practitioner program in Colorado, a U.S. Bureau of Labor study indicated that salaries of nurses at that time were woefully inadequate in comparison with other, far-less-trained American workers (Kalisch and Kalisch, 1995).

Nursing in the Sexual Revolution of the 1970s

Media images of the nurse in the 1970s were formed amid a sexual revolution and a growing antimilitary American culture. War would again provide the media backdrop. The 1976 stamp, *Clara Maas, She Gave Her Life*, commemorated the 100th birthday of Maas, a 25-year-old nurse who died after deliberately obtaining two carrier mosquito bites so that she could continue providing care to soldiers with yellow fever in the Spanish-American War (Donahue, 1985). Her modern-day counterparts would be nurses in *M*A*S*H*, the hit television series that ran from 1972 to 1983.

The nursing profession viewed *M*A*S*H* as professionally destructive because of the negative portrayal of Hot Lips Hoolihan and the nurses of the 4077th Army MASH (Mobile Army Surgical Hospital) unit in Korea. The sexual exploits of nurses and physicians and the uncaring Margaret provided few positive images. However, for the American public who were receiving a daily dose of *M*A*S*H* in the news footage of Vietnam on nightly news, *M*A*S*H* presented a glimmer of reality. Continuous front-line exposure to the massive trauma of young men did not immunize these nurses from caring or from the horrors of what they were seeing. They coped with these horrors with a sense of humor and irreverence toward "the system." Nurses serving in Vietnam would later be imaged in the television series, *China Beach*.

Nursing in the 1980s to 1990s

Portraying an actual event, the complexities of nursing are realistically described in the play and television movie, *Miss Evers' Boys*. Through the character of Miss Evers, the play tells the true story of Nurse Rivers, who was hired to recruit and retain young African-American men into the infamous Tuskegee experiment designed to describe the long-term effects of untreated syphilis. Although the study began in 1932, penicillin became the treatment of choice for syphilis in 1947. When subjects asked Nurse Rivers to obtain the new treatment of penicillin for them and she sought to do so, the physician investigators required her to discourage them from treatment. Subjects were told they would be dropped from the study and forgo the benefits of free treatment, a free ride to the clinic, one hot meal per day, and, in case of dying, $50 for their funeral. Subjects were never told they had syphilis, only that they had "bad blood." The study, which was funded for 40 years by the U.S. Public Health Service, ended in 1972 only because it became publicly known through the press. Ironically, Nurse Rivers was the only consistent staff person throughout the 40 years of the study. As the narrator of the story, Nurse Evers introduces non-nurses to the dilemmas of nursing practice during that era and the consequences of misplaced faith and trust in other health care disciplines. Notably an outcome of the Tuskegee study was the requirement for institutional review boards to prevent this from occurring again.

In 1997 three films used war and nursing as a backdrop: *The English Patient*, *Love and War*, and *Paradise Road*. In all of these films, the nurse is a knowledgeable, nonjudgmental caregiver.

Artistic views of nursing during this period focused on caring. In the *Vietnam War Women's Memorial*, the central figure is the nurse in battle fatigues cradling the head of a soldier for whom she is providing care. Evident in the bronze statue is the fatigue of the nurse and her care for this dying soldier.

Millennial Media

As Stanley (2008) noted in his review of nurses in film from 1900 to 2007, more recent films with nurses tend to portray them as thoughtful, independent, intelligent professionals. In 2000 the character of Greg Focker, RN, in the movie, *Meet the Parents*, endures his soon-to-be father-in-law's stereotyped views about men who are nurses. In the 2001 movie *Pearl Harbor*, nurses were positively portrayed as heroically providing care and order to the chaos following the bombing attack on Pearl Harbor. Although there have been a number of successful television series that take place in hospitals, such as NBC's *ER* (1994-2009), ABC's *Grey's Anatomy* (2005-), Fox's *House* (2004-), and NBC's *Scrubs* (2001-), their central characters are primarily physicians, although much of what is depicted is nursing practice provided by interns and residents. Because the primary storylines, which focus on physicians, portray the physicians negatively, the script writers' neglect of nursing may be professionally helpful to nursing.

Nurse TV is a 30-minute television show that debuted in October 2008. Each episode features the practice of two nurses (*Nurse TV —Changing the image of nursing*, 2008). Debuting in 2009 was a Fox series, *HawthoRNe*, whose primary character is a multitasking chief nursing officer who, in at least one episode, works with staff nurses who breach ethical standards and common nursing protocols. Although this series attempted to portray nurses in a positive light with strong administrative skills rather than the usual caring skills, unethical behavior such as sexual interaction between a nurse and a patient negatively affects nursing's professional image, public trust, and recruiting into the profession.

Nurse Jackie, another dark comedy that previewed in 2009 portrayed a painkiller-addicted emergency department nurse with strong clinical skills, but her own set of ethics that were definitively not in compliance with nursing professional code of ethics.

Nursing's Response

Nursing students are the future of nursing. And students have taken that responsibility seriously with two similar programs directed toward the image of nursing. In 1993 the National Student Nurses Association (NSNA) (www.nsna.org/activities/nursing.asp) developed the ongoing Image of Nursing program designed to improve and protect the image of nursing. The program logo, "Nursing: not just a job, a profession," articulated the student perspective on nursing. This program has given annual awards for Image of Nursing projects and provided information to students. An important part of the NSNA Image of Nursing program has been the media surveillance information provided to students. How to contact the television networks, how to most effectively transmit information to them, and sample letters are provided to enable the voices of students to be heard when there is negative, demeaning nursing media or advertisements (NSNA, 2006).

In April 2001, seven graduate students at the Johns Hopkins University School of Nursing founded the Center for Nursing Advocacy (www.nursingadvocacy.org). Although slated to close in 2009, during its 8-year tenure, it carefully watched the portrayal of nurses in all media venues and immediately provided feedback. In 2001 it conveyed to the directors and producers of the television show *ER* the negative ways in which nurses were being portrayed and have subsequently done so with *House, Grey's Anatomy, Jeopardy!, Law and Order*, and others. They successfully convinced Skechers to remove a "naughty nurse" televised advertisement (Center for Nursing Advocacy, 2006).

The Center for Nursing Advocacy website rated television shows, movies, and books that portray nursing. Annually, they presented the Golden Lamp Awards for the best and worst media portrayals of nursing. For example, their 2005 Golden Lamp awards recognized Suzanne Gordon's *Nursing Against the Odds: How Health Care Cost-Cutting, Media Stereotypes, and Medical Hubris Undermine Nursing and Patient Care* and two episodes of *ER*, among others (Center for Nursing Advocacy, 2006).

Leading their list of the Ten Worst Portrayals of Nursing in the Media 2005 were six episodes of *Grey's Anatomy*, five episodes of *House*, three episodes of *ER*, two episodes of *Scrubs*, and the movies, *Million Dollar Baby* and *Meet the Fockers*, among others. Also included in the Center for Nursing Advocacy's "worst portrayals list" was a Canadian Virgin Cellular advertisement that negatively portrayed nursing.

In 2009 in response to the negative portrayal of nursing in popular television series' and the ANA members' subsequent outrage, ANA posted a call to action protesting the negative portrayals of nurses and asked RNs to send letters of complaint to producers of these shows (Trossman, 2009).

Media Campaigns for Nursing

In 1990 the Tri-Council of Nursing with funding from the Pew Foundation implemented the Nurses of America (NOA) media campaign. Nurses of America was designed to convey to the public that nurses are expert clinicians who are able to interpret technical data in usable ways as well as coordinate and negotiate health care. A strategically important part of the NOA campaign raised consciousness among nurses of the invisibility of nursing in the news media. A study of sources quoted by health coverage journalists in *The New York Times, Los Angeles Times,* and the *Boston Globe* indicated that nurses accounted for only 10 of more than 900 citations, ranking nurses last after patients (Buresch, Gordon, and Bell, 1991). Sigma Theta Tau International's Woodhull study of 20,000 articles published in 16 newspapers, magazines, and other health care publications (1998) indicated that nurses were cited only 4% of the time in the more than 2000 articles about health care (Sigma Theta Tau International, 1998).

This was followed by The Nurses for a Healthier Tomorrow campaign, which led to the Johnson & Johnson $30 million Campaign for Nursing's Future and the Promise of Nursing galas to raise funds for nursing faculty scholarships. As a consequence of the Johnson & Johnson campaign, baccalaureate nursing enrollments increased by more than 8% over 2 years, and high school sophomores and juniors began to rank nursing highly as a career choice (*Johnson & Johnson Newsletter*, 2007).

THE ENDURING PUBLIC CONCERN WITH NURSING

Against this backdrop of nursing images that extend from antiquity to the latest CNN broadcast is the question of the image that will be created by nurses today.

What the Public Believes About Nursing

Since 1999 when the Gallup poll began including nursing in its annual December poll on ethics, the public has rated nursing higher than all other professions for every year except 2001 when firemen outranked nursing. In the 2008 Gallup poll on ethical professions, 84% of the public rated nurses as the most ethical; trailing RNs were pharmacists (70%), high school teachers (65%), and physicians (64%) (Gallup poll, 2008).

In December 2001, Chris Matthews of CNBC's *Hardball* was a guest on CBS's *Late Show with David Letterman*. In discussing the changes that occurred following the 2001 World Trade Center attacks, he mentioned the 2001 Gallup poll that ranked nurses second to firemen. He said, "Do you remember when we were 5 or 6 years old and we wanted to be a hero and make a difference? We all wanted to be either firemen or nurses. It's taken 9/11 to remind us of when we had big souls in little bodies" (Burnett, 2001).

From a different perspective, California college students ($n = 3000$) in California's Central Valley were surveyed about their perceptions of nursing as a career relative to a career as a high school teacher, physical therapist, or physician. Two thirds of these students believed that nursing offered a good income potential, job security, and interesting and meaningful work. However, they believed that nursing was a "woman's profession" and fell behind the other careers (high school teacher, physical therapist, and physician) for job independence (Seago et al, 2006).

THE REALITY OF THE CONTEMPORARY STAFF NURSE

The reason for the existence of the modern health care institution—the hospital, the nursing home, the mental hospital, the home care agency—is to deliver nursing. If surgery could be done safely and economically on the kitchen table, and if people could survive it, it would be. If diagnosis and management of serious medical illness could be done in office practices in 8.5-minute visits, it would be. If the chronically mentally ill could be taken care of at home, and protected from the world and from themselves, they would be. If the demented, the frail, the paralyzed, the very old could be cared for at home, they would be and it would be a whole lot cheaper because public policy would not contemplate channeling the money to family caregivers: they're supposed to want to do it anyway (Diers, 1988, pp. VIII-2 and VIII-3).

Logically it could be inferred that nurses' satisfaction with the work setting should be high because their practice settings exist to deliver their services, and new practice settings are emerging daily. The public highly values their profession. Nursing's heroic and noble public image has been etched in stone and in stained-glass windows in larger-than-life proportions. A survey of nurses indicated that those who were more likely to be satisfied with their career over time held three values: (1) the sense of professional status, (2) the belief that they made a difference (patient care rewards), and (3) pride in their profession (Mills and Blaesing, 2000). The latest National Sample Survey of Registered Nurses (NSSR) found that 78% of practicing RNs were satisfied with their job, and 78.8% were with the same employer in the preceding year (U.S. Department of Health and Human Services, 2006).

FACTS ABOUT TODAY'S REGISTERED NURSE

Forty percent of all health care professionals in the United States are registered nurses, making nursing the largest health care professional group. Sixty-five percent of all anesthesia in the United States is delivered by certified registered nurse anesthetists (CRNAs). For two thirds of all rural hospitals, CRNAs are the sole anesthesia provider and they are the main provider of anesthesia for the military and for expectant mothers (American Association of Nurse Anesthetists [AANA], 2006).

Reflecting the aging of America, nurses are older, with a mean age of 46.8 years. However, new graduates are entering the profession at younger ages—BSN graduates at 26 years, ASN graduates at 31.9 years, and diploma graduates at 31.8 years. Although nursing continues to be a female-dominated profession (only 5.7% are male), almost half (49%) of CRNAs are men. Former U.S. Surgeon General Richard Carmona entered health care as a nurse. Interestingly, 47% of female nurses obtain a baccalaureate degree in nursing as do 46% of male nurses. Although only 10.6% of nurses are minorities, African-American nurses (14.3%) were more likely than white nurses (13.3%), Hispanic nurses (10.3%), or Asian or Native Hawaiian or Pacific Islanders (9.9%) to obtain graduate education in nursing (U.S. Department of Health and Human Services [USDHHS], 2006).

Although nurses have entered the profession at different levels of education, when reporting their highest level of nursing education, the largest percentage (34.2%) have a BSN, followed by nurses with an ASN (33.7%), diploma (17%), or master's or doctorate (13%). Almost half (47.2%) of RNs have a baccalaureate or higher degree. However, between 2000 and 2004, the largest increases (37%) were found among nurses receiving a graduate degree in nursing. Conversely the highest decreases (17%) were among those receiving a diploma in nursing (USDHHS, 2006).

Slightly more than half (56%) of all nurses practice in hospitals, 14.9% in community health, 11.5% in other ambulatory settings, 8.5% in other settings, such as nursing schools, the federal government, prisons, pharmaceuticals, and durable medical equipment. The majority of nurses (78%) report satisfaction or high satisfaction with their job. Only 13.8% of nurses were dissatisfied with their job (USDHHS, 2006).

Advanced practice registered nurses (APRNs) (clinical specialists, nurse practitioners, nurse-midwives, and nurse anesthetists) are 8.6% of the nursing population. The majority (51%) of APRNs are nurse practitioners (NPs), followed by clinical nurse specialists (CNSs) (24%), CRNAs (13%), NP-CNSs (6%), and nurse-midwives (4%) (USDHHS, 2006).

The demographics of twenty-first century nursing strongly suggest that continued professional success will require attracting more students who are male and who are from ethnic and minority groups. As the data indicate, men are as likely as women and African-American nurses are more likely than their white counterparts to obtain higher degrees in nursing. However, there are not sufficient numbers entering nursing.

The American Assembly of Men in Nursing (http://aamn.org) is an organization dedicated toward positively influencing the factors affecting men in nursing. The mission of this organization of men and women is to provide a "framework for nurses to meet, discuss, and influence factors which affect men as nurses" (American Assembly of Men in Nursing, 2007). An important part of their work is their annual meeting where papers related to men in nursing and men's health are presented.

A small study of male nursing students ($n = 29$) older than age 25 in a community college program indicated that gender did not interfere with their opportunities as a student, although they did report a lack of locker facilities, absence of male faculty, and a feminine gender bias in nursing textbooks. All subjects described problems in maternity clinical rotation regarding patients who refused their care based on gender. Although describing the event as being uncomfortable for both the patient and for themselves, these students believed they had other life experiences that ameliorated any possible negative effects (Smith, 2006).

CREATING THE IMAGE OF TWENTY-FIRST CENTURY NURSING

The twenty-first century image of nursing is one that nurses create every day as they practice and describe nursing to others. Conceptually, nursing is first and foremost "knowledge work" (Bargagliotti, 2003) regardless of age, gender, ethnic background, ethical perspective, or level of job satisfaction of the nurse. Knowledge workers are people who require specialized education to do work that requires judgment (Drucker, 2002). The knowledge work of nursing counts in terms of human lives and financial costs.

The failure-to-rescue data on the loss of human life from medical error is beginning to document the human and financial cost when nursing judgment is not available. When all medical records of all Medicare hospitalized patients ($n = 37$ million) in the United States from 2000 to 2002 were surveyed for the presence of 20 patient safety indicators (PSIs) and their subsequent effects, failure-to-rescue (occurring at a rate of 155 per 1000 cases) was the most frequently occurring incident (HealthGrades, 2004). The next two highest ranking incidents, decubitus ulcer at 30 per 1000 and postoperative sepsis at 13 per 1000, are equally nurse-sensitive indicators. These top three incidents accounted for 60% of all PSIs that occurred in this population. Twenty-five percent of all Medicare patients who experienced one PSI died as a consequence (HealthGrades, 2004).

When nursing practice is conceptualized as knowledge work in which nursing judgment counts, other images of nursing fade away. Insufficient staffing is not related to an aging workforce on the one hand or a diminished work ethic of a younger generation on the other hand.

Consider the following data about the potential benefits of nursing judgment to patients. The data from 799 nonfederal acute care general hospitals in 11 states were used to change the RN staffing model in two areas: (1) raising the percentage of RN/LPNs (improving the skill mix) and (2) increasing the number of patient care hours provided by RNs to the 75th percentile. Implementing only these two changes could have reduced adverse outcomes by 70,000, hospital days by 4.1 million, and deaths by 6700. Effecting these changes would have required replacing 37,000 full time equivalent (FTE) LPNs with RNs and adding an additional 114,456 FTE RNs. Whereas the total cost to effect these changes would have been $5.7 billion, this would have amounted to only 1.5% of annual hospital expenditures (Needleman et al, 2006). Notably an earlier analysis of these same data found no relationship between increased staffing levels of LPNs or nursing aides and a reduction in adverse outcomes (Needleman et al, 2001). Similarly the data from 168 hospitals indicated that risk-adjusted mortality following common surgeries was lowest when nurses provided care to four or fewer patients and when 60% or more of the nursing staff had a baccalaureate degree in nursing (Aiken et al, 2003).

Placing a human face on the data are surveys of medical staff and anecdotal reports from nurses. A 2005 survey of licensed physicians practicing across the state of Massachusetts indicated that 19% reported patient deaths that were directly attributable to low staffing levels; 82% believed that patient care suffers from low RN staffing levels; and 74% support legislation mandating minimal nurse-patient ratios for patient safety (Massachusetts Nurses Association, 2005). An emergency department (ED) nurse published an opinion editorial in *Newsweek* describing increasing unsafe patient loads in the ED along with his enthusiasm for his work coupled with his daily gratitude for not having killed anyone today because of unsafe staffing (Duke, 2006).

Kalisch, Begeny, and Neuman (2007) found that nurses were being imaged on the Internet between 2001 and 2004 as intelligent and educated (70%) health professionals who are committed to patient care. Interestingly, they also found that the image of nurses as political advocates for health care diminished on the Internet during this time frame.

THE BASICS

At the simplest level, 3.4 million RNs create their image by ensuring that only RNs are referred to as "the nurse." Although the International Council of Nurses reserved the title of "nurse" for the RN in 1985, it is the responsibility of every nurse to ensure that the housekeeper, the untrained caregiver, the nursing assistant, and everyone else is not referred to as "the nurse." Imagine how confusing this is for patients and their families. Ensuring that patient teaching and questions about patient care are referred to "the nurse," rather than the assistant to the nurse, ensures that patients and families receive the best information possible.

Changing Nurse-Physician Interactions

An enduring mystery and common experience for nurses is how to address a medical problem with the primary customer of the hospital, the physician. Physicians are the revenue generators for hospitals, and, in exchange for hospital privileges, agree to be self-governing and to abide by a set of medical staff bylaws. All medical staff bylaws include a disciplinary process that begins with the section chief, who is required to address documented patient care problems.

All too often, when nurses practice with a physician whose practice is substandard or who is highly volatile, they believe that this behavior is a nursing problem. Rather it is a medical problem that must be addressed by medicine via their staff bylaws. Only when nurses disengage, factually document the problem in patient care terms rather than as a personality issue, and forward this in writing to a nurse manager and the appropriate section chief can the problem be resolved.

Just as nursing's involvement with medical problems is confined to appropriate notification, so should medicine's involvement with nursing be confined to the same. When a physician notifies a nurse about a nursing problem, a more positive answer is, "Thank you. Let me investigate the problem and get back to you." Lengthy detailed discussions are seldom useful. When the nurse makes an error, a simple apology and sincere statement of corrective action is sufficient. Consider the following actual clinical situations.

CASE STUDY 2-1

A nephrologist complained in a meeting with a nursing service administrator, the chief of medical staff, and the physician liaison that he was not being notified by nursing about his patients and that nurses did not know how to take care of his dialysis patients.

RESPONSE 1

Nurse 1 told the nephrologist how well prepared the nursing staff is and that his is the first complaint of this type that has been received. (The problem is denied.) However, she indicated nursing is short-staffed, and there are a lot of agency nurses. (Two excuses are provided.) She will investigate. (This is the first positive response.) However, without a specific incident and patient, she may not be able to correct the problem. (This is the third excuse.)

RESPONSE 2

Nurse 2 carefully takes notes and limits her comments to clarifying questions while the physician becomes increasingly more derogatory. She concludes that there is a need to investigate and indicates that a written report will be sent to all parties. The physician is thanked for bringing this to his or her attention.

The nurse's investigation indicates that multiple nurses over time and in different units have all phoned the nephrologist, who loudly announces that they have awakened his baby and abruptly hangs up the phone. Second, this is a difficult physician who never has time to discuss his patients when making rounds. Specific examples of unanswered questions are obtained.

The written findings are prepared, and nurse 2 poses only one question, "Since the physician is not able to 'take calls' after 5:30 PM, the patient care issue that concerns nursing is the question of who will be covering his patients."

Outcome: Within 2 weeks, the nephrologist's hospital privileges were quietly rescinded.

CASE STUDY 2-2

The nurses on a pediatric unit believed that they needed additional nursing staff.

RESPONSE 1

The nurses and nurse manager "make their case" by describing how stressed the nursing staff are to the medical staff and to nursing administration. They insist they cannot provide safe nursing care with their current level of staffing.

RESPONSE 2

The nurse manager requested data from the pharmacy about the number of medications administered by nurses on this unit for a specified period. The data indicated that nurses on this 24-bed unit had administered 84,000 medications over a 3-month period. The only unit administering more medications was a 96-bed NICU that had only administered 10,000 more medications. Additionally, the laboratory data revealed that the unit usually administered 12 units of blood products per day. This necessitated 48 additional sets of vital signs and assessments per day.

Outcome: Additional nursing staff positions were provided to the unit.

THE LOOK OF NURSING

Somewhere between the gleaming white uniform, hose, shoes, and cap of the past and the Mickey Mouse T-shirts, tattoos, nose rings, and looking as though one were going to a "come as you are party" of the present, there is a professional image for nurses. Nurses have come to realize that the "grunge" look does not encourage anyone to take them seriously and are finding more appropriate ways to express their individuality. The work attire of any professional says to the world how significant the task at hand is to that professional. Notably the wrinkled, mismatched scrubs or tank-top-over-tank-top look is far more appropriate for gardening than the knowledge work of nursing.

When some nurses and nursing students design and wear T-shirts that are sexually demeaning to the profession and to them, there is an economic demand and economic support that is being provided to companies to demean the profession. Hopefully, there might be a more appropriate way to express humor in the future.

Although inking or tattoos are popular among adolescents and gang members today, many health care organizations have decided that tattoos cannot be made visible to patients. A survey of health care providers, medical and nursing students ($n = 513$), found that no respondent group had positive attitudes toward tattooed individuals. Women's attitudes were more negative than those of their male counterparts and were extremely negative toward tattooed professional women. Ironically, this study was done to assess attitudes toward tattooed patients (Stuppy et al, 1998). There are no data that suggest that a tattoo will enhance a professional image.

Collectively the voices of nurses are heard through nursing professional associations, and nursing is imaged through participation rates in professional organizations. For example, there are approximately 50,000 members of the National Student Nurses Association (NSNA, 2009). Because 158,385 first-time takers took the NCLEX-RN® in 2008 (National Council of State Boards of Nursing, 2009), it might be estimated there are at least 300,000 to 400,000 registered nursing students in the United States. Where are the other 85% of nursing students?

These rates of participation in NSNA mirror the membership rate (5%) in the ANA. There are 3.4 million RNs; approximately 150,000 are ANA members (ANA, 2006). The influence that nursing could have in health policy and health legislation would be phenomenal if nurses participated more fully in their primary professional organization—the ANA. Whereas there are 79 or more specialty nursing organizations, the primary professional association is the ANA. At the International Council of Nursing, the national representative for U.S. nursing is the ANA.

CREATING A NEW IMAGE

Envision a new world where nurses value nursing and image it daily. Nurses take themselves seriously and dress the part. Nurses are highly visible to patients, families, and physicians because they have reclaimed their practice. Nurses are clear about the role boundaries between themselves and those who extend their practice, and others are also. Nurses are "stuck like glue" together. Negative comments about a colleague are made to the colleague and to no one else. Professional nurses recognize that their greatest benefit—and one of the most efficient and powerful uses for their money—is the less than 1% of their salary they spend for membership in the ANA, the National League for Nursing, Sigma Theta Tau International, and their specialty organization. They look forward to annual meetings because such meetings provide an excellent opportunity to meet colleagues and discuss issues and practice innovations.

Because all nursing is valued, nurses recognize the value of caring, health promotion, and health teaching in addition to the value of illness care. They celebrate that nurses save lives everyday. In the modern medical climate, nurses supervise assistive personnel and use their authority to ensure that patient care delivery is excellent. Nurses value the caring, nurturing role of the nurse because it is worn with style. To this legacy they add the astute business person, researcher, policymaker, legislator, and entrepreneur.

In this new world, nurses believe in nursing, in self, and in their colleagues. When nurses safeguard the image of nursing in local newspapers, television, media dramas, and daily practice, they realize that they play a part in forming the image of nursing on a daily basis (Box 2-1).

BOX **2-1**

Helpful Websites

American Nurses Association Press Releases
  www.nursingworld.org/pressrel
American Association of Colleges of Nursing
Press Releases
  *www.aacn.nche.edu/Media/NewsReleases/
  newslist.htm*

National League for Nursing Press Releases
  www.nln.org/pressreleases/index.htm
Sigma Theta Tau International Nursing Honor
Society—Media
  www.nursingsociety.org

SUMMARY

This chapter has described major factors that have influenced the image of nursing and how society has viewed the profession during different periods throughout history. Nursing actions that contribute to a negative view are described, as well as strategies that will lead to the public having a positive view of nursing. Nurses must be convinced that the twenty-first century image of nursing is one that they contribute to every day as they practice and describe nursing to others. Convincing the public that nursing is not just about caring but is a profession that is based on science is essential. When nurses are widely recognized as knowledge workers, job satisfaction will increase and recruitment and retention will be less of an issue for the profession.

evolve   Additional resources are available online at: http://evolve.elsevier.com/Cherry/

REFERENCES

Aides relieve nursing shortage: *LIFE* 12(1):32–34, 36, 1942.

Aiken LH, et al: Educational levels of hospital nurses and surgical patient mortality, *JAMA* 290:1617–1623, 2003.

American Assembly of Men in Nursing. Retrieved May 18, 2007 from http://aamn.org.

American Association of Nurse Anesthetists: *Nurse anesthetists at a glance.* Retrieved July 21, 2006 from: www. aana.com/becomingcrna.aspx?ucNavMenu_TSMenu TargetID=8&ucNavMenu_TSMenuTargetType=4& ucNavMenu_TSMenuID=6&id=108&.

American Nurses Association: *About ANA.* Retrieved October 21, 2006 from: www.ana.org/about/faq.htm.

Bargagliotti LA: Reframing nursing to renew the profession, *Nurs Educ Perspect* 24(1):12–16, 2003.

Biviano MB, et al: *What is behind HRSA's projected supply, demand, and shortage of registered nurses?* Washington, DC, 2004, Bureau of Health Professions, pp 1-35. Retrieved October 23, 2006 from: http://bhpr.hrsa. gov/healthworkforce/reports/behindrnprojections/5. htm.

Bureau of Labor Statistics: *Occupational outlook handbook 2008-2009,* Bureau of Labor. Washington, DC, Retrieved February, 13, 2009, from www.bls.gov/oco/o cos083.htm#outlook.

Buresch B, Gordon S, Bell N: Who counts in news coverage of health care? *Nurs Outlook* 39(5):204–208, 1991.

Burnett R, Executive Producer: *Late Show with David Letterman* [television broadcast], New York, Dec 12, 2001, CBSL, Worldwide Pants, Inc.

Center for Nursing Advocacy: *About the Center for Nursing Advocacy.* Retrieved October 25, 2006 from: www.nursingadvocacy.org/about_us/about_us.html.

Commission on Graduates of Foreign Nursing Schools: *A world of experience: 2005 Annual Report,* Philadelphia, 2006, Commission on Graduates of Foreign Nursing Schools. Retrieved October 27, 2006 from: www.cgfns.org/pdf/annualreport/2005_annual_report.pdf.

Dickens C: *Martin Chuzzlewit,* New York, 1910, Macmillan.

Diers D: *The mystery of nursing: Secretary's Commission on Nursing: support studies and background information,* vol 2, Rockville, MD, 1988, Department of Health and Human Services, pp VIII-1-VIII-10.

Donahue MP: *Nursing: the finest art: an illustrated history,* ed 3, St Louis, 2010, Mosby.

Drucker P: *Managing in the next society,* New York, 2002, St Peter's Press.

Duke P: If nurses crash, will patients follow? *Newsweek,* February 2, 2006.

Federal Reserve Bank of Minneapolis: *Consumer price index, 1913-2009,* Minneapolis, Federal Reserve Bank. Retrieved October 24, 2006 from: www.minneapolisfed.org/Research/data/us/calc/hist1913.cfm.

Gallup poll: *Nurses shine, bankers slump in ethics ratings,* 2008. Retrieved August 10, 2009 from: www.gallup.com/poll/112264/nurses-shine-while bankers-slump-ethics-ratings.aspx.

HealthGrades: HealthGrades quality study: patient safety in American hospitals, *HealthGrades,* 2004. Retrieved October 21, 2006 from: www.healthgrades.com/media/english/pdf/HG_Patient_Safety_Study_Final.pdf.

Health Resources and Services Administration: *The registered nurse population: findings from the 2004 national sample survey of registered nurses,* U.S. Department of Health and Human Services, 2006, Retrieved December 3, 2009 from bhpr.hrsa.gov/healthworkforce/rnsurvey04/.

Johnson & Johnson: *Johnson & Johnson Newsletter,* May, 2007. Retrieved May 18, 2007 from: www.discovernursing.com/newsletter_view.aspx?id=52.

Jones AH: The White Angel (1936): Hollywood's image of Florence Nightingale. In Jones AH, editor: *Images of nurses: perspectives from history, art, and literature,* Philadelphia, 1988, University of Pennsylvania Press.

Kalisch BJ, Begeny S, Neuman S: The image of the nurse on the internet, *Nurs Outlook* 55(4):182–188, 2007.

Kalisch PA, Kalisch BJ: *The advance of American nursing,* ed 3, Philadelphia, 1995, Lippincott.

Kampen MB: Before Florence Nightingale: a prehistory of nursing in painting and sculpture. In Jones AH, editor: *Images of nurses: perspectives from history, art, and literature,* Philadelphia, 1988, University of Pennsylvania Press.

Kesey K: *One flew over the cuckoo's nest,* New York, 1962, New American Library/Signet.

Longfellow HW: Santa Filomena, *Atlantic Monthly* 1(11):22–23, 1857.

Massachusetts Nurses Association: *Massachusetts physicians say nurse staffing harms patient safety and undermines patient care,* 2005, Opinion Dynamics Corp. Retrieved October 26, 2006 from: www.massnurses.org/safe_care/Safe_Staffing/news/2005/PhysSurv.htm.

Mills A, Blaesing SL: A lesson from the last nursing shortage: the influence of work values on career satisfaction with nursing, *J Nurs Admin* 30(6):309–315, 2000.

National Council of State Boards of Nursing: *Quarterly examination statistics: volume, pass rates and first-time internationally educated candidates' countries.* Retrieved April 7, 2009 from: www.ncsbn.org/2008_NCLEX_Fact_sheet.pdf.

National Student Nurses Association: *Image of nursing.* Retrieved October 30, 2006 from www.nsna.org/activities/nursing.asp.

National Student Nurses Association: Welcome to NSNA: mentoring the future of the nursing profession, 2009. Retrieved December 3, 2009 from www.nsna.org.

Needleman J, et al: Nurse-staffing levels and the quality of care in hospitals, *N Engl J Med* 346(22):1715–1722, 2001.

Needleman J, et al: Nurse staffing in hospitals: is there a business case for quality? *Health Aff* 25(1):204–211, 2006.

Norman EM: *We band of angels: the untold story of American nurses trapped on Bataan by the Japanese,* New York, 1999, Random House.

Nurse TV—Changing the image of nursing: *MedSurg Matters* 17(5):9, 2008.

Seago JA, et al: The nursing shortage: is it really about image? *J Healthcare Manage* 51(2):96–108, 2006.

Sigma Theta Tau International: *The Woodhull study on nursing and the media: health care's invisible partner,* Indianapolis, 1998, STT Center Nursing Press.

Smith JS: Exploring the challenges for nontraditional male students transitioning into a nursing program, *J Nurs Educ* 45:263–269, 2006.

Stanley DJ: Celluloid angels: a research study of nurses in feature films 1900-2007, *J Adv Nurs* 64(1):84–95, 2008.

Stuppy DJ, Armstrong ML, Casals-Ariet C: Attitudes of health care providers and students toward tattooed people, *J Adv Nurs* 27:1165–1170, 1998.

Trossman S: The reality of unreality: nurses weigh in about their portrayal in popular media, *Am Nurse,* 2009:August/September, 1 and 12.

Wachter RM: The end of the beginning: patient safety five years after "to err is human," *Health Aff*:534–545, 2004.

The Influence of Contemporary Trends and Issues on Nursing Education

Carrie B. Lenburg, EdD, RN, FAAN, ANEF

⊘volve Additional resources are available online at: http://evolve.elsevier.com/Cherry/

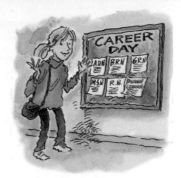

Educational diversity promotes access and career development.

VIGNETTE

Three students were having an animated discussion after class.

Mark: *I'm tired of all this lecturing! I just want to DO nursing! Why do we always have to discuss things like EBP and critical thinking? What is it anyway? And we're always having to analyze a situation when it's perfectly clear what needs to be done! I don't get it. Just do what the doc orders or what's in the procedure book. I don't need to keep looking up stuff when I've done it before. Besides, we already have way too much to read for every class!*

Katelyn: *But listen to this. I heard about a student several days ago who really got into trouble because of a big mistake she made. She did just what you said…followed the doc's orders and gave digoxin to an 80-year-old patient. She had already written a note that he was complaining of anorexia, nausea, and visual disturbances but she didn't take time to look up "dig" toxicity or to really think things through. And guess what? The patient got into a really bad situation. It was lucky that the nurse practitioner read the note, checked the patient, put the pieces together and got a stat serum "dig" level. She had to administer Digibind!—it was so life threatening, and really scary! He's not out of the woods yet. The student said the NP was nice and helped her understand what she should have done, but the instructor pulled her off the unit and really gave her a serious dress-down because she had not taken a couple of minutes to analyze the situation, to think about what things are danger signs, or to just look up the med and the patient's condition at the time—she just followed the doctor's orders. I'd be scared to be the one being grilled at the risk management meeting! She may even fail the course.*

Audrey: *That sounds like a good example of what our instructors keep telling us. Nursing is about thinking as well as doing. We can seriously harm a patient if we don't "know" what actually needs to be done. We have to learn enough so we're competent and know how to use "best practices" for all kinds of situations, and where to get the information fast. We have to really study resources, use our PDAs and whatever, to check things out first and then figure out what we need to do, and fast. Even if we're busy or just don't want to stop and look up something.*

Katelyn: *Why don't we start our own little study group, to learn how to get a better understanding of each class? Nursing is a lot more than just "doing" skills. We've got to be competent in the thinking that goes with the doing. And, there's got to be a way to organize*

41

all this information and learn how to put it together for different situations. Whadaya say? I don't want to get into trouble like that other student! Come on; let's get started on those study questions.

■ **QUESTIONS TO CONSIDER WHILE READING THIS CHAPTER:**

1 What are the major current trends in society and health care, and how do they influence nursing education and practice?

2 What are the most compelling reasons that nurses require ongoing development and validation of competencies for licensure and continuing practice?

3 What local, state, and national resources and Internet sites are available to learn about the trends and issues that influence nursing education?

4 What are the pros and cons of the many different types of nursing education programs that prepare students for current nursing practice?

5 What educational opportunities exist for graduates of various programs to advance beyond their current preparation, including traditional, mobility, and distance learning programs?

KEY TERMS

Competency outcomes The results, or end products, of planned study and experience that are focused on specific abilities required for practice.

Contemporary issues The problems, changes, and concerns that are current for the present time.

Core competencies The essential cluster of abilities and skills required for competent nursing practice.

Educational mobility The progressive movement from one type or level of education to another, often based on flexible, self-directed, or advanced placement options. Examples are progression from diploma preparation to an academic degree, such as RN to BSN or MSN; BSN to doctoral degree; or non-nursing degree to BSN, MSN, or doctoral degree.

Education trends Shifts in conditions and concerns that emerge from and influence various aspects of society; broad changes in the United States and the world that influence the education and practice of nurses and other providers.

Performance examinations Standardized evaluation based on objective demonstration of specific required competencies; used in conjunction with written tests of *knowledge about* those abilities. They may require performance in actual or simulated situations, related to physical psychomotor skills or the observable evidence of other skills such as critical thinking, communication, teaching, planning, writing, or analysis and integration of data.

LEARNING OUTCOMES

After studying this chapter, the reader will be able to:

1 Integrate knowledge of 10 current trends and issues in society and health care into a more holistic perception of their influence on nursing education, students, faculty, and nursing practice.

2 Create a personal philosophy and plan for ongoing professional development and practice that integrates knowledge of current trends and issues.

3 Access current information resources from the Internet related to evolving trends and issues as a component of ongoing learning and preparation for practice.

4 Differentiate among various types of conventional, mobility, and new nursing education programs and the issues associated with them.

CHAPTER OVERVIEW

Society as a whole is going through many significant changes, and all of them influence nursing education and health care. Nurses are becoming more important as participants in decisions about health care but to be effective they need to understand the changes that influence society, education, and health care. Our knowledge, thinking, and a broad array of skills all are critical to the kind of nursing care we provide, and they influence how we respond to changes in patients, families, and communities in times of need. Nurse educators must be vigilant in learning about these changes and integrating them into the curriculum. Students also need to be aware of evolving trends and issues and learn how they influence learning and practice.

As American society becomes increasingly diverse and complex, new trends precipitate different issues. This chapter describes 10 contemporary trends that influence the way students (and nurses) learn, become competent practitioners, and meet the needs of patients. Competent nurses integrate these changes into their way of being, to become "thinking" nurses as well as "doing" nurses; they learn to integrate essential knowledge, attitudes, and skills—the evolving best practices that promote patient safety and quality care. Some of these trends and related issues include the following: the extreme and rapid changes in technology in patient care and education, significant changes in the demographics of our society, the economic crisis and its consequences, the globalization of knowledge and diseases, the requirement for competent health care providers, the increase in domestic abuse and violence of all sorts, ethical issues, and the shortage of nursing faculty and nurses. It also describes the types of nursing education programs, their contribution to the profession, the expansion of innovative nursing programs, degrees and specialties available, and multiple technologic learning methods used. Tables illustrate online resources, important organizations and associations, and some statistics related to types of programs.

INTRODUCTION

Authors identify different lists of trends related to nursing education and practice depending on their experiences and perspectives (Baer, D'Antonio, and Rinker, 2000; Porter-O'Grady, 2001; Speziale and Jacobson, 2005). Speziale and Jacobson reviewed findings from two national faculty surveys to highlight trends in nursing education; they compared data in the 1998 and the 2004 surveys and observed how each reflects trend changes in society. Lenburg (2002, 2008) used a different perspective and identified 10 trends and related issues; her list is used as the framework to organize this chapter (Table 3-1).

New skills require new programs, courses, and experiences; they pave the way for different opportunities for students to prepare for initial and continuing practice in a rapidly changing society. These trends influence the number and types of nursing programs for basic and experienced students at the undergraduate and graduate levels. Essential differences among basic education programs; innovations in new degree programs, majors, and courses; and mobility and distance learning programs are reviewed in the context of changes in national organizations and accrediting and regulatory bodies. Students who study and comprehend these trends are better prepared to cope with them as competent health care practitioners and meet the needs of patients from multicultural and demographic backgrounds.

TRENDS AND ISSUES IN CONTEMPORARY NURSING EDUCATION
Knowledge Expansion and Use of Technology and the Internet

With ever-expanding developments in electronic information and communication technology, the volume of information is growing exponentially on a global level. Informatics has become a major part of education and practice (McBride, 2005; Pravikoff, 2006; Skiba, 2005).

TABLE **3-1**

Summary of Trends and Issues That Influence Nursing Education

MAJOR CONTEMPORARY TRENDS	RELATED ISSUES FOR STUDENTS
Rapid knowledge expansion; increasing use of technology, informatics in education and practice	• Choosing most effective electronic and technology options • Information overload; virtually unlimited global resources, global research opportunities, issues • Identifying current and accurate information; material rapidly outdated • Expanded expectations, limited time, rapid response expected; little time for reflection • Expansion of nursing informatics, content and skills development
Practice-based competency: outcomes and evidence-based content	• Learning focused on core practice competency outcomes, professional skills beyond technical psychomotor skills; core practice competencies; multiple conflicting versions; which to use? • Integration of evidence-based standards, research findings into practice; emphasis on critical thinking, problem solving • Changes in standards; ensure patient safety
Performance-based competency: learning and objective assessment methods	• Multiple teaching-learning methods: interactive collaborative, in-class and out-of-class projects; problem-based learning; increasing self-responsibility; accountability for learning and competence; interprofessional learning; using electronic devices, media to access resources • Competency assessment based on performance examinations, specified portfolio documentation; standards-based assessment methods; emphasis on patient safety
Sociodemographics, cultural, diversity, economic, and political changes, and global issues	• Increased aging population; increasing multicultural, ethnic diversity requires increased learning, respect for differences, preferences, customs; generational issues • Immigration conflicts, protests; consequences for access and health care • Community, faith-based projects, service-learning projects • Global community, globalization health issues; global nursing networks • Social, economic, and political changes influence health care delivery and access to clinical experiences; influence disrespect, conflict, abuse, violence; increased poverty and need • Multidimensional content, client care, clinical learning sites
Community-focused interdisciplinary approaches	• Interprofessional collaborative learning • Diverse alternative health practices, influence of cultures • Broad scope of nursing; clinical approach; increasing use of diverse experiences throughout community; continuum from acute care to health promotion; from hospitals to home to rural to global settings • Requires more planning, travel time, expenses, arrangements; different skills, communications; critical thinking, problem-solving strategies • Multiple teachers, preceptors, staff instructors, part-time, with varying abilities; time constraints
Consumer-oriented care: engagement, safety, and privacy	• All expect value, quality, individual respect, consideration, attention; privacy issues • Consumer initiatives for involvement and protection; balance standards and preferences • Increased litigation, medical-nursing errors; focus on safe, competent patient care • Increased individual responsibility, accountability for learning and practice

TABLE **3-1**

Summary of Trends and Issues That Influence Nursing Education—cont'd

MAJOR CONTEMPORARY TRENDS	RELATED ISSUES FOR STUDENTS
Ethics and bioethical concerns	• Alternative solutions to ethical dilemmas; issues regarding diverse beliefs; disputes regarding biotechnology and bioengineering in health care • Many gray zones instead of black-and-white absolutes; separate professional practice responsibilities from personal opinions, consequences for competence, and patient safety • Integrate into professional practice acceptance of the individual's right of choice regarding life and death issues, health care methods; respect, tolerance for patient's decisions, ethical competencies for students • Standards of quality care, patient's rights issues
Increasing shortage of nurses and faculty	• Shortage of staff results in limitations in clinical learning; heavy workload; using preceptors, part-time instructors; less one-to-one help for students; consequences for learning and patient safety • Shortage of qualified faculty; aging, retiring; increased part-time instructors, clinical staff, national and global problems, influence quality education and future nursing staff; need for increased educational funding • Students need more clinical learning; more responsibility for self-directed learning, seek assistance from others • Increased use of simulation; required to validate initial and continuing competence
Disasters, violence, and terrorism	• New learning, skills required for major natural disaster events; new program options, new courses and new skills needed for emergency responders • Violence in society, homes, workplace, schools; abuse against women and children • Preparedness for terrorism; skills, programs for first responders; increased anxiety, uncertainty
Increasing professional and personal responsibility	• Lifelong learning to meet professional expectations; certification requirements • Increasing competency assessment in workplace • Changes in standards for quality care practice • High stress from competing demands of school, home, meeting competency requirements

This ability to create, access, and disseminate unlimited information rapidly has enormous benefits. From e-mails to complex research documents and telemedicine across the globe, students are communicating more frequently, with more contacts and at Internet speed; multiple digital chat rooms, blogs, and social network systems are used in nursing education (Skiba, 2009a,b). Websites are more current and interactive than print material and can be updated quickly; teachers therefore are increasingly using online methods for course content, assignments, and examinations. Using computers for written assignments reinforces development of effective writing skills and the use of standard protocols required in academic and professional documents. They also help students prepare more effectively for computerized licensure examinations. One study, however, reports that students believe they do not have the essential information technology competencies (Fetter, 2009). Students who become competent and literate in using computers and other digital devices will be more successful in their programs and in practice.

The Internet creates opportunities for distance-learning students, from local to global sites, to participate in networks, team projects, and research that expand understanding of universal health needs and cultural differences The Internet and changes in perspectives of nurse educators also makes it possible for nursing courses or entire degree programs to be delivered online.

In addition to laptops, other mobile digital technologies, such as personal digital assistants (PDAs) (Bauldoff, Kirkpatrick, and Sheets, 2008; Williams and Dittmer, 2009), MP3 players (Skiba, 2009b), and increasingly versatile smart phones, help students, faculty, and nurses access valuable current information to manage complex patient data and thus reduce stress and errors (Jeffries, 2005). These electronic advances, however, generate several issues. With almost unlimited information available, students may actually take more time to navigate online resources than traditional print-based resources and get overly engaged in following links, networking, and overusing chat rooms. Faculty and students need to work together to promote efficient and effective use of electronic learning tools and networking; reducing overload and frustration requires disciplined focus and clear guidelines and outcomes. Learning from the Internet can help students develop skills in analytic thinking, decision making, and reflective judgment that are essential for selecting valid and reliable resources; these are difficult but essential competencies for evidence-based practice (Fetter, 2009; Heye and Stevens, 2009; Lasater, 2007, 2009; Skiba, 2005). In learning to use electronic-based information systems effectively, students acquire competencies required for contemporary, information-intensive nursing practice. In spite of these advances, studies show that health literacy among students is deficient and needs more emphasis (Cormier and Kotrlik, 2009).

Practice-Based Competency Outcomes

One trend that has a powerful influence on nursing education and practice at all levels is the emphasis on competency outcomes and criteria that establish realistic expectations for clinical practice (Cronenwett et al, 2007; Lenburg, Klein, Abdur-Rahman, Spencer, et al 2009; National Council of State Boards of Nursing [NCSBN], 2006; National Organization for Nurse Practitioner Faculty [NONPF], 2006). Competency outcomes, with related criteria (critical elements), specify expected results, the destination students need to reach; they are the measurable results of time and effort spent in learning. The ability to implement realistic practice-based abilities competently therefore is the essential outcome; competence is the target, the endpoint to be reached, the purpose of study and education. The related interactive learning strategies are the road map, the means for getting there; the subsequent performance-based assessments confirm that students have arrived at the right place: They are competent for practice (Lenburg et al, 2009). The ability of graduates in practice is the proof (Candela and Bowles, 2008; Pellico, Brewer, and Kovner, 2009).

The outcomes approach requires a mental shift from trying to memorize voluminous readings and class notes (resulting in frustration and the attitude of "just tell me what I need to know") to actually learning to think like a nurse, to integrate information in problem solving and decision making and providing competent patient care (DiVito-Thomas, 2005). Typical objectives begin with words like *describe, discuss, list,* or *recognize;* they are directions for learning, not what nurses do. Outcomes convert the meaning of the content objectives to actions that nurses actually do, such as implement, integrate, plan, or conduct. This change in approach can be confusing at first, but by achieving the end-results/outcomes students are more prepared to meet the competency expectations of nursing practice with more confidence and success (Glennon, 2006; Klein, 2006). Unprepared new nurses experience stress and frustration in the workplace and require longer orientations and internships to help them gain necessary skills and confidence (Boyer, 2008; Candela and Bowles, 2008).

Nursing organizations continue to revise standards to focus on competencies (American Association of Colleges of Nursing [AACN], 2006; NCSBN, 2006; National League for Nursing [NLN], 2005d, 2008b, 2009a; NONPF, 2006). Explore the websites in Table 3-2 for the most current information for groups concerned with accreditation, licensure, certification, and practice issues.

Validation of competencies often causes anxiety and stress to some students, faculty, nurses, and others, but they are a major incentive to promote patient safety and effective care (Bargagliotti, Luttrell, and Lenburg, 1999). Practice competencies to promote patient safety have been studied extensively by nurses and physicians under federal auspices; see the 2000 report on the website: http://bhpr.hrsa.gov/nursing/nacnep/reports/first/2.htm and click on the link *Collaborative Education to Ensure Patient Safety*. In response to the Institute of Medicine (IOM, 2000) report, Finkelman and Kenner's (2009) book promotes implementation of the recommendations in nursing education. The Robert Wood Johnson Foundation funded a national initiative, Quality and Safety in Nursing Education (QSEN), to help nursing programs reorganize curricula to focus on patient safety and quality care (Cronenwett et al, 2007). Lenburg's Competency Outcomes and Performance Assessment (COPA) model has been used since the early 1990s (Lenburg, 1999, 2009). These and other efforts focus on the imperative to improve competency outcomes to promote patient safety.

Performance-Based Learning and Assessment

Trends related to learning and evaluation methods are changing fundamentally, due in part to changing technology and the increased focus on patient safety. The emphasis on competency outcomes and criteria for acceptable practice has prompted leaders in nursing education to promote innovative programs and learning methods (NLN, 2005a, 2009a) as well as more interactivity and engagement interspersed with lectures. Passively listening, reading, and passing written tests does not necessarily promote competence in the core performance skills expected in practice. Increased emphasis on critical thinking and learning to integrate principles is more effective than trying to remember "all the content," which often leads students to retreat and just want to pass the test. Competency-based learning creates an entirely different atmosphere that is focused on learning concepts and encourages collaboration between teacher and learner to achieve actual practice competencies (Lasater, 2007; Lasater and Nielson, 2009; Neuman, 2006).

Practice-based competence uses terms like interactive learning, collaborative learning, and competency-based learning. This trend requires changes in the roles of teachers and students. The teacher is less a "lecturer" and more a facilitator and coach, providing direction for learning stated outcomes; the student is more actively accountable and responsible for achieving competence in designated knowledge and practice skills. The question is, what are the most effective ways to learn such actual performance skills as assessment, communication, critical thinking, and patient teaching? Listening to lectures and reading is less effective than active engagement and application in real practice situations. Performance skills are learned more effectively through participation in interactive strategies (Clayton and Dilley, 2009; Fay, Johnson, and Selz, 2006; Giddens and Brady, 2007; Lenburg et al, 2009). In this new paradigm, instructors

TABLE **3-2**

Online References and Resources Related to Nursing Education

The list below represents examples of Internet resources as beginning points. It is not a complete or "best" list, but a suggested sampling. At the time of this writing, addresses are operational, but many are subject to change, become obsolete, or are discontinued; use them to find other helpful links. Most addresses listed below begin with "http://www," unless otherwise indicated. Note that some have hyphens or other symbols, and some are case sensitive; be certain of spelling exactly as listed. Find other sites on the Internet using Google, Yahoo, or other search engines.

NAME OF SOURCE	ADDRESS	COMMENTS
allnurses.com	allnurses.com/distance-learning-nursing	Networking site for students especially in distance learning programs; exchange information, advice, find resources
American Academy of Nursing	aannet.org	Information on nursing issues, influence on government, other organizations; promote research, national leadership
American Association of Colleges of Nursing	aacn.nche.edu	BSN and higher degree schools; multiple publications, position papers; useful Internet links
American Association for History of Nursing	aahn.org	Membership, contacts, publications regarding nursing history
American Holistic Nurses Association	ahna.org	Publications, certificate program, and continuing education course listings
American Hospital Association	hospitalconnect.com	Hospital links; nursing shortage and workforce issues
American Nurses Association	nursingworld.org	Links to organizations, publications (American Nurse, *OJIN*, books); career and job lists
American Nurses Association	smartbriefs.com	News for the nursing profession. Free email of important news.
American Nurses Credentialing Center	nursecredentialing.org/default.aspx	Information regarding certification programs, requirements, etc.
American Nursing Informatics Association	ania.org	Links to multiple sites for nursing informatics
American Organization of Nurse Executives	aone.org	Information; publications regarding nursing leadership, administration
Arizona State University	nursingandhealth.asu.edu	Center for Advancement of Evidence Based Practice
Commission on Collegiate Nursing Education	aacn.nche.edu/accreditation/index.htm	Agency that accredits BSN and higher degrees only
Commission for Graduates of Foreign Schools of Nursing	cgfsn.org	Information for and about foreign-trained nurses
Discover Nursing	discovernursing.com	Lists scholarships, other nursing resources
Distance Learning Channel	petersons.com/distancelearning	Lists hundreds of distance learning courses, programs; search, nursing
Institute of Medicine	iom.edu	Publications, other links via National Academy of Sciences
Institute for Nursing Centers	nursingcenters.org	network of organizations focused on nurse-managed health centers, data collection
International Council of Nurses	icn.ch	ICN resources and links
International Parish Nursing Resource Center	ipnrc.parishnurses.org	Information, links to congregational, parish resources

TABLE **3-2**

Online References and Resources Related to Nursing Education—cont'd

NAME OF SOURCE	ADDRESS	COMMENTS
Martindale's Health Science Guide	martindalecenter.com	Link to medical and nursing resources; virtual medical and nurse center; excellent resource
National Coalition Against Domestic Violence	ncadv.org	Information regarding actions, self-protection, policies, resources
National Council of State Boards of Nursing	ncsbn.org	Information regarding NCLEX and regulations; links to all state boards
National League for Nursing (NLN)	nln.org	Information regarding all schools of nursing testing; educator programs
National League for Nursing Accrediting Commission	nlnac.org	Agency that accredits all types of nursing schools; sets criteria
National Organization of Nurse Practitioner Faculties	nonpf.org	Publications regarding nurse practitioner competencies; other helpful links
National Student Nurses Association	nsna.org	Excellent resources, schools, organizations, career options
New York State Coalition for Educational Mobility	lpntorn.info	Mobility program for LPNs to earn ASN degrees, example
Nursing (multiple links to resources)	nursingcenter.com	Links to resources, journals, continuing education, jobs
Nursing Ethics Network	bc.edu/bc_org/avp/son/ethics	Boston College: many links regarding nursing ethics, related issues
Nursing Informatics	nursing-informatics.com	Links to informatics resources, journal, courses
Nurses.info	nurses.info/services_violence.htm.	Information and resources for Nurses Worldwide; workplace violence
Online Journal of Issues in Nursing	nursingworld.org/ojin	Free journal; via ANA and Kent State University
Online Journal of Nursing Informatics	ojni.org	Abstracts, articles regarding technology in nursing available online
Penn State University, Evidence-Based Practice Tutorial for Nurses	libraries.psu.edu/instruction/ebpt-07/index.htm	Helpful study and practice scenarios and links
VCU Libraries, Evidence-Based Nursing Resources	library.vcu.edu/tml/bibs/ebnursing.html	Very useful resource for learning about evidence-based practice; definitions and multiple links to best practice guidelines
REGIONAL NURSING SOCIETIES		Research related by four national regions
Eastern Nursing Research Society	enrs-go.org	Information regarding research in eastern states
Midwest Nursing Research Society	mnrs.org	Example of a regional nursing organization
Southern Nursing Research Society	snrs.org	Southern regional organization; research; journal
Western Institute of Nursing	ohsu.edu/son/win	Information regarding research in western states
Sigma Theta Tau International	nursingsociety.org	Honor society information; research directory
Southern Regional Electronic Campus	electroniccampus.org	Represents public and independent colleges in southern regional education board states

Continued

TABLE **3-2**

Online References and Resources Related to Nursing Education—cont'd

NAME OF SOURCE	ADDRESS	COMMENTS
U.S. GOVERNMENT RESOURCES		
Agency for Healthcare Research and Quality	aahrq.gov	For consumers and professionals; research reports; specific populations, topics
Healthy People 2010	health.gov/healthypeople	Publications; links regarding health
National Library of Medicine	nlm.nih.gov/locatorplus/	National library locator, databases, information
U.S. Government Division of Nursing	bhpr.hrsa.gov/nursing	Informatics rgarding student financial assistance, grants, databases available by state
U.S. Government resources	USAsearch.gov	Excellent links to multiple government resources, federal, state, local contacts
U.S. Government consumer	healthfinder.gov	Links to federal, state health agencies; consumer support gateway
U.S. Government search site	medlineplus.gov	Links regarding disease, health, links to resources, publications; organizations, agencies, clinical trials, groups; health library

ONLINE RESOURCES RELATED TO NURSING EDUCATION

Most colleges and universities offer some form of educational mobility, distance learning and/or online courses; some offer entire degrees. Examples of these institutions located throughout the United States are cited below with website addresses; use these as a format guide to locate others of interest. Please note: specific addresses, names, and/or offerings may change subsequent to this publication. (In most instances, the address follows "http://www.")

NAME OF SOURCE	ADDRESS	COMMENTS
California State University, Dominguez Hills	csudh.edu	Statewide mobility program; distance learning
Case Western Reserve University	cwru.edu	Multioption; international; research; nursing informatics
Excelsior College	excelsior.edu	External degrees: ADN, BSN, master's programs; online courses
George Mason University	gmu.edu	Campus and mobility programs; WANRR (research resource)
Grand Canyon University	gcu.edu	Online nursing programs; different degrees
Indiana University/Purdue University	iupui.edu	Multiple programs and sites; nursing informatics
NOVA Southeastern University	nova.edu	Multiple degree programs in nursing, campus and distance online learning
University of Alabama, Birmingham	uab.edu	Campus and distance programs
University of Colorado Health Sciences Center	uchsc.edu	Undergraduate and graduate programs, courses, on campus or Internet assisted
University of Kansas	kumc.edu	Campus and distance programs
University of Maryland	umd.edu	Multiple programs; mobility; nursing informatics
University of Phoenix	phoenix.edu	Multiple online Internet programs; courses
Virtual Nurse	virtualnurse.com	Links to websites; online programs, career, education, health resources
Western Governors University	wgu.edu	Cooperative arrangements among several states offering academic degrees; online courses, programs

focus on the most essential content; create practice-based case studies and simulations; and set the stage for students to engage in problem solving, critical thinking, and integration of concepts, knowledge, and evidence-based practice (Horan, 2009; Murphy, 2004). They provide feedback and validation that cannot be gained through books or the Internet. Memorization of basic facts is still important, but that is insufficient when nursing practice emphasizes skills, such as assessment, critical thinking, communication, patient teaching, caring and advocating for patients. The focus on practice competence helps students learn how to access and integrate ever-changing information as required in actual practice, rather than trying to remember "all the content." Learning to access and use digital resources on mobile devices is more effective.

Many nurse leaders cite critical thinking skills and implementation of evidence-based practice as the most fundamental skills for competent practice. Tanner (2000) emphasizes that this is not the nursing process, as some think. del Bueno (2005) writes about the crisis in the lack of critical thinking in nursing practice. New partnerships with agency staff are designed to promote clinical learning and how to think like a nurse (MacIntyre et al, 2009). Critical thinking is an essential part of applying evidence-based practice, using research findings to guide actual practice (Ireland, 2008). A trend in many programs is the development of study tracks or majors in evidence-based practice, such as the one implemented by Arizona State University in 2006 (www.asu.edu/graduate/studies/asucert.html).

Simulation, in various forms, is another major performance-based learning strategy. Mannequins have become more essential and incorporate sophisticated computerization to promote more realistic learning and critical thinking (Bruce et al, 2009; Hawkins, Todd, and Manz, 2008; Horan, 2009; Jeffries, 2005; Lasater, 2007; Rush et al, 2008; Smith-Stoner, 2009; Wagner, Bear, and Sander, 2009). Another form of simulation is the use of standardized patients and telemedicine technology to achieve outcomes and more recently faculty are using web-based broadcast of simulations to increase learning (Smith-Stoner, 2009). Other interactive learning strategies include portfolio learning (Schaffer, Nelson, and Litt, 2005) and peer-to-peer learning (Scott, 2005). Higgins (2006) describes how peer teaching helps students at risk. Skiba (2009a,b) describes and evaluates new learning technology methods in each issue of *Nursing Education Perspectives*.

Interactive strategies are even more important when the location of clinical learning is considered. More and more diverse settings are used because these are places where nurses' expertise is needed. In addition to hospitals and extended care facilities, clinical learning often takes place in alternative settings, such as nurse-run clinics in schools, daycare and senior centers, and prisons (Kirkham, Harwood, and Hofwegen, 2005). Over the past decade, service-learning projects have also helped students learn actual practice skills throughout the community (Bentley and Ellison, 2007; Campbell and Dudley, 2005; Clayton and Dilley, 2009; Hunt, 2007; Worrell-Carlisle, 2005). Another form is faith-based learning projects, such as nurses in churches and parish nursing (Brendtro and Leuning, 2000; Kotecki, 2002). Many interactive clinical-related learning strategies and more traditional clinical assignments increasingly engage practicing nurses as preceptors (Wieland et al, 2007; Murray, 2007).

The change to competency outcomes and practice-based learning requires changes in evaluation methods that focus on valid, actual performance of required competencies in realistic scenarios; paper-and-pencil tests and inconsistent subjective clinical observations by instructors or preceptors are not adequate. Structured, objective validation of competence requires performance examinations that specify the core skills and related critical elements (the application of mandatory principles) that must be met according to established practice standards (Boyer, 2008; Klein, 2006; Lenburg et al, 2009; Rentschler et al, 2007). In addition to performance of nursing skills, structured portfolios are used to document other competencies (Schaffer, Nelson, and Litt, 2005).

Needless to say, this more interactive approach in clinical and classroom courses is difficult for some students and creates issues; faculty and students have to change traditional habits and expectations of each other. Sometimes students think it is easier just to figure out "what the teacher wants" and "study for the test" rather than engage in learning to think and integrate best practices through teacher-assisted interactive exercises. Such exercises, however, help students learn to make effective decisions, and to collaborate in the group process, and manage time and resources. It may cause some anxiety, but performance examinations that require 100% accuracy of the mandatory critical elements (principles) provide more reliable evidence of practice competencies (Boyer, 2008; Klein, 2006; Lenburg et al, 2009). This kind of competence is what consumers need, employers expect, and practitioners must deliver. The increase in reported medical-related errors vividly emphasizes the need for more effective validation of performance competence in schools and the workplace (Boyer, 2008; IOM, 2000; Finkelman and Kenner, 2009).

Sociodemographics, Cultural Diversity, and Economic and Political Changes

From rural to metropolitan areas throughout the United States, the population is undergoing significant changes in sociodemographic, cultural, and economic composition. These trends generate serious issues and consequences for education, health care, and many aspects of the socioeconomic-political systems. The brief overview here is a framework for learning how these trends and issues affect nursing education and practice (Cagle, 2006; Sullivan, 2009).

◆ People are living longer, and the number of the very elderly is increasing more rapidly than other age groups. This means more people live with chronic disease and disability; many live in institutions, substandard conditions, or alone. All are subject to increasing needs for health care and assistance. As a result, nursing and other provider programs have increased geriatric content and clinical experiences; geriatric patients require very different care than younger populations. The current political debate about health care reform is concerned about all age groups and regardless of the outcome, nursing will continue to focus on quality care and competent practice (AACN, 2009e; Cronenwett et al, 2007; Holroyd et al, 2009; NLN, 2005c, 2008b).

◆ The number of diverse ethnic minorities and illegal immigrants is expanding throughout the United States, with multiple socioeconomic consequences. The diversity often is unwanted and leads to disrespect, intolerance, conflicts, abuse, and violence. The Southern Poverty Law Center is a national organization that promotes tolerance in schools and monitors militant hate groups and initiates law suits against violent offenders (SPLC, 2009). Increasingly, health care providers need to learn about different cultural values and health practices and integrate them into care to the extent possible. They need to incorporate, and teach, tolerance and understanding of cultural diversity as well as positive health practices (Kleiman, 2007; Sullivan, 2009). In 2008 the American Association of Colleges of Nursing (AACN, 2008b) developed end-of-program competencies for graduates of baccalaureate nursing programs for integrating cultural competencies into undergraduate education (www.aacn.nche.edu/Education/pdf/competency.pdf). *The Essentials of Baccalaureate Education for Professional Nursing Practice* (2008) mandates the inclusion of culturally diverse nursing care concepts in the curriculum. Professional ethics requires that health care providers separate their personal values and beliefs from their professional responsibilities, even to those whose beliefs are different (Cagle, 2006; Helms, 2006; Kotecki, 2002; *Online Journal of Issues in Nursing [OJIN]*, 2009a; Tippitt et al, 2009). The number of families who become uninsured, jobless, homeless, and survive in poverty is increasing. The economic crisis during the first decade of the twenty-first century has resulted in fewer financial resources for health care and ordinary expenses, and thus more people eat unhealthy diets, go without medicines or treatments, and obtain care in emergency departments. More than half of family bankruptcies are due to overwhelming health care debt. Ehrenreich (2009) describes the incredible cycle of hunger, illness, thefts, and incarcerations that poor people experience in the United States (see Table 3-1). Bentley and Ellison (2007) and Hunt (2007) describe other service-learning experiences that help students learn about providing health care to needy groups. Clayton and Dilley (2009) report an example of a service learning project that engages students in soup kitchens for the homeless. The economic crisis also has resulted in lack of funds for healthy school programs, nursing education, hospital staffing, and material support for the sick, poor, and jobless. The issues are how to provide care and improve the health of those with little means, knowledge, or will; how to fund it; and how to reverse their condition (Rose, 2009).

◆ Domestic abuse of women and children and various forms of violence are increasing in homes, schools, and public places (Esposito et al, 2005; *Stop Violence* website, 2009; see Table 3-2). The incidence of violence has increased even in nursing schools and in hospitals, including vertical abuse among nurses (American Nurses Association [ANA], 2009c; Clark, 2009; Thomas and Burk, 2009; U.S. Department of Labor [USDL], 2003). Substance abuse, long a pervasive problem in society, has become a serious problem for nursing students and nurses (Monroe, 2009). This has consequences for safety and health of nurses, patients, and others; the increase in stress and anxiety often triggers violence and mental health and economic problems.

◆ The United States is experiencing an epidemic of obesity, with major consequences on health and the health care system. It leads to the most prevalent health problems that strain health care facilities and financial resources. It is paramount for health care providers to teach prevention of obesity and its consequences in schools. Learning to help people change their dietary habits is a major role for nurses (OJIN, 2009b) and other health workers.

◆ The traditional definition of family has changed, as evident in the number of single individuals living with other singles, single-parent households, and same-sex couples (with and without children). These nontraditional families often have limited finances and lack access to nursing and health care. They also may be resented by those with more traditional values and attitudes. Nurses must learn to respect and provide essential care regardless of differences.

◆ Disrespect for others, abuse of noisy mobile devices in public, and disregard for common courtesy has changed the nature of social interactions. Nursing students who use class time to send digital messages, use cell phones, or search the Internet are disrespectful of those who want to learn and the teacher who is trying to help them learn. This is part of the larger trend of declining civility and integrity, with increased cheating and falsification in school and work (Anastasi, Capili, and Schenkman, 2009; Clark, 2009; Clark and Springer, 2007; Tippitt et al, 2009). Such incidents trigger anger and retaliation when excessive. In health care facilities, abuse of patients also is increasing. Nurses often need to mediate abusive situations, and effective communication and mental health skills are essential (Schlariet, 2009).

As suggested, an important part of nursing education includes trends in society and the issues that result. Nurses work with those in all aspects of society, and thus, course content and interactive practice-based learning that incorporates these issues is essential. One of the most significant issues for students is learning to distinguish the meaningful differences in beliefs, values, and expectations among patients and their responses to illness, treatments, and caregivers. This is why nursing programs include, and students need to learn from, those areas of study that support effective nursing care, such as sociology, cultural diversity, psychology, ethics, religion, economics, history, and literature. Learning the experiences of diverse peoples, including patients and coworkers, their customs, beliefs, health practices, and expectations not only is interesting but also expands human understanding, tolerance, compassion, and the creativity essential for effective professional practice (Southern Poverty Law Center [SPLC], 2009).

Community-Focused Interprofessional Approaches

The societal trends described here, along with the large-scale economic and political influences to reduce health care costs, may indirectly promote prevention and interprofessional initiatives. Many lay and professional health-conscious groups are working to change the national orientation from "illness care" to more efficient and effective "health care." Another contributing factor is the increasing emphasis on health of the family as a whole and on entire communities and populations. *Healthy People 2010*, as described by Zahner and Block (2006), outlines goals for a broad-based population health set by government agencies (Centers for Disease Control and Prevention [CDC] and Merck Company Foundation, 2007; see Table 3-2).

As more citizens live longer and develop acute and chronic disabilities, nurses work in a widening range of settings, such as ambulatory clinics, nursing homes, hospices, home care, assisted living facilities, faith-based initiatives, and alternative integrative health care practices (Anastasi, Capili, and Schenkman, 2009; Helms, 2006; Kirkham et al, 2005; Kotecki, 2002). Regardless of the setting, community health care involves an interprofessional team, often coordinated by nurses, and students need to learn these diverse roles. The concept of community care agencies therefore has changed. Hospitals are only one of many community health care resources, along with wellness and senior centers (Newman, 2005). These changes require a different philosophy of care and competencies that emphasize interprofessional and interagency collaboration. This health care culture incorporates concepts of shared responsibility for health promotion among individuals, family, community, and multiple care providers. Nursing education is influenced by these trends to promote family and community health and healthy lifestyles, and increased interprofessional learning and collaboration (Holroyd et al, 2009; IOM, 2003; see Table 3-2).

With extensive global travel and commerce, the health community now encompasses the world. Illness can arrive on any airplane, ship, or bus and spread throughout the country. An example is the pandemic of the A(H1N1) "swine flu," which has spread to every continent and continues to cause illness and deaths. Nurses are on the front line of care and defense and have raised concerns about sufficient protection. Similarly, other infections, such as reemerging strains of tuberculosis (Benkert et al, 2009) and methicillin-resistant *Staphylococcus aureus* (MRSA) spread rapidly and are resistant to treatment; nurses and other providers need to become even more diligent in preventing the spread of organisms (ANA, 2009a; CDC, 2007; Lashley, 2006).

Consistent with the trend toward global health, nurses are engaged in the global health community through collaborative networks, research projects, and shared publications (NLN, 2005b; Critchley, 2009). Programs incorporate global content and students learn to participate in international health research projects and communication through the Internet and have direct learning experiences in countries abroad (Bentley and Ellison, 2007; Carlton et al, 2007; Ramal, 2009). The International Council of Nurses (ICN, 2009) provides many opportunities for students to network and learn from each other; its periodic international conferences are a major resource for students and nurses to promote world health (ICN, 2009; see Table 3-2, ICN website and student bulletin board). These experiences promote cultural understanding and respect for health conditions outside, and inside, the United States; they help students integrate the influence of environment, education, and culture on health conditions regardless of location.

These trends challenge students to prepare for a wide spectrum of nursing practice that depends on competencies such as critical thinking (Turner, 2005), communication, collaboration, and leadership. Students need to learn how to manage illness and preventive health care for diverse clients dispersed throughout the community as well as to provide critical care to hospital patients who are sicker and go home quicker. Although very helpful, learning in diverse settings throughout the community presents some issues. For example, dispersed clinical learning requires more planning, travel, expense, and time; learning time is much shorter at each location; community-based group projects take more time; students have less time with instructors because faculty can be only at one location at a time. In many settings, however, students work only with preceptors or staff who help them gain the competence and confidence they need, but who also have other responsibilities.

Consumer-Oriented Care: Engagement, Safety, and Privacy

As consumers have become more knowledgeable about illness care, health promotion, and the consequences of errors in care, they have become more assertive about their right to competent care and privacy of information. The 2002 Health Insurance Portability and Accountability Act (HIPAA) law mandates protection of an individual's privacy by health care providers and throughout society and has changed many previously careless and harmful practices. The economics and politics of health care and access to comprehensive information via the Internet have promoted more consumer activism through advocacy groups and Internet connections to influence health care policy and standards. Consumers use Internet resources, sponsored by the government and private entities, to become more informed about illness and health care (see Table 3-2). As informed and engaged patients, they are better able to make effective decisions in collaboration with health care providers. This makes critical thinking, communication, and teaching essential nursing competencies. This also means that students (nurses) need to change their approach from "giving patient care" to "working with" the patient and family as members of the health care team.

Another major issue affecting nursing education is the increasing number and consequences of serious medical errors, as reported in IOM study (2000). These errors have led to an astonishing number of deaths and an increased number of expensive lawsuits, which further increase the cost of health care and tarnish the belief in the quality of available health care. Nursing faculty, administrators, and regulators therefore are increasingly concerned with ensuring the competence of students and nurses (Finkelman and Kenner, 2009; IOM, 2003). Medical-error issues have precipitated the increased requirements for competency-based education and performance assessment in schools of nursing and other health disciplines, in annual employment evaluations, and in agency accreditation criteria, all for patient safety.

Many injuries and deaths in medical institutions are preventable, and Medicare recently decided that it will no longer pay for such preventable incidents, many of which are attributed to nurses. Thus preventive care is being emphasized even more in nursing education. QSEN, the COPA model, and similar initiatives in every specialty organization, are designed to change nursing education and practice to promote competence and patient safety (AACN, 2006; Cronenwett et al, 2007; IOM, 2003; NCSBN, 2006; NLN, 2009a). An important study submitted to the U.S. Department of Health and Human Services in 2000 was conducted jointly by the Advisory Council on Nursing Education and Practice and the Council on Graduate Medical Education. Its primary focus is the collaboration between nurses and physicians to promote patient safety and reduce errors (see www.cogme.gov/jointmtg.htm and click on link: *Collaborative Education to Ensure Patient Safety*, published in 2000; and other related links.)

Ethics and Bioethical Concerns

Another trend affecting nursing education is related to the multicultural, multiethnic population and patients who have different ways of responding to illness, treatment, and care providers. This raises ethical issues of who is "right" and who has the "right to decide." This is particularly relevant for freedom of choice and end-of-life issues (AACN, 2009d, search for multiple references by Ferrell, 2000 to 2009; ANA, 2009b OJIN, 2009a; Matzo et al, 2003). As described, one difficult issue, particularly for students and novices, is the ethical necessity to differentiate personal beliefs, values, and preferences from professional practice responsibilities. Many ethical dilemmas require students, nurses, and other providers to accept the values of others and the concept of "a gray continuum of values" instead of the black-and-white interpretations based on one's own beliefs. Some of the most controversial issues relate to the right of individual choice regarding abortion, organ transplant, stem-cell research, preference in sexual partners, and the patient's right to die a dignified death. Other issues emerge from the growing use of alternative health remedies outside the mainstream of traditional Western medicine, such as herbs and acupuncture (Anastasi et al, 2009; Helms, 2006). Dishonesty among nursing students, nurses and other professionals is increasingly alarming and threatens patient safety (Fontana, 2009; McCabe, 2009; Roberson, 2009). Chapter 9 presents a comprehensive discussion about ethics in health care and important issues students should be knowledgeable about for competent nursing practice.

Shortage of Nurses and Faculty

The shortage and aging of nurses and nurse educators is a trend that has precipitated serious issues for students, teachers, and health care consumers (AACN, 2009f; Buerhaus, Auerbach, and Staiger, 2009; Falk, 2007; NLN, 2009b). Inadequate clinical staff and use of part-time and agency nurses tend to reduce the quality of overall care and increase stress and burnout. In many locations it also means fewer staff preceptors who are too burdened with their workload to spend time instructing students.

Students are assigned to multiple and diverse community clinical settings, some of which may be short staffed, making it difficult for them to find qualified preceptors. Staff nurses who act as clinical instructors or preceptors may or may not be prepared for these roles or receive adequate orientation. Students, therefore, need to learn to take more individual responsibility and initiative to gain essential core competencies. Students in distance learning and Internet-based programs who are dependent on staff nurses as preceptors and evaluators need to be even more assertive and creative (Rush et al, 2008). New methods are created in partnership with agencies to promote more effective clinical learning opportunities for students without overburdening staff (MacIntyre, 2009).

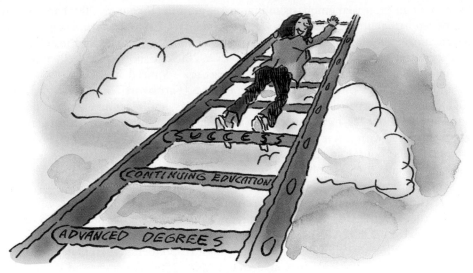

Education is the ladder to success.

Although the number of student applicants was low in recent years, the current problem is that an alarming number of well-qualified applicants are being denied admission to schools of nursing (see AACN and NLN websites for news releases and reports). The causative trends are lack of prepared nurse educators, limited space, and other administrative constraints. Faculty are aging and retiring, but the number of prospective qualified replacements is severely limited (Falk, 2007). Some schools are expanding enrollments by using more part-time, adjunct, and clinical faculty and by expanding the use of online courses and simulations. Moreover, the number of students in master of science in nursing (MSN) and doctoral programs is not adequate to meet current needs. Nursing leaders and organizations are working vigorously with state and national governments and private entities to reverse these trends by seeking increased funding and promoting recruitment and development efforts nationally (see AACN at www.aacn.nche.edu/Government/index.htm, and NLN at www.nln.org/governmentaffairs/factsandfigures.htm).

This trend presents many hardships for students, faculty, and nurses, but difficult situations promote creative initiatives and solutions. For example, many organizations and associations have initiated collaborative partnerships to improve education in all types and levels of nursing education; some are statewide or regional arrangements (Allen et al, 2007; Campbell and Dudley, 2005; Horns et al, 2007; Hunt, 2007; Murray, 2007). (See later section on flexible education programs.) NLN has implemented initiatives to improve nursing education and faculty development (see AACN and NLN websites, position statements regarding innovations and transitions in nursing education). It also initiated the NLN Centers of Excellence to recognize outstanding schools, and its national nurse educator certification program (NLN, 2005a) to promote faculty development and expertise.

Disasters, Violence, and Terrorism

Nurses have always worked in situations emanating from disasters, abuse, and violence in families and communities, and in military conflicts. Domestic violence, especially against women and children, has increased as has violence in the workplace and in schools. This has precipitated an increased emphasis in nursing education (Veenema, 2006) and in state regulations of reporting and responding to violent incidents. Criminal acts and substance abuse have become more common in hospitals and other health care agencies and in schools of nursing threatening the safety of patients and staff (ANA, 2009c; Esposito et al, 2005; Monroe, 2009). As a consequence, criminal background checks are required for all students (and employees) and by agencies providing clinical experience (Farnsworth and Springer, 2006; USDL, 2003). Population expansion, especially in urban areas, and mass disasters, such as hurricanes, floods, and earthquakes, have precipitated the need for more nurses to get prepared to function effectively along with other first responders. Adelman and Legg (2009) and Veenema (2006) describe details about preparedness and opportunities for nurses who want to learn more. State boards of nursing, such as California (ww.rn.ca.gov/pdfs/disaster.pdf), and other organizations also provide information.

Since the horrific terror attacks on September 11, 2001, in New York City, more nurses (and all other health care personnel and first responders) are more prepared to respond to acts of terrorism and disasters. Many nursing programs have added courses or even entire programs of study for specialized preparation as first responders, emergency nursing, and flight nursing (Steed et al, 2004; Weiner et al, 2005; ANA, 2006; Adelman and Legg, 2009; Whitty and Burnett, 2009). As one response to increasing mass casualty events, Vanderbilt University convened a group of nurse leaders in 2001 and subsequently developed competencies required in such events and formed the Nursing Emergency Preparedness Education Coalition as an international education site (www.nursing.vanderbilt.edu/incmce). All nurses will not become first responders, but all nurses and students should gain enough knowledge to know their limitations, who and how to notify, and how they could work with more qualified responders. Chapter 15 also provides more information about disaster preparedness for nurses.

Increasing Professional and Personal Responsibilities

In this context, another trend with multiple issues has become evident. Students, teachers, and nurses confront increasing life responsibilities and associated stressful demands on time and resources. Many cope simultaneously with the expansion of information and technology; changing health care systems; more interactive and out-of-class methods of learning; multiple care settings; higher expectations for competence; shortage of nurse preceptors and teachers; and multiple cultural, ethical, and legal aspects of an ever-changing society. Many also are responsible for the care of dependent children and aging parents.

At the same time, contemporary conditions require nurses to keep current through planned ongoing professional development. Complexities in practice, emphasis on reducing errors, and increasing consumer activism increase the need for nurses to document continuing competence for initial licensure, relicensure, and recertification. Changes in state and multistate regulations increasingly focus on the need for initial and continuing competence (NCSBN, 2006). Many states require continuing education, and some mandate a portfolio approach to validate continuing competence (see websites for NCSBN and specific states, such as California, Kentucky, Oklahoma, and Tennessee). The American Nurses Association (ANA) has cited the continuing competence of nurses as one of its focus issues of concern since the late 1990s (see ANA website and past issues of *The American Nurse*, 2000-2009).

The high stress levels associated with these professional and personal demands have consequences for one's own health and that of those around them. These issues illustrate how important it is for everyone involved in the educational process to be more caring, understanding, respectful, and helpful to each other. Teachers, students, administrators, staff nurses, employers, family, and friends need to learn anew the meaning of "a caring community" in the context of rapid and complex change.

These trends in society, nursing, and academic programs present issues of how to incorporate this additional knowledge into the already overloaded program of study. The issues for students include knowing how to access and use unlimited information, prioritize learning, implement evidence-based practice, deal with ethical dilemmas professionally, and develop competencies required for effective response to contemporary issues. Above all, students must focus on learning to think critically, reflectively, ethically, and compassionately as essential professional skills (del Bueno, 2005; Ireland, 2008; Riddell, 2007; Skiba, 2005).

DIVERSITY IN NURSING EDUCATION PROGRAMS

A brief review of the major types of education programs that prepare nurses for licensure and advanced practice sets the stage for summarizing some contemporary trends related to flexible, online, and other distance delivery methods in nursing education. A brief description of the types of programs is provided in Table 3-3 and on NLN and AACN websites (AACN, 2009a,b,c; NLN, 2008a,b). Kalisch and Kalisch (1995) and Baer and colleagues (2000) describe the historical development of all types of programs.

Licensed Practical or Vocational Nurse Programs

Practical nurse programs provide the shortest and most restricted option for individuals seeking a nursing license. Licensed practical nurse programs (LPN), named licensed vocational nurses (LVN) in California and Texas, usually are 9 to 12 months in length and may be offered by high school adult education programs, community colleges, vocational and proprietary schools, and hospitals. Each state board of nursing sets responsibilities and scopes of practice. The LPN/LVN graduate is required to work under the supervision of a registered nurse (RN) or physician, and the scope of practice focuses on technical nursing procedures. LPN/LVNs may be employed in hospitals, nursing homes, offices, and other structured settings.

In the mid-1990s, more than 1100 LPN or LVN programs produced approximately 44,000 graduates. National data on the current number of schools and graduates are not readily available because of the multiple providers of programs; however, it appears that their numbers continue to be high. Regardless of the increasing complexity of patient care, many individuals choose to begin a career in nursing as an LPN/LVN. Once licensed, many graduates continue their education in mobility programs to become RNs. Many use "1 + 1" type programs to earn an associate degree; others use the multiple entry-exit programs (MEEP). Some BSN programs accept LPN graduates based on outcomes of written and performance examinations for advanced placement.

Hospital Diploma Programs

The oldest, most traditional type of program that prepares for RN licensure is the hospital-based diploma program. These programs initially were developed in the United States in the late 1800s in general hospitals in cities such as Boston, New York, Hartford, and Philadelphia and subsequently spread across the country. They followed the Nightingale model and began as training programs taught by physicians, usually only several weeks in length. In time nurse graduates began developing and teaching courses from the nursing perspective and subsequently obtained additional education as educators and administrators. Ultimately, the length of programs was extended and by the mid-1900s, most programs were 3 years in length and had fairly uniform courses of study and clinical hours. Linda Richards and other early graduates

TABLE **3-3**

Types of Nursing Education Programs

TYPES OF PROGRAM AND CREDENTIAL	TYPE OF INSTITUTION	LENGTH OF PROGRAM	PURPOSE AND SCOPE
Practical or vocational nurse program: prepares for LVN or LPN license	High school, hospitals, vocational-technical schools; some colleges	9 to 12 months	Basic technical bedside care; hospitals, nursing homes, home care, offices in LPN positions
Diploma program: prepares for RN license	Hospitals, some in conjunction with colleges	2 to 3 years	Basic RN positions; hospitals and agency care
Associate degree in nursing: prepares for RN license	Community and junior colleges	2 years; some are 1 year bridge programs for LPN/LVN graduates	Basic technical care in RN positions, primarily in institutions
Bachelor's degree in nursing (BSN): prepares for RN license	Colleges and universities	2 to 4 years (depends on type of option); some are 1 to 2 years mobility options for graduates of PN or ADN programs or accelerated options for second-degree students	Basic professional practice as RN; management, community and public health settings; prepares for graduate school and certification; basic programs are 4 years; mobility options may be only 2 years
Master's degree in nursing (MSN)	Universities	1 to 2 years beyond BSN degree; some offer fast-track options	Advanced clinical practice, management, education, leadership positions
Doctoral degree in nursing	Universities	Varies: PhD, DSN, DNP, DNSc	Advanced nursing for research, clinical practice, education, and leadership positions

wrote initial nursing textbooks and began offering specialty training to staff hospitals and clinics (Kalisch and Kalisch, 1995). Richards also became a nurse consultant to help develop other schools in the United States and later in Japan, initiating international collaboration.

As the number of hospitals increased, the need for nurses likewise increased, and essentially, every hospital developed its own training program as its main source for nursing staff. At their peak from 1950 to 1960, more than 1300 diploma programs were operational. By 2008 only 75 diploma schools remained (NLN, 2008a). Diploma programs now are more similar to associate degree programs, typically 2 years in length; many have arrangements with colleges so that students can simultaneously earn an associate or baccalaureate degree.

Associate Degree Programs

In the late 1950s, a very different trend in nursing education emerged in response to social, political, and educational changes in society and to a growing shortage of RNs. During World War II the need for RNs who were prepared more quickly than in diploma programs became critical; the 2-year Cadet Nurse Corps was developed and proved to be very successful. From this experience some educators realized that nurses and others could be prepared in less time and still meet RN licensure and practice requirements. After the war Congress made funds available to publicly fund community colleges that offered 2-year associate degree programs in many technical fields. In addition, military benefits for college tuition allowed thousands of men and women to rise above the heritage of their parents to earn a 2-year college degree and fill jobs needed by burgeoning business and industry.

At the same time, the increasing complexity and expansion of medical care required more and better-prepared RNs. A few nurse educators began to create a new 2-year associate degree nursing program in community colleges, which required college courses in arts and sciences and a more integrated approach to nursing content and clinical learning. These pioneers reasoned that nursing belonged in a college setting, as in other disciplines, to provide a better education for nurses and to establish more respect and recognition for nursing's contribution to the community's health. As the number of community colleges grew and the need for nurses increased, associate degree nursing (ADN) programs became a logical program for development and expansion. Orsolini-Hain and Waters (2009) provide a brief and interesting historical account of ADN education.

ADN education is a vivid example of how changes in society influence the evolution of nursing education; it was another significant "first" in nursing and an important part of the evolving professionalization of nursing as a discipline. For the first time, it was possible for all RNs to be educated in a college setting and obtain a college degree. ADN programs were so successful they became the new career pathway for nurses, and now the majority of practicing RNs are ADN graduates.

In 2000 approximately 885 ADN programs were operational, and by 2007 the number increased to 1000 programs (NLN, 2008a). This trend of acceptance and growth of ADN programs along with the slowly increasing 4-year BSN programs and progressive mobility options established the educational framework for current nursing education.

Baccalaureate Degree Nursing Programs

In 1924 Yale University offered the first separate department of nursing whose graduates earned the baccalaureate degree. The 28-month program required scientific studies and clinical work and had the prestige and authority of other departments, with its own dean and budget (Kalisch and Kalisch, 1995). About the same time (1923 to 1924), a true 4-year nursing (BSN) degree program was opened at Western Reserve University (now Case Western Reserve University). The nursing school later was named after its main benefactor, Frances Payne Bolton, and today it offers many specialized programs for undergraduate and graduate students from throughout the world. This early beginning of BSN programs was another first in the history of nursing as a profession. Nurse leaders from those early years until today believe that nurses provide more comprehensive and competent care when they get a solid foundation in the arts and sciences, in addition to nursing content.

Generic BSN programs typically require 2 years of arts and sciences followed by 2 years of nursing courses. RN to BSN programs now outnumber basic BSN programs (AACN, 2009c, NLN, 2008a), and following endorsement by the AACN (2005), accelerated options for those with other degrees are growing rapidly. As in other programs, BSN courses focus on the care of patients with medical, surgical, pediatric, obstetric, and psychiatric conditions, although course sequencing and names differ considerably from school to school. BSN programs focus more emphasis on the family and community and health promotion and illness prevention; a large part of clinical experience is in diverse community settings. They also require courses such as research, management, leadership, and statistics. The AACN (2008a) reported 748 BSN programs, 610 generic, 621 RN to BSN, and 218 accelerated programs for non-nursing graduates. Graduates of BSN programs take the same NCLEX-RN® licensure examination as diploma and ADN graduates. Most specialty areas require the BSN degree for practice and as preparation for specialty certification. Admission into master's programs usually requires the BSN or other degree.

Master's Degree Nursing Programs

In the 1960s and 1970s, the number of BSN graduates increased, but so did the need for more qualified clinicians, educators, and administrators in response to the complexity of health care. The federal government responded with support for the development of MSN and BSN degree programs. Nurse leaders lobbied and obtained federal funding for building construction and increased student tuition. Traineeship and fellowship grants were made available to thousands of RNs that enabled them to earn BSN and advanced degrees to meet these needs. Different MSN program options are available; the most typical are for BSN graduates, although an increasing number are designed for graduates of non-nursing degree programs, called *accelerated* or *second-degree* programs (see the AACN website, nursing education programs for several detailed descriptions of programs and statistics (2005, 2009c).

Until the late 1960s MSN programs primarily focused on preparing educators and administrators, but then the curriculum shifted to an overwhelming emphasis on clinical practice. By the 1990s, the negative and the positive consequences of this decision became apparent with more competent clinicians but less well-prepared educators and administrators. Most MSN programs are designed to prepare advanced nurse practitioners and clinical specialists in various specialty areas. The extraordinary and rapid changes in health care since the early 1990s highlighted the cost-effective and quality care benefits of using advanced practice nurses in primary health care and other specialty areas. With intensive and persistent legal activities, nurses won battles to change state laws to permit nurse practitioners to write prescriptions, receive reimbursement for care, and operate independent nurse practices and health centers. As a result of this expanded scope of practice, an increasing number of nurses have obtained MSN degrees and advanced practice certification. Most nurses in specialty practice, managers, administrators, and educators now are required to have a master's or doctoral degree. Many universities, such as Case Western Reserve University, have developed majors that focus on flight nursing, infection control, informatics, and dual majors with business and bioethics. Many schools once again offer a major in nursing education. The AACN and NLN offer descriptions and numbers of different types of programs on their websites (see Table 3-2).

Clinical Nurse Leader

In 2000 the national movement to enhance quality and safety in health care led to discussions between the AACN, nurse executives, and other health care leaders that led to the development of a new nursing role—the clinical nurse leader (CNL). In July 2002 the AACN board created the TFER 2 (Task Force on Education and Regulation [TFER]). Its focus was the nurse competencies needed in current and future health care systems to improve patient care and what the "new nurse" role might look like. This work resulted in the publication of the White Paper on the Role of the Clinical Nurse Leader (CNL), in 2007 (AACN, 2009a). The CNL is a master's-prepared generalist clinician, not an advanced practice nurse, who oversees the care coordination of a distinct group of patients, evaluates patient outcomes, and has the decision-making authority to change care plans when necessary. The CNL actively provides direct patient care in complex situations, serves as a lateral integrator who provides centralized care coordination for a distinct group of patients, and puts evidence-based care into practice to ensure that patients benefit from the latest innovations. A CNL is a leader in the health care delivery system with expertise in quality improvement and cost-effective resource utilization (Rosseter, 2009). The Commission on Nurse Certification, an autonomous arm of AACN, began certifying CNLs in 2007 and by 2009 more than 700 CNLs were certified.

Doctoral Programs

Changes in society and health care and the trend of needing more well-educated nurse leaders and researchers led to the initiation of doctoral programs for nurses. The first doctoral program for nurses was developed at Teachers College, Columbia University, and the first nurse graduated in 1932 with a doctor of education degree (EdD). In 1934 New York University offered a PhD program for nurses. More than 30 years elapsed before doctoral programs *in nursing* (instead of *for nurses*) were offered (e.g., the doctor of nursing science degree [DNS or DNSc]).

For the past few decades, three types of doctoral degrees in nursing were available: (1) the doctor of philosophy (PhD) for those interested in research; (2) DNS or DNSc for those interested in advanced clinical nursing practice; and (3) the doctor of nursing (ND) for those with BS or higher degrees in non-nursing fields who want to pursue a career in nursing leadership. The ND degree, which prepares nurses for basic licensure (NCLEX-RN), was first offered at Case Western Reserve University in 1979. Shortly after, Rush University, the University of Colorado Health Sciences Center, and others offered this degree. Several schools also offer options combined with another major, such as business, law, informatics, or social sciences.

Beginning in 2000, AACN leaders developed and implemented a new clinical-focused doctoral degree: the doctor of nursing practice (DNP) (AACN, 2004; see AACN webpage for updated information and statistics). The DNP is conceived as preparation for contemporary advanced nurse practitioners; it is viewed as the clinical equivalent to the research-oriented PhD nursing degree. AACN has recommended that all advanced practice education programs move from the master's to the doctoral level by 2015. The DNP is still controversial although programs continue to gain support (Hathaway, et al, 2006; Kaplan and Brown, 2009; Leners, Wilson, and Sitzman, 2009). Some nurse leaders think introducing another level of preparation is not in the best interest of nursing and will exacerbate the faculty shortage further (Chase and Pruitt, 2006; Tanner, 2005). Although DNP prepares clinicians it does not formally prepare educators. However, individuals who have a DNP degree frequently serve in faculty roles. In April 2009 the AACN reported that from 2007 to 2008 the number of students enrolled in DNP programs nearly doubled from 1874 to 3415. During that same period, the number of DNP graduates increased from 122 to 361. Additionally, as of this writing, 92 DNP programs had enrolled students in schools of nursing nationwide, and an additional 102 DNP programs were in the planning stage.

FLEXIBLE EDUCATION, MOBILITY, AND DISTANCE LEARNING PROGRAMS

Various types of nontraditional mobility programs were initiated in the 1970s (Lenburg, 1975) and have evolved over the past four decades (Benjamin-Coleman, et al, 2001). Resisted for more than 20 years by more traditional educators and organizations, mobility programs now are commonplace. The websites for AACN (2006, 2008a, 2009a,c) and NLN (2008b, 2009a) attest to the growing number of programs that offer some form of flexible, alternative program, in addition to position statements on technology in nursing education, distance learning, and online programs. This well-developed trend is based on the success of these programs, the documented needs of students, the nursing shortage, and the expansion and acceptance of electronic learning technology (Shovein, Huston, Fox, et al, 2005). Distance or mobility programs include those for LPN or LVN to ADN and BSN; diploma and ADN graduates to BSN and MSN; and BSN to MSN and doctoral programs. Almost all use some form of Internet-based courses and some are entirely online. Some require periods of intensive on-campus classes or assigned clinical experiences with preceptors (see Table 3-2).

The most controversial but pace-setting distance mobility program in nursing was developed under the New York Board of Regents as "the external degree program." Initially named the NY Regents External Degree Program (NYREDP) it later was renamed Excelsior College. Its ADN program, initiated in 1972, and the BSN, in 1976, were fully accredited by NLN shortly thereafter, albeit with considerable difficulty. This innovative college provides quality degree programs in many disciplines for adult learners underserved by traditional programs by using assessment methods to document prior learning and theory and performance examinations to validate current knowledge and competence. The nursing programs enroll thousands of students and are accessible regardless of geographic location; the students primarily are LPNs or RNs, some of whom also have other degrees or health-related certificates. Early studies documented their competence in the workplace (Lenburg, 1990). It initiated a master's degree program in 2000 with two specialty options. Over the years many nursing programs have accepted and modified distance learning and assessment approach originally developed by NYREDP and continued as Excelsior College. The integration of electronic learning technology with assessment methods, makes nursing degrees accessible to an increasing number of nurses seeking additional preparation (see Table 3-2).

Career ladder programs designed as "1-plus-1" or "2-plus-2" options have been offered for many years by some schools and through several statewide programs. Multiple mobility programs are available for LPNs to obtain an ADN degree, such as one offered by the New York Coalition for Education Mobility (2004). RN to BSN programs are available in more than 600 schools as of 2009 (AACN, 2009b, 2009c). In addition, some 144 programs admit ADN graduates into MSN programs (see AACN website, education programs). With the shortage of nurses and nurse educators, some schools are finding ways to streamline RN to BSN programs.

Changes in the social, political, financial, and philosophic trends; the extensive use of communication and learning technology; verified success from past experiences; and the continuing shortage of nurses have combined to make education mobility and distance learning opportunities a necessity and a reality nationally and internationally. Whereas NLN continues to support all levels of education programs, AACN and other organizations vigorously support the BSN for "entry into practice" and the professionalization of nursing (AACN, 2000). In 2003 the New York State Board of Nursing approved a proposal that would require future graduates of diploma and ADN programs to earn a BSN degree within 10 years to be eligible for renewal of licensure; as of this writing it has not been passed. The New York Organization of Nurse Executives supports this effort and describes the rationale for it on its website (NYONE, 2006).

The escalating nursing shortage and the aging of the current nursing workforce and nurse educators have prompted more schools to offer flexible mobility options and types of programs. Some target potentially underrepresented groups, such as men, minority groups, and those with existing academic degrees. The most rapidly growing are the accelerated, fast-track, or second-degree programs, designed for non-nurses with other degrees. In 2009, the AACN reported 218 accelerated BSN programs; some schools also offer accelerated doctoral programs (AACN, 2009c).

Trends and issues that influence nursing education make it even more important to comply with quality standards that emphasize competency outcomes. Changes in number, diversity, and qualifications of students and shortage of faculty and finances make it necessary to develop more efficient and effective learning strategies for on-campus and distant students. Although mobility and electronic options are more convenient, they present issues. In addition to learning to access multiple digital resources, students also need discipline and determination to pursue courses and clinical learning when a teacher is not physically present or accessible. Regardless of methods, they must achieve required competencies in spite of other responsibilities and learn to integrate critical thinking, reflective judgment, and evidence-based practices in patient care. In contrast to previous decades, organizations and schools now require more creative, responsive programs and expect more documented competence from students and faculty (Box 3-1). Although these trends pose challenges for nursing students, faculties, and employers, they move nursing toward more competent professional practice and improved patient safety (Boyer, 2008; Lenburg et al, 2009).

BOX **3-1**

Selected Organizations Relevant to Nursing Education: General Description and Purpose

American Academy of Nursing (AAN) —The organization of leaders in all facets of nursing: practice, education, administration, research, organizations, and government; the think tank of the profession; promotes advancement of all aspects of nursing; publishes position papers, conference proceedings, and documents to advance nursing.

American Association of Colleges of Nursing (AACN)—The organization of deans and directors of baccalaureate and higher-degree nursing programs; establishes standards for programs, concerned with legislative issues that pertain to professional nursing education; publishes the *Journal of Professional Nursing, The Essentials of Baccalaureate Education* (2008), and other related documents pertaining to the BSN and higher-degree education.

American Nurses Association (ANA)—The major national nursing organization concerned with broad scope of practice issues; standard of practice, scope of practice, ethics, legal, employment; a federation of state nurses associations; publications related to array of practice issues and standards.

Commission on Collegiate Nursing Education (CCNE)—A subsidiary of AACN with responsibility for establishing and implementing standards and criteria and for accreditation of baccalaureate and graduate degree programs in nursing.

National Council of State Boards of Nursing (NCSBN)—Organization of all state boards; coordinates licensure activities on national level; creates and administers licensure examinations (NCLEX); developed computerized licensure examinations; works with other organizations to promote nursing standards and regulation and establish interstate licensure protocols.

National League for Nursing (NLN)—The national organization of nurse educators, with long-standing commitment to four types of basic programs (LPN, diploma, ADN, and BSN); includes lay citizens concerned with nursing and health care on its board. NLN also has councils for nursing informatics, research in nursing education, wellness centers, and multiple types of print publications. Initiated certification program and examination to certify excellence of nursing educators; also established Centers for Excellence for nursing programs that meet designated standards.

NLN Accreditation Commission (NLNAC)—Formed in 1997 as a subsidiary of NLN with responsibility for establishing and implementing standards and criteria and for accrediting all types of schools of nursing.

National Organization of Nurse Practitioner Faculty (NONPF)—Organization of nurse practitioners in multiple specialties; sets national standards and criteria for programs and certification.

National Student Nurses Association (NSNA)—National organization of statewide student nurse associations; concerned with education and career issues; provides student perspectives to other national nursing organizations.

SUMMARY

This chapter presented 10 major trends and related issues in nursing education programs and an overview of multiple types of nursing programs. They have a significant influence on the content, learning process, and evaluation methods used in all types of programs and have influenced the development of new degrees and majors. They have had a remarkable effect on the persistence of various types of programs for entry into practice and on the increasing acceptance of diverse mobility and distance learning programs. Regardless of the type of program, most students now use the Internet to access courses, electronic databases, and other learning resources and integrate evidence-based practice and critical thinking. As students integrate current trends and attempt to resolve issues, they create the trends for the next generation; they are participating in nursing history in the making. The most profound trend in nursing education is learning to learn, to reason, and access relevant resources to solve problems. As Alvin Toffler wrote, "The illiterate of the 21st century will not be those who cannot read and write, but those who cannot learn, unlearn, and relearn."

evolve Additional resources are available online at: http://evolve.elsevier.com/Cherry/

REFERENCES

Adelman DS, Legg TJ: *Disaster nursing: a handbook for practice*, Sudbury, MA, 2009, Jones and Bartlett.

Allen P, et al: Reinventing practice and education partnerships for capacity expansion, *J Nurs Educ* 46:170–175, 2007.

American Association of Colleges of Nursing (AACN): *Position statement: baccalaureate degree in nursing as minimal preparation for professional practice*, Washington, DC, 2000, AACN. Available at: www.aacn.nche.edu.

American Association of Colleges of Nursing (AACN): *Position statement on the practice doctorate in nursing*. 2004. Available at: www.aacn.nche.edu/DNP/DNPPosition Statement.htm.

American Association of Colleges of Nursing (AACN): *Issues bulletin: accelerated programs: the fast-track to careers in nursing*, updated 2005. Available at: www.aacn.nche. edu/publications/issues/Aug02.htm.

American Association of Colleges of Nursing (AACN): Hallmarks of quality and patient safety: recommended baccalaureate competencies and curricular guidelines to ensure high-quality and safe patient care, *J Prof Nurs* 55:329–330, 2006.

American Association of Colleges of Nursing (AACN): *The essentials of baccalaureate education for professional nursing practice*, Washington, DC, 2008a, AACN.

American Association of Colleges of Nursing (AACN): *Cultural competency in baccalaureate education*. 2008b. Available at: www.aacn.nche.edu/education/pdf/ competency.pdf.

American Association of Colleges of Nursing (AACN): *Nursing education programs*, 2008c. Available at: www.aacn. nche.edu/Education/nurse_ed/nep_index.htm.

American Association of Colleges of Nursing (AACN): *The clinical nurse leader: developing a new nurse*, Washington, DC, 2009a, AACN. Available at: www.aacn.nche.edu/ cnl/index.htm.

American Association of Colleges of Nursing (AACN): *Degree completion programs for registered nurses: RN to master's degree and RN to baccalaureate programs*. 2009b. Available at: www.aacn.nche.edu/Media/FactSheets/ DegreeCompletionProg.htm.

American Association of Colleges of Nursing (AACN): *2008-2009 Enrollment and graduations in baccalaureate and graduate programs in nursing*, Washington, DC, 2009c, AACN.

American Association of Colleges of Nursing (AACN): *End of life care*. 2009d. Available at: www.aacn.nche.edu/ ELNEC.

American Association of Colleges of Nursing (AACN): *Government affairs, nursing policy beat: healthcare reform*. 2009e. Available at: www.aacn.nche.edu/Government/index.htm. (Multiple links to shortage and strategies for change.)

American Association of Colleges of Nursing (AACN): *Nursing faculty shortage*. 2009f. Available at: www.aacn. nche.edu/Media/FactSheets/FacultyShortage.htm.

American Nurses Association (ANA): *Bioterrorism and disaster response*. 2006. Available at: www.nursingworld. org/homepage/menu.

American Nurses Association (ANA): *2009 H1N1— Information for nurses*. 2009a. Available at: www. nursingworld.org/H1N1.

American Nurses Association (ANA): *Nursing ethics: the center for ethics and human rights*. 2009b. Available at: www.nursingworld.org/MainMenuCategories/Ethics Standards.aspx:(explore links).

American Nurses Association (ANA): *Workplace violence.* 2009c. Available at: www.nursingworld.org/MainMenu Categories/ANAPoliticalPower/State/StateLegislative Agenda/WorkplaceViolence.aspx.

Anastasi JK, Capili B, Schenkman F: Developing integrative therapies in primary care program, *Nurs Educ* 34:271–275, 2009.

Baer ED, D'Antonio P, Rinker SL: *Enduring issues in American nursing,* New York, 2000, Springer.

Bargagliotti A, Luttrell M, Lenburg CB: Reducing threats to the implementation of a competency-based performance assessment system, *Online J Issues Nurs,* 1999. Available at: www.nursingworld.org/ojin.

Bauldoff GS, Kirkpatrick B, Sheets DJ, et al: Implementation of handheld devices, *Nurs Educ* 33:244–248, 2008.

Benjamin-Coleman R, et al: Distance education: a decade of distance education: RN to BSN, *Nurs Educator* 26: 9–12, 2001.

Benkert R, Resnick B, Brackley M, et al: Tuberculosis education for nursing practitioner students: where we are and where we need to go, *J Nurs Educ* 48:255–265, 2009.

Bentley R, Ellison KJ: Increasing cultural competence in nursing through international service-learning experiences, *Nurs Educ* 32:207–211, 2007.

Boyer S: Competence and innovation in preceptor development—updating our programs, *J Nurs Staff Devel* 24:E1–E6, 2008.

Brendtro MJ, Leuning C: Nurses in churches: a population-focused clinical option, *J Nurs Educ* 39:285–288, 2000.

Bruce SA, Scherer YK, Curran CC, et al: A collaborative exercise between graduate and undergraduate nursing students using a computer-assisted simulator in a mock cardiac arrest, *Nurs Educ Perspect* 30:22–27, 2009.

Buerhaus PI, Auerbach DI, Staiger DO: The recent surge in nurse employment: causes and implications, *Health Affairs* 28(4):620–624, 2009.

Cagle CA: Student understanding of culturally and ethically responsive care: implications for nursing curricula, *Nurs Educ Perspect* 27:308–314, 2006.

Campbell WE, Dudley K: Clinical partner model: benefits for education and service, *Nurs Educ* 30:271–274, 2005.

Candela L, Bowles C: Recent RN graduate perceptions of educational preparation, *Nurs Educ Perspect* 29:266–271, 2008.

Carlton KH, et al: Integration of global health concepts in nursing curricula: a national study, *Nurs Educ Perspect* 28:124–129, 2007.

Centers for Disease Control and Prevention: *Merck Company Foundation: The state of aging and health in America.* 2007. Available at: www.cdc.gov/aging/pdf/saha_2007.pdf.

Chase SK, Pruitt RH: The practice doctorate: innovation or disruption? *J Nurs Educ* 45:155–161, 2006.

Clark C: Faculty field guide for promoting student civility in the classroom, *Nurs Educ* 34:194–197, 2009.

Clark CH, Springer PJ: Thoughts on incivility: student and faculty perceptions of uncivil behavior in nursing education, *Nurs Educ Perspect* 28:93–97, 2007.

Clayton LH, Dilley KB: Service learning population-focused nursing for the homeless at a soup kitchen, *Nurs Educ* 34:137–139, 2009.

Cormier CM, Kotrlik J: Health literacy knowledge and experiences of senior baccalaureate nursing students, *J Nurs Educ* 48:237–248, 2009.

Critchley KA, et al: Student experiences with an international public health exchange project, *Nurs Educ* 34: 69–74, 2009.

Cronenwett L, et al: Quality and safety education for nurses, *Nurs Outlook* 55:122–131, 2007.

del Bueno D: A crisis in critical thinking, *Nurs Educ Perspect* 26:278–282, 2005.

DiVito-Thomas P: Nursing student stories on learning how to think like a nurse, *Nurs Educ* 30:133–136, 2005.

Ehrenreich B: Is it now a crime to be poor? *New York Times,* August 9, 2009. Available at: www.nytimes.com/2009/08/09/opinion/09ehrenreich.html.

Esposito NW, et al: Preventing violence in an academic setting: one school of nursing's approach, *Nurs Educ Perspect* 26:24–28, 2005.

Falk NL: Strategies to enhance retention and effective utilization of aging nurse faculty, *J Nurs Educ* 46:165–169, 2007.

Farnsworth J, Springer PJ: Background checks for nursing students: what are schools doing? *Nurs Educ Perspect* 27:148–153, 2006.

Fay VT, Johnson J, Selz N: Active learning in nursing education (ALINE), *Nurs Educ* 31:65–68, 2006.

Ferrell BR: *End-of-life nursing education consortium.* Available at: www.aacn.nche.edu/elnec (search for multiple other references, 2000-2009).

Fetter MS: Graduating nurses' self-evaluation of information technology competencies, *J Nurs Educ* 48:86–90, 2009.

Finkelman AW, Kenner C: *Teaching the IOM: implications of the IOM reports for nursing education,* Silver Spring, MD, 2009, American Nurses Association.

Fontana JS: Nursing faculty experiences of students' academic dishonesty, *J Nurs Educ* 48:181–185, 2009.

Giddens JF, Brady DP: Rescuing nursing education from content saturation: the case for a concept-based curriculum, *J Nurs Educ* 46:65–69, 2007.

Glennon CD: Reconceptualizing program outcomes, *J Nurs Educ* 45:55–58, 2006.

Hathaway D, et al: The practice doctorate: perspectives of early adopters, *J Nurs Educ* 45:487–496, 2006.

Hawkins K, Todd M, Manz J: A unique simulation teaching method, *J Nurs Educ* 47:524–527, 2008.

Helms JE: Complementary and alternative therapies: a new frontier for nursing education, *J Nurs Educ* 45: 117–123, 2006.

Heye ML, Stevens KR: Using new resources to teach evidence-based practice, *J Nurs Educ* 48:334–339, 2009.

Higgins B: Relationship between retention and peer tutoring for at-risk students, *J Nurs Educ* 43:319–321, 2006.

Holroyd A, et al: Attitudes toward aging: implications for a caring profession, *J Nurs Educ* 48:374–380, 2009.

Horan KM: Using the human patient simulator to foster critical thinking in critical situations, *Nurs Educ Perspect* 30:28–30, 2009.

Horns PN, et al: Leading through collaboration: a regional academic/service partnership that works, *Nurs Outlook* 55:74–78, 2007.

Hunt R: Service-learning: an eye-opening experience that provokes emotion and challenges stereotypes, *J Nurs Educ* 46:277–281, 2007.

International Council of Nurses (ICN): *Nurs Netw 2009.* Available at: icn.ch/networks.htm.

Institute of Medicine (IOM): *To err is human: building a safer health system*, Washington, DC, 2000, National Academy of Science Press. Available at: www.iom.edu. See also *Nursing response* at www.aacn.nche.edu and www.nursingworld.org.

Institute of Medicine (IOM): *Health professions education: a bridge to quality*, Washington, DC, 2003, National Academies Press.

Ireland M: Assisting students to use evidence as a part of reflection on practice, *Nurs Educ Perspect* 29:90–93, 2008.

Jeffries PR: Technology trends in nursing education: next steps, *J Nurs Educ* 44:3–4, 2005.

Kalisch PA, Kalisch BJ: *The advance of American nursing*, ed 3, Philadelphia, 1995, Lippincott.

Kaplan L, Brown M: Doctor of nursing practice program evaluation and beyond: capturing the profession's transition to the DNP, *Nurs Educ Perspect* 30:362–366, 2009.

Kirkham SR, Harwood CH, Hofwegen LV: Capturing a vision for nursing: undergraduate nursing students in alternative clinical settings, *Nurs Educ* 30:263–270, 2005.

Kleinman S: Revitalizing the humanistic imperative in nursing education, *Nurs Educ Perspect* 28:209–213, 2007.

Klein CJ: Linking competency-based assessment to successful clinical practice, *J Nurs Educ* 45:379–383, 2006.

Kotecki CN: Incorporating faith-based partnerships into the curriculum, *Nurs Educ* 27:13–15, 2002.

Lasater K: High-fidelity simulation and the development of clinical judgment: students' experiences, *J Nurs Educ* 46:269–276, 2007.

Lasater K, Nielsen A: The influence of concept-based learning activities on students' clinical judgment development, *J Nurs Educ* 48:441–446, 2009.

Lashley FR: Emerging infectious diseases at the beginning of the 21st century. 2006. Available at: www.nursingworld. org/MainMenuCategories/ANAMarketplace/ANA Periodicals/OJIN/TableofContents/Volume112006/ No1Jan06/tpc29_116054.aspx.

Lenburg CB: *Open learning and career mobility in nursing*, St Louis, 1975, Mosby.

Lenburg CB: Do external degree programs really work? *Nurs Outlook* 36:234–238, 1990.

Lenburg CB: The framework, concepts and methods of the Competency Outcomes and Performance Assessment (COPA) model, *Online J Issues Nurs* Sept 1999. Available at: www.nursingworld.org/ojin.

Lenburg CB: Changes that challenge nursing education, *TNNurse.* October 2002. Available at www.tnaonline.org/ tn-nurse-archive.html.

Lenburg CB: The influence of contemporary trends and issues on nursing education. In Cherry B, Jacob S, editors: *Contemporary Nursing: Issues, Trends, and Management*, ed 4, St Louis, 2008, Mosby.

Lenburg CB, Klein C, Abdur-Rahman V, Spencer T, et al: The COPA model: a comprehensive framework designed to promote quality care and competence for patient safety, *Nurs Educ Perspect* 30:312–317, 2009.

Leners DW, Wilson VW, Sitzman KL, : Twenty-first century doctoral education: online with a focus on nursing education, *Nurs Educ Perspect* 28:332–336, 2009.

MacIntyre RC, Murray TA, Teel CS, Karshmer JF: Five recommendations for prelicensure clinical nursing education, *J Nurs Educ* 48:447–453, 2009.

Matzo ML, et al: Communication skills for end of life nursing care: teaching strategies from the ELNEC curriculum, *Nurs Educ Perspect* 24:176–183, 2003.

McBride AB: Nursing and the informatics revolution, *Nurs Outlook* 53:183–191, 2005.

McCabe DL: Academic dishonesty in nursing schools: an empirical investigation, *J Nurs Educ* 48:614–623, 2009.

Monroe T: Addressing substance abuse among nursing students: development of a prototype alternative-to-dismissal policy, *J Nurs Educ* 48:272–278, 2009.

Murphy JI: Using focused reflection and articulation to promote clinical reasoning: an evidence-based teaching strategy, *Nurs Educ Perspect* 25:226–231, 2004.

Murray TA: Expanding educational capacity through an innovative practice-education partnership, *J Nurs Educ* 46:330–333, 2007.

National Council of State Boards of Nursing (NCSBN): *Meeting the ongoing challenge of continued competence.* 2006. Available at: www.ncsbn.org.

National League for Nursing (NLN): *NLN centers of excellence in nursing education.* 2005a. Available at: www.nln. org/Excellence/index.htm.

National League for Nursing (NLN): Headlines from NLN: creating a global community in nursing education, *Nurs Educ Perspect* 26:194, 2005b.

National League for Nursing (NLN): Task Group on Innovations in Nursing Education: Substantive innovation in nursing education: shifting the emphasis from content coverage to student learning, *Nurs Educ Perspect* 26:55–57, 2005c, 2009a.

National League for Nursing (NLN): *Annual survey of schools of nursing academic year 2006-2007: executive summary*, New York, 2008a, NLN. Available at: www. nln.org/research/slides/exec_summary.htm.

National League for Nursing (NLN): *Preparing the next generation of nurses to practice in a technology-rich environment: an informatics agenda, NLN, board of governors.* May 9, 2008b, Author.

National League for Nursing (NLN): *Public policy agenda 2009-2010: Promoting excellence in nursing education to build a strong and diverse nursing workforce.* 2009a. Available at: www.nln.org/governmentaffairs/pdf/public_policy.pdf.

National League for Nursing (NLN): *Nursing shortage info.* 2009b. Available at: www.nln.org/aboutnln/shortage_info.htm.(Many links to nursing shortage information.)

National Organization of Nurse Practitioner Faculty (2006): *2006 Domains and core competencies.* Washington, DC.

Ncuman LH: Creating new futures in nursing education: envisioning the evolution of e-nursing education, *Nurs Educ Perspect* 27:13–15, 2006.

Newman DML: A community nursing center for the health promotion of senior citizens based on the Neuman systems model, *Nurs Educ Perspect* 26:221–223, 2005.

New York Organization of Nurse Executives: *NYONE - ACTION, advancing the profession of nursing.* Retrieved September 9, 2006 from: www.nyone.org.

New York State Coalition for Educational Mobility: *LPN to ADN articulation model, 2004.* Retrieved August, 2006 from: www.lpntoadn.info.

Online Journal of Issues in Nursing (OJIN): *Ethics columns and multiple articles.* 1999-2009a. Available at: www.nursingworld.org/ojin.

Online Journal of Issues in Nursing (OJIN): *Obesity on the rise: what can nurses do?* 2009b. Available at: www.nursingworld.org/MainMenuCategories/ANAMarketplace/-ANAPeriodicals/OJIN/JournalTopics/Obesity-on-the-Rise.aspx.

Orsolini-Hain L, Waters V: Education evolution: a historical perspective of associate degree nursing, *J Nurs Educ* 48:266–271, 2009.

Pellico LH, Brewer CS, Kovner CT: What newly licensed registered nurses have to say about their first experiences, *Nurs Outlook* 57:194–203, 2009.

Porter-O'Grady T: Profound change; twenty-first century nursing, *Nurs Outlook* 49:182–186, 2001.

Pravikoff DS: Mission critical: a culture of evidence-based practice and information literacy, *Nurs Outlook* 54:254–255, 2006.

Ramal E: Integrating caring, scholarship and community engagement in Mexico, *Nurs Educ* 34:34–37, 2009.

Rentschler DD, Eaton J, Cappiello J, et al: Evaluation of undergraduate students using objective structured evaluation, *J Nurs Educ* 46:135–139, 2007.

Riddell T: Critical assumptions: thinking critically about critical thinking, *J Nurs Educ* 46:121–126, 2007.

Roberson DW: Using a student responsibility system to reduce academic cheating, *Nurs Educ* 34:60–63, 2009.

Rose JR: Nurse-run clinics offer hope to nation's tired, poor and uninsured, *Adv Nurs*, 2009. Available at: http://nursing.advanceweb.com/editorial/content/editorial.aspx?cc=204382.

Rosseter R: A new role for nurses: making room for clinical leaders, *Jt Comm Perspect* 9(8):5–7, 2009.

Rush KL, Dyches CE, Waldrop S, et al: Critical thinking among RN-to-BSN distance students participating in human patient simulation, *J Nurs Educ* 47:501–507, 2008.

Schaffer MA, Nelson P, Litt E: Using portfolios to evaluate achievement of population-based public health nursing competencies in baccalaureate nursing students, *Nurs Educ Perspect* 26:104–112, 2005.

Schlariet MC: Bioethics mediation: the role and importance of nursing advocacy, *Nurs Outlook* 57:185–193, 2009.

Scott ES: Peer-to-peer mentoring: teaching collegiality, *Nurs Educ* 30:52–56, 2005.

Shovein J, Huston C, Fox S, et al: Challenging traditional teaching and learning paradigm: online learning and emancipatory teaching, *Nurs Educ Perspect* 26:340–343, 2005.

Skiba D: Emerging technologies center: preparing for evidence-based practice: revisiting information literacy, *Nurs Educ Perspect* 26:310–311, 2005.

Skiba D: Emerging technologies center: teaching with and about technology: providing resources for nurse educators worldwide, *Nurs Educ Perspect* 30:129–131, 2009a.

Skiba D: Emerging technologies center: see column in every issue in, *Nurs Educ Perspect* , 2005-2009b. Available at: www.nln.org.

Smith-Stoner M: Using high-fidelity simulation to educate nursing students about end-of-life care, *Nurs Educ Perspect* 30:115–120, 2009.

Smith-Stoner M: Web-based broadcast of simulations expanding access to learning, *Nurs Educ* 34:266–270, 2009.

Southern Poverty Law Center, 2009. (Information re teaching tolerance; monitoring hate groups.) Available at: www.splcenter.org/index.jsp.

Speziale HJ, Jacobson L: Trends in registered nurse education programs 1998-2008, *Nurs Educ Perspect* 26: 230–235, 2005.

Steed CJ, et al: Integrating bioterrorism education into nursing school curricula, *J Nurs Educ* 43:362–367, 2004.

Stop violence against women: a project by the advocates for human rights. 2009. Available at: www.stopvaw.org.

Sullivan CH: Partnering with community agencies to provide nursing students with cultural awareness experiences and refugee health promotion access, *J Nurs Educ* 48:519–522, 2009.

Tanner CA: Critical thinking: beyond nursing process, *J Nurs Educ* 39:338–339, 2000.

Tanner CA: What are our priorities? Addressing the looming shortage of nursing faculty, *J Nurs Educ* 44:247–248, 2005.

Thomas SP, Burk R: Junior nursing students' experiences of vertical violence during clinical rotations, *Nurs Outlook* 57:226–231, 2009.

Tippitt MP, et al: Creating environments that foster academic integrity, *Nurs Educ Perspect* 30:239–244, 2009.

Turner P: Critical thinking in nursing education and practice as defined in the literature, *Nurs Educ Perspect* 26:272–277, 2005.

U.S. Department of Labor Occupational Safety and Heath Administration (USDL): *Guidelines for preventing workplace violence for health care and social service workers*, No. OSHA 3148, Washington, DC, 2003.

Veenema TG: Expanding educational opportunities in disaster response and emergency preparedness, *Nurs Educ Perspect* 27:93–99, 2006.

Wagner D, Bear M, Sander J: Turning simulation into reality: increasing student competence and confidence, *J Nurs Educ* 48:465–467, 2009.

Weiner E, et al: Emergency preparedness curriculum in nursing schools in the United States, *Nurs Educ Perspect* 26:334–339, 2005.

Whitty KK, Burnett MF: Importance of instruction on mass casualty incidents in baccalaureate nursing programs: perceptions of nursing faculty, *J Nurs Educ* 48:291–295, 2009.

Wieland DM, et al: Clinical transitions of baccalaureate nursing students during preceptored, pregraduation practicums, *Nurs Educ Perspect* 28:315–321, 2007.

Williams MG, Dittmer A: Textbooks on tap: using electronic books housed in handheld devices in nursing clinical courses, *Nurs Educ Perspect* 30:220–225, 2009.

Worrell-Carlisle PJ: Service-learning: a tool for developing cultural awareness, *Nurs Educ* 30:197–202, 2005.

Zahner SJ, Block DE: The road to population health: using *Healthy People 2010* in nursing education, *J Nurs Educ* 45:105–108, 2006.

Nursing Licensure and Certification

Susan R. Jacob, PhD, MSN, RN

evolve Additional resources are available online at: http://evolve.elsevier.com/Cherry/

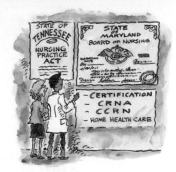

Legal regulations and professional certification ensure safe, competent nursing care.

VIGNETTE

Three nurses are discussing their nursing practice licenses. Joe Branch, a senior nursing student, is preparing for initial licensure. Mary Stone's license is due for renewal. Carmella Larkin has just moved into the state. As the three are talking about these changes in their practice, Giorgio Gonzales, a nurse practitioner, joins the group. Giorgio recently completed a certification examination and is interested in becoming certified for advanced practice. All the nurses have a general knowledge of the requirements for licensure and certification but lack the specific information needed to legally practice within the state.

Mary suggests contacting the state board of nursing. The nurses agree that this is a sensible idea, and Mary leaves to phone the board of nursing. On returning Mary informs the group that the answers to all their questions may be found in the state's nurse practice act and accompanying rules and regulations that may be accessed online on their website. She tells them that the state board of nursing office will also send free copies of both documents to individuals who request them.

The situation described here is not uncommon. Nurses need specific, current information on licensure and renewal of licensure. The most comprehensive sources for this information are the state nurse practice act and the state board of nursing. These resources provide accurate descriptions of the law governing nursing practice within each state and the U.S. territories. Every nurse and nursing student will benefit from obtaining a copy of their state's nurse practice act and becoming familiar with its contents.

■ QUESTIONS TO CONSIDER WHILE READING THIS CHAPTER

1 Who establishes the "rules" for nursing practice—the state or the employer?
2 Do graduates from different types of nursing education programs require different types of licenses?
3 If a nurse graduate passes the NCLEX-RN®, does that person still need a license?
4 What happens if a nurse's license expires? Can the nurse still practice?
5 Must a nurse complete graduate school and take an examination to be an advanced practice nurse?
6 Are the regulations governing advanced practice the same in all states?

We thank Janet C. Scherubel, PhD, RN, for her contribution to this chapter in the 4th edition.

KEY TERMS

Accreditation Voluntary process by which schools of nursing are approved to conduct nursing education programs.

Advanced practice nurse (APN) Legal title for nurses prepared by education and competence to perform independent practice.

American Nurses Association (ANA) Professional organization that represents all registered nurses.

American Nurses Credentialing Center (ANCC) An independent agency of the American Nurses Association that conducts certification examinations and certifies advanced practice nurses.

Certification Process by which nurses are recognized for advanced education and competence.

Compact state A term of law. In the context of the Nurse Licensure Compact, a state that has established an agreement with other states allowing nurses to practice within the state without an additional license. The interstate compacts are enacted by the state legislatures.

Commission on Collegiate Nursing Education (CCNE) A subsidiary of the American Association of Colleges of Nursing (AACN) with responsibility for accrediting baccalaureate and higher-degree nursing programs.

Continued competency program A variety of initiatives to ensure nurses knowledge, skills, and expertise beyond initial licensure.

Grandfathered Statutory process by which previously licensed persons are included without further action in revisions or additions in nurse practice acts.

International Council of Nursing (ICN) Professional organization that represents nurses in countries around the world.

Licensure by endorsement The original program whereby nurses licensed in one state seek licensure in another without repeat examinations. The requirements are included in state nurse practice acts or accompanying rules and regulations.

Mandatory continuing education Educational requirements imposed by individual states for renewal of a license.

Mutual recognition of nursing Program developed by the National Council of State Boards of Nursing, Inc. (2009c). The Nurse Licensure Compact program establishes interstate compacts so that nurses licensed in one jurisdiction may practice in other compact states without duplicate licensure.

National Council of State Boards of Nursing (NCSBN) Organization whose membership consists of the board of nursing of each state or territory.

National League for Nursing (NLN) Professional organization whose members represent multiple disciplines. The National League for Nursing conducts many types of programs, including accrediting nursing education programs.

Nurse practice act Statute in each state and territory that regulates the practice of nursing.

State board of nursing Appointed board within each state charged with responsibility to administer the nurse practice act of that state.

Sunset legislation Statutes that provide for revocation of laws if not reviewed and renewed within a specified time period.

LEARNING OUTCOMES

After studying this chapter, the reader will be able to:

1 Explain the development of licensure requirements in the United States.

2 Summarize current licensure requirements in the context of historical developments.

3 Analyze the various components of a nurse practice act.

4 Discuss mutual recognition of nursing practice and identify Nurse Licensure Compact states.

5 Describe the development of certification requirements for advanced practice.

6 Identify requirements for certification for advanced practice in different specialties.

7 Use appropriate resources to obtain current information on licensure and certification.

CHAPTER OVERVIEW

To practice nursing as a registered nurse (RN)! That is the goal of every student nurse. A goal achieved through study, clinical practice, and successful completion of the National Council Licensure Examination–Registered Nurse (NCLEX-RN®). This chapter discusses how and why nursing licensure developed, steps necessary to becoming licensed, licensure regulations, and the responsibilities of an RN.

After licensure as an RN, nurses must still maintain and increase their knowledge and skills. Many nurses may wish to specialize in a particular area of nursing and expand their practice. Nurses with these goals may seek certification in a specialty field. This chapter describes certification, the means to achieve certification, and the organizations that administer certifying examinations. Whether it is licensure or certification, the nursing profession is continually progressing. Legal requirements to practice are continually being revised to ensure the protection of the public. Throughout history and in the current health care environment, nurses face complex issues and new challenges as they seek to increase their competence and ensure the delivery of excellent nursing services to patients. This chapter explores issues related to licensure and certification as well as some of the challenges nurses and students will face are identified.

THE HISTORY OF NURSING LICENSURE
Recognition: Pins and Registries

The aim of caregivers throughout history has been to be recognized and acknowledged for one's skills and achievements. Early caregivers, particularly in the monasteries and convents of the medieval period, were identified by the habits they wore. Frequently special insignias designated health personnel. During the Crusades, a large Maltese cross adorned the habits of the Knights Hospitalers of St. John of Jerusalem on the battlefield (Kalisch and Kalisch, 2003). These forms of identification allowed others to recognize their particular skills in care giving and healing. More recently, nurses around the world wore a readily identifiable symbol of their school of nursing—the nursing cap.

Today, as in the past, the school of nursing pin identifies graduates from a particular school of nursing. Early in each school's history, the students and faculty crafted the pin. The pin's emblems and text symbolize the philosophy, beliefs, and aspirations of the nursing program. Students receive their own pin at graduation in a special pinning ceremony. Nurses wear their pins proudly as evidence of their achievement, learning, and skill. It is one way in which nurses distinguish themselves as distinct health care providers with a specialized body of knowledge and clinical skills.

Nursing programs also maintain a record of all graduates. Florence Nightingale started this practice in 1860 when she created a list of graduates of the St. Thomas's School of Nursing in England. This list became known as the "registry" of graduate nurses. The registry of nurses initiated by Nightingale provided institutions, as well as patients, with a system of identifying graduates of particular nursing programs. These lists proclaimed to all the skills and knowledge of graduates. These nurses could then be distinguished from lay practitioners and local citizens who provided care to the ill and infirm. Today nursing programs around the world continue the tradition started by Nightingale and maintain a registry or listing of all graduates of the nursing program. In addition, state and international agencies maintain lists of nurses practicing in their jurisdictions.

Purpose of Licensure

As nursing programs proliferated, variations developed among the programs. Entry criteria differed, and many educational programs were structured to meet specific employer needs. A simple registry of nurse graduates was no longer sufficient to ensure minimal levels of competency in all nurses, regardless of the school in which the nurses were educated. Another system was necessary to distinguish those sufficiently trained to provide nursing care from untrained or lesser-trained individuals. Graduate nurses, physicians, and hospitals met to resolve this confusion. The outcome was criteria for the licensure of nurses in the United States. Then, as now, the primary purpose of licensure was protection of the public.

Early Licensure Activities

U.S. nursing programs developed in much the same manner as was the pattern in England. As early as 1867, Dr. Henry Wentworth Acland encouraged licensure of English nurses. However, it was not until 1896 that attempts were made to license nurses in the United States. Prior to the late 1800s, many hospitals established training programs to prepare nursing staff for their own institutions. The programs varied based on the needs of the hospital, the availability of physicians and nurses for training students, and resources devoted to the training. It became apparent to many nurses that consistent minimum standards to practice across settings were necessary. These standards would provide for safety of the public and improve the mobility of nurses among institutions. A key advocate for these standards was the Nurses Associated Alumnae of the United States and Canada. This organization later became the American Nurses Association (ANA). However, the group met with resistance from hospitals, physicians, and even nurses. The early attempts at nursing licensure failed for lack of broad-based support (Joel, 2006).

Nurses worldwide mounted an extensive educational campaign explaining the purposes and safeguards inherent in licensure. Success was achieved, for in 1901 the International Council of Nurses passed a resolution that each nation and state examine and license its nurses. Several U.S. states responded shortly thereafter. In 1903 North Carolina, New Jersey, New York, and Virginia were the first to institute permissive licensure. The licensure rules were voluntary. These permissive licenses permitted but did not require nurses to become registered.

Under permissive licensure, educational standards were set at a minimum of 2 years of training for nurses. State boards of nursing were established with rules for examinations as well as revocation of the license. Nurses not passing the examination could not use the title of RN. These early regulations served two purposes: first to protect the public from unskilled practitioners, and second, the rules provided legal sanctions to protect the title of RN. The New York State Board of Regents began a registry of nurses successfully completing all requirements. In 20 years, by 1923, all states had instituted examinations for permissive licensure. Each state's licensure examinations varied in content, length, and format and included written, oral, and practice components. The early work in examinations for licensure was the forerunner of today's licensure and certification requirements (Kalisch and Kalisch, 2003).

The early state efforts in licensing nurses were commendable. Nonetheless, there was considerable variability among states in nursing education requirements, the licensure examinations, and the nurse practice acts themselves. The widespread variability in nurse practice acts prompted the ANA and later (NCSBN) to design model nurse practice acts. The model acts provided a template for states to follow. The first was published in 1915. These model practice acts are revised and updated as nursing practice advances. For example, the NCSBN approved the most recent revision of the model practice act and administrative rules in 2004 (NCSBN, 2009b).

The model nurse practice act is composed of many sections including a definition of nursing and the scope of practice for the RN, descriptions of advanced practice nursing, requirements for prescriptive authority of nurses, nursing education, compact guidelines, and processes for disciplinary actions against nurses who violate sections of the act. Separate sections of the model act provide guidelines for state boards of nursing and the necessary requirements for entry into practice. The most recent model practice act is available online at the NCSBN website (NCSBN, 2009b).

From these model acts, each state or jurisdiction developed a unique practice act. Although individual states and territories' practice acts address the needs of that jurisdiction, each includes the sections described in the model act. Students and practicing nurses may obtain the nurse practice act for any jurisdiction by contacting that state or territorial board of nursing. A listing of state boards of nursing addresses and Internet addresses is provided in Appendix B, which can be found on the Evolve website.

Mandatory Licensure

Once each state had established permissive licensure, the next movement was toward a requirement that all nurses must be licensed. This practice is termed mandatory licensure. New York was the first state to require mandatory licensure, although this requirement was not in place until 1947. At the same time nursing groups moved to standardize nursing licensure testing procedures.

After World War II the ANA formed the NCSBN. The council was composed of a representative of each state and jurisdiction in the United States. As part of its original activities, the council advocated a standardized examination for licensure. These varied activities culminated in the National League for Nursing administering the first State Board Test Pool Examination in 1950. The written examination included separate sections on medical-surgical nursing, maternity nursing, nursing of children, and psychiatric nursing. This format for examination continued for more than 30 years, and many of today's nurses took these examinations.

The next major event in licensure efforts occurred in 1982 with the development of the first NCLEX examination. The test was revised to include all nursing content within one section of the examination. In addition the format was changed to present questions in a nursing process format. Just as with previous versions of licensing examinations, the NCLEX examination has evolved over time. Paper and pencil testing was replaced with computerized adaptive testing in 1994. Extensive information on the NCLEX examination may be found in Chapter 28 of this text.

COMPONENTS OF NURSE PRACTICE ACTS

Each state develops rules and regulations to govern the practice of nursing within that state. These rules are in the nurse practice acts or in its accompanying rules and regulations to administer the act. Many nurse practice acts are patterned after the ANA or the NCSBN, Inc. model practice acts, and all contain comparable information.

Purpose of Act

Each act begins with a purpose. All nurse practice acts include two essential purposes. First, each includes statements that refer to protecting the health and safety of the citizens in the jurisdiction. The act describes the qualifications and responsibilities of those individuals covered by the regulations. Likewise the act delineates those excluded from the practice of nursing. These provisions also serve to ensure protection of the public. The second purpose is to protect the title of RN. The legal title, RN, is reserved for those meeting the requirements to practice nursing. Only those licensed may use the designation of RN. Thus unlicensed personnel are prevented from using the title RN.

Definition of Nursing and Scope of Practice

In each state or jurisdictional nurse practice act the practice of professional nursing is defined. The definition of nursing is of utmost importance because it delineates the scope of practice for nurses within the state. That is, each act outlines the activities nurses may legally perform within the jurisdiction. Many states follow the guidelines incorporated in the model practice act, although each is specific and delineates practice within that state or jurisdiction. For example, some states describe nursing as a process that includes nursing diagnosis, whereas other states list broad areas of nursing activities. To avoid becoming outdated, there are no lists of skills or procedures in the acts. As nursing knowledge and practices advance, new techniques are frequently allowable because of the comprehensive nature of the definition of nursing.

Many jurisdictions incorporate definitions of advanced practice nursing within one definition of nursing. In other states the definitions of advanced practice nursing and the scope of practice for advanced practice nurses are defined separately.

Each state or jurisdiction establishes laws regulating practice within its borders. Therefore it is imperative for the nurse to know and understand the definition of nursing in the states in which he or she practices. Further, each jurisdiction retains the right to govern practice within that jurisdiction. This right supersedes the presence of a mutual recognition agreement with other compact states. The retention of states' rights is an essential component in the mutual recognition model.

There are other important reasons for becoming familiar with the definition of nursing practice. Frequently, nurses are asked to perform in ways that are beyond the legal definition of nursing. This is illegal, and if the nurse complies, he or she could lose the privilege of practicing nursing. In other situations, labor laws or other statutes affect nurses. Definitions may include or exclude nurses based on their legal definitions of nursing practice. As nursing practice becomes more complex and sophisticated, states may revise their nurse practice acts. Nurses are accountable for knowing the definition and scope of practice within their jurisdictions and practicing accordingly. In order to know and understand the laws regulating their practice, nurses should obtain copies of and become familiar with nurse practice acts for the states or jurisdictions in which they plan to practice.

Licensure Requirements

A section of each nurse practice act describes the requirements and procedures necessary for initial entry into nursing practice, or nursing licensure. An initial requirement in all jurisdictions is graduation from high school and an accredited nursing program. Candidates for licensure must submit evidence of graduation as defined by each state.

To verify an applicant's graduation from a nursing program, frequently a transcript of coursework, a diploma, or a letter from the dean of the program is necessary. Additional requirements for licensure may include a statement regarding the mental and physical health status of the applicant. Some jurisdictions conduct a review of prior legal convictions. This is especially important in reference to felony convictions. Other states have appended provisions related to recreational drug abuse. Finally, most states require statements from the school of nursing attesting the eligibility of the candidate for licensure. The requirements for licensure are detailed in each nurse practice act and the accompanying rules and regulations for practice.

In the past it was customary for nurses to practice in only one state or territory. More than ever, nurses are practicing in more than one jurisdiction, either by their physical presence in that jurisdiction or through technological advances including telephone and computer access to patients across state and territory lines. As laws are continually being revised to reflect the current practice of nursing, it is incumbent on the individual to be cognizant of the current licensure requirements in all states and territories in which he or she intends to practice.

Regardless of individual state requirements, all nurse practice acts require candidates to successfully complete the NCLEX-RN licensure examination before they can practice. In some states it is possible to obtain a temporary permit to practice, pending receipt of success on the licensure examination. This practice was especially prevalent in past years because it took several months for results of the licensure examinations to be reported. Now, however, with computer testing and the prompt response from the testing services, the use of temporary permits to practice is becoming less frequent.

Temporary permits are still available for nurses moving from one jurisdiction to another. To obtain a license to practice in another state, the nurse applies for licensure by endorsement. Nurses licensed in one jurisdiction may apply for licensure in a second jurisdiction by submitting a letter to the second state board of nursing. Typically evidence for the new license is similar to that for initial licensure. In addition, proof of the nurse's current license to practice, as well as any restrictions imposed on the license by the first state, is required. These procedures will continue for all states not participating in the Nurse Licensure Compact (NLC). For those states designated as "compact states," the nurse should contact the state board of nursing to determine the appropriate procedures for initiating nursing practice in that jurisdiction.

Renewal of Licensure

In addition to outlining requirements for initial licensure, each nurse practice act includes the requirements and information necessary to renew one's nursing license. These regulations define the length of time a license is valid, generally from 2 to 3 years, as well as any specific requirements for renewal of licensure.

Mandatory Continuing Education

The nurse will find information on mandatory continuing education requirements for renewal of licensure in the section on license renewal. All nurses are expected to remain competent to practice through various means of continuing education. In 1976 California was the first state to institute mandatory continuing education for renewal of licensure. Since that time a number of states have instituted requirements of continuing education for renewal of licensure. The number of hours necessary varies, depending on the jurisdiction, ranging from 20 to 40 hours over a 2- to 3-year period.

A few jurisdictions require specific continuing education coursework in the areas of health care ethics, the state nurse practice act, or other content specific to that jurisdiction. Clinical course content may be designated for specific health problems such as sexually transmitted infections, human immunodeficiency virus–acquired immunodeficiency syndrome, and family violence. In other states the board of nursing allows the nurse wide latitude in meeting the requirements for renewal of licensure. Details of specific continuing education requirements are found in the nurse practice act and the accompanying rules and regulations.

ROLE OF REGULATORY BOARDS TO ENSURE SAFE PRACTICE
Membership of the Board of Nursing

An important section of every nurse practice act is the designation of a regulatory board of nurses and consumers to administer the act. Frequently this responsibility is assigned to a state board of nursing. The practice act outlines guidelines for membership on the board. In addition, procedures by which members are appointed to the board of nursing are designated. In most cases, the members are appointed by the governor's office. Interested individuals or organizations, such as the state nurses' association, may submit names to the governor for consideration.

Duties of the Board of Nursing

The responsibilities and duties of the board of nursing are delineated in detail. Specific duties of the board may be outlined in the act itself or in the enabling laws. These enabling administrative statutes are frequently designated as rules and regulations for the practice of nursing. It is through the work of the board of nursing that nursing licenses are granted and renewed and disciplinary action taken when provisions of the act are violated. Just as all nurses need to be cognizant of their nurse practice acts, nurses should also become familiar with the role of the state board of nursing.

A major responsibility of the board of nursing is addressing concerns about a nurse's practice. The review of a nurse's potential malfeasance, violation of the act, or other state and federal laws are within the responsibilities of the board of nursing. The nurse practice act describes the due process and procedures for this review. The board of nursing will then assign appropriate disciplinary action. These activities are a key responsibility of the board of nursing. Actions may include restrictions on the license or suspension or revocation of a nurse's license. Just as all nurses need to be cognizant of their nurse practice acts, nurses should become familiar with the role of the state board of nursing.

SPECIAL CASES OF LICENSURE
Military and Government Nurses

There are many nurses whose practice takes them throughout the country on a regular basis. For example, many nurses are members of the military or join the military nursing services after graduation. The Veterans Administration or U.S. Public Health Service employs thousands of nurses, who serve in many jurisdictions as well as outside the U.S. boundaries. It is not necessary for these nursing personnel to obtain a nursing license in each jurisdiction in which they practice. The graduate takes the NCLEX-RN examination in one state. On successful completion, as an employee of the U.S. government, he or she may practice in other jurisdictions without additional licensure requirements. Nurses should obtain the current requirements for licensure as rules are updated to reflect current practices.

Foreign Nurse Graduates

More than 400,000 nurses practicing in the U.S. completed their nursing education in another country. The nurses met the requirements for practice in those countries. When nurses move to the United States, they must show evidence of completing their original educational program and restrictions of their license. In addition, nurses need to demonstrate competency in English and the ability to take and pass the NCLEX-RN examination. Foreign nurses take a special examination administered by the Commission on Graduates of Foreign Nursing

Schools. The examination is given in English and tests the knowledge required to practice in this country. On successful completion the foreign nurse graduate may apply for a license to practice in this country. The intent of these regulations is not to be punitive or obstructive to the nurse. The regulations are yet another example of two key principles: first, the protection of the public and, second, the protection of the title of RN.

International Practice

In a similar manner, nurses licensed in the U.S. may want to practice in other countries. Nurses interested in these opportunities may contact either the International Council of Nurses or the nursing regulatory board of the country in which they wish to practice. The International Council of Nurses is composed of representatives of organized nursing worldwide. One function of the council is to assist nurses in obtaining licensure in other countries.

Each country has specific laws and regulations governing nursing practice that must guide the practice of the U.S. nurse. Just as a foreign nurse must demonstrate competency to practice in the United States, the U.S. nurse should be prepared to submit documentation on education, NCLEX-RN examination results, and proof of licensure and practice to officials in the foreign country. Advanced planning and contact with the appropriate regulatory agency will ease the transition for the nurse.

REVISION OF NURSE PRACTICE ACTS

Nurse practice acts, just as other sections of states' codes, are written and passed by legislators. As in any legislative endeavor, many governmental agencies, administrators, consumers, and special-interest groups seek to influence the legislation. These groups become actively involved in developing the accompanying rules and regulations. For example, physicians, dentists, pharmacists, licensed practical nurses, certified nursing assistants, emergency personnel, and physician assistants are just a few health care providers directly affected by the scope and definition of nursing practice. Likewise, organizations such as schools, hospitals, home health agencies, and extended care facilities are vitally concerned with the role of nurses today. Equally important, citizen groups are interested in determining nurses' roles and responsibilities. Because of these multiple-interest groups, the nurse practice act as finally passed or amended by the state legislature represents the aims and concerns of many individuals and groups, not only nurses.

Review of a state's practice act reveals the influential parties involved in creating the act. Each group participates in defining the scope and practice of nursing and regulations affecting nursing practice within the jurisdiction. Because of these varied interests, it is essential for nurses to understand the practice act and the additional legislation that influences and controls their practice. Further, as proposals to amend the nurse practice act are promulgated at the state level, it is imperative for all nurses to be involved in this process. The resulting laws affect their profession, their practice, and their livelihood.

Sunset Legislation

One example of legislative activity affecting nurse practice acts is sunset legislation. "Sunset laws," found in many states, are intended to ensure that legislation is current and reflects the needs of the public. When sunset provisions are included in a nurse practice act, the act must be reviewed by a specific date. If the act is not renewed, it is automatically rescinded. This review process allows for revisions to update practice acts to be consistent with current nursing practice. Many nurse practice acts contain sunset provisions. It is through these activities that the scope of nursing practice is updated and components such as the diagnosis of nursing problems have been incorporated into definitions of nursing. Other changes include changes in requirements for mandatory continuing education for licensure renewal. Equally important, sunset laws have provided the means to define advanced practice nursing and incorporate prescriptive authority for advanced practice nurses. Nurses should determine whether sunset regulations affect the nursing practice act in the state in which they practice. Likewise, nurses should be aware of, and involved in, activities to amend the nurse practice act.

DELEGATION OF AUTHORITY TO OTHERS

The rapid expansion of an array of health care providers, changes in health care delivery systems, and efforts to control health care costs have led to participation of many types of unlicensed personnel in the provision of health care. These personnel present a challenge to RNs working with them. Questions arise as to who can delegate what activities to which unlicensed provider groups. Guidelines for delegation have been developed by many nursing organizations, including the ANA and NCSBN (2009b). Although the professional organizations' guidelines are helpful, it is the nurse practice acts of individual states that establish the legal definitions of appropriate delegation practices. Because regulations differ among states, each nurse must identify and understand the regulations for the state in which he or she practices. Chapter 19 presents a detailed discussion of delegation and supervision.

CURRENT LICENSURE ACTIVITIES
Mutual Recognition Model

Efforts to provide common definitions of nursing practice, equivalent educational standards for practice, and uniform testing for entry into practice through the NCLEX examination have been very successful. Nonetheless, most nurses are still required to apply for licensure in each state in which they practice. With the increased mobility of nurses, the telehealth movement, and the necessity of caring for patients across long distances, state boards of nursing have recognized the need to provide practicing nurses with more than procedures of endorsement of their initial license. This need has led to further changes in nursing licensure.

In 1997 the Delegate Assembly of the NCSBN moved to a new level of nursing regulation. The assembly approved a resolution endorsing a mutual recognition model of nursing regulation. Through this model individual state boards formed the NLC. The first states to participate in the program were Maryland, Texas, Utah, and Wisconsin. Each year more states are developing compact laws—to date, almost half are NLC states. A listing of current compact states may be found on the website of the NCSBN (2009c). Nurses practicing in an NLC state are responsible for following the laws and regulations of each state in which they practice, although they are not required to apply for multiple individual state licenses.

A number of issues associated with mutual recognition concern nurses. On one hand, mutual recognition greatly facilitates interstate practice, telehealth programs, and movement of nurses to areas of shortage. In addition, a national database provides information on individual nurses' practice and disciplinary actions taken against nurses. The database, Nursys (NCSBN, 2009c), supports a key licensure goal—to protect the public health and safety. These advantages have resulted in support for the NLC by many nursing organizations.

On the other hand, concerns relate to monitoring nurses' practice in multiple jurisdictions, nurse privacy, and due process rights. Issues related to disciplinary action in home and distant states are still being resolved. In addition, differences in practice requirements in different states may cause nurses confusion as to their rights and responsibilities. The NLC is increasingly affecting all nurses. Nursing students and graduates must remain apprised of changing conditions. As changes occur frequently in this area, the most comprehensive and current sources of information are the websites for the ANA, the NCSBN, and the state boards of nursing for individual jurisdictions.

Continued Competency

As discussed earlier, the primary purpose of nurse licensure is protection of the public. Thus mandatory continuing education was instituted as a strategy to ensure that nurses were competent to remain in practice. These programs have continued for a number of years. However, a growing number of nurses believe that more is required than just attending seminars to demonstrate the degree of competence. Consortiums of nurses in a number of states are examining other alternatives for renewal of licensure. These requirements may include designated numbers of clinical practice hours, portfolios of achievements in clinical practice or other exemplars of practice. Nurses and students are encouraged to become aware of continued competency initiatives so that they may be prepared for changes in future licensure requirements.

There is increasing concern for patient safety and treatment in today's health care system. Models of continued competency are but one attempt by professional nurses to ensure that patients receive safe, effective nursing care. Another strategy in this quest is establishing programs of certification of advanced practice nurses.

CERTIFICATION
History of Certification

There are distinct differences between licensure and certification. At the most basic level, licensure establishes minimal levels of practice, whereas certification recognizes excellence in practice. Because of this difference, the background, requirements, and practice opportunities for licensure and certification differ markedly.

Just as with the development of nursing licensure, at its inception certification was not legally required; rather, it was voluntary. In an effort to recognize nurses who had completed additional education and demonstrated competency in clinical practice, a number of nursing graduate schools and nursing specialty organizations offered certification programs. In the 1970s and later, advanced clinical courses were designed for nurses as a certificate program. The programs varied in length and content and did not offer a full master's course of study in nursing.

A second distinct difference in licensure and certification pertains to the organizations that grant certification. Whereas licensure is granted and governed by legislation and administered through the state boards of nursing, certification is awarded by nongovernmental agencies. The first field of nursing practice to certify advanced practitioners was nurse anesthesia in 1946. Similarly in 1961 the American College of Nurse-Midwives began certifying nurse-midwives. As certificate programs developed, it became apparent that program standardization was a necessity. In 1975 the ANA convened a national study group at the University of Wisconsin–Milwaukee to explore the issue. This meeting was attended by 75 nursing specialty organizations. The report of the group recommended the formation of a central organization for certification of nurses. This report, in conjunction with efforts of many nurses, resulted in the formation of the American Nurses Credentialing Center (ANCC). At present the ANCC (2009) has certified more than 200,000 nurses in more than 40 areas of specialty practice (Box 4-1). Today, many of their examinations are open to nurses with a variety of educational backgrounds.

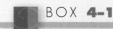

BOX **4-1**

American Nurses Credentialing Center, Certifying Examinations 2009

ADVANCED PRACTICE CERTIFICATION
Acute care nurse practitioner
Adult nurse practitioner
Adult psychiatric and mental health practitioner
Advanced diabetes management practitioner
Comprehensive care (for doctor of nursing
    practice [DNP] grads)
Family nurse practitioner
Family psychiatric and mental health practitioner
Gerontologic nurse practitioner
Neonatal nurse practitioner
Pediatric nurse practitioner
Clinical nurse specialists
    Advanced diabetes management
    Adult psychiatric and mental health
    Child and adolescent psychiatric and mental
        health
    Gerontologic nursing
    Pediatric nursing
    Public and community health

OTHER NURSING CERTIFICATION
Clinical nurse leader
Advanced nursing administration
Advanced practice palliative nurse

BACCALAUREATE-LEVEL OR HIGHER CERTIFICATION
Cardiac or vascular nurse
Gerontologic nurse
Informatics nurse
Medical-surgical nurse
Nursing administration
Nursing professional development
Pediatric nurse
Perinatal nurse
Psychiatric and mental health nurse
Public and community health

ASSOCIATE DEGREE OR DIPLOMA LEVEL CERTIFICATION
Cardiac or vascular nurse
Gerontologic nurse
Medical-surgical nurse
Pediatric nurse
Perinatal nurse
Psychiatric and mental health nurse

DIPLOMA, ASSOCIATE, BACCALAUREATE, OR HIGHER DEGREE IN NURSING
Ambulatory care nurse
Nursing case management

In addition to the ANCC, other professional specialty nursing organizations offer certification examinations. These organizations have created certification boards that are separate from the parent organization to maintain an independent role and to conform to department of education requirements. Nurses may contact these specialty nursing organizations directly for current guidelines and information. The lengths to which organized nursing has invested in certification of advanced practice in nursing are further indications of nurses' commitment to protection of the public and the patients they serve.

One of the newest certifications is available for the doctor of nursing practice (DNP) graduate through the American Board of Comprehensive Care. This certification will assure patients and the public that a nurse has achieved a standardized and advanced level of clinical competency. (The certification indicates advancement beyond the master's level certification, retrieved from www.abcc.dnpcert.org/faq.shtml on September 1, 2009.)

Certification began as a voluntary effort controlled by professional nursing organizations. State agencies were not involved in the credentialing process. This is still the case, although state nurse practice acts do include requirements for nurses to practice in advanced roles. Thus state practice acts first contained provisions requiring certification for nurse anesthetists and nurse-midwives. With the development of additional advanced practice roles, all states have included requirements of certification in their regulations for advanced practice nurses in all specialty roles.

Purpose of Certification

The purpose of advanced practice laws is first and foremost protection of the public. Within the acts are definitions of advanced practice nursing. A number of states further differentiate the advanced practice of nursing by including separate titles for nurse practitioners and clinical nurse specialists. The scope of practice of the advanced practice nurse is well defined. States describe supervisory or collaborative practice with physicians, with differences existing among states as to the regulations governing these relationships. Requirements for practice vary among states. Although many states require a master's degree in the specialty area for practice, this is not the case in all jurisdictions. All states require evidence of certification in the specialty area, and many require periods of practice in the specialty prior to awarding certification status. All states incorporate specific provisions for prescribing medications.

Steps to Certification

The best strategy for nurses wishing to practice in an expanded role is to become informed of specific requirements in their chosen field. The nurse should examine carefully the roles and responsibilities inherent in advanced practice nursing. First the nurse should contact both the ANCC and the specialty organization in his or her area of practice to determine the education, experience, and examination requirements necessary to become certified. Concurrently, every nurse should contact the state boards of nursing in the state(s) in which he or she wishes to practice and obtain information on legal requirements to practice in those jurisdictions. After gathering the requirements to practice, the nurse will be able to develop a plan of action to complete the necessary advanced coursework, clinical practice requirements, and examinations. On completion of the requirements of these agencies, the advanced practice nurse may practice in an expanded role. In addition to the certifying agencies, the nurse may wish to contact other advanced practice nurses. These nurses will serve as valuable colleagues to the new advanced practice nurse.

Current Issues in Certification

Despite tremendous strides in less than 40 years, certification processes for the advanced practice nurse continue to evolve. As with any new endeavor, advances are made in small steps and great leaps.

Nurses in advanced practice face changing educational requirements for licensure and relicensure. As the health care environment changes, so must the professional and legal issues of scope of practice and the independence of advanced nursing practice. Advanced practice nurses develop professional relationships with their physician colleagues as do all nurses. But the advanced practice nurses must define their legal relationships with physician practitioners and other caregivers as well. These issues are not uncommon to nurses in any practice setting; however, the advanced practice nurse is charting new territory.

A unique challenge of advanced practice nurses is reimbursement for nursing services. As advanced practice continues to expand, nurses have moved from secondary to independent billing for services. Federal regulations allow direct reimbursement for some nursing services, yet state and local practices vary. There are ongoing efforts at the state and national levels to resolve these issues. Advanced practice nurses are in constant communication with their peers and professional organizations. They look to all nurses to become involved in issues facing the advanced practice nurse.

A new issue in advanced nursing practice is emerging. Just as with the historical questions of which group will test and license nurses, the question is surfacing as to which organizations will credential and regulate advanced practice nursing. The NCSBN proposes that it is the appropriate agency to credential as well as license advanced practitioners in their vision for the future (2009a). Nursing professional and specialty organizations are currently responding to their draft proposal. It is incumbent for all nurses and potential nurses to become knowledge-able on this issue and participate in the professional discussions. This issue clearly illustrates the changing practice and regulation of nursing.

BOX **4-2**

Helpful Websites

American Association of Colleges of Nursing (AACN)
   www.aacn.nche.edu
American Nurses Association (ANA)
   www.nursingworld.org
American Nurses Credentialing Center (ANCC)
   www.nursingworld.org/ancc
Commission on Graduates of Foreign Nursing Schools
   www.cgfns.org
International Council of Nurses (ICN)
   www.icn.ch
National Council of State Boards of Nursing
   www.ncsbn.org
National League for Nursing (NLN)
   www.nln.org
Sigma Theta Tau International Honor Society in Nursing
   www.nursingsociety.org

SUMMARY

Nurse practice acts provide protection of the public and protection of the title of RN. This is accomplished through the development of specific regulations regarding education and examination of competence to practice. Each act contains guidelines for disciplinary action to protect both the public and professional nursing. The nurse practice act of each jurisdiction addresses the needs of the state and the responsibilities of nurses practicing within that state. It is important for all nurses and students of nursing to become familiar with the regulations guiding their own practice. Box 4-2 contains Internet addresses for nursing organizations with which RNs should become familiar.

As health care delivery evolves and nursing practice advances, new issues and initiatives arise. It is imperative to update the nurse practice act so that it remains responsive to the needs of all. Nurses must be part of this process. Collaboration with professional nursing organizations, the state boards of nursing, and individual nurses will enable nursing to continually meet the needs of patients.

evolve   Additional resources are available online at: http://evolve.elsevier.com/Cherry/

REFERENCES

American Board of Comprehensive Care: *DNP certification*. Retrieved September 1, 2009, from: www.abcc.dnpcert.org/faq.shtml.

American Nurses Credentialing Center: *Certifications available*. Retrieved May 1, 2009, from: http://www.nursecredentialing.org.

Joel LA: *The nursing experience: trends, challenges, and transitions*, ed 5, New York, 2006, McGraw-Hill.

Kalisch BJ, Kalisch PA: *The advance of American nursing*, ed 4, Philadelphia, 2003, Lippincott.

The National Council of State Boards of Nursing, Inc.: *Advanced practice registered nurses*. Retrieved May 2, 2009, from: www.ncsbn.org/170.htm, 2009a.

The National Council of State Boards of Nursing, Inc.: *Model nursing act and rules*. Retrieved May 1, 2009, from: www.ncsbn.org/1455.htm, 2009b.

The National Council of State Boards of Nursing, Inc.: *Nurse Licensure Compact*. Retrieved May 1, 2009, from: www.ncsbn.org/nlc.htm, 2009c.

Theories of Nursing Practice

Susan R. Jacob, PhD, MSN, RN

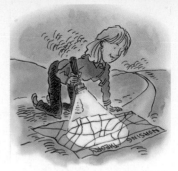

Nursing theory provides the direction for nursing practice and research.

evolve Additional resources are available online at: http://evolve.elsevier.com/Cherry/

"Science is built up with facts, as a house is with stones. But a collection of facts is no more a science than a heap of stones a house...."

JULES HENRI POINCARÉ, 1909, FRENCH SCIENTIST
AND MATHEMATICIAN

VIGNETTE

When I was a nursing student it was hard for me to understand why I needed to know anything about nursing theory, but now that I am in practice I see that theories provide a way for me to organize, deliver, and evaluate the care I provide. On our labor and delivery unit we use Roy's adaptation model to guide our practice as we provide care to laboring moms. The use of this theory allows us to assess how well they are coping and provides guidance as we plan nursing interventions that promote their successful coping.

■ QUESTIONS TO CONSIDER WHILE READING THIS CHAPTER:

1 What is nursing theory?

2 How is nursing theory different from the theory of other disciplines?

3 How does theory relate to nursing practice?

4 Why is it important to understand nursing theory?

5 Why is it important for nurses to develop theory?

KEY TERMS

Concept An idea or a general impression. Concepts are the basic ingredients of theory. Examples of nursing concepts include pain, quality of life, health, stress, and adaptation.

Conceptual model A group of concepts that are associated because of their relevance to a common theme.

Nursing science The collection and organization of data related to nursing and its associated components. The purpose of this data collection is to provide a body of scientific knowledge, which provides the basis for nursing practice.

Nursing theory The compilation of data that defines, describes, and logically relates information that will explain past nursing phenomena and predict future trends. Theories provide a foundation for developing models or frameworks for nursing practice development.

Proposition Statement that proposes the relationship between and among concepts.

Schematic model A diagram or visual representation of concepts, conceptual models, or theory.

We thank Margaret Soderstrom, PhD, RN, CS-P, APRN, and Linda C. Pugh, PhD, RNC, FAAN, for their contributions to this chapter in the 4th edition.

After studying this chapter, the reader will be able to:

1 Differentiate between a science and a theory.

2 Identify the criteria necessary for science.

3 Identify the criteria necessary for theory.

4 Explain a nursing theory and a nursing model.

5 Discuss two early and two contemporary nursing theorists and their theories.

6 Explain the effect of nursing theory on the profession of nursing.

CHAPTER OVERVIEW

Explicit, detailed knowledge is the keystone, the foundation, and the carefully laid support that are critical to the classification of a discipline. In a seminal paper The Discipline of Nursing *(1978), Donaldson and Crowley note, a discipline "is characterized by a unique perspective, a distinct way of viewing all phenomena, which ultimately defines the limits and nature of its inquiry" (p. 113). Nursing, long ranked an art and a science, is actually quite young in its continuing struggle for professional and public recognition as a matchless, expert, and commanding profession. This notion is readily supported as one marks nursing's ongoing effort to define itself as a distinct discipline that is exclusive from other disciplines, particularly the medical practice model. Only when a substantial body of nursing knowledge is collected, organized, and developed will the profession be defined and its scope of practice differentiated. Key in this accomplishment is the development and practice of nursing theory.*

It is important for nurses to study the development of nursing theory because without an idea of where you have been, how can you know how, why, when, or where to go? Nursing theory provides nurses with a focus for research and practice. You may consider using a theory as similar to using a map that provides direction while making available a variety of ways to get where you are going. As logical as this seems, the worth of studying nursing theorists and their theories and the role of responsibility these theories contribute toward the evolution of nursing science has been curiously underappreciated. Even more surprising, many of the naysayers are nursing students. Nursing theory is not usually the favorite subject of undergraduates, who would much rather learn technical hands-on skills. Whether this is a maturation issue or an issue of knowledge and experience remains undetermined by nursing faculty and the profession itself.

This chapter in no way reflects the breadth and depth of nursing theorists and their theories. There are many scholarly works devoted to this topic. Instead it is a survey, a general overview, a smattering of nursing theories, with chosen segments intended to assist in providing the idea, the notion, and indeed, the semblance of what a theory is and how it is critical to the profession of nursing. Readers interested in examining the theoretic basis for nursing practice will find resources for further exploration at the end of the chapter.

SCIENCE AND THEORY

Science is a method of bringing together facts and giving them coherence and integrity. Science assists us in understanding how the unique yet related parts of a structure fit and become more than the sum of individual parts. In the opening metaphor, the stones represent the facts,

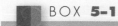

BOX **5-1**

The Five Steps of the Scientific Process

Hypothesis: Ask the question that is to be the main focus. It usually includes independent and dependent variables.

Method: Decide what data will be collected to answer the question. Decide on and identify the step-by-step procedure that will be used to collect these data. Make sure this process can be easily replicated.

Data collection: Implement the step-by-step procedure that has been determined to answer the question.

Results: On the conclusion of the data collection, statistically identify the outcomes. Establish parameters (e.g., level of significance) that will determine whether the data are relevant.

Evaluation: Examine the results to determine the relevance of outcome data in answering the hypothesis. Determine the significance and identify the potential for future research.

the process of laying the stones represents the science, and the future ideas and new directions represent the theory.

Science is dynamic and static—dynamic in figuring out how a phenomenon happens, static in describing what happens. Scientific inquiry involves five steps: (1) hypothesis, (2) method, (3) data collection, (4) results, and (5) evaluation. These five steps are described in Box 5-1.

A theory is defined as a group of related concepts that describe existing phenomena and predict outcomes (Polit and Beck, 2008). Theory development functions in a parallel manner to scientific process, although theory generally applies to a more specific area of the larger scientific process. Even though Freud and Jung each had their individual theories about the psychology of man, their theories were focused on specific ideas taken from the entire knowledge base surrounding psychology and psychotherapy and its scientific premise. Similarly, Albert Einstein's theory of relativity was but a fraction of the existing scientific knowledge base of mathematics at the time. Nevertheless, it is an undisputed fact that these theorists changed the thinking of their time and were responsible for the evolution of their philosophic and scientific interests (Anastasi, 1958). For a proposed theory to be accepted as a theory, it must meet the following six criteria: inclusiveness, consistency, accuracy, relevance, fruitfulness, and simplicity. These six criteria are further explained in Box 5-2.

The importance of theories in the evolution of science is unquestioned. Nursing has evolved as a profession and as a science in a similar manner. Nursing theories have explained, explored, defined, and delineated specific areas. Beginning with the work of Florence Nightingale in 1860, nursing theorists have taken the vast pool of scientific information available and focused on precise target areas of interest. In so doing, theoretic models have been conceptualized to guide nursing actions, interventions, and implementation. Specific nursing theories are discussed later in the chapter.

Nursing Science

As might be expected, there are several definitions of nursing science (Abdellah, 1969; Jacox, 1974). Although these definitions differ, they generally support the premise that nursing science is a collection of data related to nursing that may be applied to the practice of nursing. These data encompass a vast array of knowledge that spans all of nursing and its diversity. This knowledge guides the practice of nursing to better serve patients through healing, prevention, education, and health maintenance.

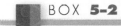
BOX **5-2**

Criteria for Theory Acceptance

Inclusiveness: Does the theory include all concepts related to the area of interest?
Consistency: Can the theory address new entities without having its founding assumptions changed?
Accuracy: Does the theory explain retrospective occurrences? Does the theory maintain its capacity to predict future outcomes?
Relevance: Does the theory relate to the scientific foundation from which it is derived? Is it reflective of the scientific base?
Fruitfulness: Does the theory generate new directions for future research?
Simplicity: Does the theory provide a road map for replication? Is it simple to follow? Does it make sense?

Theories, Models, and Frameworks

Researchers use theories and conceptual models as their primary method to organize findings into a broader conceptual context (Polit and Beck, 2008). Different terms are used in relation to conceptual contexts for research. These terms include theories, models, frameworks, schemes, and maps. Terms are often used differently by different writers, thus resulting in a blurring of distinct terms (Polit and Beck, 2008).

Theory. Theory is generally considered an abstract generalization that presents a systematic explanation about how phenomena are interrelated. Therefore traditionally a theory must have at least two concepts that are related in a way that the theory explains (Polit and Beck, 2008).

Conceptual Model. A conceptual model deals with concepts that are assembled because of their relevance to a common theme. The term conceptual framework is used interchangeably with conceptual model. Conceptual models, or frameworks, also provide a conceptual perspective regarding interrelated phenomena, but they are more loosely structured than theories. There are many conceptual models of nursing that offer broad explanations of the nursing process. Four concepts basic to nursing that are included in these models are: (1) nursing, (2) person, (3) health, and (4) environment. The various nursing models define these concepts differently, link the concepts in various ways, and emphasize differently the relationships among the concepts. For example, Roy's adaptation model emphasizes the patient's adaptation as a central phenomenon, whereas Martha Rogers emphasizes centrality of the individual as a unified whole. These models are used by nurse researchers to formulate research questions and hypotheses.

The terms *conceptual model* (or framework) and *nursing theory* are often used interchangeably. In this chapter, the nursing theories described may also be referred to as conceptual models. The term *model* is also used in reference to a diagram depicting the theory. In this chapter *model* will refer to a schematic model, which is a diagram or visual representation of the conceptual model or theory.

Nursing Theory

Theory and theoretic thinking guide research and practice. The basic ingredients of theory are concepts. Examples of nursing concepts include health, stress, and adaptation. Propositions are statements that propose the relationship between and among concepts (Polit and Beck, 2008).

TABLE **5-1**

The Language of Nursing Theory

TERM	DEFINITION	EXAMPLES
Concept	Labels given to ideas, objects, events; a summary of thoughts or a way to categorize thoughts or ideas	Comfort, fatigue, pain, depression, environment
Conceptual model	A structure to organize concepts (ideas)	Roy's adaptation model
Philosophy	Values and beliefs of the discipline	Watson's philosophy and science of caring
Theory	The organization of concepts or constructs that shows the relationship of the ideas with the intention of describing, explaining, or predicting; the purpose is to make scientific findings meaningful and generalizable; our goal in science has been to explain, predict, and control.	Self-care, adaptation, caring, behavioral system, unitary man, hierarchy of needs, interpersonal relationship, humanistic, nurse-client transactions

Theories provide us with a frame of reference, the ability to choose concepts to study, or ideas that are within one's practice. A theory helps guide research, and research helps validate theory.

In the research model, the researcher decides what to study and how and why the area of interest is important to the practice of nursing. In the practice model, the clinician decides what areas to directly assess, when to assess, and which intervention to implement. These decisions may or may not be knowingly based on a model or theory. Regardless, often the outcome supports the notion that behavior replicates a theoretic model, even though the nurse may be unaware that he or she is using a theoretic model in the practice process.

Just as in any other discipline, nursing theory has its own unique language. The words of this language identify linkages between the database of scientific nursing knowledge and the extracted information taken from this source for nursing theory. The interpretation of these words translates uniquely to the theory investigated. This application, or language of nursing theory, is the structure, or framework, from which one understands the theory. Table 5-1 presents the language of nursing theory, along with definitions and examples.

Schematic Models

A schematic model is something that demonstrates concepts, usually with a picture. It is a visual representation of ideas. The model depicts concepts and shows how the concepts are related with the use of images, such as arrows and dotted lines (Polit and Beck, 2008). For example, a blueprint is a pictorial demonstration of a particular type of house someone might build. A model airplane is a detailed miniature replication of the original full-sized version. Diagramming a sentence outlines the specific parts (adverb, adjective, verb, subject, object, phrases) that make that particular sentence complete. Similarly a nursing model gives a visual diagram or picture of concepts. Whether that is a critical pathway, decision tree, medication protocol, or other nursing-related practice, the model allows one to view the interrelated parts of the whole in picture form. A model of a nursing theory does the same thing. From the earliest model, offered by Florence Nightingale, nursing theory has been described and explained using this medium. Schematic models are used for clarifying complex concepts. The language of theory is translated into picture form, offering a comprehensive view, or model, of the theory. The schematic model shows how the concepts are related. A model, like a blueprint of a building, allows one to see the layout, including outlines of all features specific to the theory. Although it is not the same as understanding every minute detail about the structure, its intent is to provide an overview, which at a glance is informative and descriptive.

Levels of Theory

Many persons refer to the level of a nursing theory, which can range from broad in scope to a smaller, more specific scope. For example, grand theory is often broad in scope and may describe and explain large segments of human experience. Rogers's theory of unitary man describes the entire nursing process. Other levels include middle-range theory and practice theory, which are smaller in scope and may refer to a specific population, such as Jacob's grief of older women (Jacob, 1996) or to a specific situation, such as Sousa and Zauszniewski's (2005) theory of diabetic self-care management, or Tsai and colleagues' (2003) theory of chronic pain. Another example of a middle-range theory is the theory of unpleasant symptoms (Lenz and Pugh, 2003), which examines symptoms that are influenced by physiologic, psychologic, and situational factors as they relate to performance. The model of this theory is presented in Figure 5-1. Nurses often use these middle-range theories that are smaller in scope and simpler to understand to guide their daily practice.

To better illustrate the application of theory to nursing practice, Box 5-3 presents a case example of middle-range theory application using Mishel's (1997) uncertainty in illness theory. In examining nursing theories, students may be surprised to discover that they are already using some of the contained concepts in their individual practices. Nursing theories assist with further defining and organizing these concepts into an underpinning that explains, details, and claims nursing practice as a unique discipline.

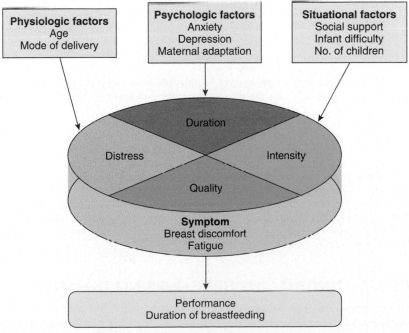

Figure 5-1 *Theory of unpleasant symptoms.*

BOX **5-3**

Case Example: Application of Theory to Practice

MISHEL'S UNCERTAINTY IN ILLNESS THEORY
Case Presentation
A 9-year-old female, Christine, is admitted to the pediatric unit for evaluation of a new onset of abdominal pain. The admission diagnosis is intermittent abdominal pain, rule out appendicitis. It is her first time as a patient in a hospital. Her father, who is a surgeon, and her mother, who is a nurse, accompany Christine to the unit. Her mother will stay with her. After talking with the parents, you the nurse are confident that Christine is well informed, well cared for, and well prepared for her admission. While her parents are speaking with Christine's attending physician in a nearby office, you talk with Christine, who goes from smiling and chatting to bursting into tears. You observe that she is quite upset as she expresses to you that she is afraid because her father told her that if she did need surgery she would not feel anything because she would be asleep. Christine tells you that when she sleeps she wakes up sometimes and that she is sure that if her appendix is "cut out" she will wake up during the operation and it "will hurt a lot." She tells you she has not told her parents she is afraid because they have told her how proud they are that she is so brave. You realize Christine is terrified. Using Mishel's uncertainty in illness theory, you apply the four-stage framework.

1. *Stimuli frame:* Inadvertently, Christine, who concretely has understood the word "sleep" using her own filter for life experience, has misinterpreted the positive intention of the language used by her father. This misinterpretation has resulted in Christine's negative cognitive schema. Christine notably does not understand "sleep" and its use (or adult misuse, in this case) as a synonym for, or definition of, surgical anesthesia. This is the root cause of Christine's current uncertainty in illness.
   Nursing intervention: Listen carefully and caringly; explain in simple understandable language what "sleep" means in the context her father presented; initiate, seek, and clarify Christine's concerns and questions; use the term "anesthesia" to differentiate it from "sleep." Inform and involve her parents in the overall process.

2. *Appraisal stage:* As a result of Christine's concrete experiential interpretation of "sleep," she has applied a negative value to the environmental conditions surrounding her abdominal pain. This is particularly so as it relates to surgical anesthesia.
   Nursing intervention: Follow-up with Christine to make sure she comprehends the newly provided information. Elicit the support of Christine's parents and staff. If there are appropriate postsurgical patients on the unit, have them talk with Christine about their positive anesthesia experience.

3. *Initiation of coping mechanisms:* Christine is 9 years old. Her coping skills are limited to those used in her 9 years of life experience.
   Nursing intervention: Check with Christine and observe verbal and nonverbal cues. Have her verbalize any uncertainties she may be experiencing. Some of this will be influenced by the progress of the illness.

4. *Adaptation:* Dependent on steps 1, 2, and 3
   Nursing intervention: As Christine accepts the idea of new information, new schema will follow. Though the outcome of her abdominal pain may initially be uncertain, her acceptance of the new schema will hopefully result in an increased comfort zone and decreased fear.

Summary: A central tenet of Mishel's theory is the core position that uncertainty in illness must be addressed. If left unheeded, negative perceptions will escalate, and clients will suffer. Their quality of life may be affected, and positive outcomes may be compromised. Nursing's responsibility in applying Mishel's theory is to reframe the client's perceived loss of control, or uncertainty, and assist the client in developing new skills of assimilation and accommodation. The client will then be able to identify, develop, and master those targets capable of control.

FLORENCE NIGHTINGALE: THE FIRST NURSING THEORIST

If theory means to put concepts in a form in which relationships are described and predictions are made, then Florence Nightingale was the first nursing theorist. Nightingale did not deliberately set out to develop theory; rather her goal was to ease the suffering of soldiers and citizens of England. However, many important influences in her life directed her toward theory development.

- A classic education (philosophy [science], French, Italian, Greek, Latin, the arts, and history)
- Upper-class background, great wealth, and a prominent social life (operas, parties, balls)
- Religion and spirituality (she spent much time daydreaming about how she could serve God and experienced four visions from God).
- Era of reform throughout England (Industrial Revolution and dichotomy among the classes)

Despite her wealth and upper-class status, Nightingale was very dissatisfied with life. In 1852 she wrote a monograph titled "Cassandra," in which she pointed out the hopelessness inherent in being a woman in her day. "The family? It is too narrow a field for the development of an immortal spirit. …The system dooms some minds to incurable infancy, others to silent misery. Marriage is the only chance [and it is but a chance] offered to women for escape from this death; and how eagerly and how ignorantly it is embraced" (Nightingale, 1992, pp. 37-38). Her diary writings have been interpreted at times to be suicidal. Often depressed, Nightingale resorted to dreams as an escape from her unhappiness and discontent. Her personality and her lifestyle (dogmatic, practical, a critical observer who was fascinated by numbers and recorded everything she saw and experienced) set her apart. She was self-willed, unhappy, and dissatisfied at times in spite of having beauty, a brilliant social career, and an education of which few men of her day could boast.

She had enjoyed the best of music and art and the companionship of charming and important people. However, in refusing marriage and the round of social gaiety, she was revolting against the restrictions placed on women of her day, and she struggled to be allowed to work in a serious way.

Florence Nightingale eventually convinced her family to allow her to attend nurses training, and so began her distinguished career in developing professional nursing. Nightingale is well remembered for her significant contributions to professional nursing in the areas of theory of practice, nursing education, scholarship, and statistics. Box 5-4 provides Nightingale's definitions of professional nursing.

Nightingale's Theory of Practice

Nightingale's theory of practice, an environmental adaptation theory, was documented for nurses and laypersons alike and served as the foundation for the promotion of health. This theory was referred to by Nightingale as the canons of nursing and guided the practice of professional nursing. A description of these canons, or standards, follows.

Ventilation and Warming. In the concept of ventilation and warming, Nightingale is very precise to "keep the air he breathes as pure as the external air without chilling him" (Nightingale,

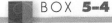

BOX **5-4**

Nightingale's Definitions of Nursing

Nursing is an art—an art requiring an organized practical and scientific training.
Nursing is putting us in the best possible conditions for nature to preserve health—to prevent or restore or to cure disease or injury.
Nursing is therefore to help the patient live.

1859, p. 8). Plenty of ventilation is necessary to carry off the noxious elements from a sick person's lungs and skin.

Noise. "Unnecessary noise, or noise that creates an expectation in the mind is that which hurts a patient" (Nightingale, 1859, p. 25). The nurse should guard against sudden noise, thoughtless chatter, and whispering in a patient's room. The effect of music may be beneficial.

Variety. Variety is another concept that helps alleviate suffering. Beautiful objects, brilliant colors, cut flowers, perhaps different things to do (e.g., handwork), and even pets may alleviate the boredom felt by those suffering.

Diet. The fourth concept is diet. "Sick cookery should half do the work of your poor patient's weak digestion" (Nightingale, 1859, p. 38). Nightingale reviews some of the common substances (gruel, arrowroot puddings, and egg flip) given to the sick.

Light. "It is the unqualified result of all my experience with the sick that second only to their need of fresh air is their need of light" (Nightingale, 1859, p. 47). Take the patient outside for direct sunlight. Keep rooms well lighted with no bed curtains or dark windows.

Chattering Hopes and Advices. According to Nightingale, chattering hopes and advices are attempts to cheer the patient by attendants and friends. Nightingale warns against this because she determines this to be false hope and hollow advice. She clearly appeals, "Leave off this practice of attempting to cheer the sick by making light of their danger and by exaggerating their probabilities of recovery" (Nightingale, 1859, p. 54).

Cleanliness (Health of Houses). Nightingale's attention to cleanliness takes up a large portion of her book. She writes that health depends on this. Describing the care of bed and bedding and of rooms and walls, she states the exact steps needed to clean each. In addition, she details how to clean the sick person so as to prevent poisoning by the skin. She describes the patient's feeling of well-being after washing and drying. The nurse needs to wash her own hands with friction as well. Some believe that Nightingale's success was based primarily on cleaning up the hospitals.

Because of these significant contributions to nursing and to improving the health of soldiers and citizens alike, Nightingale was highly recognized. Her honors, decorations, medals, and citations may be seen in the United Services Museum in Whitehall, London. She was the first woman to ever receive the British Order of Merit by King Edward VII. One of her biographers (Cook, 1942) said, "she was not only 'The Lady with a Lamp' throwing light into dark places but also a kind of galvanic battery stirring and sometimes shocking the dull and sluggish public to life and action."

SURVEY OF SELECTED NURSING THEORIES

A brief discussion of selected nursing theories follows. The date identified indicates the year in which the theory was first presented. However, most theories have continued to be refined and modified. A summary of the major nursing theorists with a brief description of their theory or conceptual model is presented in Table 5-2, which provides the reader with information to guide further exploration of nursing theory. Box 5-5 provides online resources for further investigation of nursing theories.

TABLE **5-2**

Summary of Major Nursing Theorists and Theory Description

DATE AND THEORIST	THEORY DESCRIPTION
1860: Florence Nightingale	Investigates the effect of the environment on healing
1952: Hildegard E. Peplau	Interpersonal relations model explores the interpersonal relationship of the nurse and the client and identifies the client's feelings as a predictor of positive outcomes related to health and wellness.
1960: Faye Abdellah	Twenty-one nursing problems. Client-centered interventions.
1961: Ida Jean Orlando	Theory of the nursing process. Deliberate nursing approach using nursing process, which stresses the action of the individual client in determining the action of the nurse; focus is on the present or short-term outcome.
1966: Virginia Henderson	Definition of nursing. Nursing assists patients with 14 essential functions toward independence.
1967: Myra Estrin Levine	Conservation model. Four conservation principles of inpatient client resources (energy, structural integrity, personal integrity, and social integrity).
1970: Martha E. Rogers	Science of unitary human beings: energy fields, openness, pattern, and organization; nurse promotes synchronicity between human beings and their universe or environment.
1970: Betty Neuman	Systems model: wellness-illness continuum; promotes the nurse as the agent in assisting the client in adapting to and therefore reducing stressors; supports the notion of prevention through appropriate intervention.
1971: Dorothea Orem	Self-care model. Nursing facilitates client self-care by measuring the client's deficit relative to self-care needs; the nurse implements appropriate measures to assist the client in meeting these needs by matching them with an appropriate supportive intervention.
1971: Imogene King	Goal attainment theory. Goal attainment using nurse-client transactions; addresses client systems and includes society, groups, and the individual.
1974: Sister Callista Roy	Roy's adaptation model. Client's adaptation to condition using environmental stimuli to adjust perception.
1977: Madeline Leininger	Theory of cultural care diversity and universality. Transcultural nursing and caring nursing; concepts are aimed toward caring and the components of a culture care theory; diversity, universality, worldview, and ethnohistory are essential to the four concepts (care, caring, health, and nursing).
1978: Jean Watson	Philosophy and science of caring and humanistic nursing; there are 10 "carative" factors that are core to nursing; this holistic outlook addresses the impact and importance of altruism, sensitivity, trust, and interpersonal skills.
1979: Margaret Newman	Central components of this model are health and consciousness followed by concepts of movement, time, and space; all components are summative units, described in relationship to health and to each other.
1980: Dorothy E. Johnson	Behavioral system model for nursing; separates the psychologic and the physiologic aspects of illness; role of the nurse is to provide support and comfort to attain regulation of the client's behavior.
1981: Rosemarie Rizzo Parse	Theory of human becoming (1992) proposes that quality of life from each person's individual perspective should be the goal of nursing practice. Parse first published the theory in 1981 as the "man-living-health" theory. The name was officially changed to "the human becoming theory" in 1992 to remove the term "man" after the change in the dictionary definition of the word from its former meaning of "humankind"; individual, by existing, actively participates in creating health according to environmental influences; individual is regarded as an open system wherein health is a process.

Continued

TABLE **5-2**

Summary of Major Nursing Theorists and Theory Description—cont'd

DATE AND THEORIST	THEORY DESCRIPTION
1982: Patricia Benner	Primacy of caring; the practice of nurses depends on the experience absorbed by engaging in five practice areas (novice, advanced beginner, competent, proficient, and expert) in the seven domains of nursing practice (helping, teaching-coaching, diagnostic and patient monitoring, effective management of rapid change, administration and monitoring of therapeutic interventions and regimens, monitoring and ensuring the quality of health care practices, and organizational work-role competencies).

BOX **5-5**

Helpful Websites

The following sites are excellent resources for nursing theory and information about nursing theorists, including King, Leininger, Levine, Neuman, Newman, Orem, Parse, Peplau, Rogers, Roy, Watson, and others:

    www.sandiego.edu/academics/nursing/theory
    www.nursingtheory.net

This site links to Leininger's theory of cultural care diversity and universality.

    www.tcns.org

This site brings together current knowledge and experiences with teaching, practicing, and researching comfort.

    www.thecomfortline.com

This site describes early nurse theorists and classifies nursing theories.

    www.enursecribe.com/nurse_theorists,.php# Early Nurse Theorists

Hildegard E. Peplau (1952)—Interpersonal Relations as a Nursing Process: Man as an Organism That Exists in an Unstable Equilibrium

When the client incurs an insult that renders her or him incapable of moving forward because of existing stressful environmental conditions, anxiety increases. This condition creates a situation wherein the option is to either move in a backward direction or remain on a plateau. Nursing intervention in Peplau's model focuses on reducing the related incapacitating stressors through therapeutic interpersonal interaction. Intervention involves the nurse assisting the client with mutual goal setting. These goals may address exploration of the identified problem, identification of viable options, and implementation of available resources for resolution. Nursing interpersonal process is present and interactive, using associated and appropriate nursing intervention skills, which incorporate the roles of the nurse as resource person, educator, mentor, transfer agent, and counselor. Peplau's model requires that the nurse have a self-awareness and insight regarding her or his own behaviors. This awareness may be applied in identifying and working through those behaviors unique to the client's schema. Figure 5-2 presents Peplau's psychodynamic nursing model.

Middle-Range Nursing Theory

Nurse	Stranger	Unconditional surrogate: Mother Sibling	Counselor Resource person Leadership surrogate: Mother	Adult person
Patient	Stranger	Infant	Child	Adolescent	Adult person
Phases in nursing relationship	Orientation ——— Identification ——— Exploitation ——— Resolution			

Figure 5-2 Peplau's psychodynamic nursing model. Phases and changing roles in nurse-patient relationships. (From Peplau HE: Interpersonal relations in nursing, New York, 1952, GP Putnam and Sons, p. 54.)

Martha E. Rogers (1970)—Science of Unitary Human Beings: Humans as Energy Fields That Interact Constantly with the Environment

When the client-human unit incurs an insult that renders him or her out of balance with the universe, nursing interventions must be geared toward helping the client-human unit attain an increasing complex balance and synchronicity with the universe. Essential to Rogers's theory is the belief that each being is unique and consists of more than the collective sum of parts and that each being is constantly evolving in a forward momentum as he or she interacts continually with the surrounding environmental field. Rogers's theory states that a brain integration is necessary to support the notion of human-environmental synergy, using the right side of the brain to recognize every human unit's capacity for imagery, sensation, and emotion and the left side of the brain for language, abstraction, and thought.

Dorothea Orem (1971)—Self-Care Deficit Model: Self-Care, Self-Care Deficits, and Nursing Systems

When a client incurs an insult that renders him or her incapable of fully functioning, there is a deficient self-care, which makes nursing intervention necessary. The object of Orem's theory is to restore the client's self-care capability to enable him or her to sustain structural reliability, performance, and growth through purposeful nursing intervention. The aim of such intervention is to help the client cope with unmet care needs by acquiring the maximal level of function. This would be to either regain previous function or maximize available function present after the insult, hence restoring a sense of well-being.

Sister Callista Roy (1974)—Adaptation Model: Assistance with the Adaptation to Stressors to Facilitate the Integration Process of the Client

When the client incurs an insult that renders him or her in need of environmental modification, the nurse is the change agent in assisting the individual with this adaptation. By helping the "biopsychosocial" client modify external stimuli, adaptation will occur. In the case of illness, the outcome is a diminished or absent integration of the constantly changing setting known as the illness environment with the constantly changing human, who is interacting with the existing outside surroundings. To attain wellness, adaptation must occur through this integration.

The nurse's role is to promote this adaptation by modifying and regulating peripheral stimuli to enable the client's adaptation and integration with a supportive healing environment. In so doing, the nurse is instrumental in assisting the client with the areas of health and well-being, life worth and value, and self-respect and dignity. Sister Callista Roy's adaptation model is depicted in Figure 5-3.

Jean Watson (1978)—Theory of Human Caring: Transpersonal Caring as the Fulcrum; Philosophy and Science as the Core of Nursing

When the client incurs an insult that renders him or her in need, the transpersonal process between the client and the nurse is considered a healing nursing intervention. An assumption of Watson's theory is that everyone requires human caring to quell need. Hence the transpersonal process of "caring," or the caring among nurse, environment, and client, is essential to healing. Caring promotes the notion that every human being strives for interconnectedness with other humans and with nature. The nurse who implements these carative factors is the facilitator in the goal of restoring congruence between the client's perceived self and the existent self through the promotion of health and equilibrium. The expectation is that the client will experience balance and harmony in mind, body, and soul. Harmony, or wellness, will prevail, whereas disharmony, or illness, will be altered, eliminated, or circumvented.

Margaret Newman (1979, Revised 1986)—Health as Expanding Consciousness

Margaret Newman's theory defines health as "expanding consciousness," or increasing complexity. The theory of health as expanding consciousness was stimulated by concern for those for whom health as the absence of disease or disability is not possible. Nurses often relate to such people: people facing the uncertainty, debilitation, loss, and eventual death associated with chronic illness. The theory has progressed to include the health of all persons regardless of the presence or absence of disease. The theory asserts that every person in every situation, no matter how disordered and hopeless it may seem, is part of the universal process of expanding consciousness—a process of becoming more of oneself, of finding greater meaning in life, and of reaching new dimensions of connectedness with other people and the world (retrieved August 31, 2009 from: http://healthasexpandingconsciousness.org/home/index.php?option=com_frontpage&Itemid=1).

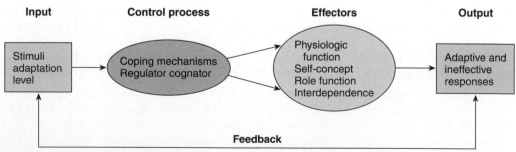

Grand Nursing Theory

Figure 5-3 Roy's adaptation model. Person as an adaptive system. (From Roy C: Introduction to nursing: an adaptation model, ed 2, Englewood Cliffs, NJ, 1984, Prentice-Hall, p. 30.)

Merle Mishel (1981, Revised 1990)—Uncertainty of Illness

Uncertainty in illness is frequently a stress-producing incident that is capable of contributing to negative physical and/or psychologic outcomes. Uncertainty exists when the client is unsure about a diagnosed illness. This uncertainty renders the client either incapable of assigning a concrete value to the illness itself or to a predictable outcome. Uncertainty can occur with a client misperceiving a diagnosed illness because of the inadequate information received, the health care provider incorrectly presuming client knowledge, or the health care informant failing to recognize the client's individual unique filtering of provided illness information. Mishel's theory is used in chronic illness and other practice settings. Mishel's model outlines a four-step approach in defining her theory. These include (1) stimuli frame: antecedents generating client uncertainty; (2) appraisal stage: client assignment of a value, positive or negative, to the uncertainty; (3) initiation of coping mechanisms: client ability to develop, improvise, and implement skills to cope with uncertainty; and (4) adaptation: positive client assimilation and accommodation to uncertainty, resulting from effective coping. Mishel's theory establishes a framework that guides nursing practice by assisting nurses to work with clients in establishing interventions that promote positive outcomes.

FUTURE OF NURSING THEORIES AND THEORISTS

At no time in history have so many health care concerns been the primary focus of federal and state legislative agendas. New questions are being asked in the twenty-first century about how health care is being conducted and managed. It is imperative that nurses be on the front lines to provide testimony in response to these queries.

The nursing shortage, scarce resources, patient safety and medical errors, managed care, Medicare, welfare-to-work plans, confidentiality issues, parity of reimbursement, advanced practice nurses and their scope of practice, mandatory overtime, whistle-blower protection, prescriptive authority, licensure, multistate compacts, telemedicine, and many other policy issues that directly affect nursing practice are coming before the U.S. Congress and individual state legislative bodies for practice-related decisions. The direct effect on nursing cannot be overemphasized.

As nursing continues to operate in an environment of ongoing change, outcome data will be analyzed in an effort to provide quality care and access to that care for all clients in need of health care services. Therefore, one may predict that established nursing theories will be reevaluated and modified accordingly. New theories will be created and developed that may help answer the health care questions of the twenty-first century. Simply put, nursing theories in the twenty-first century will embrace complex environmental changes that incorporate new technologies, such as genetics, computers, noninvasive surgery, robotics, decreasing energy sources, increasing pollutants under a thinning ozone layer, environmental hazards, new diseases, and antibiotic-resistant illness. These changes have already resulted in client needs that differ from those as recent as 5 years ago.

SUMMARY

Let the reader beware. As stated at the beginning of this chapter, the information provided here is in no manner a substitute for a comprehensive analysis of existing nursing theories and theorists. More exist than are presented here, and in fact there are several comprehensive texts that cover these theories in depth. Instead, this chapter offers an overview of theory in the attempt to familiarize readers with the idea of theory. Selected theories are described to that end. Readers should identify nursing theories as ideas that have shaped and continue to shape the nursing profession in practice and research. It is our intention to assist students with understanding that practice and theory are interdependent entities. In other words, practice and theory cannot efficiently or effectively exist one without the other. Like the metaphor at the beginning of this chapter, without the existence of the stones (scientific data), the separation into specific concentrated yet related areas (theory) could not have happened.

 Additional resources are available online at: http://evolve.elsevier.com/Cherry/

REFERENCES

Abdellah FG: The nature of nursing science, *Nurs Res* 18(5):393, 1969.

Anastasi T: Heredity, environment, and the question "how?" *Psychol Rev* 65:197–208, 1958.

Cook E: *The life of Florence Nightingale*, New York, 1942, Macmillan.

Donaldson SK, Crowley DM: The discipline of nursing, *Nurs Outlook* 26(2):113–120, 1978.

Jacob S: The grief process of older women whose husbands received hospice care, *J Adv Nurs* 24:280–286, 1996.

Jacox AK: Theory construction in nursing: an overview, *Nurs Res* 23(1):4, 1974.

Lenz ER, Pugh LC: Theory of unpleasant symptoms. In Smith MJ, Liehr P, editors: *Middle range theory for nursing*, New York, 2003, Springer.

Mishel MH: The measurement of uncertainty in illness, *Nurs Res* 30:258–263, 1981.

Mishel MH: Uncertainty in acute illness, *Ann Rev Nurs Res* 15:57–80, 1997.

Nightingale F: *Notes on nursing: what it is, and what it is not (commemorative edition)*, Philadelphia, 1992, Lippincott.

Nightingale F: *Notes on nursing: what it is, and what it is not*, London, 1859, Harrison and Sons.

Polit D, Beck C: *Nursing research*, ed 8, Philadelphia, 2008, Lippincott Williams & Wilkins.

Sousa VD, Zauszniewski JA: Toward a theory of diabetes self-care management, *J Theory Construct Test* 9(2):61–67, 2005.

Tsai P, Tak S, Moore C, Palercia I: Testing a theory of chronic pain, *J Adv Nurs* 43(2):159–169, 2003.

ADDITIONAL RESOURCES

Benner P: *From novice to expert: excellence in power in clinical nursing practice*, Menlo Park, CA, 1984, Addison-Wesley.

Chinn P, Kramer M: *Theory and nursing: integrated knowledge development*, St Louis, 1999, Mosby.

Health as Expanding Consciousness: Retrieved August 31, 2009, from: http://healthasexpandingconsciousness.org/home/index.php?option=com_frontpage&Itemid=1.

Johnson BM, Webber PB: *An introduction to theory and reasoning in nursing*, Philadelphia, 2001, Lippincott.

King I: *Toward a theory for nursing: general concepts of human behavior*, New York, 1971, John Wiley & Sons.

Kolcaba K, Schirm V, Steiner R: Effects of hand massage on comfort of nursing home residents, *Geriatr Nurs* 27(2):85–91, 2006.

Kolcaba K, Tilton C, Drouin C: Comfort theory: a unifying framework to enhance the practice environment, *J Nurs Adm* 36(11):538–544, 2006.

Leddy S, Pepper J: *Conceptual bases in professional nursing*, Philadelphia, 1998, Lippincott.

Leininger MM: *Transcultural nursing: concepts, theories and practices*, New York, 1978, John Wiley & Sons.

Levine M: The four conservation principles of nursing, *Nurs Forum* 6:93, 1967.

Newman MA: *Health as expanding consciousness*, St Louis, 1986, Mosby.

Nicoll L: *Perspectives on nursing theory*, Philadelphia, 1997, Lippincott.

Orem DE: *Nursing concepts of practice*, ed 6, New York, 1971, McGraw-Hill.

Parse RR: *Man-living-health: a theory of nursing*, New York, 1981, John Wiley & Sons.

Peplau HE: *International relations in nursing*, New York, 1952, GP Putnam.

Tomey AM, Alligood MR: *Nursing theorists and their work*, ed 5, St Louis, 2002, Mosby.

Nursing Research and Evidence-Based Practice

Jill J. Webb, PhD, MSN, RN, CS

e)volve Additional resources are available online at: http://evolve.elsevier.com/Cherry/

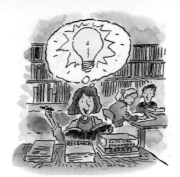

Nursing research provides the foundation for evidence-based nursing practice.

VIGNETTE

I did not understand why I had to take a research class when all I wanted to do was be a staff nurse in a critical care unit. Research? Evidence-based practice? Why are these topics in the nursing program? I have enough to do just learning all the content in my clinical courses. What do research and evidence have to do with developing my nursing abilities? I trust the faculty, the textbooks, and clinical experience to prepare me for nursing. I'm already getting what I need to know. That was my earlier attitude. Now that I am practicing, I have a new appreciation for nursing research and the evidence it provides for application to practice. I have an entirely different way of addressing clinical questions. I'm starting to ask questions about how I can improve the care I give to patients and how I can be involved in my workplace's efforts to improve care for the patients it serves. I have discovered by purposeful reading in my practice area that research reports and research summaries contain many implications that apply to practice in the critical care unit.

■ QUESTIONS TO CONSIDER WHILE READING THIS CHAPTER:

1 How can faculty encourage students to read research journals?
2 How does research affect nursing practice?
3 How can nurses motivate colleagues to base their practice on research?

KEY TERMS

Clinical nurse researcher (CNR) An advanced practice nurse who is doctorally prepared and directs and participates in clinical research.
Clinical nurse specialist (CNS) An advanced practice nurse who provides direct care to clients and participates in health education and research.
Clinical practice guideline (CPG) an evidence-based guide to clinical practice developed by experts in a particular field for direct application in clinical environments.
Control group Subjects in an experiment who do not receive the experimental treatment and whose performance provides a baseline against which the effects of the treatment can be measured. When a true experimental design is not used, this group is usually called a comparison group.
Data collection The process of acquiring existing information or developing new information.

Empirical Having a foundation based on data gathered through the senses (e.g., observation or experience) rather than purely through theorizing or logic.

Ethnography A qualitative research method for the purpose of investigating cultures that involves data collection, description, and analysis of data to develop a theory of cultural behavior.

Evidence-based practice The process of systematically finding, appraising, and using research findings as the basis for clinical practice.

Experimental design A design that includes randomization, a control group, and manipulation between or among variables to examine probability and causality among selected variables for the purpose of predicting and controlling phenomena.

Generalizability The inference that findings can be generalized from the sample to the entire population.

Grant Proposal developed to seek research funding from private or public agencies.

Grounded theory A qualitative research design used to collect and analyze data with the aim of developing theories grounded in real-world observations. This method is used to study a social process.

Meta-analysis Quantitative merging of findings from several studies to determine what is known about a phenomenon.

Methodologic design A research design used to develop the validity and reliability of instruments that measure research concepts and variables.

Naturalistic paradigm A holistic view of nature and the direction of science that guides qualitative research.

Needs assessment A study in which the researcher collects data for estimating the needs of a group, usually for resource allocation.

Phenomenology A qualitative research design that uses inductive descriptive methodology to describe the lived experiences of study participants.

Pilot study A smaller version of a proposed study conducted to develop or refine methodology, such as treatment, instruments, or data collection process to be used in a larger study.

Qualitative research A systematic, subjective approach used to describe life experiences and give them meaning.

Quantitative research A formal, objective, systematic process used to describe and test relationships and examine cause-and-effect interactions among variables.

Quasi-experimental research A type of quantitative research study design that lacks one of the components (randomization, control group, manipulation of one or more variables) of an experimental design.

Randomization The assignment of subjects to treatment conditions in a random manner (determined by chance alone).

Secondary analysis A research design in which data previously collected in another study are analyzed.

State-of-the-science summary A merging of findings from several studies concerning the same topic. Examples include meta-analysis with a quantitative approach and integrative review with a descriptive approach.

Survey A nonexperimental research design that focuses on obtaining information regarding the status quo of a situation, often through direct questioning of participants.

Triangulation The use of a variety of methods to collect data on the same concept.

LEARNING OUTCOMES

After studying this chapter, the reader will be able to:

1 Summarize major points in the evolution of nursing research in relation to contemporary nursing.
2 Evaluate the influence of nursing research on current nursing and health care practices.
3 Differentiate among nursing research methods.
4 Evaluate the quality of research studies using established criteria.
5 Participate in the research process.
6 Use research findings to improve nursing practice.

CHAPTER OVERVIEW

This chapter provides basic knowledge regarding the research process and the ultimate importance of evidence-based nursing practice. The intent is to inspire an appreciation for nursing research and to show how it can improve nursing practice and how results can be translated into health policy. Nursing research is defined as a systematic approach used to examine phenomena important to nursing and nurses. A summary of major points in the evolution of nursing research in relation to contemporary nursing is presented. A description of private and public organizations that fund research is given, and their research priorities are listed. Major research designs are briefly described, and examples of each are given. Nurses of all educational levels are encouraged to participate in and promote nursing research at varying degrees. The process of locating research and evidence for practice is reviewed. Students are introduced to the research process and guided in the process of critically appraising published research and research syntheses. Ethical issues related to research are examined, and historical examples of unethical research are given. The functions of the institutional review board (IRB) and the use of informed consent in protecting the rights of human subjects are emphasized.

DEFINITION OF NURSING RESEARCH

Research is a process of systematic inquiry or study to build knowledge in a discipline. The purpose of research is to develop an empirical body of knowledge for a discipline or profession. Specifically, research validates and refines existing knowledge and develops new knowledge (Burns and Grove, 2007). The results of research process provide a foundation on which practice decisions and behaviors are laid. Research results create a strong scientific base for nursing practice, especially when deliberately and carefully evaluated for application to specific clinical topics (Melnyk and Fineout-Overholt, 2005). In recent decades the nursing discipline has begun to pay much greater attention to the necessity of participating in research.

Nursing research is a systematic approach used to examine phenomena important to nursing and nurses. Because nursing is a practice profession, it is important that clinical practice be based on scientific knowledge. Evidence generated by nursing research provides support for the quality and cost-effectiveness of nursing interventions. Thus recipients of health care—and particularly nursing care—reap benefits when nurses attend to research evidence and introduce change based on that evidence into nursing practice. The introduction of evidence-based change into the direct provision of nursing care may occur at the individual level of a particular nurse or at varied organizational or social levels.

In addition to nursing research aimed at affecting the direct provision of nursing and health care to recipients of nursing care, nursing research also is needed to generate knowledge in areas that affect nursing care processes indirectly. Research within the realms of nursing education, nursing administration, health services, characteristics of nurses, and nursing roles provides evidence for effectively changing these supporting areas of nursing knowledge (Burns and Grove, 2007). Today the importance of nursing research to the discipline is recognized. However, much nursing history underlies the current state of acceptance.

EVOLUTION OF NURSING RESEARCH

Nursing research began with the work of Florence Nightingale during the Crimean War. After Florence Nightingale's work, the pattern that nursing research followed was closely related to the problems confronting nurses. For example, nursing education was the focus of most research studies between 1900 and 1940. As more nurses received their education in a university setting, studies regarding student characteristics and satisfactions were conducted. As more nurses pursued a college education, staffing patterns in hospitals changed because students were not as readily available as when more students were enrolled in hospital-affiliated diploma programs. During this period, researchers became interested in studying nurses. Questions such as what type of person enters nursing and how are nurses perceived by other groups guided research investigations. Teaching, administration, and curriculum were studies that dominated nursing research until the 1970s. By the 1970s more doctorally prepared nurses were conducting research, and there was a shift to studies that focused on the improvement of patient care.

The 1980s brought nursing research to a new stage of development. There were many more qualified nurse researchers than ever, widespread availability of computers for collection and analysis of data, and a realization that research is a vital part of professional nursing (Polit and Beck, 2006). Nurse researchers began conducting studies based on the naturalistic paradigm. These studies were qualitative rather than quantitative. In addition, instead of conducting many small, unrelated research studies, teams of researchers, often interdisciplinary, began conducting programs of research to build bodies of knowledge related to specific topics, such as urinary incontinence, decubitus ulcers, pain, and quality of life. The 1990s brought increasing concern about health care reform, and now in the twenty-first century, research studies focus on important health care delivery issues, such as cost, quality, and access.

Research findings are being used increasingly as the basis for clinical decisions. Evidence-based practice (EBP) can be defined as the process of systematically finding, appraising, and using research findings as a basis for making decisions about patient care. The rise of technology and the worldwide access and flow of information have transformed the decision-making processes of practitioners. Helpful informational websites for busy practitioners are listed in Box 6-1. No longer do nurses simply compare outcomes of patient care with other units in the

BOX **6-1**

Helpful Websites

National Guideline Clearinghouse—resource for evidence-based clinical practice guidelines
   www.guidelines.gov
U.S. Department of Veterans Affairs Clinical Practice Guidelines
   www.healthquality.va.gov
AHRQ Healthcare Innovations Exchange—innovations and tools to improve health care
   www.innovations.ahrq.gov/index.aspx
The Evidence-Based Medicine Education Center of Excellence—extensive list of databases, journals, and textbooks
   http://library.ncahec.net/ebm/pages/resources.htm
U.S. National Institute for Health Consensus statements
   http://consensus.nih.gov
Centre for Evidence-Based Nursing, based at University of York—United Kingdom
   www.york.ac.uk/healthsciences/centres/evidence/cebn.htm
The Joanna Briggs Institute, based at Royal Adelaide Hospital and the University of Adelaide, Australia—multiple evidence resources for practice
   www.joannabriggs.edu.au
Cochrane Center—resource for evidence-based clinical practice guidelines
   www.cochrane.org

same hospital. Nurses and other health care professionals are more likely to look for solutions, choices, and outcomes for patients that represent the best available knowledge internationally (Hamer and Collinson, 2005).

RESEARCH PRIORITIES

Why set priorities for research in the nursing discipline? Can nurses do research in areas that match personal areas of interest? The answer to the second question is, yes, certainly. But nursing exists to provide high-quality nursing care to individuals in need of health-promoting, health-sustaining, and health-restoring strategies. The main outcome of research activity for a nurse is to eventually put the knowledge gained to work in health care delivery. Research priorities, often set by groups that fund research, encourage nurse researchers to invest effort and money into those areas of research likely to generate the most benefit to recipients of care. Of course the funding opportunities offered by such groups do not hurt the research enterprise either. Research costs money. Thus nurses engaged in research often match personal interests with funding opportunities that are available during the planning phase for a proposed investigation.

Two major sources of funding for nursing research are the National Institute of Nursing Research (NINR) and the Agency for Healthcare Research and Quality (AHRQ) (formerly known as the Agency for Health Care Policy and Research [AHCPR] and reauthorized as AHRQ by Congress in 1999). Both of these organizations are funded by federal congressional appropriations. Private foundations and nursing organizations also provide funding for nursing research.

National Institute of Nursing Research

As part of the National Institutes of Health (NIH), the NINR supports research on the biologic and behavioral aspects of critical health problems that confront the nation. The NINR's research focus encompasses "health promotion and disease prevention, quality of life, health disparities, and end-of-life" (NINR Strategic Plan 2006-2010, 2006). A small sampling of potentially supported research topics includes those aimed at:

- Determining disease risk and treatment through utilizing genetic information
- Determining effective health-promotion strategies for individuals, families, and communities
- Discovering approaches that encourage people to effectively take responsibility for symptom management and health promotion
- Assisting in identification and effective management of symptoms related to acute and chronic disease
- Improving clinical settings in which care is provided
- Improving the quality of care giving in settings such as long-term care facilities, the home, and the community
- Understanding predisposition to disease, socioeconomic factors that influence health, and cultural health practices that either protect from or expose to risk for health problems
- Improving symptom management for those at end of life

The areas of research emphasis published by the NINR are useful guides for investigators developing proposals but are not considered to be prescriptive in nature. Investigators bring to bear their own unique expertise and creativity when proposing research in harmony with NINR priority research areas.

Annually the NINR conducts a roundtable discussion with multiple nursing organizations to obtain the feedback of the disciplines regarding the need for continued or new research emphases. Information obtained is used in setting future research agendas and making decisions about funding of proposals submitted by researchers (Office of Science Policy and Public Liaison, NINR, 2009). The NINR website details current announcements regarding research priorities (www.ninr.nih.gov/ResearchAndFunding).

Agency for Healthcare Research and Quality

The AHRQ broadly defines its mission as "improving the quality, safety, efficiency, and effectiveness of health care for all Americans" (AHRQ, 2009a). As an agency of the U.S. Department of Health and Human Services, the AHRQ's health-related aims are to reduce the risk of harm by promoting delivery of the best possible health care, improve health care outcomes by encouraging the use of evidence to make informed health care decisions, transform research into practice to facilitate wider access to effective health care services, and reduce unnecessary costs (AHRQ, 2009a). Since the inception of the agency in 1989, strategic goals have centered on supporting improvements in health outcomes, strengthening measurement of health care quality indicators, and fostering access to and cost-effectiveness of health care. The 1999 reauthorizing legislation expanded the role of the agency by directing the AHRQ to:

- Improve the quality of health care through scientific inquiry, dissemination of findings, and facilitation of public access to information.
- Promote patient safety and reduce medical errors through scientific inquiry, building partnerships with health care providers, and establishment of centers for education and research on therapeutics (CERTs).
- Advance the use of information technology for coordinating patient care and conducting quality and outcomes research.
- Establish an office on priority populations to ensure that the needs of low-income groups, minorities, women, children, the elderly, and individuals with special health care needs are addressed by the agency's research efforts.

The research-related activities of the AHRQ are quite varied, but a recent shift emphasizes a more deliberate translation of research evidence into practice. In a process similar to that used by the NIH, investigators are invited to submit research proposals for possible funding through grant announcements. A listing of current areas of the agency's research interests can be found online at www.ahrq.gov/fund/portfolio.htm.

The AHRQ actively promotes EBP, partially through the establishment of 14 EBP centers (EPCs) in the United States and Canada. EPCs conduct research on assigned clinical care topics and generate reports on the effectiveness of health care methodologies. Health care providers may then use the evidence in developing site-specific guidelines that direct clinical practice. AHRQ also actively maintains the National Guideline Clearinghouse (www.guidelines.gov), a website that makes available to health care professionals a wide array of clinical practice guidelines that may be considered in health care decision making. Another recent addition to AHRQ's initiatives is the Healthcare Innovations Exchange (2009b), which provides a public source of information about innovations taking place in health care delivery. Submitted innovations are reviewed for the quality of achieved outcomes, providing evidence as a foundation for decision making by others who may be searching for or considering similar innovations. Although most AHRQ activities are intended to support health care professionals and institutions, the agency supports health care recipients by designing some information specifically for dissemination to the lay public (AHRQ, 2009a).

Private Foundations

Federal funding is available through the NIH and the AHRQ. However, because obtaining money for research is becoming increasingly competitive, voluntary foundations and private and community-based organizations should be investigated as possible funding sources. Many foundations and corporate direct-giving programs are interested in funding health care projects and research. Computer databases and guides to funding are available in local libraries. In addition, grant-seeking enterprises often purchase subscriptions that allow computer access to enhanced listings of funding foundations that include information about the types of projects those foundations typically fund. Though subscriptions are expensive, costs are often balanced by the efficiency with which suitable funding prospects are identified. An example of such a service is Prospect Research Online (www.iwave.com).

Private foundations, such as the Robert Wood Johnson Foundation (2009a,b) or the W.K. Kellogg Foundation (2009), offer program funding for health-related research. Investigators should be encouraged to pursue funding for small projects through local sources or private foundations until a track record is established in research design and implementation. After several years of experience in the research arena, investigators are more likely to be successful in securing funding through federal sources, such as the NIH.

Nursing Organizations

Sigma Theta Tau International (STTI), the American Nurses Association (ANA), and the Oncology Nurses Society (ONS), are a few of the nursing organizations that fund research studies. STTI makes research grant awards to increase scientific knowledge related to nursing practice. STTI supports creative interdisciplinary research and places importance on identifying "best practices" and benchmark innovations. Awards are made at the international and local chapter levels. The ANA awards small grants through the American Nurses Foundation. Specialty nursing organizations offer grants to support research related to their specialty. For example, the ONS awards grants that focus on issues related to oncology.

To summarize, multiple potential sources of funding are available for research projects. The individual or group wishing to conduct research will need to carefully develop a proposal, search for a possible funding source, and submit the proposal. Libraries and the Internet provide ample information about the many foundations and organizations interested in funding research endeavors. Most research institutions establish offices that help in the search and procurement of funding. Thus researchers are supported in their work of knowledge building.

COMPONENTS OF THE RESEARCH PROCESS

The research process involves conceptualizing a research study, planning and implementing that study, and communicating the findings. The process involves a logical flow as each step builds on the previous steps. These steps should be included in published research reports so that the reader has a basis for understanding and critiquing the study (Box 6-2).

STUDY DESIGNS

Study designs are plans that tell a researcher how data are to be collected, from whom data are to be collected, and how data will be analyzed to answer specific research questions. Research studies are classified into two basic methods: quantitative and qualitative, two distinctly different approaches to conducting research. The researcher chooses the method based on the research question and the current level of knowledge about the phenomena and the problem to be studied. Quantitative research is a formal, objective, systematic process in which numeric

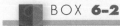

BOX **6-2**

Components of the Research Process

Research is a process that takes place in a series of steps:

1. Formulating the research question or problem
2. Defining the purpose of the study
3. Reviewing related literature
4. Formulating hypotheses and defining variables
5. Selecting the research design
6. Selecting the population, sample, and setting
7. Conducting a pilot study
8. Collecting the data
9. Analyzing the data
10. Communicating conclusions

data are used. Qualitative research is a systematic approach used to describe and promote understanding of human experiences related to health. Concepts such as pain, caring, caregiving, and depression are of primary importance to nursing (Speziale and Carpenter, 2007); thus qualitative research design provides a dimension of understanding to nursing science that adds to traditional quantitative methodology.

Quantitative Designs

Arising from early scientific models for doing research, the nursing discipline directly adopted the quantitative method of conducting research. Thus quantitative design has traditionally been prevalent in nursing research studies. Deriving meaning from the statistical analysis of numerical data obtained from samples and populations has yielded significant contributions to nursing knowledge. The usual intent of quantitative study is to apply or generalize knowledge from a smaller sample of subjects to a larger population. Quantitative studies usually produce knowledge about very precise topics, creating a need for multiple studies over multiple years before conclusive knowledge is yielded. The most common quantitative designs used in health care research are survey, needs assessment, experimental, quasi-experimental, methodologic, meta-analysis, and secondary analysis. A brief overview of these mostly quantitative study designs is given in Table 6-1. For in-depth understanding of particular methods and their suitability for studying particular phenomena, consult research methods texts.

Qualitative Designs

Qualitative research is a method of research designed for discovery rather than verification. It is used to explore little-known or ambiguous phenomena. The researcher is looking to explain phenomena or process rather than to verify a cause and effect. Qualitative methods can be important to the complex study of humans. Concepts that are important to health care professionals often are difficult to reduce in a quantitative way. Interviewing is the main technique used in qualitative methods to explore the meaning of certain experiences to individuals. This method is time consuming and costly and uses small samples; therefore, generalizations cannot be made from findings. However, when exploring issues, such as caregiver strain or hardiness, it might be more appropriate to interview participants to get their perspective than to send out a standard questionnaire that might not encompass everything the researcher would discover from personally interviewing the participant. The main types of qualitative research designs include phenomenology, ethnography, and grounded theory. Table 6-2 provides brief

TABLE **6-1**

A Sample of Quantitative Research Methodologies

METHOD	DESCRIPTION
Survey	Survey research designs are popular in nursing research studies that are designed to obtain information regarding the prevalence, distribution, and interrelationships of variables within a population. Surveys are a good design to use when collecting demographic information, social characteristics, behavioral patterns, and information bases.
Needs assessment	Needs assessments are used to determine what is most beneficial to a specific aggregate group. This design can be used by organizations, communities, or groups to establish priorities for their respective client groups (Polit and Beck, 2008).
Methodologic	Methodologic research focuses on the development of data collection instruments, such as surveys or questionnaires. The goal is to improve the reliability and validity of instruments. This work is time consuming and tedious, but necessary for the implementation of research studies. However, when quality instruments are developed, they can be used in multiple studies.
Meta-analysis	Meta-analysis is an advanced process whereby multiple research studies on a specific topic are reviewed and the findings of these multiple studies are statistically analyzed. Meta-analysis synthesizes quantitative data from multiple similar studies, thus enlarging the power of the results and allowing more confident generalizations than a single study.
Experimental study	Experimental studies, having several subtypes, include the manipulation of one or more independent variables, random assignment to either a control or treatment group, and observation of the outcome or effect that is presumably a result of the independent variable. Rigor and control of extraneous variables allow researchers to establish cause-and-effect relationships, testing causal relationships (Polit and Beck, 2006).
Quasi-experimental design	A quasi-experimental design lacking one of the required components of the experimental design. When randomization, a control group, or the manipulation of one or more variables is not possible, this is a useful design. Several subtypes exist.
Secondary analysis	Secondary analysis involves asking new questions of data collected previously. The data may have been generated from previous formal research or may have resulted from any prior systematic collection of data. Examples of prior nonresearch data include the many inevitable records generated as a by-product of health care delivery systems.

TABLE **6-2**

A Sample of Qualitative Research Methodologies

METHOD	DESCRIPTION
Phenomenology	Phenomenology is designed to provide understanding of the participants' "lived experience." Phenomenology is a valuable approach for studying intangible experiences, such as grief, hope, and risk taking.
Ethnography	Ethnography is a method used to study phenomena from a cultural perspective. Ethnographers spend time in the cultural setting with the research participants to observe and better understand their experience.
Grounded theory	Grounded theory is designed to explore and describe a social process. It is a method used to explore a process that people use to deal with problematic areas of their lives, such as coping with a terminal illness or adjusting to bereavement.

descriptions of these methods. For more complete understanding, refer to qualitative research texts.

Although there is a need for qualitative research studies in health care research, qualitative one-on-one interviews take time; they must be recorded, typed, transcribed, and analyzed. Data analysis is conducted by the researcher, who reviews each transcribed interview line by line to group common conceptual meanings. Concepts are combined to describe the experience for the particular group being studied. Qualitative studies usually have small samples, and results are not generalizable to the whole population. The researcher cannot assert that findings from a small unique sample would be the same in a large diverse population. However, findings should be transferable. The researcher should give a thorough description of the sample and setting so that findings could be expected to occur in similar individuals in a similar setting. In addition, triangulation studies that involve both quantitative and qualitative methods might provide the strength needed to recommend change based on qualitative research findings.

Triangulation

Triangulation is the use of various research methods or different data collection techniques in the same study. Triangulation commonly refers to the use of qualitative and quantitative methods in the same study. This method can be useful when data from multiple sources and methods are necessary to provide a relatively complete understanding of the subject matter.

Pilot Studies

Pilot studies are small-scale studies often referred to as feasibility studies. The purpose of the pilot study is to identify the strengths and limitations of a planned larger-scale study. Pilot work is preliminary research that can be used to assess the design, methodology, and feasibility of a study and typically includes participants who are similar to those who will be used in the larger research study. By performing each step of the procedures to be used in a planned larger-scale study, the researcher can evaluate the effectiveness of the proposed data collection methods. Information can be gained that will aid the improvement of the study and help assess the feasibility of the study (Polit and Beck, 2006).

Pilot studies can serve to determine the feasibility of using interventions and to discover preliminary trends in outcomes for a particular agency, personnel, and clients. Most funding agencies favor research that is based on pilot work, although a pilot study may not be warranted if the researcher has used the same techniques, instruments, and participants in the same or similar setting.

EVIDENCE-BASED PRACTICE AND RESEARCH UTILIZATION

From the beginnings of the nursing research endeavor, nurses have been interested in using nursing research to effectively impact the care of individuals and aggregate groups. Despite other incentives for the conduct of research, none is more powerful for a nurse than the difference that might be made in the lives of individuals and aggregates for the betterment of health. Thus early emphasis in the 1980s on research utilization has been expanded, with the increasing emphasis on EBP. Though the two terms, research utilization and EBP, are related, research utilization has been described as a subset of EBP (LoBiondo-Wood and Haber, 2006). EBP encompasses multiple types of evidence such as research findings, research reviews and evidence-based theory, and the integration of that evidence with clinical expertise and patient preferences and values (Melnyk and Fineout-Overholt, 2005).

In the approaching second decade of the twenty-first century, EBP is positioned to become a major driving force in the disciplinary life of clinicians, students, educators, administrators, and policymakers. Historically, there was concern that nurses have failed to realize the potential for using research findings as a basis for making decisions and developing nursing interventions. Discussion on those aspects of individuals and organizations that create barriers to research utilization and EBP has shifted to how to actively overcome barriers to the implementation of EBP. The gap between the discovery of knowledge and its use in practice remains (LoBiondo-Wood and Haber, 2006), but specific overcoming strategies are already being shared. Extensive work is being done on the best ways to translate research into practice, spawning a new area of health care science called translation science. Eventually the promise of translation science is to provide evidence on the best ways to incorporate best evidence into health care, including nursing. Whole texts are now available that explain the multiple aspects of EBP (Dawes et al, 2005; Hamer and Collinson, 2005; Larrabee, 2009a; Malloch and Porter-O'Grady, 2010; Melnyk and Fineout-Overholt, 2005), and various models have been proposed that more carefully detail the process of incorporating evidence into practice (Larrabee, 2009b; Mackay, 1998; Newhouse et al, 2007; Stetler, 1994; Titler et al, 2001). Within these named resources and many others resides a treasure trove of EBP history, resources, processes, examples, and results.

Advancing Evidence-Based Practice

How does one get started with EBP? A list of strategies for encouraging a climate of EBP is likely to look somewhat different depending on the context of care: Is the context of care delivery a clinic, a hospital, or a conglomerate? A short list of broad strategies suggested by Melnyk and Fineout-Overholt (2005) applies regardless of the setting:

- Assessment of barriers to EBP
- Correction of misperceptions about EBP goals and processes
- Questioning of current clinical practices

Assessment should be as comprehensive as possible in order to identify the knowledge, beliefs, and behaviors that are common in the existing system and to raise the awareness of a need for shifting decision making about clinical care toward a consideration of current best evidence. Misperceptions about EBP may include doubts about the feasibility of EBP initiatives within a busy clinical environment or the idea that EBP is a one-size-fits-all approach to patient care; both of these may be addressed by a learning process. Raising questions about current clinical practices provides a strategy for getting the critical thinking juices flowing about particular clinical practices and problems. Individuals with common interests may form collaborative groups that further strengthen the EBP culture through bonding around specific patient problems and the discovery of evidence-based solutions. The specific tactics, processes, and events that undergird an EBP initiative require allocation of resources, creativity, and dedication. Of particular significance to EBP initiatives is the availability of individuals in clinical environments who have the specific responsibility and expertise to understand and translate evidence into practice (Malloch and Porter-O'Grady, 2010).

Nurse Researcher and Evidence-Based Practice Roles

Two nursing roles are specifically focused on research and EBP: CNS and the CNR.

Clinical Nurse Specialist. The CNS is a registered nurse with graduate preparation in a specialized area of nursing practice and an expert clinician with additional responsibility for education and research. A CNS is in an ideal position to link research to practice by assessing an agency's readiness for research utilization, consulting with staff to identify clinical problems, and helping staff to discover, implement, and evaluate findings that improve health care delivery (National Association of Clinical Nurse Specialists, 2003, 2004). CNSs are educated in the research process and can conduct their own investigations and collaborate with doctorally prepared nurses.

Clinical Nurse Researcher. The CNR should be a doctorally prepared nurse with clinical and research experience. Terminology used to refer to this type of position tends to vary among countries, settings, and agencies. One might see position postings for clinical nurse scientist, nurse scientist, director of nursing research, and others. A CNR can focus either on the conduct or facilitation of research and should possess knowledge of statistics, grantsmanship, evaluation research, and administration. Interpersonal skills, such as patience, flexibility, and approachability, are imperative. A CNR employed by a hospital or home health agency must develop relationships with staff nurses to identify the research questions that staff nurses see as most significant in the particular setting. The CNR is responsible for designing studies and assisting staff nurses with understanding the implications of the study. In addition, the CNR provides guidance to the staff regarding their role in the research process. This role could involve patient recruitment for studies or actual data collection. The CNR also is responsible for disseminating findings of the research not only to staff nurses but also to administrators of the agency so that findings can be incorporated into practice.

The CNR also may need to communicate results to legislators or other policymakers if the results potentially affect health policy. Research evidence is important to policymaking because it provides a logical foundation for policy change. The process of writing brief summaries of evidence or personally testifying about particular topics should be approached carefully. One should know the exact policy issue, the background of the issue, and the full range of pertinent evidence (Melnyk and Fineout-Overholt, 2005).

If agencies do not have a CNR, they should be encouraged to develop relationships with researchers in university settings or other agencies. Professors in academic settings are expected to conduct research and often are interested in collaborating with health care agencies that might serve as a site. These agencies often have the patient population that can serve as a study sample. For example, a university professor interested in home health care issues might collaborate with an agency to examine the efficacy of various health care delivery models for patients with congestive heart failure. In a managed care environment, it would be essential for the agency to offer care that is the most effective and efficient. Therefore this collaborative relationship would have benefits for the researcher and the health care agency.

The following case study is an illustration of how a CNR led efforts to use research findings to improve practice.

CASE STUDY

Mary, a CNR in a medical center, asks the staff nurses on a pediatric oncology unit to identify patient care problems that need to be investigated. The nurses identify pain control as a major problem for the children admitted to the unit. In talking with the nurses on the unit, Mary discovers that the nurses routinely use physiologic measures, such as heart rate and blood pressure, as indicators of pain. Occasionally the nurses rely on parents' reports, but rarely do they consult the child. Mary conducts a review of the literature to determine proven ways to assess pain in children. In the *Western Journal of Nursing Research*, Mary discovers a meta-analysis of pediatric pain assessment techniques. Findings from this

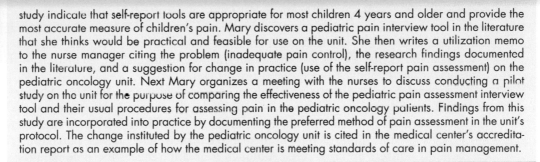

CASE STUDY—cont'd

study indicate that self-report tools are appropriate for most children 4 years and older and provide the most accurate measure of children's pain. Mary discovers a pediatric pain interview tool in the literature that she thinks would be practical and feasible for use on the unit. She then writes a utilization memo to the nurse manager citing the problem (inadequate pain control), the research findings documented in the literature, and a suggestion for change in practice (use of the self-report pain assessment) on the pediatric oncology unit. Next Mary organizes a meeting with the nurses to discuss conducting a pilot study on the unit for the purpose of comparing the effectiveness of the pediatric pain assessment interview tool and their usual procedures for assessing pain in the pediatric oncology patients. Findings from this study are incorporated into practice by documenting the preferred method of pain assessment in the unit's protocol. The change instituted by the pediatric oncology unit is cited in the medical center's accreditation report as an example of how the medical center is meeting standards of care in pain management.

Emerging Roles. In addition to the CNS and CNR, there are emerging role definitions for those of the clinical nurse leader (CNL) and the doctorate in nursing practice (DNP). Because of their newness and the sparse literature describing role development outcomes, the concrete research and EBP effect of individuals prepared for these roles is yet to be determined. Given the specified role definitions published by the American Association of Colleges of Nursing (AACN), the CNL and DNP are potential major contributors to the advancement of nursing research and EBP (AACN, 2006, 2007). Regardless of official role definition, nurses at the point of care and nursing division leaders may increasingly be called upon to lead and contribute to collaborative research and EBP initiatives at the health care agency level (Larrabee, 2009a).

About the Evidence

Some years ago, the author received a gift, a lapel button reading "Show me the evidence." The button underscored the practical expectation that practice decisions made from a foundation of evidence are more likely to be clear, rational, and motivational than those decisions made from the foundation of mere authority. Serving others within the discipline of nursing involves assent to authority. However, the idea of adhering to an authority-based practice or policy without the benefit of knowing the evidence behind it is less likely to persuade clinicians. Clinicians serve patients who value the benefit of a nurse who is able to differentiate between those clinical approaches derived from the best evidence and those based on tradition or authority. The questions then become, where and what is the best evidence?

Locating Published Research and Evidence Summaries for Evidence-Based Practice

Many health care practitioners may routinely read clinical practice journals, but are unfamiliar with research or EBP journals. Other than reading the occasional research report that may be disseminated through a practice journal, busy clinicians may not spend time browsing the library for research or evidence summaries. Computerized databases have aided the process of locating research and evidence summaries relevant to current practice. The number, scope, and ownerships of computerized databases change over time, making database access an important ongoing task for academic and heath care libraries. A consumer of health care literature is well served when he or she maintains working relationships with librarians at academic institutions and the workplace. CINAHL Information Systems (formerly the Cumulative Index to Nursing and Allied Health Literature, or CINAHL), historically has been a significant access point for nurses engaged in literature search (www.ebscohost.com/cinahl). CINAHL Information

Systems has undergone significantly enhanced services in recent years including the provision of online full-text articles, and multiple other record types. MEDLINE (Medical Literature Analysis and Retrieval System Online) is the most comprehensive online resource for national and international medical literature (U.S. National Library of Medicine, 2008). Multiple other useful databases may be available from academic and health care libraries. Computerized literature databases may simply list article information, include short summaries of the article contents, or provide linked access to full-text articles.

Traditionally, printed journal articles have been available on the shelves of libraries in paper or microfiche format. If articles are not available locally, users may request that their library acquire the articles from another library (interlibrary loan). Increasingly, in the past few years, university and public libraries have been able to enhance collections by purchasing electronic databases of full-text online articles. Although it greatly reduces the time required to access certain articles, this feature is expensive for libraries to obtain and maintain. Many journals are available online through prescription, or articles may be purchased online directly from publishers. Because of online availability through libraries or individual purchase, there is a temptation to novice users to limit searches to only those articles that are available online as full text. This is a serious mistake that any investigator of published literature should avoid.

Literature searches should be conducted with the intent of procuring all or most of the current articles appropriate to the topic of interest, regardless of the ease of obtaining sources. A truly comprehensive reading of the literature may include all articles of current and historical relevance to the topic. Therefore, a relatively comprehensive literature search must anticipate by many weeks the time when the researcher needs the articles in hand.

Even though nurses may have access to computerized databases to assist with a literature search, they often are unaware of the journals that are devoted entirely to the publication of research studies and the summaries derived from them. Box 6-3 contains a list of research journals and other health-related journals that publish research and evidence summaries.

BOX **6-3**

Nursing and Health-Related Research and EBP Journals

NURSING	HEALTH
Advances in Nursing Science	*American Journal of Public Health*
Applied Nursing Research	*Hastings Center Report*
Biological Research for Nursing	*Health Affairs*
Clinical Nursing Research	*Health Care Management Review*
Evidence-Based Nursing	*Health Services Research*
International Journal of Nursing Studies	*Heart & Lung*
Journal of Nursing Scholarship	*Journal of Pain & Palliative Care*
Journal of Advanced Nursing	*Pharmacotherapy*
Journal of Transcultural Nursing	*International Journal of Evidence-Based*
Nursing Clinics of North America	*Healthcare*
Nursing Economics	*Journal of Health Economics*
Nursing Research	*Journal of the American Medical*
Nursing Science Quarterly	*Association*
Qualitative Health Research	*New England Journal of Medicine*
Research in Nursing and Health	*Oncology Nursing Forum*
Western Journal of Nursing Research	*Social Science and Medicine*
Worldviews on Evidence-Based Nursing	

Another important publication is the *Annual Review of Nursing Research*. As of 2008, the book was in its twenty-sixth volume. The purpose of this annual publication is to conduct systematic reviews of nursing literature, to provide guidance to graduate students and faculty in specific fields for research, and to provide critical evaluations for health policymakers (Abdellah and Levine, 1994). These volumes are an excellent resource for nurses involved in the development and use of research. For example, if a nurse wants to study children's responses to cancer, a good starting point in the literature review stage is to read the review of "Research on Child Health and Pediatric Issues" in the *Annual Review of Nursing Research*, volume 21, that includes studies such as "Symptom Experiences of Children and Adolescents with Cancer" authored by Sharron Docherty (Fitzpatrick, Miles, and Holditch-Davis, 2003). This review gives a summary of published studies focusing on symptoms experienced by children living with cancer. In 2008 the focus of the *Annual Review of Nursing Research* was rural health (Fitzpatrick and Merwin, 2008). From the sampling, one can see that the clinical topics vary broadly. Important information includes study designs, variables considered, instruments, important clinical evidence from each of the reviewed studies, and gaps that exist in the body of research that has already been conducted. Reviews usually include suggestions for further study on the particular topic reviewed.

Types and Levels of Evidence

Evidence exists in many forms. Perhaps the most obvious form is the journal article describing a single research study. When a particular topic has been studied extensively, the set of research articles available for knowledge building may also be extensive. Prior to the current disciplinary emphasis on EBP, it would have been the responsibility of the reader of these reports to critique each article and decide which, if any of the research findings, could be used in practice (research utilization). Though this technique of logical narrative summary continues to be somewhat useful, more systematic methods have been developed for synthesizing multiple research reports on a single topic. These systematic review methods include meta-analysis (already referred to in the CNR case study) and meta-synthesis, as well as other forms of systematic review. In a meta-analysis, the findings of multiple quantitative studies on a single topic are statistically analyzed to produce a summary statistic. A meta-synthesis takes the findings of multiple qualitative studies on a single topic and synthesizes and amplifies the narrative information contained in the reports. The importance of such reviews is that they represent a meticulous integration of the best evidence available at the time the review was conducted (Polit and Beck, 2008). Therefore, individuals or agencies with clinical questions are able to consult well-prepared knowledge syntheses for possible application in the practice arena.

In the United Kingdom, which played a major role in the development of EBP, the Cochrane Collaboration (www.cochrane.org) has published hundreds of intervention guidelines based on meta-analyses and research reviews of important health care practice areas. These guidelines are mainly medical in nature, but not exclusively so. For example, in a review of 29 studies comparing nursing intervention for smoking cessation with comparison groups, nurse counseling on smoking cessation significantly increased the likelihood of quitting (Rice and Stead, 2007). Also Gray and Flenady (2001) reviewed clinical trials that compared modified open-cot nursing for preterm infants with incubator care. The review concluded that there was not enough information to recommend cot nursing as an alternative to incubator care. Therefore, research reviews do not automatically yield consensus or recommendations for a practice guideline. In the health care environment, where costs are an important factor, care alternatives are likely to be suggested and subsequently undergo trial and evaluation. Research reviews may then have a role in preventing scientifically unfounded alternatives from being promoted in clinical care.

Although research evidence forms the backbone of EBP, other evidence types such as patient values and preferences, expert opinion, theory-based information, evidence-based theories, and compiled database information are usefully included in the evidence pool when clinical decisions are at issue (Fawcett and Garity, 2009; Malloch and Porter-O'Grady, 2010; Melnyk and Fineout-Overholt, 2005). At the point when care is being delivered to an individual, evidence regarding patient assessment and resource availability must also be considered (Melnyk and Fineout-Overholt, 2005).

With such an array of evidence types, it is not surprising that evidence is viewed as requiring an assessment of just how strong it is. The terms, evidence hierarchy, levels of evidence or strength of evidence are used to refer to the categorical classifications that have been proposed to rate evidence along a continuum of best evidence to worst evidence. Most rating schemes rate meta-analyses of well-conducted randomized clinical trials (RCTs) as best evidence, with other evidence types sitting lower in the hierarchy (Polit and Beck, 2008). One of the tasks of the consumer of evidence is to attend to the strength of various evidence types used for decision making about care and care processes.

Critical Appraisal

Nurses of all levels of educational preparation should critically read research journal articles and research summary articles. Research reports and research summaries are published in research or specialty journals. These articles are accepted on a competitive basis and are peer reviewed. Researchers who are doing work in the particular field of study are asked to review the article and recommend whether the journal should publish the article. The review is called a blind review because the reviewers are unaware of who wrote the article. Therefore, readers generally can assume that experts have scrutinized it for merit and relevance to nursing. If the article is reporting the results of a research study that has been funded by a grant, this is acknowledged in the credits of the article. This is added verification for the reader that the study has gone through review and probably is valid. However, readers cannot assume that findings are valid; therefore, articles must be critically appraised. Critical appraisal of the validity of research findings through detailed analysis of study design and measurement strategies is another layer of evaluation that must be incorporated into appraisal of research evidence for possible use in practice. The abstract section of the article gives an overview of the study, and the discussion section offers suggestions for nursing practice based on the findings of the research study. These two sections often are the easiest for the novice to interpret. If sections on methods or statistics are confusing, the reader should consult a CNR to help interpret results.

Pre-appraised evidence such as systematic reviews also require appraisal but the emphasis is on whether the review provides ample and trustworthy evidence for answering a particular clinical question and the strength of that evidence. The appraisal of various types of research and research summary articles for application to practice are best approached through using defined appraisal guidelines. EBP textbooks are an excellent source of these guidelines. Careful appraisal may or may not lead one to make a change in practice. If change is implemented, there is an ethical responsibility to evaluate the quality of patient outcomes derived from the change.

Rather than being a simple process of implementing the practice suggestions found at the end of a research report, use of research requires careful and complex analysis, wise implementation, and patient outcome assessment. On the way to becoming seasoned evidence-based nurses, novice nurses should avail themselves of expert guidance from CNRs, CNSs, and other experienced health care professionals. Novice nurses can also develop skill in EBP by reviewing and digesting some of the various proposed models for research utilization and EBP.

Evolution of Evidence-Based Practice: Some Examples

Though much work remains to be done, the potential effect of research on health care knowledge and practice can be demonstrated by three examples.

The use of heparinized saline for flushing capped peripheral intravenous catheters was compared with saline only. Saline only was found to be clinically effective in maintaining patency of peripheral catheters (Goode et al, 1991, 1993). As a result of this research, many acute care facilities revised their institutional policies to recommend saline only as a flush for peripheral intravenous catheters. In contrast Shah, Ng, and Sinha (2006), in a review of heparin use in neonates with peripheral intravenous catheters, concluded that the evidence is still insufficient for making a recommendation for the neonate population.

Research on cancer-related fatigue has been ongoing for the past decade. Mock (2003), an oncology nurse, described a set of four studies conducted to ascertain the effects of moderate exercise on individuals undergoing active cancer treatment. Results indicated that the prescribed exercise had beneficial effects on fatigue, sleep, functional capacity, and activity levels. From that foundational research arose multiple other studies by multiple investigators. By 2008 there was a sufficient research evidence base to support systematic review. Cramp and Daniel (2009) conducted a systematic review of randomized controlled trials that investigated the effect of exercise on cancer-related fatigue in adults. The conclusion was that exercise is beneficial for individuals during and after cancer treatment. In this particular context, the notion that rest is the simple remedy for fatigue is refuted. Thus research evidence plays a role in supporting or refuting common and logically held notions.

Pressure ulcers are a significant problem for multiple populations. It should not be surprising that many groups are interested in their prevention and treatment. An online search of the National Guideline Clearinghouse (NGC) yielded multiple clinical guideline statements contributed by groups, public and private, nursing and medical. The national identities of those contributing included New Zealand, Singapore, the United States, and the United Kingdom. In the case of pressure ulcers, a significant amount of research evidence is available for implementing prevention and management strategies.

From the three examples it can be seen that research evidence can play a significant role in health care practice. However, the process of spreading the "good news" about new or refined practice-related knowledge is a complex one. Researchers must make the knowledge they generate available and understandable. Practitioners must access, digest, interpret, and carefully apply research evidence to the unique contexts presented by individual patients and by patient populations. Different persons and populations need not respond similarly to interventions. Also there can be honest disagreement among experts about the evidence required to support a practice change. The scientific process may take years to yield enough data to make clinical recommendations and more years to evaluate the effect of evidence-based changes through outcomes research. Although these difficulties exist, nursing and other health care disciplines will continue to be held accountable by the public for developing and using the best available evidence for providing health care. A specific methodology for condensing and disseminating evidence is through the development of clinical practice guidelines.

Clinical Practice Guidelines

A clinical practice guideline (CPG) is an evidence-based guide to clinical practice developed by experts in a particular field for direct application in clinical environments (definition derived from Polit and Beck, 2008). In 1992 the federal government demonstrated support for research utilization activities when the AHCPR within the U.S. Department of Health and Human Services (USDHHS) convened panels of experts to summarize research and develop CPGs. These panels summarized research findings and developed practice guidelines in the following three areas:

- Acute pain care management in infants, children, and adolescents
- Prediction and prevention of pressure ulcers in adults
- Identification and treatment of urinary incontinence in adults

Under the reauthorization of 1999, the AHRQ (formerly AHCPR) continues to support research utilization through its oversight of the NGC. Although AHRQ is no longer mandated to directly develop practice guidelines, the agency continues to carefully compile guidelines submitted from a wide variety of groups. NGC guidelines are freely and publicly accessible, making them a valuable source for the public, health care professionals, and agencies seeking guidance on clinical practices.

In the past decade, the development of CPGs by various groups has greatly increased. This is a positive development for EBP, even though the strictness of the process of synthesis used by guideline developers tends to vary. Thus end users of CPGs should carefully appraise them before accepting or adapting the recommendations for local implementation (Melnyk and Fineout-Overholt, 2005; Polit and Beck, 2008). CPGs can be found through Internet search or directly from the websites of multiple specialty organizations and through library database searches. Accessing the full text of CPGs is not straightforward because many organizations make guidelines accessible only to members, to paid subscribers, or through direct purchase. Despite this access difficulty, acquiring CPGs can be worth the effort for individuals and organizations intent on creating an evidence-based culture.

ETHICAL ISSUES RELATED TO RESEARCH
Institutional Review

In institutional review, a committee called an IRB or human subjects committee examines research proposals to make sure that the ethical rights of those individuals participating in the research study are protected. Persons participating in research must be assured that their right to privacy, confidentiality, fair treatment, and freedom from harm is protected. They must sign an informed consent that explains the study and assures them of their rights, including their right to refuse to participate or to withdraw from the study. Institutions that receive federal funding or conduct drug or medical device research regulated by the U.S. Food and Drug Administration (FDA) are required by federal regulations to establish an IRB. Studies that are funded federally have to meet strict guidelines to ensure the protection of the human rights of subjects, such as self-determination, privacy, anonymity and confidentiality, fair treatment, and protection from discomfort and harm. The IRB is responsible for reviewing the study procedures and process of informed consent to ensure the protection of subjects. The informed consent must include essential study information and statements about potential risks and benefits, protection of anonymity and confidentiality, voluntary participation, compensation, alternative treatment, and specific information on how to contact the investigator (Polit and Beck, 2008).

Historical Examples of Unethical Research

In addition to the institutional review process, a number of codes and regulations have been implemented to ensure ethical conduct in research. The two historical documents are the Nuremberg Code and the Declaration of Helsinki, which were developed in response to unethical acts, such as the Nazi experiments. These experiments occurred in the 1930s and 1940s and included experiments with untested drugs, sterilization, and euthanasia on prisoners of war. These experiments were unethical not only because they caused harm to the subjects but also because the subjects were not given the opportunity to refuse participation (Polit and Beck, 2006).

Another famous incident of unethical research that prompted the need to oversee the conduct of research is the famous Tuskegee syphilis study. This study, which was initiated by the U.S. Public Health Service, continued for 40 years. The study was conducted to determine the natural course of syphilis in African-American men. Many participants were not adequately informed about the purpose and procedures of the study. The subjects were examined periodically, but did not receive treatment for syphilis, even after penicillin was determined to be effective. The study was not stopped until 1972, when public outrage was sparked by published reports of the study (CDC, 2009). *Bad Blood* (Jones, 1993), a comprehensive documentary account of the Tuskegee syphilis study, clearly relates the study's adverse effects on research participation by African-Americans and on race relations in the United States.

As late as the 1960s, another famous study that violated human rights took place. The Jewish Chronic Disease Hospital in New York was the setting for a study to determine patients' rejection of liver cancer cells. Twenty-two patients were injected with liver cancer cells without being informed that they were taking part in the research. In addition, the physician directing the study did not have institutional approval for a study that had the potential to cause the subjects harm or even death (Polit and Beck, 2006).

In institutions in which IRB approval is not required for nonfederally funded programs, the researcher should seek external advice regarding ethical considerations. When IRB approval is an option, researchers should seek it because IRB approval demonstrates scientific rigor to the audience when the research is disseminated either through presentation or publication.

SUMMARY

Educators must prepare health care professionals to have an appreciation of research and to participate in research design implementation and evaluation at the level of their preparation. Practicing nurses of various educational levels must actively seek, develop, and adopt EBP protocols while encouraging affiliated institutions to support this effort. Health care administrators must facilitate an environment that fosters intellectual curiosity and supports research efforts. Collaborative arrangements between health care agencies and universities must be developed for such activities as student projects, continuing education, development of clinical practice guidelines, and research endeavors. Consumers must be educated about the value of health care research, and policymakers must be informed of pertinent findings so that results can be translated into health policy.

⊝volve   Additional resources are available online at: http://evolve.elsevier.com/Cherry/

REFERENCES

American Association of Colleges of Nursing: *The essentials of doctoral education for advanced nursing practice*. 2006. Available online at: www.aacn.nche.edu/DNP/pdf/Essentials.pdf.

American Association of Colleges of Nursing: *White paper on the education and role of the clinical nurse leader*. 2007. Available online at: www.aacn.nche.edu/Publications/WhitePapers/ClinicalNurseLeader07.pdf.

Abdellah F, Levine E: *Preparing nursing research for the 21st century*, New York, 1994, Springer.

Agency for Healthcare Research and Quality: *Mission and budget*. 2009a. Available online at: www.ahrq.gov/about/budgtix.htm.

Agency for Healthcare Research and Quality: *Healthcare innovations exchange*. 2009b. Available online at: www.innovations.ahrq.gov/index.aspx.

Brown S: *Knowledge for health care practice: a guide to using research evidence*, Philadelphia, 1999, Saunders.

Burns N, Grove S: *Understanding nursing research: building an evidence-based practice*, ed 4, St. Louis, 2007, Saunders.

Caramanica L, Cousino JA, Peterson S: Four elements of a successful quality program: alignment, collaboration, evidence-based practice, and excellence, *Nurs Adm Q* 27:336–343, 2003.

Centers for Disease Control and Prevention: *U.S. Public Health Service syphilis study at Tuskegee*. 2009. Available online at: www.cdc.gov/tuskegee/timeline.htm.

CINAHL Information Systems: *Products and services*. 2006. Available online at: www.cinahl.com/prodsvcs/prodsvcs.htm.

Cramp F, Daniel J: Exercise for the management of cancer-related fatigue in adults. Cochrane Database of Systematic Reviews [serial online]. Available from: CINAHL, Ipswich, MA. Accessed June 24, 2009.

CURN Project: *Using research to improve nursing practice, series of clinical protocols: clean intermittent catheterization (1982), closed urinary drainage patient care (1982), pain: deliberative nursing interventions (1982), preventing decubitus ulcers (1982), reducing diarrhea in tube-fed patients (1981), structured preoperative teaching (1981)*, New York, 1981, 1982, Grune and Stratton.

Dawes M, et al: *Evidence-based practice: a primer for health care professionals*, Philadelphia, 2005, Elsevier.

Fain JA: *Reading, understanding, and applying nursing research*, ed 2, Philadelphia, 2004, FA Davis.

Fawcett J, Garity J: *Evaluating research for evidence-based nursing practice*, Philadelphia, 2009, FA Davis.

Fitzpatrick JJ, Merwin E: *Annual review of nursing research: focus on rural health*, New York, 2008, Springer.

Fitzpatrick JJ, Miles MS, Holditch-Davis D: *Annual review of nursing research: research on child health and pediatric issues*, New York, 2003, Springer.

Goode CJ, et al: A meta-analysis of effects of heparin flush and saline flush: quality and cost implications, *Nurs Res* 40:324–330, 1991.

Goode CJ, et al: Improving practice through research: the case of heparin vs. saline for peripheral intermittent infusion devices, *Medsurg Nurs* 2(1):23–27, 1993.

Gray PH, Flenady V: Cot-nursing versus incubator care for preterm infants (Cochrane Database of Systematic Reviews). In *The Cochrane Library*, Issue 2, 2001. Last updated Jan 20, 2003, Chichester, UK, John Wiley & Sons, Ltd.

Hamer S, Collinson G: *Achieving evidence-based practice: handbook for practitioners*, ed 2, Philadelphia, 2005, Ballière Tindall.

Horsley JA, Crane J, Bingle JD: Research utilization as an organizational process, *J Nurs Adm* 8(7):4–6, 1978.

Horsley JA, et al: *Using research to improve nursing practice: a guide, CURN project*, New York, 1983, Grune and Stratton.

Jones J: *Bad blood: the Tuskegee syphilis experiment*, rev ed, New York, 1993, Free Press.

Krueger J: Utilization of nursing research: the planning process, *J Nurs Adm* 8(1):6–9, 1978.

Krueger JC, Nelson AH, Wolanin MO: *Nursing research: development, collaboration, and utilization*, Germantown, MD, 1978, Aspen.

Larrabee J: *Nurse to nurse: evidence-based practice*, New York, 2009a, McGraw-Hill.

Larrabee J: The model for evidence-based practice change. In *Nurse to nurse: evidence-based practice*, New York, 2009b, McGraw-Hill.

LoBiondo-Wood G, Haber J: *Nursing Research: methods and critical appraisal for evidence-based practice*, ed 6, St. Louis, 2006, Elsevier.

Mackay M: Research utilization and the CNS: confronting the issues, *Clin Nurse Spec* 12:233–237, 1998.

Malloch K, Porter-O'Grady T: *Introduction to evidence-based practice in nursing and health care*, ed 2, Sudbury, MA, 2010, Jones and Bartlett.

Melnyk BM, Fineout-Overholt E: *Evidence-based practice in nursing and healthcare*, Philadelphia, 2005, Lippincott Williams & Wilkins.

Mock V: Clinical excellence through evidence based practice: fatigue management as a model, *Oncol Nurs Forum* 30:790–796, 2003.

National Association of Clinical Nurse Specialists: *What is a clinical nurse specialist?* 2003. Available online at: www.nacns.org/faqs.shtml.

National Association of Clinical Nurse Specialists: *Statement on clinical nurse specialist practice and education*, Harrisburg, PA, 2004, Author.

National Institute of Nursing Research: *NINR Strategic Plan*. 2006. Available as pdf download online at: www.ninr.nih.gov.

Newhouse RP, et al: *Johns Hopkins nursing evidence-based practice model and guidelines*, Indianapolis, IN, 2007, Sigma Theta Tau International.

Office of Science Policy and Public Liaison: Personal communication, *NINR*, May 27, 2009.

Polit D, Beck C: *Essentials of nursing research: methods, appraisal and utilization*, ed 6, Philadelphia, 2006, Lippincott Williams & Wilkins.

Polit D, Beck C: *Nursing research: generating and assessing evidence for nursing practice*, ed 8, Philadelphia, 2008, Lippincott Williams & Wilkins.

Prospect Research Online: *How do I subscribe?* 2009. Available online at: www.iwave.com.

Rice VH, Stead LF: Nursing interventions for smoking cessation (Cochrane Database of Systematic Reviews). In *The Cochrane Library*, Issue 1, 2004. Last updated October 21, 2007, Chichester, UK, John Wiley & Sons, Ltd.

Robert Wood Johnson Foundation: *About us*. 2009a. Available online at: www.rwjf.org/about.

Robert Wood Johnson Foundation: *What we fund*. 2009b. Available online at: www.rwjf.org/applications/whatwefund.jsp.

Shah PS, Ng E, Sinha AK: Heparin for prolonging peripheral intravenous catheter use in neonates (Cochrane Database of Systematic Reviews). In *The Cochrane Library*, Issue 4, 2006. Last updated June 1, 2005, Chichester, UK, John Wiley & Sons, Ltd.

Speziale H, Carpenter D. *Qualitative research in nursing: advancing the humanistic imperative*, ed 4, Philadelphia, 2007, Lippincott Williams & Wilkins.

Stetler CB: Refinement of the Stetler/Marram model for the application of research findings to practice, *Nurs Outlook* 42:15-25, 1994.

Titler MG, et al: The Iowa model of evidence-based practice to promote quality care, *Crit Care Nurs Clin North Am* 13(4):497-509, 2001.

U.S. National Library of Medicine: *Fact sheet MEDLINE*. 2008. Available online at: www.nlm.nih.gov/pubs/factsheets/medline.

WK Kellogg Foundation: *Our work*. 2009. Available online at: www.wkkf.org.

CHAPTER

7

Paying for Health Care in America: Rising Costs and Challenges

Marylane Wade Koch, MSN, RN

(e)volve   Additional resources are available online at: http://evolve.elsevier.com/Cherry/

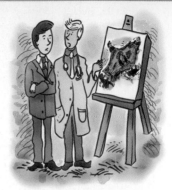

There is a tug of war for the shrinking health care dollar.

VIGNETTE

As a home care nurse for many years, Callie Thompson's patients were primarily older adults. Knowledge of Medicare coverage guidelines for service was critical to the financial success of the home care agency. Today in the home care agency she cares for patients of all ages with varying reimbursement guidelines. These guidelines, which affect the types of services she provides for her patients, differ among managed care organizations (MCOs), government-provided coverage, and insurance companies. When she first took this job, understanding Medicare coverage guidelines was a new challenge. Now even more is required. Callie knows that today's nurse needs extensive knowledge of health care reimbursement guidelines and the economic influences on professional practice to provide quality patient care.

■ QUESTIONS TO CONSIDER WHILE READING THIS CHAPTER:

1 Often the role of the professional nurse is influenced by the employer's ability to pay for the costs associated with staffing and providing quality health care services. Is this likely to continue in today's evolving health care environment?

2 What do health care economics have to do with me as I provide patient care?

3 Why do I need to understand health care economics and its implications for my practice? Is that not the role of the finance department or business office at my workplace?

4 With so many variations in health care insurance, I have a hard time understanding my own policy coverage. What role do I have in assisting my patients in understanding their insurance or coverage options? Can being a more informed consumer add value to my practice?

KEY TERMS

Capitation A method of reimbursing providers (usually primary care providers, such as physicians or nurse practitioners) in which the insurance company pays the provider a set amount of money each month to provide a defined set of health care services for the patient enrolled in the insurance company's health plan. The payment is typically expressed as a per-member-per-month payment. The defined health care services generally include preventive, diagnostic, and treatment services.

Centers for Medicare & Medicaid Services (CMS) The federal government agency that administers Medicare and Medicaid.

DRGs (diagnosis-related groups) Refers to reimbursement for health care services based on a predetermined fixed price-per-case or diagnosis in 468 categories.

Effectiveness Production of a desired outcome; take the right action to achieve the expected result.

Efficiency The extent to which resources, such as energy, time, and money, are used to produce the intended result.

GDP (gross domestic product) The measure of the total value of goods and services produced within a country; the most comprehensive overall measure of economic output; provides key insight to the driving forces of the economy.

Marginal An economic term that refers to a small or insignificant change in some variable (e.g., the number of tests performed).

Medicaid A jointly sponsored state and federal program that pays for medical services for persons who are elderly, poor, blind, or disabled and for certain families with dependent children who meet specified income guidelines.

Medicare A federally funded health insurance program for the disabled, persons with end-stage renal disease, and persons 65 years of age and older who qualify for social security benefits.

Prospective payment system A method of reimbursing health care providers (i.e., physicians, hospitals) in which the total amount of payment for care is predetermined based on the patient's diagnosis; provides for a "set price per diagnosis" payment system in contrast to the retrospective or "fee-for-service" system; encourages increased efficiency in the use of health care services because providers are reimbursed at a set level regardless of how many services are rendered or procedures performed to treat a particular diagnostic category; most common method of payment in today's health care system.

Private health insurance A method for individuals to maintain insurance coverage for health care costs through a contract with a health insurance company that agrees to pay all or a portion of the cost of a set of defined healthcare services such as routine, preventive, and emergency health care; hospitalizations; medical procedures; and/or prescription drugs. Typically the private insurance is provided through an individual's employer with a portion of the cost paid by the employer and a portion paid by the employee. Private insurance policies can also be purchased by individuals but are generally much more expensive than when provided through an employer's group plan.

Provider An individual (such as a physician or nurse practitioner) or an organization (such as a hospital) that receives reimbursement for providing health care services.

Retrospective payment system A method of reimbursing health care providers (i.e., physicians, hospitals) in which professional services are rendered and charges are billed based on each individual service provided; also known as the "fee-for-service" payment system. This system may encourage overuse of health care services because the more services rendered or procedures performed, the more revenue received by providers.

Single payer system A method of reimbursement in which one payer, usually the government, pays all health care expenses for citizens, funded by taxes. Decisions about covered treatments, drugs, and services are made by the government. Though the terms *universal health care* and *single payer system* are sometimes used interchangeably, universal health care could be administered by many different payer groups; both offer all citizens health insurance coverage.

Third-party payer An organization other than the patient and the supplier (hospital or physician), such as an insurance company, that assumes responsibility for payment of health care charges. An individual's health insurance plan provided by his or her employer is considered a third-party payer.

After studying this chapter, the reader will be able to:

1 Analyze major factors that have influenced health care access and financing since the middle of the twentieth century.

2 Analyze the relationship between market issues and health care resource allocation.

3 Integrate knowledge of health care resources, access, and financing into managing professional nursing care.

4 Critique the relationship between contemporary economic issues and trends and professional nursing practice.

CHAPTER OVERVIEW

In the past several decades the costs of health care have continued to increase, with economic issues taking a central role in health care decision making. Hospital managers know that for most patients the hospital will receive a predetermined payment, regardless of length of stay and specific treatments. Physicians and nurse practitioners recognize that the prescribed course of treatment for their patients may be analyzed by a peer review committee; the costs their patients incur may be compared with those of other providers or against cost benchmarks. Businesses require employees to cover larger amounts of their health insurance premiums or pay larger deductibles and copayments. Health insurance companies "manage" care, sometimes placing limits on medical care coverage or on the site of care delivery. These practices are the result of the evolving economics of health care.

The objective of this chapter is to provide an overview of the major economic issues and trends driving changes in health care delivery, how health care is paid for, and how these issues affect nursing practice. The chapter presents information about historical trends in health care finance, the problem of the uninsured and underinsured, allocation of health care resources, methods of paying for health care, and the effect of health care finance on professional nursing practice.

HISTORY OF HEALTH CARE FINANCING

The high costs of health care did not occur overnight. To understand current health care financing, it is necessary to understand its history (Table 7-1). Historically, several underlying themes have driven health care financing in the United States. Among these are:

◆ The physician's role as being primarily responsible for health care decision making

◆ The broad objective of providing the "best" possible care to everyone

◆ The rapidly increasing sophistication and cost of medical technology

◆ Economic incentives and the fee-for-service payment method that encouraged overuse of health care services

For many years, physician domination in decision making and the fee-for-service payment method were intertwined and contributed to the lack of cost consciousness in health care. Physicians made all decisions about what health care services were needed; costs were rarely discussed between physician and patient, so the cost of care was not considered until bill-paying time. Medical tests or procedures were provided if the physician determined that they offered even marginal aid or diagnostic information.

TABLE **7-1**

Historical Highlights of Health Care Finance

1847	Massachusetts Health Insurance of Boston offers group policy.
1861-1865	Insurance plans available during the Civil War.
1890	Individual disability and/or illness policies available.
1929	First group health coverage for a monthly charge; teachers in Dallas, Texas, contract with Baylor Hospital. This is the beginning of Blue Cross/Blue Shield Insurance.
1932	Blue Cross insurance formed.
1934	Hospitals receive payment through Blue Cross, prepaid health insurance plan to protect hospitals during the Great Depression.
1945	Blue Cross captured 50% of insurance market.
1946	California Physician Service ensures physician payment through Blue Shield plans.
1950s	Employee benefit packages initiated to attract workers.
1954	Government disability program available with social security coverage.
1965	Medicare and Medicaid programs created, making comprehensive health care available to millions of Americans.
1977	Health Care Financing Administration (HCFA) created to manage Medicare and Medicaid separately from the Social Security Administration.
1980-1990	Managed care plans emerge.
1983	Hospitals come under diagnosis-related groups (DRGs).
2001-2003	The Centers for Medicare & Medicaid Services is created, replacing the HCFA.
2003	Enactment of the Medicare Prescription Drug Improvement, and Modernization Act of 2003, the most significant expansion of Medicare since its enactment, including a prescription drug benefit.
2006	Blue Cross/Blue Shield plans cover more than 94 million Americans (1 in 3 Americans). Pay-for-performance is introduced as a model of reimbursement for health care services.

Sources:
www.hhs.gov/about/hhshist.html.
www.lieberson.com/en/medical_history_and_ethics/history/history_of_health_insurance.htm.
www.wpri.org/Reports/Volume19/Vol19no10.pdf.

Beginning in the 1960s, "if it might help, do it" flourished as the rapid pace of sophisticated technologies enhanced physicians' abilities to provide treatment. The more tests or procedures physicians performed, the greater their earnings because physicians were paid according to the number of procedures performed or services provided. Instead of attempting to allocate medical resources to the highest medical need, the financial incentive was to provide as much care as possible using the most technically advanced methods of care. Overuse of health services and rapid cost inflation resulted.

Yet consumers of health care remained insulated from cost inflation. Most patients had some form of insurance or "third-party payment" and did not pay the full cost for their care or even for their health insurance premiums. The full cost of care remained hidden from consumers because costs were subsidized by employers or by taxpayers through such programs as Medicare and Medicaid. Providers had little incentive to contain costs so the demand for medical care generated "perverse" economic incentives in which providers received more income for using more services with no financial risk for their use of additional resources.

These perverse economic incentives had a drastic effect on the Medicare program. Medicare was established by the U.S. Congress in 1965 to provide health insurance coverage for people age 65 and older who are eligible for social security benefits, people with end-stage renal disease, and the eligible disabled population. By the early 1980s, increased medical usage (increased intensity of care) and high inflation combined with a growing older adult population generated substantial increases in Medicare costs. The rapid growth of Medicare expenditures became a major factor in the federal budget deficit, causing the Centers for Medicare & Medicaid Services (CMS) to rethink the entire Medicare payment system and led to a revolution in how the government and private insurance companies paid for health care.

Health Care Financing Revolution

In 1965 health care expenditures in the United States were $202 per person; in 2004 health care expenditures had risen to $6280 per person. National health expenditures as a percentage of gross domestic product (GDP) rose to 17% in 2008, which means that for every dollar a person spends buying products or services in the United States, 17 cents goes to pay for health care. In contrast health care spending was 10.9 % of the GDP in Switzerland, 10.7% in Germany, 9.7% in Canada, and 9.5% in France, and each of these countries provide health coverage for all their citizens (National Coalition on Health Care, 2009). Health care spending increased from $1.3 trillion in 2000 to $2.4 trillion in 2008. Projections show that by 2017, health care in the United States will reach $4.3 trillion and consume 20% of the GDP (National Coalition on Health Care, 2009). The rising cost of health care is a dangerous trend that poses a significant threat to the U.S. economy.

To control rapidly rising health care costs, a health care financing revolution began in 1983, when Medicare moved from a retrospective (fee-for-service) reimbursement to a prospective payment system (PPS) based on diagnosis-related groups (DRGs). This shift was critical for hospitals because Medicare is the largest single payer of hospital charges. Under DRGs each Medicare patient is assigned to a diagnostic grouping based on his or her primary diagnosis at hospital admission. Medicare limits total payment to the hospital to the amount preestablished for that DRG, unlike the previous approach in which hospital patients incurred costs and Medicare reimbursed these charges with a generous payment schedule.

Since 1983, if hospital costs exceed the DRG payment for a patient's treatment, the hospital incurs a loss, but if costs are less than the DRG amount, the hospital makes a profit. Thus hospitals face a strong financial incentive to reduce the patient's length of stay and minimize procedures performed. Although DRGs originally applied only to hospital payments for Medicare patients, similar reimbursement arrangements were initiated by private insurance companies.

Implementation of the DRG system expanded the role of hospital management, including nurse administrators. First, financial gains were made from careful diagnosis of patients according to their highest potential DRG classification. Hospital-based utilization management nurses reviewed medical records to determine the most appropriate DRG for patients. Second, hospital record keeping and accounting methodologies were revolutionized by specific Medicare cost accounting procedures. Experienced nurses with business knowledge brought needed technical background and skills to these new accounting and utilization management tasks, expanding opportunities for nurse managers and nurse administrators.

By the early 1990s the financing revolution extended to physician reimbursement. The previous Medicare physician fee system was replaced with the resource-based relative value scale (RBRVS) reimbursement system. The objective was to bring payments for medical services in line with the physician skills required and the actual time spent on specific procedures. For example, when Medicare initially covered payment for cataract surgery, it was a relatively rare and lengthy procedure. However, over time cataract correction became a frequently performed Medicare surgical procedure, viewed by CMS as overpaid. The RBRVS system corrected the disparity between Medicare's high payments for this type of procedure and relatively low payments for more hands-on primary care.

The Development of Managed Care

With the shift to prospective payment under Medicare, private insurance companies followed Medicare's lead and developed managed care. MCOs encompass several different approaches, such as health maintenance organizations (HMOs), preferred provider organizations (PPOs), and point-of-service (POS) plans (Table 7-2). The primary commonality among each of these health plans is that they use some method to review and provide oversight for the use of health care services. In this review process, the patient's medical options are reviewed by a nurse or physician employed by the health insurance company and a judgment is made as to the necessity of the service being considered. Coverage may be denied for unnecessary, excessive, or experimental procedures, in strong contrast to the previous "if it might help, do it" approach. The goal of managed care is to minimize payment of charges for inappropriate or excessive health care services.

By the late 1980s, the increasing costs for businesses to provide health insurance for their employees were passed to consumers by increasing the price for their products or services. U.S. businesses struggled to compete in an international market, where health care costs were significantly lower. Large businesses, such as automobile manufacturers, pushed health insurance companies to decrease the rapid rise of insurance premiums. Employer health insurance markets moved rapidly from conventional insurance plans to MCOs. The Employer Health Benefits 2008 Annual Survey conducted by the Kaiser Family Foundation showed the percentage of workers who are offered a PPO option increased from 45% in 1996 to 89% in 2008 (Kaiser Family Foundation, 2008). With managed care, the private insurance market initially slowed growth in health care costs. Unfortunately, this accomplishment was short-lived.

ACCESS TO HEALTH CARE—THE PROBLEM OF THE UNINSURED AND UNDERINSURED

As health care costs continue to rise dramatically in the United States, one major issue that needs to be addressed is access to health care for the uninsured or underinsured. Lack of access to health care today primarily reflects a lack of insurance coverage, so access is an issue of financial access. In 2006 the population without insurance coverage rose to nearly 47 million but declined to 45.7 million in 2007 (U.S. Census Bureau, 2007). The uninsured and underinsured include the working poor employed by small firms without insurance coverage, part-time workers, and unemployed people. See Table 7-3 for an idea of the average costs of some health care services and consider this in light of a family with an annual income of $25,000 and no health insurance.

Medicaid, a federal health insurance program administered by each state, is intended to improve access to health care for the poor, covering approximately 43 million people. However, even with improved access as compared with the uninsured, Medicaid recipients are not as likely to obtain needed health services. The poor are more likely to lack a usual source of care, less likely to use preventive services, and more likely to be hospitalized for avoidable conditions than those who are not poor.

Lack of insurance is a serious problem for households and presents problems for providers and for insurers as well. The uninsured and underinsured populations generate uncompensated or indigent care costs and bad debt for health care providers. Unpaid costs must be covered by those who do pay so the hospital can continue operating, a process known as cost shifting. Providers increase their charges against households and public and private

TABLE **7-2**

Common Types of Health Insurance Plans in America

Fee-for-service (FFS)/ indemnity plan	• Member (covered individual) pays a premium for fixed percentage of expense covered. • Includes deductible and copayment. • Allows member to choose physician and specialists without restraint. • May only cover usual or reasonable and customary charges for treatment and services, with member responsible for charges above that payment. • May or may not pay for preventive care.
PPO (preferred provider organization)	• Member (covered individual) pays a premium for fixed percentage of expense covered. • Includes deductible and copayment. • Member may select physician, but pays less for physicians and facilities on the plan's preferred list. • May or may not pay for preventive care.
POS (point of service)	• Offered by HMO or FFS. • Allows use of providers outside plan's preferred list or network, but requires higher premiums and copayments for services.
HMO (health maintenance organization)	• Member (covered individual) pays a premium. • Has a fixed copayment. • Member must select primary care physician approved by HMO. • Member must be referred for treatments, specialists, and services by primary care physician. • Services outside of "network" must be preapproved for payment. • Plan may refuse to pay for services not recommended by primary care physician. • Encourages use of preventive care.
Medicare	• Federal health insurance plan for Americans 65 and older and certain disabled people. • Client must be eligible for social security or railroad retirement. • Part A covers hospital stays. • Part B requires payment of a premium and covers physician services and supplies. • Carries a prescription drug benefit.
Medicaid	• Health care coverage for low-income people who are aged, blind, disabled, or certain families with dependent children. • Federal program is delivered and managed by each state for eligibility and scope of services offered.
TRICARE: military health insurance (formerly CHAMPUS)	• Civilian health and medical health insurance program for military, spouses, dependents, and beneficiaries. • Program offered through Military Health Services System.

Sources:
Checkup on health insurance choices available at: www.ahrq.gov/consumer/insuranceqa/insuranceqa.pdf.
Medicare and you 2009 available at: www.medicare.gov/Publications/Pubs/pdf/10050.pdf.
TRICARE: military health insurance (formerly CHAMPUS) available at: www.ha.osd.mil.

insurers who pay for their own care plus make some contribution for the care of the uninsured population. This increases insurance premiums, making it even more difficult for many households and businesses to afford coverage. Experts in California estimate that cost shifting caused by the uninsured population costs each family in that state approximately $1,186

TABLE **7-3**

What Health Care Costs

Typical adult physician office visit	$60-$170
Adult Emergency room visit	$383-$700
Magnetic resonance imaging (MRI)	$500-$3500
Vaginal delivery of a baby average hospital bill	$5000-$10,000
Cesarean section	Add at least $2000
Baby born premature or with health problems needing neonatal care	Ranges from a few thousand to $200,000
Total knee replacement	$45,000
Balloon angioplasty	$29,000-$43,000
Coronary bypass surgery	$20,000- $44,820
Bone marrow transplant	$100,000-$250,000

Sources:
www.bcbstx.com/employer/hccc/topic6.htm
http://www.bluecrossma.com/common/en_US/pdfs/SampleMedicalCosts.pdf
http://ezinearticles.com/?Cost-of-MRI-Procedures-Affording-Medical-Care&id=1996703.
www.pregnancy.lovetoknow.com/wiki/Cost_of_Having_a_Baby.
www.marchofdimes.com/aboutus/14458_15365.asp.
www.progenyhealth.com/public/Clinical%20and%20Financial%20Perspectives%20in%20NICU%20Care%20Management.pdf.
www.wockhardthospitals.net/knee-replacement.asp.
www.bcbst.com/learn/treatment-options/balloon_angioplasty_medical_technology_rating.shtm.
www.drcranton.com/chelation/angioplasty.htm.
www.consumeraffairs.com/news04/2005/bypass.html.
www.acor.org/ped-onc/treatment/BMT/BMT.html.

in annual premiums (Klein, 2006). The problem of uncompensated care and cost shifting is a major reason that many people advocate some form of national or universal health insurance coverage.

In February 2009, President Obama issued a call to Congress to enact major health care reform to include a mechanism to provide health insurance for America's uninsured populations. Massachusetts passed the nation's first near-universal health care plan, creating a mechanism that covers at least 95% of its citizens. Clearly, some form of government health care coverage is on the horizon to address the serious problems of uninsured U.S. citizens.

ALLOCATION OF HEALTH CARE RESOURCES

The health care system of any society consists of its financing mechanisms, its health and medical institutions, and any additional resources that affect health. Health care resources can be allocated in a limited number of ways. The following sections describe considerations for resource allocation and economic approaches to resource allocation.

Health Care Resources

Health care resources include the inputs devoted to producing health care: (1) "labor," such as nurses, physicians, technicians, pharmacists, and administrators, with their education, skills, and training; (2) "capital" including medical facilities and equipment; (3) "land," the land area for hospitals and other facilities; and (4) "entrepreneurship," skills and risk taking of health businesses and new ventures. Because health care resources are "scarce" or limited in the amounts available at any given time, decisions (choices) must be made about how to best use them. Health care resources must be allocated based on such decisions and choices made by government and society.

Resource Allocation Questions

Each society decides how to allocate its health care resources. The following questions are important for resource allocation decision making:

◆ How much or what share of all goods and services should be devoted to health care?

◆ If the share of expenditures devoted to health care increases, what non-health goods and services can be eliminated to transfer those resources to health care?

◆ What combination of specific health care services should be produced?

◆ Will high-tech institution-based health services emphasizing crisis-oriented medical care be preferred, or will a prevention-oriented health system emphasizing primary care and wellness be chosen? For example, if the society decides to allocate more scarce health resources to hip replacements for older adult osteoporosis patients, then there may be fewer health care resources to allocate to other areas, such as prenatal care or child health screenings.

◆ Who should receive the medical goods and services? This depends largely on who has the health insurance coverage to finance the purchase of health care.

If the society has some form of national health insurance, then all citizens should have financial access to available medical care. In contrast in the United States, federal or state funding is only provided for defined groups that have eligibility for specific programs, such as Medicare and Medicaid. Some groups, such as veterans, have established (or legislated) "rights" to medical care, but the overall entire population does not. The way a society answers these basic questions defines that society's type of health care system.

Economic Approaches to Allocating Health Care

To understand economic approaches to health care, it is necessary to have some understanding about market systems and the nature of competitive market systems. The next important point to understand is how the third-party payment system for health care that currently exists in the United States violates the economic principles of competitive market systems.

Market System. A market system is a means by which a buyer and a seller come together so that the buyer can purchase products or services from the seller. A market system implies (1) private ownership of resources and (2) private decision making by consumers about their purchases and by businesses about their products and sales. Decisions are largely based on the prices of goods and services. To function effectively and efficiently, the market system should be competitive. The U.S. economy is founded on the principles of a competitive market system, which are:

◆ Numerous buyers and sellers are in the market, so no single seller can manipulate the price.

◆ Products of all suppliers in similar markets are similar.

◆ Consumers and sellers are well informed about market conditions and prices.

◆ New resources are free to enter or leave this market.

No advanced industrial country has a purely competitive market system for the allocation of health care resources. The United States and South Africa are the only industrialized Western countries without a national health insurance system covering all of their citizens. Most European countries have a substantial amount of central government planning in their health systems, with Great Britain being a primary example of a fully centralized or nationalized system. Almost all of the health care resources in the British National Health Service (e.g., hospitals, clinics, nursing homes) are owned and run by the government.

Regulated market systems imply some sort of government control over the business owners and sellers in the market. The U.S. health care system is considered a regulated market system because it is regulated to some extent by federal or state legislation. Examples of a regulated market system for health care include requirements of minimal nurse staffing in long-term care facilities, laws regarding the disposal of medical waste products, and regulations affecting the conduct of medical laboratories. In addition, all licensure and certification laws or qualifying examinations represent regulation of medical professionals.

Although the United States has a regulated health care market system, these markets are not really competitive and thus are out of sync with the rest of the U.S. economy. Consider how the health care market system violates the principles of a competitive market system previously discussed:

- Consumers may not know what health care to purchase without a provider's diagnosis.
- Consumers do not get information about the prices of services until after the services are provided.
- Once the patient visits the provider for health care services, that provider is likely to be in charge of numerous subsequent decisions, so the provider becomes an "agent" for the patient.
- The provider's reimbursement incentives may encourage overuse or underuse of treatment options.

Third-Party Payers. Another issue affecting health care markets is "third-party payers," which are entities other than the patient that assume responsibility for payment of health care charges. The health insurance company that makes payments for health care is the most common type of third-party payer in the United States. Third-party payers interfere with common principles of a competitive market system. A competitive market system assumes that people make their decisions to purchase something on the basis of its price, but health care consumers often pay less than the "full price" because their insurance pays some or all of the cost. Consider the following scenario. If an employer bought "shoe insurance" for employees so they only had to pay a coinsurance payment of perhaps $10 (or possibly only 20% of the full price) for shoes, how many pairs would an employee buy? And would the employee buy more expensive or cheaper shoes? This demonstrates that insurance coverage, or third-party payment, adds to the confusion of health care markets. Remember that the cost of the "shoe insurance"—or health insurance—is passed on to consumers in the form of price increases for the products or services offered by the business paying the health insurance premiums for its employees. Because of these "hidden" health care costs, the patient perceives health care as much cheaper than it actually is and may not be motivated to make informed decisions about the cost of various health care options.

HOW HEALTH CARE IS PAID

A combination of private and public sources pays for health care services and supplies for individuals in the United States. Most individual health care is paid either by households through direct out-of-pocket payments or by third-party public or private insurers (Table 7-4). Third-party payers include private insurance companies and government health programs (Medicare, Medicaid, and the Veterans health system).

Private Insurance

Private insurance accounts for the largest percentage of coverage for health care with the cost of providing health insurance to employees passed on by the employer to the consumer in the pricing of goods and services. This means that everyone pays a part of the country's health

TABLE **7-4**

Health Insurance Coverage in America (2008)

People with health insurance in America	255.1 million or approximately 84% of population
People without health insurance	46.3 million or 15.4% of population
Children under age 18 without health care coverage	7.3 million or 9.9% of children
People covered by employer plans	176.3 million or 58.5% of population
People with government insurance	87.4 million or 29% of population (42.6 million Medicaid; 43.0 million Medicare, other military)

Source: U.S. Census Bureau: http://www.census.gov/hhes/www/hlthins/hlthin08/hlth08asc.html.

care costs in every purchase made. Individuals still must pay a portion of their health care costs directly from their own pockets through payments for insurance premiums, deductibles, and copayments.

With managed care products, such as HMOs, PPOs, and POS arrangements, the premium the consumer pays for coverage has continued to rise. The Kaiser Health Survey 2008 demonstrates this point with a 5% increase in consumer premiums over those in 2007 and documents an 119% increase in family plan premiums since 1999 (Kaiser Family Foundation, 2008). In response to these concerns, some companies now offer their employees high-deductible health plans (HDHPs), health reimbursement accounts (HRAs), health savings accounts (HSAs), or a combination of these. These plans offer more flexibility and consumer discretion over their health care dollars and provides a tax-free way to save for future health care needs (U.S. Office of Personnel Management, 2006).

Public Insurance: Medicare and Medicaid

Government is the biggest influence in the health insurance market, generating half of hospital revenues and more than one fourth of physician incomes. The largest health insurance program is Medicare. Since enactment of the program by the federal government in 1965, the population covered by Medicare has doubled. Medicare is an entitlement program based on age or disability criteria rather than on need. Medicare Part A covers inpatient hospital services, skilled nursing facilities (SNFs), and home health benefits. Hospital coverage has deductible and coinsurance requirements and some coverage limitations. In January 2006, Medicare added access to a prescription medication benefit, a noted and costly change from previous benefits.

Medicaid is a joint federal-state program to provide health insurance coverage for impoverished families, particularly those with children. States establish Medicaid eligibility criteria based on their Aid to Families with Dependent Children (AFDC) income eligibility levels. The federal government establishes minimum coverage that states may supplement. Medicaid covers primarily disabled persons, AFDC households, and those in nursing homes who qualify based on their low income level. Medicaid is the primary payer of long-term care nationwide, covering almost half of all nursing home costs. In addition, Medicaid is required to cover the deductibles and copayments for Medicare beneficiaries who are impoverished and thus termed dual eligible (i.e., dual eligible for both Medicare and Medicaid). For most states, Medicaid represents the fastest growing component in the state budget.

Effect of Payment Modes

New methods of reimbursing providers for health care services are emerging because of the rapid growth in health care costs combined with concerns about the safety and quality of health care. For the first time in the history of health care payment systems, hospitals can be rewarded for achieving improved health outcomes and will not be paid for certain medical errors. As described here, two new payment methods—(1) pay-for-performance and (2) "never events"—are focused on aligning reimbursement with patient outcomes. Nurses are at the very center of helping hospitals and other health care organizations successfully manage these new payment mechanisms by ensuring that health outcomes are achieved and errors are prevented.

Pay-for-Performance. Medicare and private insurance companies are showing success with various methods of reimbursing providers based on the quality of care provided with an emphasis on prevention and reducing complications from chronic diseases. Such programs, known as "pay-for-performance" or P4P, provide financial and nonfinancial incentives to promote high-quality care. Hospitals and other providers are rewarded for meeting standards of care for certain conditions such as diabetes, myocardial infarction, pneumonia, and heart failure. Studies suggest that the verdict is still out on the value of P4P payment systems, but there is evidence of modest improvement in care processes in hospitals participating in P4P programs as compared to hospitals receiving standard Medicare reimbursement (Mehrotra et al, 2009). There is definitely a need for continued research into the value and effectiveness of P4P payment methods. Nurses need to stay alert for developments in P4P because they will have a very significant effect on quality patient outcomes and successful P4P reimbursement.

Never Events. In an effort to save lives and millions of dollars, Medicare adopted a policy effective October 1, 2008, that it will no longer pay hospitals for the extra costs of treating preventable errors. Commonly referred to as never events, hospitals will no longer be paid by Medicare for the cost of treating 28 medical errors that are largely preventable and have serious consequences for patients. The purpose of the never events payment policy is to eliminate payments for certain medical errors and encourage hospitals to direct resources to preventing errors rather than being paid for them. Never events include hospital-acquired infections, injuries from falls, wrong site surgery, and mismatched blood transfusions. A full list of never events is available online at www.cms.hhs.gov/apps/media/press/factsheet.asp?Counter=3043. It is also important to note that most private insurance companies typically follow Medicare's lead in payment methods so "never events" for private insurance companies are sure to be on the horizon.

IMPLICATIONS FOR NURSES: MANAGING COST-EFFECTIVE, HIGH-QUALITY CARE

Nurses represent a major professional force in the delivery of health care services in the United States and are absolutely essential to the delivery of high-quality and efficient health care (Needleman & Hassmiller, 2009). Never has there been greater opportunity to advance the practice of professional nursing and affect health care financial reimbursement. Innovation and excellence in all nursing practice is needed to contain costs while attaining positive, measurable outcomes. As the reader can see from the new methods of reimbursement discussed earlier, nurses are at the center of ensuring positive patient outcomes and maximizing reimbursement.

BOX **7-1**

Economic Issues and Trends

FROM		TO
Illness emphasis	→	Preventive emphasis
Acute care	→	Preventive, home care
Hospital or institution based	→	Noninstitution based (clinic or home)
Fee-for-service (cost based)	→	Prospective payment and managed care
Physician directed	→	Diverse decision makers and managed care
If it might help, use it	→	Outcomes measurement and cost-effectiveness
Independent decisions (practice variation)	→	Protocols and guidelines (best practice)
Local perspective (practice variation, standards, and benchmarking)	→	Global perspective (protocols/guidelines/ practice)
Introduction of new technologies (regardless of cost)	→	Outcomes measurement and cost-effectiveness
Paper records, medical charts	→	Information systems, computer records

Every setting in which professional nurses practice holds challenges in providing and managing care that is efficient, affordable, and of high quality. Box 7-1 summarizes the trends occurring in health care that affect professional nurses. These trends mandate that nurses have a clear understanding of the economic and financing issues underlying the continually developing roles of nurses.

The American Nurses Association (ANA) published its Health System Reform Agenda in 2008. The highlights of this agenda include ANA's support for quality health care as a basic human right and universal access to health care for all U.S. citizens, preferably with a single payer approach. This agenda also confirms that the health care policies must be outcomes based and reflect the six quality aims of the Institute of Medicine: health care that is safe, effective, efficient, timely, patient-centered, and equitable. Care provided should be targeted toward primary care to lower dependence on costly secondary and tertiary care. ANA advocates a team approach that includes consumers, providers, policymakers, and industry leaders to solve the U.S crisis with an affordable health care system. Access this agenda at: www.nursing world.org/MainMenuCategories/HealthcareandPolicyIssues/HealthSystemReform/Agenda/ ANAsHealthSystemReformAgenda.aspx.

Nursing Practice and Health Care Finance Decisions

Many opportunities for nurses in today's health care environment are economically and politically driven. Changes in the financing of health care services directly affect professional nursing practice. Following are several reasons why payment reform is important to nursing:
- ◆ The rules of payment are important as a reflection of the value and worth society places on health care services for the public.
- ◆ Government policy influences the public's openness to secure services from various professionals, such as nurse practitioners.
- ◆ Financing affects salaried employees because health care providers build job opportunities based on payment sources. For instance, if a professional service is covered under reimbursed allowances, jobs in that service will be offered by the provider.
- ◆ Payment modes will determine whether a particular nursing role will be reimbursed, affecting specialties and professional autonomy.

As national health care concerns change, the financing rules will reflect the attitudes of policymakers and hopefully the public at large. In particular, Medicare payment changes will increasingly affect nursing practice as the number of older adults depending on Medicare for their primary health insurance increases. Nurses must be proactive and position themselves educationally and professionally to work with the economic challenges of health care.

Efficiency and Effectiveness of Care

Nurses provide services as a resource in the health care delivery system to produce patient care and care management. As such, nurses are key to achieving efficiency (using the right combination of resources—energy, time, and money—to accomplish a task) and effectiveness (do the right thing right) in health care. Nurses can affect the cost and quality of care by care coordination, case management, disease management, and outcomes management. Because resources are limited and decisions are based on service costs, administrators may combine non-nursing resources with limited nursing resources to decrease the total cost of services. Thus professional nurses are pressured to demonstrate excellent clinical resource management and to design care delivery that provides a less costly service that satisfies the customer requirements.

Care Coordination. Integrated or coordinated care is one way to decrease duplication of services and reduce wasted health care resources. This type of care uses case management and integration of services for cost-efficient care. More care is delivered in the community through home care, outpatient clinics, and ambulatory care centers at less costly rates; more expensive inpatient hospital-based care decreases. Changes in the health care environment require professional nurses to understand basic principles of financial and resource management and to take a leadership role to ensure the effective and efficient use of resources.

Case Management. Case management offers nurses the opportunity to demonstrate cost-effectiveness by ensuring that patients get effective treatment in the appropriate level of care across the continuum of care. Opportunities exist for nurses who understand the overall structure and processes of the health care industry and who bring skills of critical thinking and patient advocacy. Understanding current health care economics is critical to this role. The American Association of Managed Care Nurses (www.aamcn.org) provides excellent resources for nurses interested in advancing their case management skills.

Disease Management. This coordinated process is designed to manage and to improve the health status of a defined patient population over the course of a disease. Professional nurses can impact effectiveness and efficiency of health care services through disease management. Some controversy exists about whether these programs consistently deliver improved care in a cost-effective way, but reports continue to be positive. For example, Bray and colleagues (2008) described positive results in a study about use of diabetes life coaches in disease management. Participants experienced decreased complications from their diabetes with this program, with statistically significant improvements in seven targeted areas. The Disease Management Association of America (DMAA) is committed to disease management research and support as a way to decrease health care costs in this county. Their 2009 almanac states that $1.7 trillion was spent in 2007 treating chronic illness in the United States. This group advocates health promotion and disease prevention with disease care management for those Americans at risk and those with chronic disease (DMAA, 2009).

Outcomes Management. Nurses are most successful when they can demonstrate efficiency of care with measurable, effective outcomes. Nurses should know how much their services cost, at what price services can be offered, and how effective patient care outcomes can be achieved. They must minimize resource use, demonstrate a decrease in costs, and respond to the economic incentives of prospective payment and capitation. Rewards will come to those health care professionals who can manage the costs of disease and teach the value of good health.

Expansion of Technology

Improved technology for diagnostic and therapeutic practice is under examination for cost-efficiency versus outcome delivery. Leaders must balance the health contributions of the improved technology and the accompanying costs with issues of quality of life, access to care, risk-benefit analysis, and individual consumer choice.

U.S. consumers have had access to high levels of technology with little concern for costs. Nurses are key players in educating patients and families about the cost-to-benefit ratio of certain technologies and can assist in selecting alternative treatment options. One example is found in the increased use of pharmaceuticals; more advanced drugs are marketed with varying degrees of actual documented benefit over existing, less-expensive drugs. Patients may not trust generic drugs, although they are less expensive. The nurse can be a link to educating the public regarding the potential and implications of using a less expensive drug instead of a more expensive alternative.

The technology of the Internet offers promise for information and education that will allow consumers (or patients) to access health care resources more effectively. Some health care plans offer subscribers free newsletters that highlight ways to prevent disease and to manage chronic illness for improved quality of life and lower costs.

Information technology provides the professional nurse the ability to gather and analyze health-related information and data for improved care. Health care information systems are expensive, but they offer many opportunities for managing health care costs. Combining clinical skills with information technology skills can provide a significant advantage to the success of professional nurses because they demonstrate their ability to provide cost-effective outcomes measurement.

Consumer Empowerment

Health care customers are demanding quality health care services at affordable rates. Economic forces are motivating the shift toward a model of health promotion and preventive care to achieve cost-effectiveness. This brings a new relationship with the consumer, emphasizing cost sharing through individual choices in health practices. For instance the insurance rate may be higher, and/or benefits may vary, based on the presence of unhealthy personal practices, such as smoking, illegal drug use, or sedentary lifestyle. Smokers may pay higher rates and have to be smoke-free for 1 year to qualify for lower rates. Excess body weight may cost the subscriber more in premiums because this poses additional health concerns and potential increased health costs. See Box 7-2 for ways to help consumers reduce their health care costs.

Hawaii was recognized by the U.S. Department of Health and Human Services for the state's Healthy Hawaii program started in 1999. This statewide initiative, funded in part by tobacco settlement funds, includes healthier vending machine options in schools, funded walking trails, health promotion campaigns, and school education programs for healthier lifestyles (Healthy Hawaii Initiative, 2007). In January 2009 the Hawaii Medical Services Association launched the first "real-time online care system" designed to connect patients/consumers and

BOX **7-2**

Ways to Reduce Health Care Costs as a Consumer

- Take good care of yourself. Manage minor illnesses yourself at home.
- Use the Internet to learn more about your health and preventing disease.
- Recognize early warning signs of disease and get prompt treatment from your health care provider.
- Practice preventive health with health screenings and routine self-examination. Take advantage of free screenings offered at community sites, at hospitals, or at churches.
- Develop an active relationship with health care providers to improve communication. Ask providers to explain the purpose of all prescribed tests and medications. Become an informed consumer.
- Use emergency care only in emergencies. See your health care provider during office hours.
- Know health risks for lifestyle choices, such as alcohol and drug use, dietary habits, sedentary behaviors, and safety at home and while driving.
- Understand and use the health care benefits of the insurance plan you have to stay healthy. Take advantage of all preventive benefits offered.
- Choose nonhospital alternatives for treatment whenever possible. Take a conservative approach to health care. Comparison shop for health care alternatives.
- Choose generic drugs whenever possible. Ask your health care provider to prescribe the least expensive drugs that will provide positive outcomes.
- Review your health care bills carefully and notify provider and/or facility and/or agency of errors.

Sources:
www.missourifamilies.org/FEATURES/healtharticles/health38.htm.
www.bankrate.com/brm/news/insurance/20061204_care_cost_health_a1.asp.
www.nfib.com/object/4287945.html.

physicians and to lower health care costs with convenient information and improved access to physicians (IIMSA, 2008; to learn more go to www.iimsa.com/mediacenter/print/assets/annu alreport2008.pdf).

Nurses have many opportunities in a consumer-empowered marketplace. Nurse practitioners have demonstrated their ability and skills to deliver customer-focused primary care at reasonable costs as a cost-effective alternative to physician services. Opportunities for advanced practice nurses include primary care, case management, utilization management, quality improvement, patient advocacy, triage, education, and resource management. Nurses must take the lead in demonstrating the value of wellness and teaching health consciousness. Written materials for all levels of education will be needed, providing yet another opportunity for nurses who want to publish.

SUMMARY

Changes in the focus of the U.S. health care delivery system bring new challenges for professional nurses. Health care has moved from an emphasis on illness to an emphasis on wellness and prevention and is shifting from acute care services to preventive and community-based services, such as ambulatory care and home care. Financing of health care services has gone from retrospective, fee-for-service payment systems to prospective payment and managed care and continues to evolve to new models, such as pay-for-performance and never events. Today technology is viewed as important to health care delivery, but its value is based on having the appropriate service at the right price.

U.S. leaders and legislators agree that health care costs are too high, but they differ in the best ways to stop the increased cost of health care and insurance premiums. Some favor government control of health care for all citizens, whereas others believe a free market approach is preferred. Few think the current approach can support the escalating costs for consumers as well as employers. Most agree that when citizens practice healthy lifestyles, they require less health care and enjoy a better quality of life. However, what will motivate people to make healthier choices and practice disease prevention?

What do these changes in health care delivery mean to professional nursing? Nursing practice in a cost- and quality-conscious environment is here to stay. Nurses must constantly challenge current practice for quality improvement and cost-effectiveness. Accurate data must be collected to show cost containment and positive patient outcomes. Nurses need to be leaders and have a voice in the ever-changing economic and political environment that determines payment for services. Roles on clinical teams, in administration, with insurance companies, and with the government hold promise for empowered change. Professional nurses can prepare for these evolving careers with a commitment to lifelong learning. (Box 7-3 lists online resources to learn more about health care costs and finance.) Nurses can take the lead by being healthy role models, educating consumers, and encouraging personal responsibility for improved health practices. Managing care brings nurses back to the basics as society recognizes that healthy people are good business.

 Additional resources are available online at: http://evolve.elsevier.com/Cherry/

BOX **7-3**

Helpful Websites and Online Resources

American Association of Managed Care Nurses
    www.aamcn.org
American Case Management Association
    www.acmaweb.org
Centers for Disease Control and Prevention
    www.cdc.gov/nchs/fastats/hexpense.htm
Health Care Financing Review—sponsored by
Centers for Medicare & Medicaid Services
    www.cms.hhs.gov/HealthCareFinancingReview
    www.healthierUS.gov

Healthcare Financial Management Association
    www.hfma.org
Managed Care Magazine Online
    www.managedcaremag.com
Pay for Performance—Centers for Medicare &
Medicaid Services
    www.cms.hhs.gov/MedicaidSCHIPQualPrac/
    03_P4P.asp
U.S. Census Bureau
    www.census.gov

REFERENCES

ANA Health System Reform Agenda. 2008. www.nursingworld.org/MainMenuCategories/Healthcareand PolicyIssues/HealthSystemReform/Agenda/ANAsHealth SystemReformAgenda.aspx.

Bray K, et al: Defining success in diabetes disease management: digging deeper in the data, *Dis Manag* 11(2): 19–128, 2008. Retrieved from: www.liebertonline.com/doi/abs/10.1089/dis.2008.112722.

Disease Management Association of America. www.dmaa.org.

Hawaii Medical Service Association: *Annual report.* 2008. Available online at: www.hmsa.com/mediacenter/print/assets/annualreport2008.pdf.

Healthy Hawaii Initiative, Hawaii State Department of Health.2007.www.healthyhawaii.com/about_hhi/about_start_living_healthy/about_the_healthy_hawaii_initiative.htm.

Kaiser Commission on Medicaid: *Medicaid and the uninsured.* 2008. Available online at: www.kff.org/medicaid/upload/7235_03-2.pdf.

Kaiser Family Foundation: *Employer health benefits 2008 annual survey.* 2008. Available online at: http://ehbs.kff.org/images/abstract/7791.pdf.

Klein E: *Going universal: the American healthcare system is, simply put, a mess, but we may finally be ready to fix it,* latimes.com. Retrieved December 26, 2006, from: www.latimes.com/news/opinion/la-oe-klein26dec26,0,5461327.story?coll=la-opinion-rightrail.

Mehrotra A, et al: Pay-for-performance in the hospital setting: what is the state of the evidence? *Am J Med Qual* 24(1):19–28, 2009.

National Coalition on Health Care: *Health insurance costs.* 2009. Available online at: www.nchc.org/facts/cost.shtml.

Needleman J, Hassmiller S: The role of nurses in improving hospital quality and efficiency: real-world results, *Health Affairs* 28(4):w625–w633, 2009.

U.S. Census Bureau: *Income, poverty, and health insurance coverage in the United States.* 2007. Retrieved 2008 from: www.census.gov/prod/2008pubs/p60-235.pdf.

U.S. Office of Personnel Management: *High deductible health plans (HDHP) with health savings accounts (HSA).* 2006. Available online at: www.opm.gov/hsa.

Legal Issues in Nursing and Health Care

Laura R. Mahlmeister, PhD, RN

*e*volve Additional resources are available online at: http://evolve.elsevier.com/Cherry/

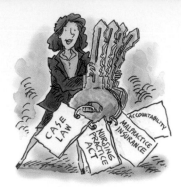

Knowledge of the law enhances the nurse's ability to provide safe and effective care.

VIGNETTE

Mary Clark is a registered nurse (RN) employed in the emergency department (ED) of a large for-profit hospital. The facility treats clients who are privately insured and individuals with Medicare coverage. Nurse Clark is the assigned triage nurse when Mr. Jones, a 48-year-old, walks in for evaluation. He states that he has persistent, mild substernal pain that is now radiating laterally toward both shoulders. His skin is pink and dry, and he does not appear to be in obvious distress. His vital signs, taken at the triage desk, are within normal parameters. He reports eating half of a garlic pizza and drinking three beers 1 hour ago. "I'm pretty sure it's just indigestion. This happened before when I ate garlic." He also tells the nurse, "I know I'm supposed to go to Community Hospital; I have 'feel-well' insurance, but I'm miserable and don't want to drive 10 miles across town in rush hour traffic with this much pain."

Mr. Jones is enrolled in a health maintenance organization (HMO). The HMO may not reimburse the for-profit hospital for Mr. Jones's visit if it is determined that his condition was not a true emergency after review by the HMO's utilization review department. In that case Mr. Jones will have to pay out of pocket for the medical evaluation and care received in the ED. In this cost-conscious health care environment, the nurses in the ED are well aware of the financial losses their hospital has recently suffered as a result of unpaid emergency services. Nurses in this facility are expected to contribute to the facility's success in reducing operating costs.

■ QUESTIONS TO CONSIDER WHILE READING THIS CHAPTER:

1 What is nurse Clark's legal duty in this situation?

2 What legal principles underlie the nurse's obligations to the patient?

3 What laws, if any, would govern the nurse's decision-making process in this case?

4 If Mr. Jones is not evaluated or treated and suffers a myocardial infarction while driving to Community Hospital, who would be legally accountable for his injuries? The nurse? The for-profit hospital? The HMO that may not have reimbursed for services?

Accountability Being responsible for one's actions; a sense of duty in performing nursing tasks and activities.

Advance directives Written or verbal instructions created by the patient describing specific wishes about medical care in the event he or she becomes incapacitated or incompetent. Examples include living wills and durable powers of attorney.

Case law Body of written opinions created by judges in federal and state appellate cases; also known as judge-made law and common law.

Civil law A category of law (tort law) that deals with conduct considered unacceptable. It is based on societal expectations regarding interpersonal conduct. Common causes of civil litigation include professional malpractice, negligence, and assault and battery.

Common law Law that is created through the decision of judges as opposed to laws enacted by legislative bodies (i.e., Congress).

Comparative negligence A type of liability in which damages may be apportioned among two or more defendants in a malpractice case. The extent of liability depends on the defendant's relative contribution to the patient's injury.

Criminal negligence Negligence that indicates "reckless and wanton" disregard for the safety, well-being, or life of an individual; behavior that demonstrates a complete disregard for another, such that death is likely.

Damages Monetary compensation the court orders paid to a person who has sustained a loss or injury to his or her person or property through the misconduct (intentional or unintentional) of another.

Defendant The individual who is named in a person's (plaintiff's) complaint as responsible for an injury; the person who the plaintiff claims committed a negligent act or malpractice.

Disclosure A process in which the patient's primary provider (physician or advanced practice nurse) gives the patient, and when applicable, family members, complete information about unanticipated adverse outcomes of treatment and care.

Durable power of attorney for health care An instrument that authorizes another person to act as one's agent in decisions regarding health care if the person becomes incompetent to make his or her own decisions.

Error A failure of a planned action to be completed as intended or the use of a wrong plan to achieve a specific aim.

Gross negligence A legal concept that means extreme carelessness showing willful or reckless disregard for the consequences to a person (patient).

Immunity Legal doctrine by which a person is protected from a lawsuit for negligent acts or an institution is protected from a suit for the negligent acts of its employees.

Liability Being legally responsible for harm caused to another person or property as a result of one's actions; compensation for harm normally is paid in monetary damages.

Licensing laws Laws that establish the qualifications for obtaining and maintaining a license to perform particular services. Persons and institutions may be required to obtain a license to provide particular health care services.

Malpractice Failure of a professional to meet the standard of conduct that a reasonable and prudent member of his or her profession would exercise in similar circumstances that results in harm. The professional's misconduct is unintentional.

Negligence Failure to act in a manner that an ordinary, prudent person (either layperson or professional) would act in similar circumstances, resulting in harm. The failure to act in a reasonable and prudent manner is unintentional.

Plaintiff The complaining person in a lawsuit; the person who claims he or she was injured by the acts of another.

Preventable adverse event An injury caused by medical management rather than the patient's underlying condition. An adverse event attributable to error is a preventable adverse event.

Punitive damages Monetary compensation awarded to an injured person (patient) that goes beyond that which is necessary to compensate for losses (e.g., the ability to function, death, income), and is intended to punish the wrongdoer.

Res ipsa loquitur Legal doctrine applicable to cases in which the provider (i.e., the physician) had exclusive control of events that resulted in the patient's injury; the injury would not have occurred ordinarily without a negligent act; a Latin phrase meaning "the thing speaks for itself."

Respondeat superior Legal doctrine that holds an employer indirectly responsible for the negligent acts of employees carried out within the scope of employment; a Latin phrase meaning "let the master answer."

Risk management Process of identifying, analyzing, and controlling risks posed to patients; involves human factor and incident analysis, changes in systems operations, and loss control and prevention.

Sentinel event As defined by The Joint Commission, an unintended adverse outcome that results in death, paralysis, coma, or other major permanent loss of function. Examples of sentinel events include patient suicide while in a licensed health care facility, surgical procedure on the wrong organ or body side, or a patient fall.

Standard of care In civil cases, the legal criteria against which the nurse's (and physician's) conduct is compared to determine whether a negligent act or malpractice occurred; commonly defined as the knowledge and skill that an ordinary, reasonably prudent person would possess and exercise in the same or similar circumstances.

Statute or statutory law Law enacted by a legislative body; separate from judge-made or common law.

Strict liability A legal doctrine, sometimes referred to as absolute liability, that can be imposed on a person or entity (e.g., a hospital) without proof of carelessness or negligence.

Vicarious liability Legal doctrine in which a person or institution is liable for the negligent acts of another because of a special relationship between the two parties; a substituted liability.

LEARNING OUTCOMES

After studying this chapter, the reader will be able to:

1 Differentiate among the three major categories of law on which nursing practice is established and governed.

2 Analyze the relationship between accountability and liability for one's actions in professional nursing practice.

3 Outline the essential elements that must be proven to establish a claim of negligence or malpractice.

4 Distinguish between intentional and unintentional torts in relation to nursing practice.

5 Identify causes of nursing error and patient injury that have led to claims of criminal negligence.

6 Incorporate fundamental laws and statutory regulations that establish the patient's right to autonomy, self-determination, and informed decision making in the health care setting.

7 Incorporate laws and statutory regulations that establish the patient's right to privacy and privacy of health records.

8 Complete the critical thinking exercises at the end of the chapter to consolidate understanding of the relationship between nursing practice and the law.

CHAPTER OVERVIEW

The preceding vignette highlighted a growing clinical dilemma that nurses face in the complex ever-changing health care system. Financial considerations may conflict with clinical concerns for patient well-being. In an increasingly complex health care environment, the nurse's ability to make appropriate decisions about the provision of patient care services is assisted by a sound knowledge of the laws governing practice. In the case of Mr. Jones, triage, assessment, medical evaluation, and treatment are regulated by a federal law known as the Emergency Medical Treatment and Active Labor Act (EMTALA) (COBRA, 42 U.S.C. 1395dd). There also may be a specific state law regarding essential care and transport of patients in EDs. Additionally, sections of the state's nurse practice act) describing the professional conduct of the RN would assist nurse Clark in managing this clinical problem. Financial concerns, such as pressure exerted on the nurse to reduce the cost of care become a secondary consideration for the nurse with this baseline knowledge of the law.

Each nurse must be able to describe his or her professional duty to the patient or client under the law and to recognize legal risks in practice. Knowledge of the law enhances the nurse's ability to provide safe, effective, and humane care in all settings. This chapter examines legal aspects of nursing practice. The concepts of law, professional accountability, legal liability, negligence, malpractice, and criminal offense are defined. Specific laws or statutes governing nursing practice are also reviewed. The reader is introduced to current, relevant information about case law, also known as common law or judge-made law, as it applies to professional nursing practice. Patients' rights are explored within the context of law and court opinions. Finally the ongoing reports published by the organizations, such as the Institute of Medicine (IOM), The Joint Commission (TJC), and the Agency for Healthcare Research and Quality (AHRQ), about medical errors are discussed, and specific strategies to reduce errors and legal risk are detailed.

SOURCES OF LAW AND NURSING PRACTICE

The actions of all individuals are regulated through two systems of principles known as laws and ethics. Laws enforce a minimal level of conduct by imposing penalties for violations of acceptable behavior (Griffith and Tengnah, 2008). Laws are expressed in terms of "must" and "shall" and are based on a society's interest in prohibiting or controlling certain behaviors. Ethics are described in terms of "should" and "may" and address beliefs about appropriate behaviors within a societal context (Westrick and Dempski, 2008). Chapter 9 presents an in-depth discussion about nursing ethics. Along with ethics, professional nursing conduct also is regulated by a variety of laws. There are two major sources of law:

◆ Statutory law
◆ Common law

The standards for professional nursing practice are in great part derived from statutory as well as common law. The following section of the chapter deals with statutory law and describes how it governs and indirectly influences nursing practice.

STATUTORY LAW

The terms "law" and "statute" are used interchangeably in this chapter. Laws that are written by legislative bodies, such as Congress or state legislatures, are enacted as statutes. The previously mentioned law, EMTALA, is an example of a federal statute. Violation of law is a criminal offense against the general public and is prosecuted by government authorities. Crimes are punishable by fines or imprisonment. The list of federal and state statutes that govern nursing practice has multiplied over the past 25 years. Nurses at all levels of practice must develop a greater depth and breadth of knowledge about laws related to patient safety, professional practice, their specific practice setting (i.e., the ED in the case of EMTALA), and health care systems in general. Ignorance of the law is never a defense when a nurse violates a health care statute. A nurse who violates the law is subject to penalties, including monetary fines, suspension or revocation of his or her license, and even imprisonment in some instances (Kazmier, 2008).

Federal Statutes

Federal laws have a major effect on nursing practice, mandating a minimal standard of care in all health care settings that receive federal funds (i.e., reimbursement for treatment of Medicare patients). Medicare is administered by the Centers for Medicare & Medicaid Services (CMS) and has the authority to establish new rules and regulations to enhance patient safety and quality, and reduce the cost of care. In 2008, the CMS issued new rules that halt payment to hospitals for treatment of preventable patient complications and injuries, often referred to as "never events". The CMS identified 10 categories of hospital-acquired conditions that studies have demonstrated are "reasonably preventable" (ECRI, 2008). Box 8-1 lists the 10 categories of adverse events that are subject to nonpayment. The new rules were enacted in 2009, and will have a tremendous effect on hospital nursing practice because they involve intensive nursing care to prevent complications such as falls, infections, and the development of stage III and stage IV pressure ulcers. Furthermore, legal concerns have been raised about an increase in malpractice claims related to hospital-acquired conditions as the public becomes aware of the new CMS rules. Risk managers and other legal professionals also fear that a hospital could not defend a malpractice claim if "strict liability" is applied to these hospital-acquired events (Vonwinkel, 2008). Strict liability imposes legal responsibility for damages or injury, even if the person (the hospital in the case of hospital-acquired conditions) is not "strictly" at fault or negligent.

Nursing homes are another highly regulated industry that must meet federal and state requirements to operate. Federal laws have also established rules and regulations to ensure the confidentiality of patients' personal health information (Health Insurance Portability and Accountability Act, or HIPAA). Several federal laws protect the rights of patients who participate as subjects in research by mandating the creation of institutional review boards and an appropriate informed consent process. The Federal False Claims Act makes it an offense to submit a false claim to the government for payment of health care services. Furthermore the person who reports the false or fraudulent claim (often a whistle-blower) is entitled to 15% to 25% of any monetary amount recovered by the federal government if the government wins the case in court. Nurses have been the recipients of these "bounties" in several recent false claim cases in which the federal government recovered several million dollars. The Americans with Disabilities Act (ADA) requires health care entities to provide interpreter services and communication devices when patients are unable to effectively communicate their needs or wishes.

BOX **8-1**

Categories of Hospital-Acquired Conditions Subject to Nonpayment

1. Foreign object retained after surgery (i.e., instruments, surgical sponges)
2. Air embolism
3. Blood incompatibility (blood transfusion error)
4. Stage III and stage IV pressure ulcer development
5. Falls and trauma
   - Fractures
   - Joint dislocation
   - Intracranial injuries
   - Crushing injuries
   - Burns
   - Electric shock
6. Manifestations of poor glycemic control
   - Diabetic ketoacidosis
   - Nonketotic hyperosmolar coma
   - Hypoglycemic coma
   - Secondary diabetes with ketoacidosis
   - Secondary diabetes with hyperosmolarity
7. Catheter-associated urinary tract infection (UTI)
8. Vascular catheter-associated infection
9. Surgical site infection following:
   - Coronary artery bypass graft—mediastinitis
   - Bariatric surgery
   - Orthopedic procedures
10. Deep vein thrombosis (DVT)/pulmonary embolism (PE)

Source: Centers for Medicare & Medicaid Services (CMS): Medicare program: changes to the hospital inpatient prospective payment system and fiscal year 2009 rates (final rule). 42 CFR Parts 411, 412, 413, 489. Retrieved January 2009 from: http://edocket.access.gpo.gov/2008/pdf/E8-17914.pdf.

Three federal statutes that nurses must be familiar with and clearly understand are discussed in this section. The list is not comprehensive, but it includes examples of federal laws that directly affect nursing practice. Many federal laws are relevant to specific health care settings (i.e., mental health, nursing homes, EDs, maternity settings). When nurses are knowledgeable about the federal laws applicable to their area of practice, they are able to more effectively advocate for patients in that setting. Unfortunately, most nurses are unfamiliar with health care law and rely on authorities in their employment setting to know what is legal and therefore permissible. Automatically deferring to administrators or nurse managers about the legality of a particular issue is no longer acceptable behavior for the professional nurse. Each RN must take accountability for knowing the law and understanding how it relates to patient care and nursing practice.

Emergency Medical Treatment and Active Labor Law (COBRA, 42 U.S.C. 1395dd). This federal statute, often referred to as the "antidumping" law, was enacted in 1986 to prohibit the refusal of care for indigent and uninsured patients seeking medical assistance in an ED (Moy, 2009). This law also prohibits the transfer of unstable patients, including women in labor, from one facility to another. The law states:

> "All persons presenting for care must receive the same medical screening examination and be stabilized, regardless of their financial status or insurance coverage, before discharge or transfer."

EMTALA is applicable to people coming to non-ED settings, such as urgent care clinics. It even governs the transfer of patients from an inpatient setting to a lower level of care in some parts of the United States (*Roberts v. Galen of Virginia, Inc.*, 1997). Significant penalties can be levied against a facility that violates the EMTALA, including a $25,000 to $50,000 fine (not covered by liability insurance). The federal government also can revoke the facility's Medicare contract, and this could result in a major loss of revenue for the institution or even insolvency. Many legitimate concerns that nurses have about the discharge or transfer of patients could be promptly addressed if the nurse had a solid understanding of the EMTALA. A recent case illustrates the importance of understanding the EMTALA. In *Love v. Rancocas Hospital* (2006), a woman was transported by ambulance to the ED after losing consciousness at home. She had a history of hypertension and continued to have high blood pressure readings in the ED. The woman also fell off the bed twice while being monitored, but the ED nurse did not report this to the physician. The nurse received a discharge order from the physician, and sent the woman home in an *unstable* condition, thus violating the stabilization requirement of the EMTALA. The woman returned 2 days later after experiencing a stroke. Understanding the EMTALA is not a daunting task for nurses engaged in the triage and medical screening of patients presenting to the ED or obstetric triage department. Nursing journals have published many articles about the EMTALA and the nurse's role in upholding this statute (Angelini and Mahlmeister, 2005; Bond, 2008; Caliendo et al, 2004).

Americans with Disabilities Act of 1990 (Public Law No. 101-336, 42 U.S.C. Section 12101). The intent of this law is to end discrimination against qualified persons with disabilities by removing barriers that prevent them from enjoying the same opportunities available to persons without disabilities. Court cases have established that as a place of public accommodation, a health care facility must provide reasonable accommodation to patients (and family members) with sensory disabilities, such as vision and hearing impairment (*Abernathy v. Valley Medical Center*, 2006; *Boyer v. Tift County Hospital*, 2008). In another case (*Parco v. Pacifica Hospital*,

2007), a nurse was caring for a ventilator-dependent quadriplegic patient who was unable to speak or use his call light. She requested a special pillow that activated the patient's call light when he turned his head, but was told that all the pillows were in use. The patient subsequently experienced three episodes of respiratory distress that he was unable to alert the nurse about, and could only hope that someone would discover his problem before he suffered brain damage or died (Snyder, 2007a). The patient sued for emotional distress and mental anguish. The court affirmed that the ADA requires hospitals to provide assistive devices to patients with communication problems related to a disability. The hospital settled the lawsuit for $295,000.

This statute has relevance for all nurses. As patient advocates, nurses have a legal and ethical duty to provide appropriate patient and family education and to support the process of informed consent. In *Parco v. Pacifica Hospital*, the court noted that it was a basic tenet of nursing practice that patients be given the ability to communicate with caregivers. The health care facility must have a policy that defines how it will meet the client's needs for education and information, when there are vision or hearing disabilities. The policy also describes how a nurse can obtain translators and special types of equipment needed to facilitate communication when there are physical disabilities or language barriers.

Patient Self-Determination Act (PSDA) of 1990; Omnibus Budget Reconciliation Act of 1990 (Public Law No. 101-508, Sections 4206 and 4751). This federal statute is a Medicare and Medicaid amendment intended to support individuals in expressing their preferences about medical treatment and making decisions about end-of-life care. The law requires all federally funded hospitals to give patients written notice on admission to the health care facility of their decision-making rights and policies regarding advance health care directives in their state and in the institution to which they have been admitted. Patient rights under the PSDA include the right to:

- Participate in their own health care decisions
- Accept or refuse medical treatment
- Make advance health care directives

These choices include collaborating with the physician in formulating "do not resuscitate" (DNR) orders. Facilities must inquire as to whether the patient already has an advance health care directive, and must make note of this in the patient's medical record. The institution must also provide education to their staff about advance health care directives. The law provides guidance to nurses who often are in the best position to discuss these issues with the patient (e.g., while completing a comprehensive admission assessment). (Legal considerations related to living wills, durable power of attorney, and DNR orders are discussed in the last section of this chapter.)

Health Insurance Portability and Accountability Act of 1996 (Public Law No. 104-191). The intent of this law is to ensure confidentiality of the patient's health information. Legitimate concerns regarding the uses of and release of medical information, particularly to private entities, such as insurance companies, led to the passage of this law. The introduction of electronic medical records has provided additional impetus for introduction of this legislation. The statute sets guidelines for maintaining the privacy of health data. It provides explicit guidelines for nurses who are in a position to release health information. To maintain confidentiality of the patient's health information, all nurses must have a basic understanding of this federal law. Nurses should also take note that HIPAA confers whistle-blower protection for individuals who report in good faith any illegal disclosure of patients' health. In 2005 a federal statute,

The Patient Safety and Quality Improvement Act, was enacted to allow certain disclosures of patient safety data. The law permits a provider to disclose *nonidentifiable* patient data to a qualified patient safety organization (PSO) for the purpose of analyzing medical errors. The law prohibits an accreditation body, such as TJC, from taking any action against a provider who reports patient safety data to an approved PSO (Public Law No. 109-41).

State Statutes

In addition to federal laws, nursing practice is governed by state laws that delineate the conduct of licensed nurses and define behaviors of all health care professionals in promoting public health and welfare.

State Nurse Practice Act and Board of Nursing Rules and Regulations. One of the most important state laws governing nursing practice is a nurse practice act (NPA), which defines the scope and limitations of professional nursing practice. The aim of regulating practice in this manner is to protect the public and make the individual nurse accountable for his or her actions. State legislatures authorize the nurses' licensing board to promulgate administrative rules and regulations necessary to implement the NPA. Once these administrative rules and regulations are formally adopted, they have the same force and effect as any other law.

Although NPAs vary from state to state, they usually contain the following information:
- Definition of the term "RN"
- Description of professional nursing functions
- Standards of competent performance
- Behaviors that represent misconduct or prohibited practices
- Grounds for disciplinary action
- Fines and penalties the licensing board may levy when an NPA is violated

For further exploration, excerpts from three separate state NPAs can be found online (http://evolve.elsevier.com/Cherry/) to illustrate how an NPA defines the scope of practice for nurses.

Surprisingly, many nurses are not even aware that the NPA is a law, and they unknowingly violate aspects of this statute (Wright, 2005). They are not familiar with the administrative rules and regulations enacted by the licensing board. This is an unfortunate lapse because these administrative rules and regulations answer crucial questions that nurses have about the day-to-day aspects of practice and unusual occurrences. For example, the increasing complexity of health care requires effective communication, collaboration, and planning of care among many licensed health team members. Rules promulgated by the Ohio Board of Nursing Section 4723.03 related to the competent practice as an RN direct the nurse in appropriate reporting and consultation.

"A registered nurse shall in a timely manner:
(1) Implement any order for a client unless the registered nurse believes or should have reason to believe the order is:
   (a) Inaccurate
   (b) Not properly authorized
   (c) Not current or valid
   (d) Harmful, or potentially harmful to a client
   (e) Contraindicated by other documented information; and
(2) Clarify any order for a client when the registered nurse believes or should have reason to believe the order is: [a through e as delineated in (1)]"
OHIO ADMINISTRATIVE CODE, SECTION 4723-4-03, E, 2009

Based on this, an RN in Ohio who does not clarify a questionable order, before administering a medication or carrying out the prescribed action, is in violation of the law.

Each nurse should own a current copy of the NPA and the licensing board's administrative rules and regulations. The nurse also must know how to access the licensing board online and by telephone in order to clarify issues related to nursing practice. The dramatic changes occurring in health care often lead to uncertainty among nurses about which functions constitute the exclusive practice of registered nursing and which patient care tasks may be lawfully delegated to a licensed practical nurse/licensed vocational nurse (LPN/LVN), or unlicensed assistive personnel. The NPA and licensing board rules and regulations provide essential information that clarifies these important questions. In 2008 the Texas Board of Nursing approved a new rule requiring all nurses to take and pass a Nursing Jurisprudence Exam prior to initial licensure. The exam tests knowledge regarding nursing board statutes, rules, position statements, disciplinary action, and other resource documents accessible on the Texas board website (http://bon. state.tx.us/index.html).

Nurses may also have questions and concerns regarding the legal aspects of floating to unfamiliar units. An NPA provides information regarding the scope of practice, required competencies, and the responsibilities of a nurse who accepts an assignment or agrees to carry out any task or activity in the clinical setting. The NPA broadly defines the practice of registered nursing in accordance with nursing's rapidly evolving functions. In recent years, with the expansion of basic nursing functions and the development of advanced nursing practice, many states have revised their NPAs. Licensing boards also have been authorized in some states to provide guidelines for the development of "standardized procedures." Standardized procedures are a legal means by which RNs may expand their practice into areas traditionally considered to be within the realm of medicine. The standardized procedure actually is developed within the facility where the expanded nursing functions have been approved. It is developed in collaboration with nursing, medicine, and administration. An example of a standardized procedure is a written protocol authorizing a nurse to implement a peripherally inserted venous catheter for patients in the neonatal intensive care unit.

Violations of an NPA. State legislatures have given licensing boards the authority to hear and decide administrative cases against nurses when there is an alleged violation of an NPA or the nursing board's rules and regulations. Nurses who violate the NPA or board's administrative rules and regulations are subject to disciplinary action by the board. Research indicates that there has been an increase in the number of consumer complaints to licensing boards related to nursing misconduct, and disciplinary actions more than doubled from 1996 to 2006 (Kenward, 2008. Table 8-1 provides a synopsis of the licensing board procedure when a complaint is made about a nurse.

Box 8-2 presents the more common grounds for disciplinary action by state boards of nursing. Penalties that licensing boards may impose for violations of an NPA include:
- Issuing a formal reprimand
- Establishing a period of probation
- Levying fines
- Limiting, suspending, or revoking a nurse's license

An estimated 8% to 10% of RNs in the United States are chemically dependent (Willis, 2008). The majority of disciplinary actions by licensing boards are related to misconduct resulting from chemical impairment, including the misappropriation of drugs for personal use and the sale of drugs and drug paraphernalia to support the nurse's addiction. When a nurse's license is limited or suspended because of problems related to chemical impairment, the ability to practice in the future often is predicated on successful completion of a drug rehabilitation program and evidence of abstinence. An increasing number of state licensing boards have established programs to guide nurses through the process of rehabilitation to reestablish licensure.

TABLE **8-1**

Licensing Board Procedure When a Complaint Is Filed

ACTION	CONSEQUENCE
Complaint is made (initial complaint may be lodged by a telephone call or a letter mailed to the licensing board) by: • Consumer (patient) • Family member • Nurse or nurse manager or employer • Professional nursing organization • State board of nursing • Federal or state authority (i.e., CMS or Department of Health and Human Services)	Sworn complaints must be filed
Licensing board reviews complaint: • Examines evidence • Review of reports	Insufficient evidence—no action Administrative review scheduled • Nurse notified
Determination made by board	Nurse summoned • Rules of proceeding explained • Witnesses called to testify • Further evidence examined
Licensing board makes decision	Nurse exonerated Nurse guilty of violating NPA
Board takes disciplinary action	Possible actions • Board issues formal reprimand • Fines levied against nurse • Nurse placed on probation • License suspended or revoked • License not renewed
Nurse may challenge licensing board's actions	Nurse must file appeal in court
Court reviews case (court action is dependent on jurisdiction) • Reviews conduct of proceedings • Review's board's decision	Licensing board ruling is reversed
Licensing board can appeal ruling	Court reviews case
Court renders a decision	Licensing board ruling is upheld
OR	OR
Court renders a decision	Licensing board ruling overturned
	Licensing board can appeal to a higher court
Case scheduled for trial	Licensing board ruling upheld OR Licensing board ruling reversed

CMS, Centers for Medicare & Medicaid Services; *NPA,* nurse practice act.

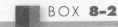

BOX **8-2**

Grounds for Disciplinary Action by State Boards of Nursing

- Practicing without a valid license
- Failure to use appropriate nursing judgment
- Guilty of a felony
- Falsification of records
- Failure to complete nursing documentation
- Incorrect nursing documentation

- Failure to practice in accordance with nursing standards
- Inappropriate behavior or occurrence at work
- Medicare fraud
- Misappropriation of personal items

Nurse-Patient Ratios and Mandatory Overtime Statutes

Inadequate and often unsafe nurse-patient ratios continue to plague nursing. A growing body of evidence confirms a strong association between nurse-patient ratios and patient outcomes (Clarke and Donaldson, 2009; Kane et al, 2007). The American Nurses Association (ANA) has launched the Safe Staffing Saves Lives Campaign, and has published the results of a poll conducted in 2008 to examine nurses' perceptions of staffing problems (ANA, 2009). More than half of respondents were considering leaving their current nursing position and 42% indicated the reason for leaving was associated with inadequate staffing. Another study surveyed direct care nurses about nursing errors of omission. Greater than 70% of respondents reported the inability at times to plan and implement required care and intervene in a timely manner. Forty-four percent of respondents missed essential assessments (Kalisch, Landstrom, and Williams, 2009). Eighty-five percent of the nurses indicated that lack of human resources (nurse and support staff) was the primary reason for omissions in essential components of the nursing process.

As I travel across the United States speaking with nurses about the rapid and often daunting changes in health care, a common question I hear is, "Isn't there a law prohibiting this reduction in RN staff? Floating? The use of nurse aides in this patient care situation? Mandatory overtime?" Nurse staffing is influenced to some degree by federal law, through the rules for participation in Medicare, and increasingly, by state laws. When concerns about work-related issues arise (e.g., a change in scope of practice for unlicensed staff or a reduction in RN staffing), the first question the nurse asks and answers should be, "Is this legal?" (Brooke, 2009). In 1999 California became the first state to enact a law (California Assembly Bill 394) that mandates the establishment of minimum nurse-patient ratios in acute care facilities. The law took effect in January 2004 and sets minimum nurse-patient ratios in critical care units, step-down and medical-surgical units, and maternity departments. On July 1, 2009, a Pennsylvania statute (Act 102) was enacted that prohibits mandatory overtime for nurses, with the exception of natural disasters, a state or municipal emergency, or major accident. (The law can be retrieved at: www.dli.state.pa.us/landi/cwp/view.asp?a=185&q=252605.)

An increasing number of lawsuits against health care facilities have set forth claims of corporate negligence for inadequate staffing or "understaffing" when adverse outcomes occur. A jury awarded a $1.7 million verdict against a nursing home for the death of a resident who fell from her wheelchair. Evidence revealed that there was a widespread pattern of understaffing at the nursing home (*Sunbridge Healthcare Corp. v. Penny*, 2005). In a second case, *Penalver v. Living Centers of Texas* (2004), the director of nursing and the facility's administrator were found negligent in the death of a resident who fell from her wheelchair. Evidence was presented during the trial that there had been more than 800 other falls in the facility as a result of severe and chronic understaffing (Snyder, 2004a). The jury awarded her family $856,000. In 2006, another jury awarded $240,000 in punitive damages (out of a total award of $400,000) against a nursing home because understaffing at the facility was considered an aggravating factor in a patient's death (*Miller v. Levering Regional Healthcare Center*, 2006). The patient was 91 years old and suffering from Alzheimer's disease. The resident (patient) was left unattended and fell, hitting her head, and subsequently died of her injuries. The court records contained adequate evidence that the facility knew it had a chronic understaffing problem and that the problem directly led to the woman's death (Snyder, 2006a). The director of nursing was also found negligent for failing to comply with Medicare guidelines that required the facility to provide sufficient staffing.

Reporting Statutes

The federal government and states seek to protect at-risk individuals (children and older adults) by requiring nurses and other health care providers to report specific types of suspected or actual patient-client injury, abuse, or neglect (Buppert and Klein, 2008). This is also the case with boards of nursing, created to protect the public from unethical, incompetent, or impaired nursing practice. Some states have enacted statutes that *mandate* nurses report unsafe, illegal, or unethical practices of nursing colleagues. The types of conduct the boards of nursing require nurses to report vary from state to state. Nurses can access the specific requirements for reporting nurse coworkers at their board of nursing website. Two states, Kentucky and California, require nurses and providers to report victims of domestic or interpersonal violence, whether or not the victim (patient) consents (National District Attorneys Association, 2006). Certain specifiable communicable diseases must also be reported to the Centers for Disease Control and Prevention (CDC) such as bubonic plague, anthrax, and botulism. (The list of reportable diseases can be retrieved from: www.cdc.gov/ncphi/od/AI/phs/infdis2008.htm.) State law may also require nurses to report injuries resulting from the use of weapons, attempts to harm oneself, or impaired driving (Buppert and Klein, 2008). Nurse managers and administrators are responsible for ensuring that reports made by direct care nurses are forwarded to the appropriate legal authorities. Nurse leaders who fail in this duty may face criminal charges, claims of negligence, and disciplinary action by the nursing board (Hudspeth, 2008).

Child Abuse Reporting Statutes. In 1973 the U.S. Congress enacted the Child Abuse Prevention and Treatment Act, which mandates all states to meet specific uniform guidelines to qualify for federal funding of child abuse programs. All 50 states and the District of Columbia have created laws that require reporting of specific health problems and the suspected or confirmed abuse of infants or children. Nurses often are explicitly named within the context of these statutes as one of the groups of designated health professionals who must report the specified problems under penalty of fine or imprisonment. Nurses need not fear legal reprisal from individuals or families who are reported to authorities in suspected cases of abuse. Most legislatures have granted immunity from suit within the context of the mandatory reporting statute. A court decision in the case of *Heinrich v. Conemaugh Valley Memorial Hospital* (1994) upheld this doctrine of immunity. The family of an injured child initiated a lawsuit against a hospital that reported suspected child abuse after a state investigation found them innocent of the charge. The court ruled that the hospital and the physician who made the report in "good faith" were immune from litigation under the Pennsylvania Child Protective Service Law that required reports of suspected child abuse.

It is crucial that nurses understand the requirements of abuse reporting statutes as they apply to their practice setting. For example, ED and pediatric nurses must have in-depth knowledge regarding child abuse reporting laws. Agency policies and procedures in the work setting may provide guidance in regard to reporting duties. If in doubt, the nurse should immediately contact his or her supervisor, an administrator, or the agency's compliance officer (the individual responsible for understanding and ensuring adherence to federal and state statutes) for additional guidance in the matter. In rare situations, when information is not available within the institution, the nurse may consult with the state department of health or the state nurses' licensing board for guidance in obtaining these reporting statutes. There are serious ramifications for failing to report as required by the state's specific statute, and could result in criminal charge and claims of negligence.

In a Missouri case, a nurse failed to report a suspected case of child abuse to that state's division of family services and to the physician in charge of her ED as required by law. She was charged with two misdemeanors that could have resulted in punishment of up to 2 years in prison and $2000 in fines, if she was convicted (Goldsmith, 2003). In 2004, the Supreme Court of Missouri reversed a lower court decision to dismiss the case, and the nurse *still* faced misdemeanor charges. Finally, in October 2004, the county prosecutor dropped all charges against the nurse. Although this case settled favorably for the nurse, 2 years were spent defending the charges with the assistance of attorneys. (Details of the case can be retrieved from: http://springfield.news-leader.com/ specialreports/dominicjames/0804-NurseinDom-148351.html and http://springfield.news-leader.com/columnists/overstreet/1107-FriendsofL-220780.html.)

Institutional Licensing Laws

All facilities (i.e., hospitals, nursing homes, rehabilitation centers) providing health care services must comply with licensing laws promulgated by state legislatures. These laws are created to protect the public and ensure the safe and effective provision of health care services. Specific language usually is contained within health facility licensing statutes regarding the following issues:

- ◆ Minimal standards for the maintenance of the physical plant
- ◆ Basic operational aspects of major departments (nursing, dietary, clinical laboratories, and pharmacy)
- ◆ Essential aspects of patients' rights and the informed consent process

Many state licensing laws mandate minimal levels of education, experience, or credentialing for department administrators, such as nurses, anesthesia personnel, pediatricians, and obstetricians. Several states also require minimum nurse-patient ratios in critical care units and other specialty departments, such as the operating room, nursery, or ED.

Health care redesign and cost-reduction efforts have led to many changes in the way health care services are provided and the settings in which care is rendered. Not all change has been positive, and some redesign schemes have resulted in adverse outcomes for patients (Mahlmeister, 2009a). Investigations by state authorities on reports of patient injuries or death have discovered that in some cases health facilities have operated in violation of existing licensing laws. In the past, direct-care RNs generally could rely on their nurse managers to have a comprehensive knowledge of health facility licensing law and to create policies and procedures that implement and enforce applicable aspects of the law. The trend toward flattened management and reduction in role development for leaders has altered this picture. In an increasing number of settings, nurse managers have been replaced with non-nurse administrators, who may have minimal knowledge of the health facilities' licensing laws.

In light of these changes, direct-care nurses should have a working knowledge of current licensing laws as they relate to nursing care and patient care services. The nurse also is guided by the ANA Scope and Standards of Practice, which states: "The registered nurse systematically enhances the quality and effectiveness of nursing practice" (ANA, 2004). In many instances, nurses who have serious questions regarding quality of care in their employment setting have been able to resolve these concerns once they have read applicable sections of the health facility licensing law relevant to their setting. Bringing the pertinent section of the law to the attention of managers, administrators, a compliance officer, or the risk management department often is the most effective strategy to resolve problems. In settings in which nurses are represented by union contracts, potential violations of health facility licensing laws may be most effectively addressed through union representatives.

Internet access has allowed nurses to obtain rapid information about current institutional licensing laws. Information can be downloaded and printed quickly. Nurses also can obtain a copy of the health facility's licensing law for their employment setting through the state department of health or public health, division of licensing and certification. Other states provide the statute and address questions through the department of health, division of facilities regulations or division of health facilities inspection, or division of health quality assurance. The telephone number for this agency can be found in the white pages of the local telephone directory under the heading "State of " (e.g., Michigan). Nurses may call their licensing board or the state nursing association for guidance in reaching the appropriate authority to obtain a copy of the licensing law and to speak to a consultant about concerns.

COMMON LAW

In addition to statutory law, nursing practice is guided by common law, also known as decisional or judge-made law. Common law is created through cases heard and decided in federal and state appellate courts. Throughout the years judge-made law regarding nursing practice has accumulated in the form of written opinions. These opinions eventually contribute to the expected standard of nursing conduct (Griffith and Tengnah, 2008). The body of written opinions about nurses also is known as nursing case law. The importance of nursing case law in establishing the current standard of practice cannot be overstated.

One of the most important cases to establish the expected conduct of nurses was *Utter v. United Hospital Center, Inc.* (1977). This West Virginia case affirmed that nurses were required to exercise independent judgments to prevent harm when caring for patients. Before the 1970s, the issue of whether nurses were licensed professionals who made independent judgments was not clearly established. In the Utter case, a patient whose arm was casted had signs and symptoms of compartment syndrome. The affected limb became progressively more edematous and eventually turned black. The nurses failed to activate the chain of command when the primary providers did not respond to their reports and requests for medical reevaluation. The patient's arm eventually had to be amputated. The court wrote:

> Nurses are specialists in hospital care who, in the final analysis, hold the well-being, in fact in some instances, the very lives of patients in their hands. In the dim hours of the night, as well as in the light of day, nurses are frequently charged with the duty to observe the condition of the ill and infirm in their care. If the patient, helpless and wholly dependent, shows signs of worsening, the nurse is charged with the obligation of taking some positive action…there was evidence that certain nurses did not fulfill their obligation.

The duty to prevent harm, known as the nurse's "affirmative duty," has been supported in numerous court decisions. In *Rowe v. Sisters of Pallottine Missionary Society* (2001), a hospital and its ED nurses were found negligent for failing to question a physician's discharge order. A 17-year-old motorcyclist was admitted to the ED for an injury to his left leg. He complained of severe pain in his left knee and numbness in his left foot. The nurses were unable to find a pulse in the left leg or foot. The physician issued a discharge order and gave instructions that included the application of ice and elevation of the affected leg. The next day the man sought emergency care at another hospital for worsening pain and swelling of his leg. An examination revealed a lacerated popliteal artery and dislocated knee. He underwent extensive surgery and suffers permanent impairment of the affected limb. The physician settled the suit against him for $275,000. The jury returned a verdict for the patient in excess of $880,000 and found the nurses negligent for failing to question the discharge order and invoke the chain of command to obtain additional medical consultation and advice.

The nurse's role as a patient advocate has been reaffirmed in more recent cases. In *Martin v. Abilene Regional Medical Center* (2006), a patient was discharged from the hospital after placement of a coronary artery stent. The discharge instructions, formulated by the cardiologist, included teaching about the use of Plavix, a drug given to inhibit thrombus formation; however, there was no prescription written for the medication. The nurse did not question the absence of a prescription for Plavix and sent the patient home. The coronary artery stent occluded after the patient was discharged, and he subsequently sued the hospital. The nursing expert witness in the case asserted that the discharge nurse breached the applicable standard of care in failing to question the absence of an order for Plavix. The Texas Nursing Practice Act was used as the basis for this opinion. The Texas Nursing Practice Act states the nurse will "clarify any order or treatment regimen that the nurse has reason to believe is inaccurate." The Texas Court of Appeals confirmed that the nurse should have questioned why there was no order written for the take-home medication.

Every nurse should understand the effect that nursing case law has on his or her current practice. Case law made in appellate court decisions has addressed a range of vital issues related to professional nursing, including:

- Nursing malpractice cases
- Questions concerning labor law and collective bargaining
- Lawsuits alleging wrongful termination
- Legal challenges to state board of nursing disciplinary action against a nurse's license
- Legal actions against the nurse instituted by medical licensing boards
- "Practicing medicine without a license" claims
- Lawsuits claiming violation of the nurse's civil rights, including free-speech issues and reasonable accommodation for nurses with disabilities

Efforts should be made by professional nurses to review case law as it is published and discussed in nursing journals. There has been a trend to incorporate "legal advice" columns into many practice journals, and journals often include discussions about nursing case law. There also has been a proliferation of nursing journals dedicated solely to legal issues in nursing practice. Table 8-2 lists examples of these publications.

TABLE **8-2**

Examples of Journals Dedicated to Legal Issues in Nursing Practice

JOURNAL	PUBLISHER
Nursing Law's Regan Report (formerly Regan Report on Nursing Law)	Medica Press Inc., Providence, RI
Journal of Nursing Law	KRM Information Services, Inc., Eau Claire, WI
Legal Eagle Eye Newsletter for the Nursing Professions	Legal Eagle Eye Newsletter, Seattle, WA
Journal of Legal Nurse Consulting	American Association of Legal Nurse Consultants, Glenview, IL
JONA's Healthcare Law, Ethics and Regulation	Lippincott Williams & Wilkins

Nurse managers in particular should have knowledge regarding the disposition of cases in their jurisdiction. A risk manager or agency attorney may assist any nurse in understanding how judge-made law in his or her state relates to expectations for nursing practice in the local community. Many medical libraries also subscribe to publications that review federal or appellate court decisions in health care law that are relevant to the local community. Although local jury verdicts do not contribute to common law, it is useful for managers and interested nurses to periodically review published reports of malpractice cases in the state and their immediate community. Medical libraries also often subscribe to a local "jury verdicts" publication. (More information on finding nursing case law is available online at http://evolve.elsevier.com/Cherry/.)

CIVIL LAW

Two major categories of law have been created to deal with conduct that is considered unacceptable—criminal law and civil law. Nurses generally are more familiar with civil law and, in particular, the branch of civil law that deals with torts. Tort law is discussed first, with a discussion of criminal law following.

A tort is a civil wrong or injury committed by one person against another person or a property. The wrong results from a breach in one's legal duty regarding interpersonal relationships between private persons. This duty is established through societal expectations regarding interpersonal conduct (Iyer and Levin, 2007). Civil suits almost always are brought by one person against another and generally are based on the concept of "fault." The person who initiates the civil lawsuit, the plaintiff, seeks damages for the wrongful behavior from the offending person, known as the defendant. The determination of whether wrongful behavior has occurred usually is determined by a jury, although in certain cases the right to a trial by jury can be waived by the private parties in the suit. In that case the judge considers the facts and determines the outcome. If the plaintiff succeeds in the civil lawsuit (plaintiff verdict), damages generally are awarded in the form of monetary compensation. Damages may include "hard" damages—financial reimbursement for treatment of injuries, loss of wages, rehabilitation services, or special equipment—and "soft" damages—monetary compensation for pain and suffering, loss of companionship, or mental anguish, among others (Griffith and Tengnah, 2008).

Negligence and Malpractice

There are two types of torts: an unintentional tort or wrong and an intentional tort. An unintentional tort is an unintended wrong against another person. The two most common unintentional torts are negligence and malpractice.

Negligence is defined as the failure to act in a reasonable and prudent manner. The claim of negligence is based on the accepted principle that everyone is expected to conduct themselves in a reasonable and prudent fashion. This is true of laypersons, student nurses, and licensed professionals. A more formal definition of negligence is the failure of a person to use the care that a reasonably prudent and careful person would use under similar circumstances (Griffith and Tengnah, 2008).

Malpractice is a special type of negligence (i.e., the failure of a professional, a person with specialized education and training, to act in a reasonable and prudent manner) (Iyer and Levin, 2007). As state NPAs have evolved to reflect the increasing professionalism of RNs, courts have begun to recognize the negligent acts of nurses as malpractice. Evidence of this change in perceptions is apparent in the increasing use of RNs as expert witnesses in malpractice cases.

In general, expert testimony is not needed in cases of "simple negligence," when the actions of the defendant are so obviously careless that even a layperson would recognize the conduct as negligent. In contrast, if the jury does not possess the special knowledge and information that professionals ordinarily have, an expert witness is required to establish whether the person breached the expected standard of care. In that case the breach in duty is not simple negligence but malpractice.

Elements Essential to Prove Negligence or Malpractice. Although any patient (or surviving family member, in the case of a patient death) may sue the nurse and his or her employer, the following elements must be proved for the plaintiff to succeed in the case.

1. The nurse owed the patient or client a special duty of care based on the establishment of a nurse-patient relationship. When the nurse accepts a patient assignment, it establishes the relationship and requires the nurse to meet his or her duty to the patient. The duty of the nurse is to possess the knowledge and skill that a reasonable and prudent nurse would possess and exercise in the same or similar patient care situation. The duty of the nurse as described, is the standard of care. A nurse-patient relationship also may be established through telephone communication in the case of a nurse who performs telephone triage and advice or via computer or audiovisual systems that are being introduced in some health care settings (Austin, 2008; Tammelleo, 2006).
2. The nurse has breached his or her duty to the patient or client. Evidence is presented that proves the nurse breached the standard of care. The standard of care is derived from a multiplicity of sources; these are described in Box 8-3.
3. Actual harm or damage is suffered by the patient.
4. There is proximate cause or a causal connection between the breach in the standard of care by the nurse and the patient's injury.
   - No intervening event is responsible for the injury.
   - A direct cause and effect can be demonstrated.
   - In some jurisdictions, the nurse's breach in duty must only be proven to be a substantial cause of the patient's injury.

This last element merits further discussion. The relationship between the nurse's breach in the standard of care and the patient's injury must be established by the plaintiff. To prove proximate cause, there must be a direct causal link. For example, a patient reports that he has an allergy to penicillin and wears a MedicAlert bracelet to that effect. A physician orders penicillin to treat the patient's infection. The nurse fails to check or ask the patient about allergies. The nurse administers the penicillin, and the patient suffers an anaphylactic reaction and dies. There is a direct connection between the nurse's actions and the patient's death. Proximate cause has been established.

One may ask what the physician's liability is in this case. The physician also owes a duty to the patient and may be found negligent for ordering penicillin, if he or she had knowledge of, or should have had knowledge of the allergy. However, even in the case of a physician's negligence—"I knew about the penicillin allergy, but forgot"—the nurse has a separate and independent duty to the patient to prevent harm. The nurse must review the patient's medical record for information about allergies, ask the patient about allergies, and check the patient's identification band before administering a drug.

In some jurisdictions it only is necessary to prove that the nurse's actions were a substantial cause of the injury or harm to prove negligence. For example, in a large teaching hospital, a nurse notes a significant change in a patient's vital signs, suggesting deterioration in his

BOX **8-3**

Sources That Contribute to the Standard of Nursing Care

FEDERAL LAWS
Emergency medical treatment and active labor law
Americans with Disabilities Act
Patient Self-Determination Act
Occupational Health and Safety Act
The Patient Safety and Quality Improvement Act

FEDERAL ADMINISTRATIVE RULES AND REGULATIONS
Rules and regulations for participation in Medicare

FEDERAL AGENCIES
U.S. Food and Drug Administration
Agency for Healthcare Research and Quality clinical guidelines
National Institutes of Health publications
Centers for Disease Control and Prevention publications *(Morbidity and Mortality Weekly Report)*

STATE STATUTES
Nurse practice act
State reporting statutes
• Child abuse/elder abuse reporting statutes
• Domestic violence reporting statutes
• Health facility licensing laws

STATE ADMINISTRATIVE RULES AND REGULATIONS
Licensing board rules

BOARD OF NURSING
Position statements and advisories

NURSING CASE LAW
Appellate court decisions

PROFESSIONAL ORGANIZATIONS
Standards and guidelines for practice
Nursing journals
Position statements
Technical bulletins and practice resources
Code of ethics

MANUFACTURER GUIDELINES
Durable medical equipment
Drugs and solutions
Disposable equipment and supplies

AGENCY POLICIES AND PROCEDURES
Job descriptions
Agency-specific documents
Nursing care plans
Care maps or critical pathways
Unit- or department-based standards of practice
Medical bylaws

condition. A first-year resident is called to the bedside and made aware of the patient's status. The resident orders the nurse to simply continue observing the patient. The first-year resident remains immediately available in the unit and receives repeated reports of a continued decline in the patient's condition. There is a clear chain of command policy established in the hospital, which takes into account varying levels of skill and expertise of the residents in training. There is also a chain of command policy to deal with unresolved disagreements between health care professionals and nonresponsive providers. Despite the existence of these policies, the nurse does not activate the chain of command.

The patient suffers hypovolemic shock caused by internal bleeding, and this leads to permanent anoxic brain damage. In this case the nurse's failure to obtain additional medical advice and consultation (a senior resident was physically present and available in the hospital) was a substantial cause of the patient's injury. These two examples illustrate that negligence may constitute a commission (inappropriate penicillin administration) or an omission (failure to activate chain of command) in care.

Negligence and the Doctrine of *Res Ipsa Loquitur*. In the majority of cases, a plaintiff must retain a nurse expert witness because the jury does not ordinarily possess the scientific and technologic knowledge necessary to determine the required standard of care. When the negligent act clearly lies within the range of a jury's common knowledge and experience, the doctrine of *res ipsa loquitur* ("the thing speaks for itself") may be applied. For example, recent studies have confirmed that approximately 2000 to 2500 foreign bodies (instruments, needles, surgical sponges) are inadvertently left in a patient's body following surgery each year, resulting in approximately $42,000 in additional care costs (Lincourt et al, 2007; Shah and Lander, 2009; West, 2006). Leaving a surgical instrument in the patient's body after an operation is one case in which the doctrine of *res ipsa loquitur* may apply. It would be obvious to any layperson that it is below that standard of care not to remove a surgical instrument.

Dickerson v. Fatehi (1997) illustrates this point. A woman who underwent neck surgery experienced severe pain in her right arm, hand, and neck after the procedure. Approximately 20 months later a second surgery was performed to determine the cause of the patient's continued pain. An 18-gauge hypodermic needle with a plastic attachment for a syringe was discovered in her neck and removed. The woman sued the surgeon and nurses involved in the original surgical procedure. The claims against the nurses included a failure to maintain a proper needle count and a failure to ensure the removal of the needle after surgery. The court hearing this case dismissed the suit. On appeal the Supreme Court of Virginia reversed the lower court's decision and directed the case for trial. The Supreme Court held that in this particular case expert testimony was not necessary to establish the applicable standard of care and that the doctrine of *res ipsa loquitur* applied. A jury would be able to determine whether a reasonably prudent circulating nurse and scrub nurse should have made and reported an accurate needle count.

Gross Negligence. In some cases the negligent act of the nurse is so reckless and reflects such a conscious disregard for the patient's welfare that it represents gross negligence. When the nurse acts with complete indifference to the consequences for his or her patient, the court may award special damages meant to punish the nurse for the outrageous conduct. These damages are referred to as punitive damages. Each state has established standards to determine when punitive damages may be awarded. In *Mobile Infirmary Medical Center v. Hodgen* (2003), the jury awarded $2.5 million in punitive damages (later reduced to $1.5 million) when a new graduate, not yet licensed, administered five times the ordered dose of digoxin. The jury found that the new graduate had been improperly supervised by the novice nurse assigned as her preceptor by the shift charge nurse. The charge nurse was also found liable for failing to properly direct the preceptor in her role responsibilities. The Supreme Court of Alabama found, among other things, that the nurses acted callously and wantonly, the legal threshold that must be crossed before punitive damages can be awarded (Snyder, 2003b).

Another landmark case is *Stogsdill v. Healthmark Partners, L.L.C.* (2004). A resident of a nursing home died as a consequence of multiorgan system failure secondary to sepsis from a ruptured bowel. The nursing home staff had failed to promptly report the patient's failure to have a bowel movement or complaints of severe abdominal pain and abdominal swelling. The nursing home staff also failed to follow the physician's standing orders to provide appropriate therapy for constipation, including enemas and milk of magnesia. When a family member expressed concern about the resident's severe constipation and abdominal pain, a nurse told the relative that they did not call the physician every time "somebody gets a bellyache." The jury awarded $500,000 in compensatory damages and $5 million in punitive damages. The U.S. Circuit Court of Appeals for the Eighth Circuit ruled that the nurses' conduct was so outrageous that punitive damages were appropriate (Tammelleo, 2004a).

Claims of Negligence and Student Nurses

Claims of negligence may arise in situations in which student nurses provide care. The emphasis on patient safety and reporting preventable adverse outcomes has brought an increasing number of student errors to light (Institute for Safe Medication Practices [ISMP], 2007; Mahlmeister, 2008; Wolf et al, 2009). Because the student is not yet a licensed professional, the faculty member or licensed nurse who is supervising the student is often named in the lawsuit. The agency or hospital in which the student is practicing also may be named under the legal doctrine of vicarious liability. *Dimora v. Cleveland Clinic Foundation* (1996) is a case in point. A student nurse was assigned to care for a patient who had serious difficulty with maintaining her balance and required close supervision when standing, walking, and transferring. The student nurse testified that she knew the patient had an unsteady gait, but still left her unattended on a commode. The patient fell and was injured. The hospital was named in the lawsuit and appealed, claiming the student was not an employee. The Ohio Court of Appeals ruled that a hospital was held to the same legal standard of care for a student nurse's error as for the same error committed by a licensed professional nurse.

Several recent cases reinforce the importance of informing the patient that a student is providing the care, and documenting that he or she agrees to the care. In *Lovett v. Lorain Community Hospital* (2004), a student nurse, under the direct supervision of an instructor, administered Demerol and Vistaril by the intramuscular route and punctured the sciatic nerve. The patient sued the hospital for negligence. A lower court dismissed the initial lawsuit because the student and the instructor were not employees of the hospital. The Ohio Court of Appeals reversed the lower court's decision. The higher court affirmed that a patient may assume that the care he or she receives in a hospital is provided by that institution. The patient can assume the student and instructor are agents of the hospital, unless the patient has been specifically informed and has agreed to receive care from the student (Snyder, 2004b). In a case involving an RN training to become a certified registered nurse anesthetist (CRNA), the court again affirmed the fundamental right of the patient to give informed consent when a student is providing the care. The student CRNA accidentally tore the patient's esophagus while performing a tracheal intubation (*Luettke v. St. Vincent Mercy Medical Center*, 2006). The legal standard of care requires patients to be informed of the identities of persons providing care and treatment, and told who will be supervising a student (Snyder, 2006b).

Because a student nurse is not yet a licensed professional, if a lawsuit is filed the alleged claim is usually "ordinary negligence" rather than "professional malpractice." In one case, however, the Michigan Court of Appeals permitted a claim of professional malpractice when a student nurse committed a medication error resulting in the patient's death (*Dennis v. Specialty Select Hospital—Flint*, 2005). In the case, a physician ordered an oral antifungal agent (Nystatin). The student nurse erroneously administered the drug intravenously. The patient died shortly thereafter. The court ruled, among other things, that the student should have possessed the requisite knowledge and clinical judgment to administer the drug safely. The actions of the student were not "ordinary negligence," but "professional malpractice" (Tammelleo, 2005). The court also ruled that both the student nurse and the hospital in which the patient death occurred could be subjected to the claim for malpractice.

Criminal Negligence. Criminal negligence represents a case in which the negligent acts of the nurse (normally an unintentional civil wrong) also constitute a crime. In most states, a nurse can be prosecuted when the conduct is deemed so reckless that the action results in serious harm or death to the patient. In 1997 two RNs and an advanced practice nurse licensed in Colorado were charged with criminal negligent homicide in the death of a newborn resulting from a medication error (Kowalski and Horner, 1998). In this case an oil-based form of penicillin was erroneously administered to the infant. The drug was administered at 10 times the physician's prescribed dose. This case is detailed in a 1998 article by Kowalski and Horner titled "A Legal Nightmare: Denver Nurses Indicted" (see References). This article should be read by every student and graduate nurse.

The Colorado case reflects the changing perspective of our justice system when negligent acts of health care professionals result in patient death. In the event of an unanticipated patient death, it is more likely that the conduct of basic as well as advanced practice nurses will be scrutinized by the criminal justice system (Iyer and Levin, 2007). This shift may in part be a result of the public's increasing awareness of the magnitude of error in health care. It also may stem from consumer demands for greater accountability by health care systems and workers when injury or death occurs. Conservative estimates suggest that as many as 98,000 patients die each year as a result of the negligence and malpractice of health care providers (Institute of Medicine, 2000), and another 90,000 deaths per year are attributed to hospital-acquired infections (National Nosocomial Infections Surveillance [NNIS], 2004). Recent data derived from surveillance activities conducted under the auspices of the National Healthcare Safety Network [NHSN] (Edwards et al, 2007) support earlier estimates for hospital-acquired infections.

Other negative consequences that a nurse faces when criminal charges are filed include the loss of his or her job and disciplinary action by the state licensing board. Even when the criminal charges are not supported, the nurse's license can be suspended or revoked and out-of-pocket fines levied by the board if there is evidence of violation of the NPA. An attorney may have to be retained to represent the nurse at considerable personal expense when criminal charges are filed. The nurse's malpractice insurance generally does not cover the attorney's fees in this case. Neither is the nurse's employer obligated to pay the legal fees of a nurse charged with a felony. In the Colorado case, the nurse practitioner was immediately terminated. The two direct-care nurses were permitted to work in nonpatient care areas of the hospital. The costs of the criminal defense of all three nurses were paid by the hospital.

Nursing care that is deemed "deplorable" by the courts may result in disqualification of the nurse's employer from participation in the federal government's Medicare or Medicaid programs. Essentially the facility will be without adequate funding to continue operating, and the nursing staff will lose their jobs. A case in point is *Barbourville Nursing Home v. U.S. Department of Health and Human Services* (USDHHS) (2006). During a compliance survey visit to the facility by the DHHS, major infractions of nursing home regulations were discovered. A fine in excess of $24,000 was levied by the federal government, and because the actions of the nurses placed the patients in immediate jeopardy (e.g., contaminating wounds with feces during dressing changes and inadequate skin care resulting in severe pressure sores), the nursing home was disqualified from participating in Medicare.

Defenses Against Claims of Negligence. In some cases a nurse can use certain legal doctrines as a defense against a claim of negligence. These standard defenses are discussed in the next section. In no case may a nurse provide a defense of "only following the provider's orders" against allegations of negligence (ANA, 2006; Snyder, 2007b). The NPA, licensing board rules and regulations, and nursing case law have delineated the nurse's independent duty to evaluate all provider orders before implementing them. In doing so, the nurse must consider two points: (1) is the order lawful and (2) is the order in this particular patient's best interest?

Each nurse has an absolute duty to take some positive action to prevent harm when orders are inappropriate or incomplete or when the actions of another health care provider endanger the patient's well-being. This principle of affirmative duty is well recognized in law and in ethics. The ANA Code of Ethics for Nurses (2001) and the American Medical Association's Code of Medical Ethics (2008-2009) recognize the central role of nurses in preventing patient harm.

In *Columbia Medical Center of Las Colinas v. Bush* (2003), a jury awarded $13.1 million to a patient who suffered permanent brain damage and has no independent motor function or capacity for speech after receiving the wrong medication for a cardiac dysrhythmia. After consulting with a cardiologist, the ED physician ordered verapamil for treatment of the patient's ventricular tachycardia. The ED nurse, certified in advanced life support and her nursing supervisor who was present, knew the drug was contraindicated for ventricular tachycardia. The two nurses did not question the order and permitted an emergency medical technician (EMT) to give the drug. The patient suffered profound hypotension and a cardiopulmonary arrest. The Texas Court of Appeals opined that the nurse and her supervisor had a duty, when they had serious questions about a medication involving extreme risk to the patient, to activate the chain of command to obtain additional medical consultation and advice (Tammelleo, 2004b).

Emergency Situations. Nursing care rendered in a life-threatening emergency may breach the standard of care required under ordinary circumstances. For instance, a woman who is 8 months' pregnant arrives in the labor and delivery suite. She is hemorrhaging because of a premature separation of the placenta (abruptio placentae). An emergency cesarean delivery is ordered by the physician. The woman is near death as a result of blood loss. There also are clear signs of fetal distress. To expedite the surgical delivery, the operating room team does not observe the strict aseptic technique normally required during insertion of a Foley catheter into the woman's bladder and forgoes the lengthy abdominal scrub normally performed with an iodine solution.

The mother and infant are brought through the crisis safely, although the woman develops a skin infection at the site of the abdominal incision, which causes noticeable scarring. She also must be treated for a bladder infection, which resolves by discharge on the fourth postpartum day. She sues the nurses and physician. In this case the defense could argue that to save the life of the mother and baby, the methods used were reasonable and prudent. Even a delay of seconds could have resulted in the death of the woman or her infant. Expert witnesses are produced to support the defense assertion that it would breach the standard of care in this particular situation to follow customary procedures in preparing the woman for surgery.

Governmental Immunity. For nurses working in federal or state health care facilities, a defense of governmental immunity may be used. Laws have been enacted that shield individual health care workers employed in federal or (some) state facilities from personal responsibility for damages awarded in malpractice cases. Nurses employed by the Department of Veterans Affairs, the U.S. Public Health Service, the National Aeronautics and Space Administration, and the Department of Defense are shielded from civil suits in the performance of professional duties. This immunity was granted through enactment of specific federal statutes, including the Federal Tort Claims Act of 1946 and the Federal Employees Liability Reform and Tort Compensation Act of 1988. The intent of these laws was to substitute the U.S. government as the defendant in a malpractice suit. The government has waived its sovereign immunity against suit and pays the damages for injuries caused by the negligent acts of health care professionals employed in the aforementioned federal agencies.

State immunity statutes vary. In some instances individual states have not waived their sovereign immunity from lawsuits. In those cases the state is *not* substituted for the individual health care provider in malpractice cases. Nurses and physicians are liable for their negligent acts in these states and are personally responsible for damages awarded. It may be imperative in this circumstance for the health care professional to have individual malpractice insurance. The nurse should seek the advice of an attorney to determine whether it would be prudent to purchase malpractice insurance (Ashley, 2005; Buppert, 2008).

Good Samaritan Immunity. Good Samaritan laws may limit a nurse's liability or shield the nurse from a malpractice claim if the nurse renders assistance in an emergency that occurs outside of the employment setting. Although in most states the nurse owes no legal duty to an accident victim, once the nurse makes a decision to stop and render aid (an ethical decision), a nurse-patient relationship is established. (Some states, including Vermont, Minnesota, and Wisconsin, have enacted "duty to rescue" or "compulsory assistance" laws.)

When the nurse renders care at the scene of an accident, he or she is required to render the standard of care that any reasonable and prudent nurse would render in a similar situation. To prevail in a malpractice suit under the Good Samaritan laws, the plaintiff must prove that the nurse intentionally caused the injury or was grossly negligent. Therefore, each nurse should be familiar with his or her state-specific Good Samaritan statute. Nurses also should be reassured by the fact that the preponderance of malpractice cases that invoke the Good Samaritan defense are settled in favor of the nurse.

Statutes of Limitation in Malpractice Cases

Each state has established a time limit in which a person may initiate a lawsuit. Although many states have established a time limit of 2 or 3 years from the date of the patient's injury or death in which the plaintiff must sue, statutes of limitation vary widely from state to state. In some jurisdictions a "termination of treatment" rule exists. It is predicated on the assumption that some injuries result from a series of treatments over time. In this case the statute of limitation does not begin to run until the treatment ends.

Other rules and regulations govern the "tolling" or running of the statutes of limitation. The court recognizes that an injured party cannot initiate a malpractice case until he or she discovers that some harm was done (discovery rule). This can occur when health care providers actually hide the facts in the case of an injury through fraud, deceit, or concealment, as in the following:

◆ Fraudulent or misleading entries in the medical record
◆ Destruction of evidence
◆ Destruction of the medical record

The statute of limitation also is altered when a foreign object is left in the patient's body. Until the foreign object is discovered, the statute of limitation does not begin to run. States have rules that regulate the tolling of the statute of limitation in cases involving mentally incompetent adults and minors. In the case of an adult patient who is so severely injured that there is a loss of mental capacity, the statute of limitation may not begin to toll until mental competence is regained. The statute of limitation varies in the case of minors and may only expire when the child reaches the age of majority (age 18 or 21 years) (Westrick and Dempski, 2008).

Each nurse should be familiar with the statute of limitation for his or her state. If the nurse suspects that some form of fraud or deceit has occurred relative to a patient's injury, the agency's risk manager or attorney should be contacted immediately. Major penalties and fines are applicable in cases in which health care providers deliberately deceive the patient or destroy evidence. These acts rise to the level of criminal misconduct and can result in loss of one's professional license and possible incarceration.

Transparency and Disclosure of Error. When errors occur in practice, studies repeatedly confirm that telling the patient (and family) about the mistake (voluntary disclosure) results in far less severe ramifications for the clinicians and healthcare facility (American Society for Healthcare Risk Management [ASHRM], 2006; Woods and Rozovsky, 2003). In 2001 TJC established a new patient safety care standard requiring that institutions have a process in place to disclose unanticipated outcomes to patients. Disclosure of errors and unanticipated adverse outcomes is a key element of the national patient safety movement (Riley et al, 2008). The process of disclosure has been delineated by the National Quality Forum [NQF] in its publication, "Safe Practices for Better Healthcare" (2009). Safe Practice Number 7 states,

> "Following serious unanticipated outcomes, including those that are clearly caused by systems failures, the patient, and as appropriate, the family should receive timely, transparent, and clear communication concerning what is known about the event" (p. vi).

When an unanticipated outcome occurs, the provider is generally responsible for discussing the situation with the patient and or family members. Other agency representatives may be involved in the disclosure process, including administrators, risk managers, or attorneys. The nurse should not assume responsibility for disclosure before speaking to the provider and agency leaders. It should be determined in advance who will speak with the patient (or family) and how questions and concerns about the patient's condition, subsequent treatment, and the cost of any required care will be addressed. Fear that disclosure will lead to a malpractice claim is a significant barrier to voluntary disclosure, despite research findings to the contrary. In fact patients sue for many reasons, including withdrawal of health team members after the event, silence, mishandling of information about unanticipated outcomes, delayed communication about adverse events, and anger when they believe they have not been told the truth about events (Kachalia, 2009; Stewart et al, 2006). If a nurse believes that providers have not disclosed essential information to the patient, concerns should be taken to the managers, administrators through the agency's line of authority. Research conducted by Shannon and associates (2009) on nurses' perceptions regarding disclosure found that nurses conceived of disclosure as a team event, rather than a physician-patient discussion. Nurses felt they were excluded from the disclosure process. Furthermore, nurses in the study focus groups admitted to routinely and independently disclosing nursing errors that did not involve serious injury, but believed that when systems flaws or team mistakes contributed to the error and injury, the physician should serve as the team leader in the disclosure discussion.

Nursing Malpractice Insurance

With more states recognizing nursing malpractice as a legitimate claim in a civil suit, the question of whether nurses should carry malpractice insurance has become increasingly important. Nursing journals have published a number of articles that either address this question or describe the types of malpractice coverage the nurse should consider (Buppert, 2008); textbooks also discuss the issue of liability insurance (Westrick and Dempski, 2008). An increasing consensus appears to recommend that all nurses purchase malpractice insurance as a result of changes in the health care system, civil law, and insurance company policies. Legal authors also are quick to note the fallacy of the assumption that having malpractice insurance increases the risk that the nurse will be targeted in a malpractice case. Lack of coverage will not discourage a lawsuit when there is a legitimate claim. Reasons given for the purchase of malpractice insurance by RNs include:

- Expanding functions of RNs and advanced practice nurses
- Floating and cross-training mandates
- Increasing responsibility for supervising subordinate staff
- Failure of some employers to initiate an adequate defense for nurses
- Insurance coverage limits that are lower than the actual judgment made against the nurse in a lawsuit

Other considerations that the nurse must take into account when considering malpractice insurance include whether he or she is employed by the federal government. In this case the nurse may be shielded from personal liability by federal tort statutes, although some states still uphold the doctrine of "sovereign immunity," making it impossible to sue a state-run medical facility for negligence. In those states, it is a virtual necessity for nurses to purchase malpractice insurance because health care workers become the only available targets in a malpractice case.

Liability

Closely tied to the concepts of negligence and malpractice is that of liability. Liability asserts that every person is responsible for the wrong or injury done to another resulting from carelessness.

Personal Liability

Within the context of nursing practice, the nurse is always accountable for the outcomes of his or her actions in carrying out nursing duties. The rule of personal liability requires the professional nurse to assume responsibility for patient harm or injury that is a result of his or her negligent acts. The nurse cannot be relieved of personal liability by another professional, such as a provider or nurse manager, who asserts, "Don't worry; I'll take responsibility for the consequences."

The principle of personal liability is illustrated in a Connecticut case, *Osiecki v. Bridgeport Health Care Center, Inc.* (2005). A jury found that a nurse caring for a patient with a tracheostomy failed to provide proper tracheostomy care, assessment of breath sounds, and reevaluation of the patient's pulmonary status at appropriate intervals. The patient died secondary to a pulmonary hemorrhage, and the breaches in the standard of nursing care were found to be a substantial factor contributing to the patient's death. Had the nurse properly assessed the patient and at frequent intervals, early identification of pulmonary congestion would have permitted timely treatment. The surviving spouse was awarded $827,000 for the nurse's negligent actions.

An earlier case, *Gladney v. Sneed* (1999), also affirmed the nurse's duty to serve as a patient advocate and invoke the chain of command when a physician's orders appear inappropriate based on the patient's condition. Following a motor vehicle accident a woman was taken to the ED of a hospital with signs of hypovolemic shock. The physician ordered morphine and Valium despite the patient's deteriorating condition, and the nurse administered the drugs. The patient coded and expired 3 hours later. The court ruled that the hospital, as the nurse's employer, was negligent for the patient's death. A reasonable and prudent ED nurse should have recognized the signs and symptoms of worsening shock, refused to give the medications, promptly instituted resuscitative measures, and invoked the chain of command to obtain additional medical assistance (Snyder, 2000a).

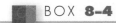

BOX **8-4**

Most Frequent Allegations of Nursing Negligence

- Failure to communicate and report*
- Failure to monitor the patient and report significant findings
- Failure to ensure patient safety
- Failure to rescue
- Improper treatment or negligent performance of the treatment

- Medication errors
- Failure to follow the agency's policies and procedures
- Failure to invoke the chain of command/access the line of authority

*The Joint Commission found that communication failures (i.e., reporting, SBAR communication, and shift hand-offs) were the number one contributing cause of medical error and preventable adverse outcomes (Joint Commission guide to improving staff communication, Oakbrook Terrace, IL, TJC, 2005).
Adapted from Nursing Service Organization (NSO): *CNA Healthpro nursing claims study: an analysis of claims with risk management recommendations 1997-2007*, Hatboro, PA, 2008, NSO. Retrieved April 2009 from: www.nso.com/pdfs/db/rnclaimstudy.pdf?fileName=rnclaimstudy.pdf&folder=pdfs/db&isLiveStr=Y&refID=rnclaim.

In 1989 the ANA summarized the most frequent allegations of negligence leveled against nurses in malpractice cases (Box 8-4). These charges have not substantially changed in the ensuing decades (Iyer and Levin, 2007; Nursing Service Organization [NSO], 2009). Nurses may be educated to implement effective risk control strategies that reduce these claims. These personal and system-wide strategies are discussed in the next section.

Many nurses practice under the misconception that they are protected from personal liability when employed by a health care entity, such as a hospital. I have heard nurses say, "Why would a patient sue me personally? I don't have the financial resources of this [hospital, nursing home, home health care agency]!" Nurses can and have been individually named in lawsuits and found negligent. Damages can be levied against the nurse's current assets and future earnings for negligent acts. Furthermore as Snyder (2003b) reports, hospitals have sued nurses to recoup financial losses suffered when they were required to pay damages for the alleged negligence of the nurses named in the malpractice case. Personal liability is illustrated in the case of *Siegel v. Long Island Jewish Medical Center* (2003). A hospital nurse and two private-duty nurses erroneously administered a lethal hypertonic saline solution to a 33-year-old woman. The New York Supreme Court, Appellate Division ruled that after the hospital settled with the deceased woman's father, the hospital could continue its suit from the nurses to recoup the money the hospital paid to the family.

Personal Liability with Floating and Cross-Training

New models of patient care often mandate floating and cross-training of patient care staff to enhance efficiency and reduce staffing costs. These models of care have increased the personal liability of nurses (Westrick and Dempski, 2008). Professional nurses must be cognizant of state statutes and case law when asked to perform services outside of their usual area of practice. In no case is a nurse ever permitted to perform tasks or render services when he or she lacks the requisite knowledge and skill to act competently.

The NPA and the administrative rules and regulations of the licensing board provide explicit statutory language regarding a nurse's duty to provide safe and competent care. For example, the Administrative Rules of the Tennessee Board of Nursing (revised, 2007) state:

"Each individual is responsible for personal acts of negligence under the law. RNs are liable if they perform delegated functions they are not prepared to handle by education and experience, and for which supervision is not provided. In any patient care situation, the RN should perform only those acts for which each has been prepared and has demonstrated ability to perform, bearing in mind the individual person's responsibility under the law."

—TENNESSEE RULES AND REGULATIONS OF REGISTERED NURSES RULE 1000-1-04 (3)(a): RESPONSIBILITY

In addition to the laws governing practice in floating and cross-training situations, an increasing body of nursing case law also defines the limitation of assignments. Appellate court decisions have addressed the issue of when a nurse may safely refuse an assignment to float without risk of job termination. A landmark case, *Winkelman v. Beloit Memorial Hospital* (1992), addressed the legal issues surrounding floating. The Supreme Court of Wisconsin ruled that under certain circumstances a nurse had a right to refuse floating assignments without fear of reprisal.

Nurse Winkelman was a skilled maternity nurse who was employed for 16 years at Beloit Memorial Hospital, working exclusively in the nursery. In 1987 the hospital created a policy that required nurses in the maternity setting to float when the patient census was low in their unit. Nurse Winkelman was asked to float to an adult floor dedicated to the care of postoperative and geriatric patients. She notified her immediate supervisor that she did not feel qualified to float to that unit and that attempting to provide care in that setting would place the patients at risk. In her testimony the nurse said that she was given three choices: float, find another nurse who would float in her place, or take an unexcused absence day. She subsequently went home, and her employer construed her actions as "voluntary resignation of her employment." Nurse Winkelman then filed a complaint for wrongful discharge and breach of contract. A jury verdict was rendered in favor of Nurse Winkelman on the charge of wrongful discharge. The case was appealed and affirmed by the Supreme Court of Wisconsin. The court found that the nurse had identified a fundamental and well-defined public policy in the Wisconsin Administrative Code, which stated that a nurse should not offer or perform services for which he or she is not qualified by education, training, or experience.

The nurse's right to refuse a floating assignment has not been supported in all cases. Courts have affirmed the right of a health care facility to redirect staff to meet the needs of patients. The New Mexico Supreme Court, in *Francis v. Memorial General Hospital* (1986), held that the hospital was not prohibited from discharging a nurse who refused to float when the employer had made a reasonable offer to train the nurse for new responsibilities.

Nurse Francis, a critical care nurse, refused to float to an orthopedic unit, stating he did not feel qualified to care for orthopedic patients. The hospital then offered to provide him with an orientation to the floors where he might float in the future. When he refused the opportunity for orientation, he was terminated. The court upheld his discharge.

Although it is clear that nurses have a legal duty to refuse specific tasks that they cannot perform safely and competently, the prudent nurse should carefully consider the consequences of not floating. Careful negotiation with the nursing supervisor and the team leader making the actual assignment often can result in a satisfactory compromise. The floated nurse should clarify what aspects of professional nursing care he or she can safely carry out and which tasks are beyond his or her current capabilities. A reasonable supervisor will not insist that a nurse attempt to perform a task that he or she has no education, training, or current expertise to implement.

Another important strategy that may reduce the nurse's personal liability is to request that the team leader appoint a resource nurse who is skilled in the care of the patients on the unit. The resource nurse can assist the floated nurse as needed. It also is prudent practice for the floated nurse to enter a note in the medical record naming the resource or support nurse who will be available and responsible to assist with planning and evaluating care. For instance:

> "Assumed care of Mrs. Jones after report completed. L. Doe, RN, will co-manage patient and assist with procedures, planning, and evaluation of care as needed"
>
> **—J. SMITH, RN (FLOATER)**

An NPA affirms that an RN ultimately is responsible for the quality of care provided to each patient, regardless of who actually is delegated the responsibility of carrying out the task. A claim of negligence may be leveled against the team leader who does not assign a competent "backup" or resource nurse to assist the floater. Only a nurse who is competent in the care of the patients normally treated in the setting (hospital, clinic, or home) can properly supervise a lesser-skilled worker and evaluate the outcomes of care. The point is so critical that professional nursing organizations in California joined together to affirm this concept in law.

A section of the California Health Facilities Licensing for Hospitals (California Code of Regulations, Title 22, 1996; revised 2005) mandates:

> "No hospital shall assign a licensed nurse to a nursing unit or clinical area unless that hospital determines that the licensed nurse has demonstrated current competence in that area, and has also received orientation to that hospital's clinical area sufficient to provide competent care."
>
> **—SECTION 70217, NURSING SERVICE STAFF: (a)**

Furthermore, TJC requires accredited organizations to ensure that all staff providing patient care, including float staff and agency or registry nurses, are properly oriented to their jobs and the work environment before providing care (TJC, 2006). Chapter 12 provides additional information about floating and accepting assignments.

Personal Liability for Team Leaders and Managers

The concept of personal liability extends to nurses who function as team leaders, supervisors, and upper-level managers. Team leaders, charge nurses, and managers are held to the standard of care of the reasonably prudent nurse employed in that role (Mahlmeister, 2006). Claims of negligence leveled against charge nurses generally surround:

- ◆ Functioning as a first responder in emergencies
- ◆ Triage of patients and allocation of staff and equipment
- ◆ Delegation of patient care tasks
- ◆ Supervision of orientees, float staff, and subordinates
- ◆ Reporting performance deficits in team members
- ◆ Supporting or invoking the chain of command process when indicated

Nurse managers and administrators at the upper end of the management ladder also may be held liable for the following:

- ◆ Inadequate training
- ◆ Failure to periodically reevaluate staff competencies
- ◆ Failure to discipline or terminate unsafe workers
- ◆ Negligence in developing appropriate policies and procedures
- ◆ Failure to uphold institutional licensing laws and state and federal statutes

The implementation of new models of care that alter staffing patterns and mixes may place managers at the same risk for liability as the health care providers delivering the actual bedside care (Hudspeth, 2008; Snyder, 2004b). The ANA affirms this view in the Code of Ethics for Nurses (2001):

> "Although nurses in administration, education, and research have relationships with patients that are less direct, in assuming the responsibilities of a particular role, they share responsibility for the care provided by those whom they supervise and instruct." (p. 17)

The appropriate standard of care is established in the case of team leaders, charge nurses, managers, and leaders by expert nurse witnesses who function in those positions. An increasing body of case law in malpractice suits also is contributing to expectations about team leader and manager conduct. Although nurse managers and administrators generally are well aware of their particular liability risks, direct-care nurses who are relatively unfamiliar with the expanding role of team leaders or charge nurses may be particularly vulnerable to claims of negligence. Health care redesign has resulted in considerable flattening of the chain of command for nursing departments (Tammelleo, 2004c).

In September 2003, the American Organization of Nurse Executives, the American Hospital Association, and other health-related organizations submitted an amicus curiae (friend of the court) brief in support of the unique role of the charge nurse (brief amici curiae, July 24, 2003). These associations responded to a National Labor Relations Board invitation to file briefs to provide guidance on the meaning of the term "independent judgment" and the scope of discretion required for independent judgment with respect to the charge nurse. The brief asserts that:

> "The charge nurse's background in the hospital's organization and in nursing practice enables him or her to step in when there is crisis or conflict, quickly to assess the situation and identify needed resources. Charge nurses also direct other employees, sometimes making split-second decisions that can literally be a matter of life or death." (pp. 6-7)

Team leaders, regardless of their title or designation, have assumed greater responsibility for unit- or department-based functions, such as those listed in Box 8-5.

Any RN functioning in the role of team leader or charge nurse should review the following documents from administration:
- Detailed job description for the role, including how responsibilities are limited when the nurse is asked to lead a team or serve as a charge nurse on an unfamiliar floor or department
- Job descriptions for the team members assigned delegated tasks
- Formal period of training and mentoring in the role
- Validated proof of competence before team leading independently
- Guidelines regarding personal patient care assignment when also serving as team leader
- Chain of command model for the facility, department, or unit

Administrators and nurse managers should be aware of landmark case laws regarding incompetent charge nurses and team leaders. A jury directed a verdict in excess of $7 million against a hospital in a 1995 Illinois case, *Holston v. Sisters of the Third Order* (1995).

A charge nurse repeatedly refused a direct-care nurse's requests to personally evaluate a patient whose vital signs were rapidly deteriorating after gastric bypass surgery. The charge nurse also refused to call the patient's physician until the patient experienced cardiopulmonary collapse. Emergency surgery revealed that a central venous pressure catheter had migrated and perforated the cardiac muscle. The patient experienced cardiac tamponade and died approximately 1 week after this critical incident.

BOX **8-5**

Professional Role Functions of the Team Leader or Charge Nurse

Regardless of the term used for the unit-based coordinator of care, a registered nurse on each shift is generally accountable for the following:

1. Assignment of nursing team members based on:
   - Unit census
   - Patient acuity
   - Complexity of care
   - Skill mix of team members
   - Anticipated admissions and discharges
2. Planning for supervision of:
   - Licensed practical or vocational nurses
   - Unlicensed assistive personnel
   - Temporary staff (floats, agency, or registry nurses)
   - Students
3. Surveillance of unit conditions, patient status, team activities
   - Periodic patient rounds
   - Ongoing communication with team members and providers
   - Periodic team "huddles" to identify new problems and needs
4. Monitoring team member performance
   - Provides positive feedback
   - Identifies knowledge or skill deficits and directs performance as needed to protect patients
   - Reports knowledge or skill deficits to appropriate managers
5. Consultant for clinical problems

6. Anticipatory planning for unusual situations or emergencies
7. First responder in clinical emergencies/disaster response coordinator for unit
8. Reassignment of staff based on changing unit conditions or patient status
9. Management of the flow of traffic through the unit
10. Arbitrator in clinical disputes or conflicts
11. Directing team members to appropriate resources including policies and procedures, standards of care, and evidence-based practice guidelines
12. Status updates to managers and administrators
    - Alerts leadership team about patient or family concerns or complaints
    - Reports acute shortage of staff or essential equipment and supplies
    - Invokes chain of command when indicated
13. Assists in planning for smooth transition at shift change
    - Obtains team member reports before shift change
    - Identifies staffing needs for next shift and works with management to ensure safe staffing
    - Completes an accurate and concise shift hand-off to oncoming charge nurse

In a second case, *Justin and Michelle Malovic v. Santa Monica Hospital Medical Center* (1995), a California jury found a nurse manager negligent for failing to implement the chain of command. The case is described as follows:

> The nurse manager failed to summon the chief of obstetrics when the primary obstetrician was unresponsive to a nonreassuring fetal heart rate. The primary nurse asked the nurse manager to personally evaluate the electronic fetal heart rate pattern. The manager did so, but decided there was no need to call the chief of the department. This case was complicated by the fact that the managing obstetrician's practice already was under investigation, and the nurse manager was aware of this fact. The primary obstetrician eventually attempted a forceps birth over an unacceptably long period of time (1 hour). A subsequent cesarean delivery resulted in the birth of an infant who is now neurologically damaged. The plaintiff's attorney successfully argued that had the nurse manager called the chief of obstetrics he would have effectively intervened, and the infant would have been born without damage.

These cases illustrate the necessity of validating the strong clinical skill of all RNs who are being considered for a leadership role that includes clinical supervision and consultation. Effective risk management of an unresolved clinical problem requires direct-care nurses to consult early and frequently with team leaders or managers. Each consultation with the team leader or manager should be carefully documented in the patient's medical record to demonstrate that appropriate chain of command process has occurred. The employer will likely be named in any lawsuit under the rule of vicarious liability if the team leader or manager offers negligent advice. Vicarious liability is discussed later in this chapter.

Personal Liability in Delegation and Supervision of Team Members

Team leaders and charge nurses who are responsible for delegation and supervision of team members must be absolutely clear about the legality of patient care assignments. They must determine whether it is reasonable and prudent to delegate a particular task based on their knowledge of the worker, the patient's status, and the current conditions in the work setting. The determination of whether a team leader or charge nurse has been negligent in delegating any particular patient care task or supervising subordinates will be based on these aforementioned considerations.

Mobile Infirmary Medical Center v. Hodgen (2003) is a case in point. A patient with cardiac problems sued after suffering catastrophic physical and mental disabilities when a graduate nurse, not yet licensed, administered five times the ordered dose of digoxin. The shift charge nurse assigned another nurse with only 7 months' experience to act as the graduate nurse's preceptor. The preceptor did not supervise the new graduate when she administered the drug. The jury found all three nurses negligent. The court criticized the shift charge nurse for assigning a novice nurse as a preceptor and for failing to give her explicit directions regarding the level of supervision required in the circumstances. The court also faulted the preceptor, who had never worked with the new graduate, for inadequate supervision. The jury awarded $2.5 million in punitive damages.

Criteria for lawful and safe delegation have been spelled out by state boards of nursing and professional organizations, such as the ANA, the American Association of Critical-Care Nurses, and the National Council of State Boards of Nursing (AACN, 2004; ANA, 2005; ANA-NCSBN, 2005; NCSBN, 2005). These guidelines and a growing body of case law assist the nurse in making decisions about safe delegation of patient care. *Singleton v. AAA Home Health, Inc.* (2000) illustrates the professional duties of the RN and the legal risks inherent in delegating nursing care to unlicensed assistive personnel.

Rhea Polk, a patient with cardiac and renal disease, was released from the hospital with a discharge plan for home health care to be provided by skilled nursing staff. Orders were issued to provide treatment for a right hip decubitus ulcer, including packing with Betadine gauze. The wound did not heal, and surgical debridement was required. The surgeon discovered gauze embedded in the ulcerated wound, and this was determined to be the cause of the problem. On behalf of Ms. Polk, Ms. Singleton sued the home health agency. Evidence uncovered during the trial indicated that the RN responsible for Ms. Polk's care had instructed home health aides in packing the wound and inappropriately delegated the task to them. The expert witness in the case asserted that the failure of an RN to properly inspect, clean, and treat the wound was the cause of the ulceration and need for surgery. The trial court rendered a verdict in favor of Ms. Singleton. The Louisiana Court of Appeals affirmed the verdict of the lower court on appeal.

It is important to note that in addition to acting negligently in delegating the wound packing to a home health aide, the nurse had violated the state's NPA. Although this issue was not addressed in the Singleton case, courts have ruled in previous malpractice cases that a failure to adhere to the NPA (a law) and the administrative rules and regulations of the licensing board constitutes negligence per se (negligence as a matter of law).

In *Williams v. West Virginia Board of Examiners* (2004), the Supreme Court of Appeals of West Virginia upheld the Kentucky Board of Nursing disciplinary action of an RN. The nurse was responsible for supervising the care of home health aides. Inspectors found numerous violations of the nurse's duty to delegate and supervise care given by the aides. Furthermore, there was evidence that the nurse falsified patients' records, indicating that home health aides were present, when in fact they were absent from the home. The nursing board suspended the nurse's license for 1 year.

Employer Liability

Although a nurse is never relieved of personal liability, the doctrine of vicarious or substituted liability permits a person to also sue the employer for the negligent conduct of nurses within the scope of their employment. Vicarious liability is based on the legal principle of *respondeat superior*, a Latin term that means "let the master answer" (for the actions of subordinates or servants). Because the employer has some control over the worker, the courts have affirmed that the employer may be held responsible for the employee's negligent acts when injury occurs.

In a New York case, *Pedraza v. Wyckoff Heights Medical Center* (2002), a hospital was found liable for the negligence of its nurses when they failed to adhere to the explicit policy it had established that bedrails were to be raised at all times for a particular category of high-risk patients. An 86-year-old patient with Alzheimer's disease was admitted to the hospital for pulmonary problems. Because the woman had Alzheimer's disease, she was classified as high risk for falling, and a fall-injury prevention protocol was to be implemented per hospital policy. A safety alert sign was to be posted above the bed, the patient was to be checked every 2 hours, the bed was to be kept in the lowest position, and all bedrails were to be up at all times. This protocol was not followed. A nurse found the patient face down on the floor in the hallway. One bedrail was down when the nurse had put the patient to bed after ambulating her. The hospital argued, in its defense, that keeping all four bedrails raised amounted to physical restraints and that restraints could not be applied without a physician's order. The court ruled in favor of the injured patient. The court opined that when a hospital employee expressly violates the institution's own internal policy, it is evidence of negligence. A further discussion about the legal aspects related to the use of restraints is presented later in this chapter.

In another case, *Johannessen v. Salem Hospital* (2003), the Supreme Court of Oregon ruled in a maternal death case that the husband of the deceased woman could claim punitive damages from the hospital for the egregious misconduct of the nurses. The patient exhibited symptoms of preeclampsia, a hypertensive disease of pregnancy. The physician failed to prescribe the customary medications ordinarily administered to prevent seizures and to lower the woman's high blood pressure. All the while the nurses did not question the lack of orders or advocate for the woman by invoking the chain of command. The court viewed this as reckless indifference to the patient's health and safety and held both the nurses and hospital liable for the woman's death (Snyder, 2004c)

Corporate Liability

Hospitals and other health care facilities have evolved into dynamic systems that coordinate the care provided by a range of health care professionals. As a consequence of these changes, the courts have expanded the concept of corporate negligence in verdicts rendered against health care giants. In *Brodowski v. Ryave* (2005), the Pennsylvania Superior Court ruled that there was sufficient evidence that a systematic breakdown in communication caused an improper diagnosis, and led to the patient's admission to a psychiatric unit before a stroke had been ruled out (Passarella, 2005). The patient was not properly treated, is now partially paralyzed, and has brain damage. The "standard of care" required of a health care corporation has been established through these cases, but varies from state to state. Some jurisdictions have permitted TJC standards or state department of health licensing laws to define the "corporate standard of care." An agency's own medical bylaws or policies and procedures have been admitted as evidence of the appropriate corporate standard of care. In *Thompson v. Nason Hospital* (1991), the court elaborated four duties of a health care corporation:

1. Maintain safe and adequate physical facilities and equipment.
2. Select and retain competent physicians.
3. Oversee the acts of all persons who practice medicine within the facility as they relate to patient care.
4. Formulate, adopt, and enforce rules and policies to ensure quality of care.

The court in the Brodowski case based its ruling on the doctrine of corporate liability outlined in the Thompson case.

In another case, *Rodebush v. Oklahoma Nursing Homes, Ltd.* (1993), the court found a nursing home liable for negligent hiring and supervision of a staff member, a nurse aide, who had a previous conviction of a violent felony: assault and battery with the intent to kill. The criminal record was discovered only after the family of a patient in the nursing home filed a lawsuit. The suit was initiated when the family's elderly parent was injured by the nurse aide, who was intoxicated at the time of the incident. The jury awarded $50,000 in actual damages and $1.2 million in punitive damages against the corporation for failing to follow its own policies in hiring, training, and supervising employees and in investigating employee misconduct.

Health care facilities also have been found corporately liable for failing to have adequate numbers of qualified nursing staff assigned on each shift to meet the needs of patients. In a landmark case, *HCA Health Services v. National Bank* (1988), an unattended infant experienced a respiratory arrest and suffered permanent anoxic brain damage. The jury rendered a verdict for the plaintiff, and awarded $2 million in compensatory damages (for the cost of ongoing care) and $2 million in punitive damages for failing to provide an adequate number of qualified staff.

The current nursing shortage is anticipated to grow in the first decades of this century. Nurses must develop a clear understanding of principles of safe staffing and advocate for appropriate staffing levels. Guidelines published by the ANA (2005) can assist nurses to ensure the efficient use of human resources. Nurses should review position statements published by the board of nursing as well as their specialty nursing organizations (i.e., Association of periOperative Registered Nurses [AORN] or the Association of Women's Health, Obstetric and Neonatal Nurses [AWHONN]). Staffing guidelines promulgated by these organizations may assist the nurse in articulating concerns and formulating recommendations for improved staffing levels. Another useful strategy is to provide managers and administrators with journal articles that discuss the liability of hospitals when they do not provide sufficient numbers of qualified team members to meet patient needs (Iyer & and Levin, 2007; Kalisch et al, 2009).

A similar finding of hospital negligence for failing to provide adequate staffing was found in *Merritt v. Karcloglu* (1996), in which a Louisiana hospital was found negligent for failing to have sufficient nursing staff to provide essential care. The hospital had a written policy that directed a nurse in the cardiac care unit to respond to "codes" called in other areas of the hospital. A nurse assigned exclusively to a disoriented older adult patient in the critical care unit was required to respond to a code. While she was out of the unit, her patient attempted to get out of bed, fell, and fractured her hip. She subsequently died, in part because of complications of her fall (pneumonia, decubitus development, sepsis). Her family sued and was awarded $500,000. The verdict was upheld on appeal. The hospital had a policy that required a nurse to be in "two places at one time," an impossible standard to meet.

As more nurses become independent contractors, working for temporary staffing agencies, courts have been asked to determine whether a hospital using temporary nursing staff was liable for the acts of an agency nurse (*Ruelas v. Staff Builders Personnel Services, Inc.*, [2001]). An agency nurse was alleged to have abused a patient during administration of an enema. (The precise nature of the abuse was not delineated.) The court affirmed that as a general rule, the employer (in this case Staff Builders) is legally liable for an employee's wrongful conduct. However, in this case, the agency had no practical or even theoretical right to control how its nurses carried out their clinical responsibilities in a particular setting. Although the agency is responsible for ensuring that the nurse has the requisite license, education, experience, and certifications, the hospital has direct control and supervision of the nurse's actions. Staff Builders was dismissed from the lawsuit.

The TJC has developed detailed standards related to the orientation, training, and education of agency (contracted) staff (TJC, 2009). Courts have affirmed that facilities have a duty to provide a targeted orientation for agency nurses. A job-based or unit-based handout, if readily available, can be a useful reference for the agency nurse (TJC, 2006). A mentor or resource nurse should be provided during the targeted orientation and thereafter as needed when a new task or problem is encountered. Team members should have an opportunity to evaluate the agency nurse and provide written feedback about performance.

REDUCING LEGAL LIABILITY
Risk Management Systems

One of the most powerful allies the nurse has in any health care setting to facilitate positive change and reduce personal and corporate liability is the risk manager. The risk manager is a professional who tracks accidents and injuries that occur in the facility. The job of the risk manager is to establish and strengthen systems within the agency to reduce preventable patient injuries or deaths and to eliminate the loss of revenues as fines or the payment of damages through the insurance carrier. The risk manager may assist nurse managers in the development of effective policies and procedures to improve practice. The risk manager also is knowledgeable about federal and state administrative rules and regulations affecting health care systems, health care licensing laws, and health care case law. This knowledge is essential to prevent inadvertent violation of health care laws and to reduce claims of negligence and malpractice within the institution.

The IOM report *To Err Is Human* (2000) recommends a proactive approach to risk management. Nurses are encouraged to anticipate the potential for errors, report "near misses," and work closely with the risk manager to reduce preventable adverse events. All health care providers are urged to develop high-reliability operating systems. This concept is derived from the airline and nuclear energy industries. Both have established excellent safety records despite the highly complex and dangerous nature of their operations. The IOM recommends creation of a nationwide mandatory reporting system for collection of information about adverse events and the development of performance standards that focus on patient safety. Nurses will play a central role in this process.

Incident Reports or Unusual Occurrence Reports

Nurses are legally bound to report critical incidents to their nurse managers, agency administration, and the risk manager through a formal intra-agency document titled the "Unusual Occurrence Report" or "Incident Report." Emphasis on patient safety and quality has resulted in renaming of the Incident Report in many health care settings. The document is frequently referred to as the "Unusual Occurrence Form" but is also known by other titles, such as the "Quality Variance Report." This form often is directed to the risk management department through the nurse's immediate manager. The nurse manager has an opportunity to review the written report and begin the process of collecting information and mitigating any identified systems flaws in a timely fashion, depending on the nature of the incident. The report then is forwarded (usually within 24 hours) to the risk manager. If an ongoing problem does not appear to be any closer to resolution as the nurse works through the formal chain of command, the nurse may speak directly to the risk manager for guidance and advice. However, in the usual course of events, the nurse would first address concerns with his or her immediate nurse manager. Unfortunately, studies indicate that the rate of incident reporting still remains relatively low, particularly among physician providers (AACN, 2005; Kaldjian et al, 2008). Nurses are more likely to report unusual occurrences, and unanticipated adverse outcomes, but improvement is required to proactively prevent error and patient injury.

Critical incidents that result in patient injury or death eventually may lead to a malpractice claim. Because state laws vary as to whether the incident report may be "discovered" by the plaintiff's attorney in a lawsuit, it is essential that the nurse follow appropriate procedures when completing and filing this document.

1. The nurse should describe all events objectively; avoid subjective comments, personal opinions about why the incident occurred, or assumptions about events that were not witnessed. For example, if a patient was found lying on the floor at the foot of the bed, the nurse should avoid the statement, "Patient fell out of bed—found on floor." That the patient fell out of bed is an unfounded assumption. The nurse should instead state, "Entered room. Patient discovered lying prone at the foot of the bed. Both upper and lower side rails were raised."

2. The nurse should never note in the patient's medical record that an incident report has been completed and filed. This may alter the protection from discovery normally provided the document in some states. The jury also will be made aware that an incident report has been filed because they have access to nurses' notes submitted in evidence during the trial.

3. The nurse should never photocopy the incident report for his or her personal files. Photocopying an incident report generally is prohibited by agency policy and may be expressly prohibited in writing on the incident report itself. Photocopying the incident report and taking it out of the agency violates patient confidentiality. It may fall into the hands of individuals who are not authorized to read any information about the patient. It may fall into the hands of the plaintiff's attorney, should a lawsuit be filed, with damaging effects on the agency's ability to defend against the claims of negligence.

4. Physicians and advanced practice nurses should not write an order for an incident report to be filed. This brings the existence of an incident report to the attention of the plaintiff's attorney.

5. Report every unusual occurrence or incident. Do not assume that "everyone knows about the problem or event." Box 8-6 lists circumstances under which incident reports should be filed.

INTENTIONAL TORTS IN NURSING PRACTICE

Ordinarily, in the course of carrying out one's nursing duties, breaches in the applicable standard of care are assumed to be unintentional acts. In other words, the nurse did not intend to harm the patient. As noted, this civil wrong is referred to as an unintentional tort. An intentional tort is a second category of civil wrong. It involves the direct violation of a person's legal rights. In this case the nurse intends to perform the offensive act, although normally most nurses do not mean to harm the patient. The following acts are intentional torts:

- Assault
- Battery
- Defamation of character
- False imprisonment

BOX **8-6**

Circumstances Under Which the Incident Report Should Be Filed*

- Patient or client injury
- Unanticipated patient death
- Malfunction or failure of durable medical equipment
- Significant or unanticipated adverse reactions to ordered therapy or care
- Inability to meet a patient need(s) ordered therapy, medications, or treatments after consultation with appropriate nurse mangers or providers. This may be related to:
  - System problems (e.g., pharmacy closed, drug not available)
  - Unresolved problem with order (e.g., incomplete or illegible order)
  - Lack of qualified staff to implement order to provide needed care (e.g., registered nurse [RN] not available to perform task, and law stipulates that only an RN may perform the task
  - Patient or family refusal of care (e.g., request for do-not-resuscitate [DNR] orders)
- Unresolved problems with physical plant that jeopardize patient well-being (e.g., electrical hazard, loose carpet section, delay in repair of essential equipment)
- Unethical, illegal, or incompetent practice that is witnessed or reported
- Patient complaint about provider or health care worker
- Toxic spills, fires, other environmental emergencies
- Violent behavior on part of family or patient

*This list is not comprehensive but is a representative list of occurrences that should be reported.

♦ Invasion of privacy
♦ Intentional infliction of emotional distress

In the case of intentional torts, the plaintiff does not have to prove that the nurse breached a special duty or was negligent. The duty is implied in law (e.g., the duty to respect a patient's right to privacy). Generally, legal remedies for intentional torts include fines and punitive damages, although some intentional torts rise to the level of a criminal act (such as battery) and may result in a jail sentence. Some states, such as California, also have enacted penalties that include a term of imprisonment for willful and malicious breach of confidentiality in releasing information about a patient's human immunodeficiency virus (HIV) status.

Assault and Battery

Patients who agree to treatment or nursing care do not surrender their rights to determine who touches them. Assault is causing the person to fear that he or she will be touched without consent. Battery is the unauthorized or the actual harmful or offensive touching of a person. It is important to note that a charge of battery does not require proof of harm or injury. Nurses engaged in therapeutic procedures may face charges of battery if they touch a patient without consent. It is essential that the nurse ask the patient's permission to proceed before initiating any procedure, particularly those of an invasive nature. Nurses also should document that the patient has given permission for the treatment or procedure. Consider the following situation:

A woman in active labor cries out through each contraction. The nurse has a standing order from the obstetrician for administration of an intravenous narcotic should the woman request pain relief. However, the woman refuses, being determined to experience a medication-free birth. As labor progresses, the woman's cries become so loud that other laboring women and visitors in the unit express concern and anxiety. Repeated efforts to assist the woman with breathing and relaxation exercises to reduce her vocalization have failed. The nurse finally says to the patient, "Look, if you don't stop screaming and making those horrible noises, I'm going to give you the pain medication your doctor has ordered, whether you want it or not. You're frightening the other patients!" She repeats this threat several times and in the presence of the woman's family. Although the woman continues to cry out, the nurse does not give the medication. The delivery of the infant is uneventful and without problems. After discharge from the hospital, the patient retains a lawyer, claiming she was threatened with being sedated against her will. She further asserts that the nurse's repeated threats to inject her with a narcotic created an unbearable level of anxiety that interfered with her ability to cooperate with other necessary procedures during the birth. This assertion could result in a charge of negligence or intentional infliction of emotional distress.

In this case the nurse is charged with assault (i.e., threatening the patient with unauthorized touching). Had the nurse actually carried out her threat of giving the medication, the charge could be expanded to assault and battery. Consequences for the nurse charged with assault may include the following:

- Imposition of fines and punitive damages
- State board of nursing disciplinary action
- Termination by the employer

When battery occurs, the nature of the touching may raise the offense to the level of a crime. In the aforementioned scenario, assume that the nurse decides to give the narcotic against the woman's will. She engages the assistance of a scrub technician to physically restrain the woman so that she can access a vein for the injection. The technician, becoming frustrated with the woman's resistance to the procedure, says, "You're going to be sorry if you don't stop struggling." The technician purposefully hyperextends the woman's arm and says, "There, maybe if it hurts enough, you'll stop this nonsense." A loud snapping sound is heard, and tests indicate that the technician has fractured the woman's arm. The charge of battery in this case may result in more serious ramifications, including punitive damages and a term of imprisonment. Both of these cases are fact-based events known to this author. Unfortunately, similar cases are noted in the nursing and legal literature each month.

In *Duncan v. Scottsdale Medical Imaging, Ltd.* (2003), a court affirmed that a patient could sue a nurse for battery when she gave an injection of a narcotic, fentanyl, despite a direct, verbal refusal by the patient. The patient told the nurse that she would only accept meperidine (Demerol) or morphine for pain control during a diagnostic procedure. The nurse lied, telling her that the medication was indeed Demerol, but instead gave the fentanyl. The patient suffered serious complications including breathing difficulties, vocal cord dysfunction, and posttraumatic stress disorder. Such conduct by the nurse could also result in disciplinary action by the state licensing board; however, this was not addressed by the court.

Defamation of Character

A person has a right to be free from attacks on his or her reputation (defamation of character). Libel is a form of defamation caused by written work. Slander refers to an injury to one's reputation caused by the spoken word. Nurses may be subject to a charge of libel for subjective comments meant to denigrate the patient that are placed in the medical record or in other written materials read by others. For example, a patient suffering from extreme pain who requested narcotics frequently was labeled as a "whiner," a "liar," and a "drug seeker" with an "addictive" personality. These comments were noted on the medical record, on the nursing Kardex, and in nurse's notes attached to a clipboard, which was kept on a wall peg outside the patient's room.

The patient subsequently was found to have a severe intraabdominal infection that accounted for the intense pain he experienced. The patient sued for failure of the medical staff to identify and treat the infection. In the process of discovery, the patient, his family, and the attorney he had retained read the defamatory comments about his character. It was a distinct possibility that other family members, coworkers, and the patient's employer who visited may have read these subjective comments on the clipboard. A charge of libel was leveled against the nursing staff.

Nurses also may face charges of slander when they repeat similar types of subjective comments about patients in public places, such as elevators or hospital cafeterias. All patient care staff must be extremely cautious about discussing the patient or their opinions about the patient in public places. Even in report rooms or conference rooms, nurses should consider who in the immediate vicinity could inadvertently overhear the conversation. In all circumstances, only objective, professional language should be used in discussing patients.

False Imprisonment

False imprisonment is defined as the unlawful restraint or detention of another person against his or her wishes. Actual force is not necessary to support a charge of false imprisonment. An adult of sound mind (mentally competent) has a right to refuse any treatment that has previously been agreed to (Grace and McLaughlin, 2005; Iyer and Levin, 2007). If he or she refuses, the person may leave the facility (i.e., hospital, rehabilitation center, long-term care facility) whenever he or she chooses. The nurse has no authority to detain the patient, even if there is a likelihood of harm or injury as a result of discontinuing therapy.

The nurse has a duty to immediately notify the provider and appropriate nursing supervisors when a competent patient intends to leave "against medical advice" (AMA) but may not in any way prevent the individual from leaving the facility. Many agencies request that a patient sign an AMA form when they intend to leave in contradiction to the plan of care and despite the absence of a discharge order. The form may provide the facility with a reasonable defense against a malpractice claim if the patient's condition worsens or an injury is sustained and a malpractice claim is filed. A more detailed discussion follows later in this chapter.

Intentional Infliction of Emotional Distress

When the nurse's behavior is so outrageous that it leads to the emotional shock of a patient, the court can compensate the patient for emotional distress. A recent case in the area of maternity nursing illustrates the potential for a claim of intentional infliction of emotional distress. In *Roddy v. Tanner Medical Center* (2003), a woman brought suit against the hospital after she was treated in the ED for a miscarriage at approximately 10 weeks' gestation. While en route to the hospital, Ms. Roddy felt something large extrude from her vagina, and she bled heavily. She reported to the ED nurse that whatever she had passed was still in her underpants with a great deal of blood. Ms. Roddy indicated that the nurse told her she would take whatever she could out of her clothes, and then the nurse placed the soiled clothes in a plastic bag.

Ms. Roddy was subsequently discharged home in stable condition after a gynecologic examination confirmed that she had passed the products of conception. When she returned home and began to remove her clothes from the plastic bag to launder them, the intact fetus dropped to the floor. Ms. Roddy claimed intentional infliction of emotional distress. The court permitted the case to go forward, indicating that there was evidence of "reckless disregard" of the rights of the patient.

Invasion of Privacy

Another basic right is to be free from interference with one's personal life. An invasion of privacy occurs when a person's private affairs (including health history and status) is made public without consent. The nurse has a legal and ethical duty to maintain patient confidentiality, and there may be serious repercussions when the nurse breaches this duty and violates this fundamental patient right.

With the explosion in electronic information systems, issues related to patient confidentiality and invasion of privacy are now being addressed by the federal and state legislatures. Statutes, including the federal law HIPAA, have been enacted to control access to electronic health data. Nurses are given passwords to access a patient's electronic medical record. Nurses should never share passwords with colleagues because this increases the risk of unauthorized access to the patient's record.

In certain circumstances the law permits divulging information contained in a patient's medical record. These situations include reporting certain communicable diseases, child abuse, and gunshot wounds to the proper authorities. If a nurse is asked to provide information to any sources, the matter should immediately be referred to the agency's administrator or risk manager. In no case should the nurse personally divulge the information or provide copies of the patient's record to another person or agency. Another fact-based case known to this author illustrates the intentional torts of invasion of privacy and intentional infliction of emotional distress. Consider the following situation:

> A nurse works in a physician's office in a small, semirural community. The majority of the town's residents know each other. A patient being treated for several opportunistic infections has an HIV test performed. The nurse also is aware that the patient has been questioned by the physician about his sexual activities and that he has divulged that he is gay and has had unprotected sex with several male partners. When the test results are reported as positive, the nurse calls several close friends (who also know the patient) and reports the finding and information about the patient's sexual conduct. Before the patient is informed about his diagnosis by the physician, the man encounters two of the people who have been told about the HIV test result. They tell him that they know he is gay and infected with the HIV virus. He then discovers that the nurse has informed them about his condition. Suffering from intense shock and emotional pain, the man unsuccessfully attempts suicide.

In this case the nurse's actions rise to the level of willful, malicious, and intentional infliction of emotional distress. The nurse faces serious charges and, in some states with HIV confidentiality laws, could face a prison sentence for intentionally violating the patient's confidentiality in a manner meant to harm the patient. It is likely that the nurse's license also will be revoked for her actions, and the board may impose a significant fine.

The Nurse and Criminal Law

A crime is an offense against society, defined through written criminal statutes or codes. A criminal act is deemed to be conduct so offensive that the state is responsible for prosecuting the offending individual on behalf of society. Legal remedies for crimes include fines, imprisonment, and in some states, execution (death penalty). Criminal acts are classified as either minor (misdemeanors) or major (felonies) offenses. Misdemeanor offenses that nurses are commonly charged with include the following:

◆ Illegal practice of medicine
◆ Failing to report child or elder abuse
◆ Falsification of the patient's medical record
◆ Assault and battery and physical abuse of patients

Felony acts may be committed against the federal government and generally involve drug trafficking offenses and, increasingly, fraud in billing for services of Medicare patients. Other serious criminal acts include theft, rape, and murder. A nurse found guilty of a felony generally serves time in prison and usually suffers the permanent revocation of his or her nursing license.

Five RNs were indicted on 21 counts, including falsification of records, alteration of forms filed with the state department of health, and tampering with physical evidence in the death of a 97-year-old nursing home patient (Kelley, 2000). The woman died after being fed through a stomach tube attached to an enema bag. The nurses used the enema bag in lieu of the appropriate feeding equipment that was not available. The nursing director was found guilty on three counts and also surrendered her nursing license.

THE LAW AND PATIENT RIGHTS
Advance Directives

Society now recognizes the individual's right to die with dignity rather than be kept alive indefinitely by artificial life support. As a consequence, the majority of states have enacted "right-to-die" laws. These statutes grant competent adults the right to refuse extraordinary medical treatment when there is no hope of recovery. The term "advance directive" refers to an individual's desires regarding end-of-life care. These wishes generally are made through the execution of a formal document known as a living will. Right-to-die statutes vary from state to state; therefore, nurses must become familiar with their state-specific statute. Agency policies and procedures in the nurse's employment setting also will guide the nurse in an understanding of the patient's rights in this matter.

Living Wills

A living will is a legal document, a type of advance directive, in which a competent adult makes known his or her wishes regarding care that will be provided in the final stages of a terminal illness. A living will generally contains the following:

- Designation of the individual (proxy or surrogate) who is permitted to make decisions once the patient is incapacitated and no longer able to make decisions (often referred to as "decisionally incompetent" or "decisionally incapacitated")
- Specific stipulations regarding what care is acceptable and which procedures or treatments are not to be implemented
- Authorization of the patient's physician to withhold or discontinue certain life-sustaining procedures under specific conditions

Although living wills are legal in every state, they may not be legally binding. In some cases, a proxy is not recognized or sanctioned by the state statute. Living wills have been overturned, particularly when disputes arise among family members or significant others when the terminally ill patient is no longer able to make decisions. A living will may be revoked under any of the following conditions:

- There is evidence that the patient was not competent when the living will was executed.
- The patient's condition is not terminal.
- A state-imposed time for enforcement of the will has expired, and a new living will must be executed.
- The patient's condition has changed substantially, and the stipulations of the will no longer apply.

A living will must be written (in some cases, using a state-specific document), dated, signed, and witnessed. If asked to witness a patient's living will, the nurse should refer the matter to the agency's risk manager. It may not be lawful in a particular state for the nurse to witness this document.

Medical or Physician Directives and DNR Orders. A more specific type of living will that the patient may execute is known as the medical or physician directive. This document lists the desire of the patient in a particular scenario, such as whether he or she would want to be resuscitated if cardiopulmonary arrest occurs. DNR orders would be written by the physician based on written medical directives dictated by the patient. The medical directive, if properly executed, provides the physician with immunity from claims of negligence or intentional wrongdoing in the patient's death. The physician must also follow any state-specific statute and the agency's policies and procedures before writing a DNR order. Research has discovered a serious lack of uniformity among and within health care facilities in making certain that direct-care nurses and providers are aware of a patient's DNR status (Sehgal and Wachter, 2007). This can result in a significant risk for confusion and error and contribute to claims of negligence.

The nurse has an absolute duty to respect the patient's wishes in the case of DNR orders. A lawfully executed DNR order must be followed. Nurses have been sued for failure to observe DNR orders (Iyer and Levin, 2007). Claims against the nurse include battery, negligent infliction of pain and suffering, and "wrongful life" (*Anderson v. St. Francis–St. George Hospital*, 1992). Three problems may arise regarding a DNR order: A physician refuses to comply with the patient's wishes and initiates resuscitation, the patient revokes consent to the DNR order, or a family member demands that the DNR order be rescinded, despite the patient's continued objection to resuscitation (Teno, 2008). If one of these issues arises, the nurse must act promptly to enlist the assistance of the nursing supervisor or a hospital administrator. Remember that a patient may revoke a living will, including a DNR order, at any time.

The agency's ethics committee may be helpful in resolving disagreements between a physician and the patient, or between the family and the patient regarding DNR orders. After notifying the appropriate administrative team members, the nurse should document in detail any comments made by the patient or family regarding a change in DNR status, or comments, actions or orders issued by a physician who will not respect the patient's stated wishes.

Durable Power of Attorney for Health Care. In 1993, the Uniform Health-Care Decisions Act was approved. The Act recognizes an individual's right to make decisions about healthcare and enables a patient to accept or refuse treatment. The Act is also designed to provide autonomy when making end-of-life decisions. Durable power of attorney is a legal document that authorizes the patient to name the person (the health care proxy) who will make the day-to-day and final end-of-life decisions once he or she is decisionally incompetent. Naming a proxy who is intimately knowledgeable about the person's true wishes is important to ensure that the patient's desires will be carried out when he or she is no longer able to make decisions. Health care law experts recommend that individuals interested in naming a proxy seek legal assistance with executing a durable power of attorney for health care.

Nurses may be asked questions about living wills and durable power of attorney for health care by patients and their families. An important aspect of speaking to the patient about these issues is to provide the written materials about advance directives that are required under the federal statute, the Patient Self-Determination Act.

Informed Consent

For any patient to make meaningful choices about a particular procedure or treatment, the provider must convey certain material information. Under the doctrine of informed consent, the physician or advanced practice nurse has a duty to disclose information so that the patient can make intelligent decisions. This duty is mandated by federal statute (in the case of Medicare and Medicaid patients) and state law and is grounded as well in common law. In the case of routine as well as specialized care, the primary provider must disclose the following:

- Nature of the therapy or procedure
- Expected benefits and outcomes of the therapy or procedure
- Potential risks of the therapy or procedure
- Alternative therapies to the intended procedure and their risks and benefits
- Risks of not having the procedure

This duty to disclose rests with the provider and cannot be delegated to the RN. When the nurse has reason to believe that the patient has not given informed consent for a procedure, the provider should be immediately notified. In no case should the nurse proceed with initiating any part of the therapy that he or she is responsible for implementing. The patient's questions or concerns should be documented in the medical record to indicate why there has been a delay in carrying out the procedure (Mahlmeister, 2009b). If the nurse is responsible for witnessing the patient's signature on a consent form for the specified procedure, this process also should be deferred until the provider has had an opportunity to clarify the patient's questions.

A variety of negligence claims arise out of the informed consent process. The provider may be alleged negligent for failure to obtain informed consent. Court decisions generally have upheld the provider's duty to obtain informed consent and have dismissed cases that have claimed hospitals and its nurses were negligent for "failing to obtain informed consent." With adoption in some states of the corporate negligence doctrine, an increasing number of appellate courts have ruled that hospitals and nurses may be liable for failure to ensure that informed consent was given to the provider (*Karibjanian v. Thomas Jefferson University Hospital*, 1989; *Keel v. St. Elizabeth Medical Center*, 1992). Nurses have a duty to discuss concerns about informed consent with the primary provider. Should the nurse be unable to resolve the issue, the chain of command should be invoked to clarify questions or concerns.

In some cases, timely notification of a nursing manager may be essential to prevent violation of the patient's right to give consent. For instance, an RN is circulating during a surgical procedure, intended to debride and clean a severe leg wound. The consent form signed by the patient explicitly lists "wound debridement" as the procedure to be performed. On beginning the procedure, the surgeon asks for additional instruments, indicating that the wound is so infected that the leg will have to be amputated below the knee. Because the patient has received general anesthesia and is unable to give consent, and the consent form itself does not authorize an amputation procedure, the nurse must question the surgeon's intention to remove the leg. If the surgeon refuses to discuss the matter, or again requests the instruments necessary for the procedure, the nurse must obtain immediate assistant from her supervisor and if possible, the medical administrator (chief of surgery). The instruments for surgical amputation should not be placed on the sterile table, and in compliance with intraoperative communication standards, all other team members should be alerted that there is a unresolved question about the procedure, and that a manager or administrator is on the way to evaluate the surgical plan.

Communication Barriers and Informed Consent. Health care organizations that receive federal funds are required to meet the language access provision of the Culturally and Linguistically Appropriate Services [CLAS] Standards for Health. The standards were issued in 2001 by the USDHHS. The standards require that the organization must:

- Offer and provide free and timely language assistance services, including bilingual staff and interpreter services at all points of contact at all hours of operation.

◆ Provide verbal and written notices (in the individual's preferred language), of the right to receive language assistance services.

◆ Ensure competence of language assistance provided by interpreters and bilingual staff.

Family and friends should *not* be used as interpreters except at the care recipient's request. The duty to ensure appropriate communication is also established by the ADA (discussed previously). When an interpreter is used to facilitate communication, the nurse should document this process. The medical record should contain the name of the interpreter, the topic of the educational session, or substance of the informed consent discussion, and the patient's questions and consent, if given (Smith, 2007).

TJC Comprehensive Accreditation Manual for Hospitals (2009) requires the facility to respect a patient's right to and need for effective communication. Written materials, including consent forms and discharge instructions, should be available in the patient's preferred language. Educational materials should be culturally sensitive, and at a reading level that recognizes literacy limitations. TJC (2008) provides detailed information and guidance for development of a central office to coordinate all communication services, including the availability of interpreters fluent in medical terminology for informed consent discussions between the provider and patient. Language access also includes access to interpreters skilled in signing for hearing-impaired patients and materials in Braille for vision-impaired individuals.

A New Jersey case (*Borngesser v. Jersey Shore Medical Center* [2001]) illustrates the duty to provide an interpreter before informed consent is given for an invasive procedure. A female patient was admitted to the hospital with severe cardiac disease. She was also completely deaf and mute. Notes in the medical record stated, "Patient deaf and dumb and difficult to assess." The nurses established a diagnosis of "Sensory deficit: hearing impaired" and recorded that it was difficult to communicate with the patient. Providers and nurses documented continued difficulty with assessments, patient education, and obtaining informed consent. The patient's 17-year-old daughter was not deaf and could sign, but was not a trained medical interpreter. Ms. Borngesser subsequently died due to her severe cardiac disease and associated complications. Her daughter sued the hospital, claiming that the facility failed to make reasonable accommodation for her deaf and mute mother. *There were no claims of medical or nursing negligence.* The Superior Appellate Court of New Jersey affirmed that the case against the hospital could go forward. The court stated, among other things, that when a hearing-impaired patient is asked to give informed consent, the hospital has a duty to ensure that communication is effective by providing an interpreter fluent in American Sign Language (ASL).

The unique legal requirements related to informed consent in minors is a complex issue. All 50 states and the District of Columbia explicitly allow a minor to consent to testing and treatments for sexually transmitted diseases, except HIV testing and treatment. All other statutes regarding informed consent in adolescents vary widely from state to state (Tillett, 2005). As noted earlier, when dealing with minors, the nurse must use agency resources including social workers, managers, administrators, and risk managers when facilitating an appropriate informed consent process between the provider and adolescent or older child.

The Right to Refuse Diagnostic Testing, Treatment, and Care

As noted, an adult of sound mind has a right to refuse any treatment that has previously been agreed to. A Connecticut Supreme Court decision affirmed the fundamental right of adults to refuse medical treatment. In the case of *Stamford Hospital v. Vega* (1996), a woman who hemorrhaged after the birth of her infant refused blood on the grounds that it violated her beliefs as a Jehovah's Witness. The hospital obtained an emergency court order authorizing the facility to administer blood. The woman survived and was discharged in good health. Although it was a moot point (the blood already had been given), the family appealed the initial court decision authorizing the blood transfusion. The Supreme Court decided to hear the case and reversed the lower court's decision, stating the hospital did not have a right to substitute its decision for that of the patient.

In a more recent case, *Jiosi v. Township of Nutley* (2000), a man arrested on suspicion of driving under the influence was taken to an ED to have a blood sample drawn to provide evidence against him in court. The Superior Court of New Jersey ruled that the police were acting properly up to this point. The ED physician told the police that the blood sample could only be tested for alcohol and that a urine specimen would be required to perform a toxicology screening test for other illicit substances. The court noted that it was the physician, not the police, who initiated the idea of getting a urine sample. Under orders from the physician, the nurses were directed to have the man drink at least eight glasses of water, and then taunted him with a urinary catheter to intimidate him into urinating (Snyder, 2000b). Two minutes after the man finished the last glass of water, the nurses had the police hold the man down (who was literally kicking and screaming) and catheterized him. The man sued the hospital for violation of his constitutional rights, battery, and negligence. The New Jersey Appellate Court ruled that the man had a right to move forward with the lawsuit against the nurses, physician, and hospital.

If a patient under the nurse's care refuses treatment, the nurse has a duty to notify the primary provider. The same principles pertaining to the informed consent process apply to situations when the patient refuses care. The physician or advanced practice nurse should provide the patient with information about the consequences, risks, and benefits of refusing therapy. The provider also must explore any alternative treatments that may be available to the patient. Hospitals have a right to seek a judicial review when patients refuse specific types of lifesaving treatments, but current case law falls squarely in favor of the patient's right to self-determination.

Leaving AMA. A common allegation made when a patient self-discharges AMA, and then is subsequently injured, is that the patient was not fully apprised of the risks inherent in leaving the facility. If a patient intends to leave the facility without a written order, the nurse must act promptly to notify the provider. When circumstances suggest that the person may suffer immediate physical harm, the nurse must clearly articulate the dangers inherent in leaving. This precautionary statement is reserved for situations in which the life and limb of the patient are at risk and the appropriate providers (physicians or advanced practice nurses) are not available to address the direct and indirect consequences with the patient. The nurse should document all these actions and any communication with the aforementioned parties.

If the primary provider has not arrived before the patient leaves, the nurse's notes should reflect the specific advice given the patient, which should include the fact that leaving the facility could:

- Aggravate the current condition and complicate future care
- Result in permanent physical or mental impairment or disability
- Result in complications leading to death
- In the case of a competent elder, prompt notification of the immediate family also would be a reasonable and prudent action.

Lyons v. Walker Regional Medical Center (2000) is a case in point. An ED nurse was found negligent for failing to warn a patient who was leaving AMA that his laboratory results indicated a state of diabetic ketoacidosis, a condition that could be lethal. When the "panic" value laboratory findings were displayed on the computer, the nurse did not bring the results to the physician or patient's attention. Instead she directed the unit secretary to complete the patient's discharge paperwork. The patient left, and died 3 days later.

A study of patient characteristics associated with discharge AMA has found that low socioeconomic status, substance abuse, sickness within the family, underlying (and often untreated) psychiatric disorders, anger and anxiety about the admission diagnosis, and lack of effective communication with team members correlated with self-discharge (Alfandre, 2009). Nurses and providers should collaborate to address immediate patient concerns, communicate a time-limited plan of care, and advocate for appropriate consultations (i.e., psychiatry, social work, pastoral services, pain management) to reduce the likelihood of patient self-discharge.

Almost all health care facilities have an AMA form that patients are asked to sign when they decide to refuse or discontinue ordered therapy or intend to leave the facility. The value of the document in countering a claim of negligence should the patient or family later sue will depend in great part on the quality of the nurse's charting.

Nurses have also been charged with a variety of offenses when unlawfully detaining patients, including assault, battery, and false imprisonment (Snyder, 2001). These charges generally arise when well-meaning nurses try to prevent the patient from carrying out his or her intent. Actions that lead to a claim of false imprisonment include applying restraints, refusing to give the patient his or her clothes or access to a telephone, intimidating the patient by assigning a security person to guard his or her room, and sedating the patient against his or her will. As can be expected, in addition to civil penalties, the nurse faces disciplinary action by the licensing board when charges of false imprisonment are reported.

The Use of Physical Restraints

One last but equally important area of patient rights to be discussed is the right of a competent adult to be free of restraint. Even patients with mental illness cannot be incarcerated or restrained without due process, and the institution must have the treatment and rehabilitation services necessary to reintegrate the individual into society (Iyer and Levin, 2007). Restraint of any kind is a form of imprisonment, and the reasonable and prudent nurse will closely adhere to all laws, rules, and policies pertaining to the use of restraints. The goal when restraints are clinically indicated is to use the least restrictive restraint and only when all other strategies to ensure patient safety have been exhausted. Patients may never be restrained physically or chemically because there is not enough staff to properly monitor them. Nurses have a legal and ethical duty to report institutions or individuals who violate patient rights through unlawful restraint.

As noted, one of the most common allegations leveled against nurses is a failure to ensure patient safety. Nurses in many practice settings must balance the right of patients to unrestricted control of their bodies and movements against the need to keep vulnerable patients safe from harm. The use of seclusion, chemical restraints, and physical restraints, including vests, mittens, belts, and wrist restraints, is governed by federal and state statutes and accrediting bodies, such as TJC. Many nurses do not realize that even bedrails and chair trays fall under the category of physical restraints; these articles may not be used indiscriminately.

Violation of restraint statutes and the administrative rules and regulations promulgated to enact these laws can result in stiff penalties. The institution can lose its Medicare contract (decertification) and TJC accreditation, effectively putting it out of business. Patients and family members may initiate civil suits for unlawful restraints, resulting in monetary damages if the plaintiff succeeds in the suit. Charges of assault, battery, and/or false imprisonment may be leveled against nurses who use restraints improperly. Claims of negligence may arise from improper monitoring of the patient who has been appropriately placed in restraints in compliance with applicable laws and hospital policy.

Careful nursing documentation is essential when restraints are applied. The patient's mental and physical status must be assessed at regular and frequent intervals as prescribed by law and the agency's policies. The chart must reflect these assessments and the frequency with which restraints are removed. Neurovascular and skin assessments of limbs or other body parts covered by the restraints also must be entered in the medical record. Written physician orders for restraints must be timed and dated, and renewal of orders must be accompanied by evidence of medical evaluations and nursing reassessments.

Based on the aforementioned information, some nurses are under the misconception that current law prohibits restraining patients until a written order is obtained. Nurses may lawfully apply restraints in an emergency, when in their independent judgment no other strategies are effective in protecting the patient from harm. The physician must be contacted promptly to discuss the patient's condition and the need to restrain and to obtain an order for temporary continuance of restraints. The nurse is guided in the decision to restrain by knowledge of the laws, the agency's policies and procedures, qualifications of the staff, and conditions on the unit or in the department. In *Estate of Hendrickson v. Genesis Health Ventures, Inc.* (2002), the jury awarded a family more than $1 million when it decided that the nursing home staff had failed to appropriately restrain a family member who had suffered a stroke. The patient had been admitted to a nursing home following a severe stroke and was paralyzed on her right side. Despite the hemiplegia, the patient was able to slide from one side of the bed to the other and had been found trapped between the mattress and side rail on previous occasions. Subsequently the patient was found dead, with her head wedged between the side of the mattress and the bed side rail. The jury noted that the patient's death had been foreseeable, based on the staff previously finding the patient precariously trapped between the mattress and side rail but had taken no protective action to prevent harm.

SUMMARY

Professional nursing practice is governed by an ever-widening circle of federal and state statutes and is constantly evolving in great part because of an accumulating body of nursing case law. The law provides guidance for every aspect of practice and can assist the nurse in managing the complexities of practice in a rapidly changing health care system. Knowledge is power, and the nurse who possesses a sound understanding of the law as it pertains to professional practice is empowered. Box 8-7 provides a list of Internet resources that can be accessed to learn more about legal issues in nursing.

This chapter has reviewed the major sources and categories of law influencing nursing practice. The reader has been introduced to the doctrines of civil and criminal law that affect all nurses. The chapter has explored issues related to the legal rights of patients who are served by professional nurses. As patient advocates, all nurses should keep these fundamental rights uppermost in their minds as they attempt to provide safe, effective, quality care in all settings.

evolve   Additional resources are available online at: http://evolve.elsevier.com/Cherry/

BOX **8-7**

Helpful Websites

American Association of Legal Nurse Consultants:
www.aalnc.org.
Provides information about legal nurse consultants: credentialing process, standards of practice, publications, networking opportunities, continuing education

American Society for Healthcare Risk Management:
www.ashrm.org
Provides information to consumers and members about risk management and risk control in health care settings, publications, news regarding health care laws and regulations

U.S. Food and Drug Administration:
www.fda.gov
Provides information about adverse events related to medication administration and use of durable medical equipment

The Joint Commission:
www.jointcommission.org
Provides information regarding health care standards, sentinel event alerts, related health care law

National Council of State Boards of Nursing:
www.ncsbn.org
Provides general information regarding nursing practice, position statements regarding nursing conduct, such as delegation of nursing tasks

The American Association of Nurse Attorneys:
www.taana.org
Website of the association of nurse attorneys; provides information on select laws; provides guidance for nurses interested in becoming attorneys

Centers for Medicare & Medicaid Services (CMS):
www.cms.hhs.gov
Provides information about a wide range of health care law, Medicare program; offers access to other websites in health care law

REFERENCES

Abernathy v. Valley Medical Center, WL 3754792 (W.D. Wash., 2006).

Alfandre D: "I'm going home": discharges against medical advice, *Mayo Clin Proc* 84(3):255–260, 2009.

American Association of Critical-Care Nurses (AACN): *AACN delegation handbook*, ed 2, Aliso Viejo, CA, 2004, AACN.

American Association of Critical-Care Nurses and Vital-Smarts: *Silence kills; the several crucial conversations for healthcare*, Aliso Viejo, CA, 2005, AACN and Vital-Smarts.

American Medical Association (AMA): *Code of medical ethics*, Chicago, 2008-2009, AMA.

American Nurses Association (ANA): *Code of ethics for nurses*, Washington, DC, 2001, ANA.

American Nurses Association (ANA): *Nursing: scope and standards of practice*, Washington, DC, 2004, ANA.

American Nurses Association (ANA): *Principles of delegation*, Washington, DC, 2005, ANA. Retrieved August 2005 from: www.nursingworld.org/MainMenuCategories/ThePracticeofProfessionalNursing/workplace/PrinciplesofDelegation.aspx.

American Nurses Association (ANA): *The American Nurses Association comments on the Wisconsin Department of Justice decision to pursue criminal charges against an RN in Wisconsin*. Retrieved November 2006 from: www.nursingworld.org.

American Nurses Association (ANA): *Safe staffing saves lives*, Washington, DC, 2009, ANA. Retrieved July 2009 from: www.safestaffingsaveslives.org/WhatisANADoing/PollResults.aspx.

American Nurses Association and National Council of State Boards of Nursing: *Joint statement on delegation*. 2005. Retrieved June 2007 from: www.ncsbn.org/Joint_statement.pdf.

American Society for Healthcare Risk Management (ASHRM): *Risk management pearls on disclosure of adverse events*, Chicago, 2006, ASHRM.

Anderson v. St Francis–St George Hospital, 614 NE 2d 841 (OH, 1992).

Angelini D, Mahlmeister L: Liability in triage: management of EMTALA regulations and managing obstetric risks, *J Midwifery Womens Health* 50(6):472–478, 2005.

Ashley R: Is malpractice insurance important? *Crit Care Nurs* 25(6):54, 2005.

Austin S: Are you liable for telephone advice? *Nursing* 38:6–7, 2008.

Barbourville Nursing Home v. USDHHS, No 05-3421 (6 Cir 04/06/2006) F3d-KY.

Bond P: Implications of EMTALA on nursing triage and ED staff education, *J Emerg Nurs* 34(3):205–206, 2008.

Borngesser v. Jersey Shore Medical Center, 774 A. 2d 615 (N.J. App. Ct., 2001).

Boyer v. Tift County Hospital. WL 2986283 (M.D. Ga., 2008).

Brief amici curiae American Hospital Association, American Organization of Nurse Executives, American Society for Healthcare Human Resources Administration, Michigan Health and Hospital Association in response to the National Labor Relations Board's July 24, 2003. Notice and invitation to file briefs. Filed Sept 22, 2003 United States of America before the National Labor Relations Board.

Brodowski v. Ryave, 885 A.2d 1045 (PA Supr Ct. 2005).

Brooke P: When can you say no? *Nursing 2009* 39(7): 43–47, 2009.

Buppert C: *Frequently asked questions and answers about malpractice insurance*. 2008. Retrieved April 208 from: http://findarticles.com/p/articles/mi_hb6366/is_5_20/ai_n309 72427/pg_2/?tag=content;col1.

Buppert C, Klein T: Dilemmas in mandatory reporting for nurses, *Medscape Top Adv Pract Nurs eJournal* 1–17, 2008. Retrieved February 2009 from: http://cme.medscape.com /viewprogram/18738.

Caliendo C, et al: Obstetric triage and EMTALA regulations. Practice strategies for labor and delivery nursing units, *AWHONN Lifelines* 8(5):442–448, 2004.

City of Irving v. Pak, 885 SW 2d 189 (Tex, 1994).

Clarke S, Donaldson N: *Nurse staffing and patient care quality and safety. In Patient safety and quality—an evidence-based handbook for nurses*. Retrieved August 2009 from: www.ahrq.gov/qual/nurseshdbk.

Columbia Medical Center of Las Colinas v. Bush, WL 22725001 WW3d (Tex., 2003).

Convalescent Services, Inc v. Schultz, 921 SW 2d 731 (Tex. App, 1996).

Dennis v. Specialty Select Hospital—Flint, WL 2402454 NW2d (Mich., 2005).

Dickerson v. Fatehi, 84 SE 2d 880 (Va., 1997).

Dimora v. Cleveland Clinic Foundation, 683 NE 2d 1175 (Ohio App, 1996).

Duncan v. Scottsdale Medical Imaging, Ltd, 70 P 3d 435 WL 21382470 (Ariz., 2003).

ECRI Institute: *List of CMS hospital-acquired conditions expanded under new final rule. ECRI Special Advisory*. 2008, ECRI Institute. Retrieved November 2008 from: www. ecri.org/Documents/Patient_Safety_Center/CMS_ New_Final_Rule.pdf.

Edwards J, et al: National Healthcare Safety Network (NHSN) report, data summary for 2006, issued June 2007, *Am J Infect Contr* 36(5):290–301, 2007.

Estate of Hendrickson v. Genesis Health Ventures, Inc, SE. 2d WL1462267 (N.C. App, 2002).

Francis v. Memorial General Hospital, 726 P 2d 852 (N.M., 1986).

Gladney v. Sneed, 742 So. 2d 642 (La. App. Ct., 1999).

Goldsmith J: Negligent nurse or scapegoat? *Am J Nurs* 103(6):23, 2003.

Grace P, McLaughlin M: When consent isn't informed enough, *Am J Nurs* 105(4):90–84, 2005.

Griffith R, Tengnah C: *Law and professional nursing*, Exeter, UK, 2008, Learning Matters, Ltd.

HCA Health Services v. National Bank, 745 SW 2d 120 (Ark., 1988).

Heinrich v. Conemaugh Valley Memorial Hospital, 648 A 2d 53 (Pa., 1994).

Holston v. Sisters of the Third Order, 650 NE 2d 985 (Ill., 1995).

Hudspeth R: Failing the duty to report: disciplinary risk for the chief nursing officer, *Nurs Adm Q* 32:3491–3500, 2008.

Institute for Safe Medication Practices (ISMP): *Error-prone conditions that lead to student nurse-related errors. ISMP Safety Alert!* 2007. Retrieved July 2008 from: www.ismp. org/Newsletters/acutecare/articles/20071018.asp.

Institute of Medicine: *To err is human: building a safer health system*, Washington, DC, 2000, National Academy Press.

Iyer P, Levin B: *Nursing malpractice*, ed 3, Tucson, AZ, 2007, Lawyers & Judges Publishing.

Jiosi v. Township of Nutley, 753 A 2d 132 (N.J. App, 2000).

Johannessen v. Salem Hospital, 336 Or 211, 82 P3d 139 (Ore., 2003)

Justin and Michelle Malovic v. Santa Monica Hospital Medical Center, Los Angeles County Superior Court, Case No SC019 167 (Calif., 1995).

Kachalia A: *Disclosure of medical error. Agency for Healthcare Research and Quality (AHRQ)*. January 2009. Retrieved May 2009 from: www.webmm.ahrq.gov/perspective.aspx? perspectiveID=70.

Kaldjian L, et al: Reporting medical errors to improve patient safety, *Arch Intern Med* 168(1):40–46, 2008.

Kalisch B, Landstrom G, Willams R: Missed nursing care: errors of omission, *Nurs Outlook* 57(1):3–9, 2009.

Kane R, et al: The association of registered nurse staffing levels and patient outcomes: systematic review and meta-analysis, *Med Care* 45(12):1195–1204, 2007.

Karibjanian v. Thomas Jefferson University Hospital, 717 F Supp 1081, 1083-84 (ED Pa., 1989).

Kazmier J: *Health care law*, Florence, KY, 2008, Delmar Cengage Learning.

Keel v. St. Elizabeth Medical Center, 842 SW 2d 869 (Ky., 1992).

Kelley T: Death at a nursing home leads to indictment of five, *New York Times* , Nov 7, 2000, p. B-1.

Kenward K: Discipline of nurses: a review of disciplinary data 1996-2006, *JONAS Healthc Law Ethics Regul* 10(3):81–84, 2008.

Kowalski K, Horner M: A legal nightmare: Denver nurses indicted, *MCN* 23(3):125–129, 1998.

Lincourt A, et al: Retained foreign bodies after surgery, *J Surg Res* 138(2):170–174, 2007.

Love v. Rancocas Hospital, WL1541052 (Distr Ct New Jersey, 2006).

Lovett v. Lorain Community Hospital, WL239927 N.E. 2d. (Ohio, 2004).

Luettke v. St. Vincent Mercy Medical Center, WL 2105049 (Ohio App. Ct., 2006).

Lyons v. Walker Regional Medical Center, 791 So. 2d 937 (Ala., 2000).

Mahlmeister L: Best practices in perinatal nursing: professional role development for charge nurses, *J Perinat Neonat Nurs* 20(2):122–124, 2006.

Mahlmeister L: Best practices in perinatal nursing: collaborating with student nurses to ensure high-reliability, *J Perinat Neonat Nurs* 22(1):8–11, 2008.

Mahlmeister L: Best practices in perinatal care: maintaining safe and cost-effective staffing models in an during the current economic downturn, *J Perinat Neonat Nurs* 23(2):111–114, 2009a.

Mahlmeister L: Best practices in perinatal nursing: partnering with patients to enhance informed decision-making, *J Perinat Neonat Nurs* 20(2):122–124, 2009b.

Mahlmeister L: Best practices in perinatal nursing: collaborating with student nurses to ensure high-reliability, *J Perinat Neonat Nurs* 22(1):8–11, 2008.

Mahlmeister L: Best practices in perinatal nursing: professional role development for charge nurses, *J Perinat Neonat Nurs* 20(2):122–124, 2006.

Martin v. Abilene Regional Medical Center, WL 241509 (Tex. App, Feb 2, 2006).

Merritt v. Karcloglu, 668 So 2d 469 (La., 1996).

Miller v. Levering Regional Healthcare Center, S.W. 3d. WL1889883 (MO Mo. App. Ct., 2006).

Mobile Infirmary Medical Center v. Hodgen, So 2d, WL 22463340 (Ala., 2003).

Moy M: *The EMTALA answer book*, 2009 ed, Gaithersburg, Md, 2009, Aspen Publishers.

National Council of State Boards of Nursing (NCSBN): *Working with others; a position paper*, Chicago, 2005, NCSBN, Retrieved November 24, 2006 from: www. ncsbn.org/Working_with_Others.pdf.

National District Attorneys Association: *Reporting requirements for competent adult victims of domestic violence*. 2006. Retrieved April 20, 2009 from: www.ndaa.org/pdf/ dv_summary.pdf.

National Nosocomial Infections Surveillance (NNIS): NNIS System Report, data summary from January 1992 through June 2004, issued October 2004, *J Infect Control* 32(8):470–485, 2004.

National Quality Forum (NQF): *Safe practices for better healthcare—2009 update. Executive summary*, Washington, DC, NQF, 2009, Retrieved May, 2009 from: www.qual ityforum.org/Publications/2009/03/Safe_Practices_for_ Better_Healthcare–2009_Update.aspx.

National Quality Forum (NQF): *Serious reportable events in healthcare*, Washington DC, NQF, 2002. Retrieved July 2, 2003 from: http://www.qualityforum.org/Publications/ 2002/Serious_Reportable_Events_in_Healthcare.aspx.

Nursing Service Organization (NSO): *CNA Healthpro Nursing Claims Study: an analysis of claims with risk management recommendations 1997-2007*, Hatboro, Pa, 2009, NSO, Retrieved April 2009 from: www.nso.com/pdfs/d b/rnclaimstudy.pdf?fileName=rnclaimstudy.pdf&folder =pdfs/db&isLiveStr=Y&refID=rnclaim.

Osiecki v. Bridgeport Health Care Center, Inc., 2005 WL 1331225 (Conn. Super, May 12, 2005).

Parco v. Pacifica Hospital, WL 2491516 (Supr Ct. Los Angeles County, Calif., 2007).

Passarella G: Hospital faces trial on corporate negligence claim, *Legal Intelligencer*, October 31, 2005:Retrieved July 2007 from: www.law.com/jsp/ihc/PubArticle FriendlyIHC.jsp?id=900005440117.

Pedraza v. Wyckoff Heights Medical Center, NYS2d, 2002 NY Slip Op 22094, 2002 WL 1364153 (N.Y. Sup, June 4, 2002).

Penalver v. Living Centers of Texas, Inc., 2004 WL 1392268 (Tex. App., June 23, 2004).

Riley W, et al: The Patient Safety and Quality Improvement Act of 2005: developing an error reporting system to improve patient safety, *J Patient Saf* 4(1):13–17, 2008.

Roberts v. Galen of Virginia, Inc, 111 F 3d 405 (6 Cir, 1997).

Rodebush v. Oklahoma Nursing Homes, Ltd, 867 P 2d 1241 (Okla., 1993).

Roddy v. Tanner Medical Center, 585 SE 2d 175 (Ga., 2003).

Rowe v. Sisters of Pallottine Missionary Society, WL 1585453 SE 2d (W.Va., 2001).

Ruelas v. Staff Builders Personnel Services, Inc., 18 P 3d 138 (Ariz. App, 2001).

Sehgal N, Wachter R: Identification of inpatient DNR status: a safety hazard begging for standardization, *J Hosp Med* 2(6):366–371, 2007.

Shah R, Lander L: Retained foreign body during surgery in pediatric patients: a national perspective, *J Pediatr Surg* 44(4):738–742, 2009.

Shannon S, et al: Disclosing errors to patients: perspectives of registered nurses, *Jt Comm J Qual Patient Saf* 35(1):5–12, 2009.

Siegel v. Long Island Jewish Medical Center, NYS 2d NY Slip Op 17790 WL 22439814 (N.Y., 2003).

Singleton v. AAA Home Health, Inc., WL 1693814, So 2d (La., 2000).

Smith L: Documenting use of an interpreter, *Nursing 2007* 37(7):25, 2007.

Snyder E: Chain of command: court rules nurses should have gone over doctor's head, *Leg Eagle Eye Newslett Nurs Profession* 8(2):1, 2000a.

Snyder E: Nurses forcibly catheterized patient: court willing to find civil rights violation, *Leg Eagle Eye Newsletter Nurs Profession* 8(9):2, 2000b.

Snyder E: Automatic blood pressure cuff: nurses ignored the patient, committed battery, *Leg Eagle Eye Newsletter Nurs Profession* 9(4):1, 2001.

Snyder E: Hypertonic saline solution: nursing negligence in wrongful death, *Leg Eagle Eye Newslett Nurs Profession* 11(12):8, 2003a.

Snyder E: Digoxin overdose: $1.5 million punitive damages, *Leg Eagle Eye Newslett Nurs Profession* 11(12):1, 4–5, 2003b.

Snyder E: Understaffing: court blames DON for death, aide did not have time to read care plan, *Leg Eagle Eye Newslett Nurs Profession* 12(8):1, 2004a.

Snyder E: Student nurse/instructor: court discusses host hospital's legal liability, *Leg Eagle Eye Newslett Nurs Profession* 14(3):4, 2004b.

Snyder E: Preeclampsia: nurses failed to advocate for patient, punitive damages allowed, *Leg Eagle Eye Newslett Nurs Profession* 12(2):5, 2004c.

Snyder E: Understaffing, fall, no neuro assessment, epidural hemorrhage, death: nurses faulted, *Leg Eagle Eye Newslett Nurs Profession* 14(8):6, 2006a.

Snyder E: Informed consent: patient has a right to know extent of student participation, *Leg Eagle Eye Newslett Nurs Profession* 12(3):4, 2006b.

Snyder E: Disability discrimination: Quad on ventilator could not communicate with his caregivers, *Leg Eagle Eye Newslett Nurs Profession* 15(10):1, 2007a.

Snyder E: Medication ordered is contraindicated: court discusses nurse's legal responsibilities, *Leg Eagle Eye Newsletter Nurs Profession* 15(1):1, 2007b.

Stamford Hospital v. Vega, 674 A 2d 821 (Conn., 1996).

Stewart R, et al: Transparent and open discussion of errors does not increase malpractice risk in trauma patients, *Ann Surg* 243(5):645–651, 2006.

Stogsdill v. Healthmark Partners, LLC F 3d, 2004 WL 1636426 (8 Cir, July 23, 2004).

Sunbridge Healthcare Corp. v. Penny, SW3d, 2005 WL 562763 (Tex. App, March 11, 2005).

Tammelleo A: Constipation/impaction: nurses failed to report significant change in health status. Punitive damages upheld, *Nurs Law Regan Rep* 45(9):2, 2004a.

Tammelleo A: Wrong drug ordered: nurses must intervene, *Nurs Law Regan Rep* 45(1):1, 2004b.

Tammelleo A: Nurse manager subjected to disciplinary action, *Nurs Law Regan Rep* 45(2):1, 2004c.

Tammelleo A: Student nurse gives antibiotic IV—death results, *Nurs Law Regan Rep* 46(5):1, 2005.

Tammelleo A: Telephone triage is a "risky business" for nurses, *Nurs Law Regan Rep* 46(10):4, 2006.

Teno J: *The wrongful resuscitation. Cases from Agency for Healthcare Research and Quality (AHRQ)*. Retrieved November 2008 from: http://cme.medscape.com/view article/575601.

The Joint Commission: Contracted staff: ensuring safety in clinical and nonclinical departments, *Jt Comm Source* 4(7):5–6, 2006.

The Joint Commission: Promoting effective communication—language access services in health care, *Jt Comm Perspect* 26(2):8–11, 2008.

The Joint Commission: *Comprehensive accreditation manual for hospitals*, Oakbrook Terrace, IL, 2009, TJC.

Thompson v. Nason Hospital, 591 A 2d 703, 707 (Pa., 1991).

Tillett J: Adolescents and informed consent, *J Perinat Neonat Nurs* 19(2):112–121, 2005.

Utter v. United Hospital Center, Inc., 236 SE 2d 213 (W.Va, 1977).

Vonwinkel P: *The never ever eleven*. Retrieved October 2008 from: www.riskandinsurance.com/story.jsp?storyId= 130246047.

West J: Surgical "never events": how common are adverse occurrences? *ASHRM J* 26(1):15–21, 2006.

Westrick S, Dempski K: *Essentials of nursing law and ethics*, Sudbury, MA, 2008, Jones and Bartlett.

Williams v. West Virginia Board of Examiners, S.E. 2d WL1432298 (W.Va., 2004).

Willis MJ: *Is your nursing colleague impaired?* Nursing Education and Technology (NEAT), 2008. University of Madison–Wisconsin. Retrieved May 2009 from: www. neatproject.org/learning_objects/test/Option4.swf.

Winkelman v. Beloit Memorial Hospital, 483 NW 2d 211 (Wis., 1992).

Wolf Z, et al: Nursing student medication errors involving tubing and catheters: a descriptive study, *Nurse Educ Today* 29(8):681–688, 2009.

Woods J, Rozovsky F: *What do I say? Communicating intended or unanticipated outcomes in obstetrics*, San Francisco, 2003, Jossey-Bass Inc.

Wright L: Bill of rights for nurses in licensure matters, *J Nurs Law* 10(3):177–181, 2005.

Ethical and Bioethical Issues in Nursing and Health Care

Carla D. Sanderson, PhD, RN

evolve Additional resources are available online at: http://evolve.elsevier.com/Cherry/

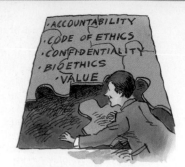

Ethical dilemmas are the puzzles of life.

VIGNETTE

Joe Smith has accepted a position as the nurse manager in a very busy inner-city emergency department serving patients from diverse cultures. Among Joe's many responsibilities is developing the 24-hour, 7-day-week work schedules of the department's nursing workforce in which he has 10 unfilled positions. Another responsibility is implementing the hospital's policy of offering all patients, regardless of cultural beliefs, the right to an advance directive for end-of-life care. At the same time Joe must ensure that each patient who enters the emergency department receives appropriate high-quality care from competent professional care providers who respect and respond to patients' individual needs and desires. With these responsibilities come challenges, sometimes so significant that the nurse manager is faced with an ethical dilemma.

■ QUESTIONS TO CONSIDER WHILE READING THIS CHAPTER:

1 How will ethical and bioethical issues in nursing and health care affect my professional nursing practice?

2 What ethical theories and principles serve as a basis for nursing practice?

3 What goals can I establish to move me toward excellence in moral and ethical reasoning?

4 How can I assist patients and families who face difficult ethical decisions?

KEY TERMS

Accountability An ethical duty stating that one should be answerable legally, morally, ethically, or socially for one's activities.

Autonomy Personal freedom and right to make choices.

Beneficence An ethical principle stating that one should do good and prevent or avoid doing harm.

Bioethics The study of ethical problems resulting from scientific advances.

Code of ethics Set of statements encompassing rules that apply to people in professional roles.

Deontology An ethical theory stating that moral rule is binding.

Ethical sensitivity The capacity to decide with intelligence and compassion, given uncertainty in a care situation, with an additional ability to anticipate consequences and the courage to act (Weaver, Morse, and Mitcham, 2008).

Ethics Science or study of moral values.

Ethics acculturation The didactic and experiential process of developing ethical reasoning abilities as a part of ongoing professional preparation

Nonmaleficence An ethical principle stating the duty not to inflict harm.
Utilitarianism An ethical theory stating that the best decision is one that brings about the greatest good for the most people.
Values Ideas of life, customs, and ways of behaving that society regards as desirable.
Veracity An ethical duty to tell the truth.

LEARNING OUTCOMES

After studying this chapter, the reader will be able to:

1 Integrate basic concepts of human values that are essential for ethical decision making.

2 Analyze selected ethical theories and principles as a basis for ethical decision making.

3 Analyze the relationship between ethics and morality in relation to nursing practice.

4 Use an ethical decision-making framework for resolving ethical problems in health care.

5 Apply the ethical decision-making process to specific ethical issues encountered in clinical practice.

CHAPTER OVERVIEW

In a nursing education program, nursing students only begin to embrace the complex and dynamic profession of nursing. Prelicensure nursing education is only an introduction to a discipline in which there are no knowledge boundaries. The abundance of nursing practice information is evident from a quick glance across the nursing textbook selections in the campus or online bookstore.

Most of that information addresses the "how-to" aspects of nursing care. The scientific aspects of nursing care are evolving more rapidly than ever as a host of nurse researchers delve into questions about the safe, competent, and therapeutic aspects of professional nursing care. As quickly as nursing science produces new nursing knowledge, how-to information is shared through professional journals, textbooks, and electronically through Internet resources. The scientific aspects of care evolve constantly through how-to research.

Myriad potential questions surpass the how-to body of knowledge that is inherent in the profession of nursing. Everywhere in today's health care delivery system are potential questions of another nature—the "how should" questions, which are challenging and sometimes evolve into ethical dilemmas. The "how should" questions that the emergency department nurse manager faces may sound something like this:

◆ *How should I determine the competency of an acutely ill 80-year-old patient who comes to the emergency department without an advance directive? Is her competency intact? How should I determine whether she is capable of giving an informed advance directive?*

◆ *How should I act if her decision for her own end-of-life care is not consistent with what her family wants for her? Or how should I respond if the family, because of cultural beliefs, will not even allow information about end-of-life care to be shared with their loved one?*

◆ *How should I view the care of this 80-year-old patient? Is an emergency resuscitation effort for an 80-year-old considered ordinary and routine, or is it considered extraordinary and heroic?*

◆ *How should I respond to her if, in the course of efforts to stabilize her, she calls me in to ask me whether she is dying?*

◆ *How much of the truth is warranted?*

◆ *How should I decide when the availability of one-on-one trauma care beds becomes threatened and the decision must be made to move someone out of one bed to make room for this 80-year-old woman whose condition is rapidly deteriorating?*

◆ *Is the life of this 80-year-old woman any less significant than that of the 40-year-old father of four who has just been admitted after a tragic car accident?*

◆ *How should I feel when this 80-year-old patient is entered into a research study designed to test a new drug for flash pulmonary edema from congestive heart failure that has previously only been tested on a younger population?*

◆ *How should I make staffing assignments when the number of nurses on a given shift is insufficient to provide effective and adequate emergency department care to all?*

◆ *How should I respond when one of the few nurses reporting to work on a given day refuses to accept the care of patients because of inadequate staffing?*

This chapter introduces the nursing student to a different aspect of nursing care—the "how should" aspect, or as it is more appropriately called, the ethical aspect. Ethics is a system for deciding, based on principles, what should be done. With the goal of developing excellence in moral and reasoning ability, the nursing student begins a career-long process of ethics acculturation. This process allows the professional nurse to practice with an increasing level of understanding that goes beyond the scientific and moves toward a more complete and whole understanding of human existence.

NURSING ETHICS

Nursing ethics is a system of principles concerning the actions of the nurse in his or her relationships with patients, patients' family members, other health care providers, policymakers, and society as a whole. A profession is characterized by its relationship to society. The results of the 2008 Gallup poll on professional honesty and ethics as reported in a number of news outlets indicate that the public ranks nursing as the most ethical of all professions. Codes of ethics provide implicit standards and values for the professions. A nursing code of ethics was first introduced in the late nineteenth century and has evolved through the years as the profession itself has evolved and as changes in society and health have come about. Current dynamics, such as the emerging genetic interventions associated with therapeutic and reproductive cloning, debates about securing stem cells for research and treatment, evolving legal definitions of family, ongoing questions about euthanasia and assisted suicide, and the escalating threats to the effective delivery of health care as a result of significant nursing shortages, now being called ethical climate in the workplace, bring nursing's code of ethics into the forefront (Boxes 9-1 and 9-2).

BIOETHICS

Nursing ethics is part of a broader system known as bioethics. Bioethics is an interdisciplinary field within the health care organization that has developed only in the past four decades. Whereas ethics has been discussed since there was written language, bioethics has developed with the age of modern medicine, specifically with the development of hemodialysis and organ transplantation. New questions surface as science and technology produce new ways of knowing. Think of the questions that come from stem cell research, sexual reassignment, and reproductive-assisting technologies such as donor insemination, in vitro fertilization, removal of unused zygotes, surrogate parenting, and the ever-evolving practice of organ transplantation. Bioethical questions have emerged from experiences with natural disasters such as Hurricane Katrina in 2005. Bioethics is a response to these and other contemporary advances and challenges in health care. It is difficult to imagine a time when answers will be more plentiful than bioethical questions.

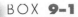

BOX **9-1**

American Nurses Association Code of Ethics

- The nurse, in all professional relationships, practices with compassion and respect for the inherent dignity, worth, and uniqueness of every individual, unrestricted by considerations of social or economic status, personal attributes, or the nature of health problems.
- The nurse's primary commitment is to the patient, whether an individual, family, group, or community.
- The nurse promotes, advocates for, and strives to protect the health, safety, and rights of the patient.
- The nurse is responsible and accountable for individual nursing practice and determines the appropriate delegation of tasks consistent with the nurse's obligation to provide optimum patient care.
- The nurse owes the same duties to self as to others, including the responsibility to preserve integrity and safety, to maintain competence, and to continue personal and professional growth.
- The nurse participates in establishing, maintaining, and improving health care environments and conditions of employment conducive to the provision of quality health care and consistent with the values of the profession through individual and collective action.
- The nurse participates in the advancement of the profession through contributions to practice, education, administration, and knowledge development.
- The nurse collaborates with other professionals and the public in promoting community, national, and international efforts to meet health needs.
- The profession of nursing, as represented by associations and their members, is responsible for articulating nursing values, for maintaining the integrity of the profession and its practice, and for shaping social policy.

Reprinted with permission from American Nurses Association: *Code of ethics for nurses with interpretive statements,* Washington, DC, 2001, American Nurses Publishing, American Nurses Foundation, American Nurses Association. Available online at: www.nursingworld.org/about/01action.htm#code.

Dilemmas for Health Professionals

Physicians, nurses, social workers, psychiatrists, epidemiologists, clergy, philosophers, theologians, researchers, and policymakers are joining to address ethical questions, difficult questions, and right-versus-wrong questions. As they seek to deliver quality health care, these professionals debate situations that pose dilemmas. They are confronting situations for which there are no clear right or wrong answers. Because of the diverse society in which health care is practiced, there are at least two sides to almost every issue faced.

Every specialization in health care has its own set of questions. Life and death, the margin of viability, quality of life, design of life, one life offering cure for another, right to decide, informed consent, medical confidentiality, and alternative treatment issues prevail in every field of health care from maternal-child to geriatric care; from acute episodic to intensive, highly specialized care; and from hospital-based to community-based care. Questions about the economics of nursing care and the use of technologies in the diagnosis and treatment of illness abound. In every aspect of the nursing profession lies the more subtle and intricate questions of how should this care be delivered and how should one decide when choices are in conflict.

Many nursing students do not consider health care and the practice of nursing in terms of the personal, truthful, honest, faithful (keeping promises to patients), qualitative, and subjective side; rather they look at it only in terms of the technical, quantitative, and objective side. Yet there most definitely are factors that influence the way patients actually are treated, or at least the way they perceive their treatment, that go beyond the data-driven aspect. In many ways, advanced technology has changed the face of health care and created the troubling questions that have become central in the delivery of care.

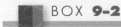

BOX **9-2**

International Council of Nurses Code for Nurses

- The fundamental responsibility of the nurse is fourfold: to promote health, to prevent illness, to restore health, and to alleviate suffering.
- The need for nursing is universal. Inherent in nursing is respect for life, dignity, and rights of humans. It is unrestricted by considerations of nationality, race, creed, color, age, sex, politics, or social status.
- Nurses render health services to the individual, the family, and the community and coordinate their services with those of related groups.

NURSES AND PEOPLE
- The nurse's primary responsibility is to those people who require nursing care.
- The nurse, in providing care, promotes an environment in which the values, customs, and spiritual beliefs of the patient are respected.
- The nurse holds in confidence personal information and uses judgment in sharing this information.

NURSES AND PRACTICE
- The nurse carries personal responsibility for nursing practice and for maintaining competence by continual learning. The nurse maintains the highest standards of nursing care possible within the reality of a specific situation.
- The nurse uses judgment in relation to individual competence when accepting and delegating responsibilities.
- The nurse, when acting in a professional capacity, should at all times maintain standards of personal conduct that reflect credit on the profession.

NURSES AND SOCIETY
- The nurse shares with other citizens the responsibility for initiating and supporting action to meet the health and social needs of the public.

NURSES AND COWORKERS
- The nurse sustains a cooperative relationship with co-workers in nursing and other fields.
- The nurse takes appropriate action to safeguard the patient when his or her care is endangered by a co-worker or any other person.

NURSES AND THE PROFESSION
- The nurse plays a major role in determining and implementing desirable standards of nursing practice and nursing education.
- The nurse is active in developing a core of professional knowledge.
- The nurse, acting through the professional organization, participates in establishing and maintaining equitable social and economic working conditions in nursing.

From International Council of Nurses: *ICN code for nurses: ethical concepts applied to nursing,* Geneva, 2005, Imprimiéres Populaires.

Dilemmas Created by Technology

Advances in health care through technology have created new situations for health care professionals and their patients. For the very young and old and for generations in between, illnesses once leading to mortality have become manageable and are classified as high-risk or chronic illness. Although people can now be saved, they are not being saved readily or inexpensively. Care of the acutely or chronically ill person sometimes creates hard questions for which there are no easy or apparent answers. Mortality for most will be a long drawn-out phenomenon, laced with a lifetime of potential conflicts about what ought to be done.

Even the nature of life itself and the technical manipulation of deoxyribonucleic acid (DNA) are under investigation. Health care professionals who adhere to an exclusively scientific or technologic approach to care will be seen as insensitive and will fail to meet the genuine needs of the patient, needs that include assistance with these more subjective concerns, such as how to think about the many advanced care choices laid before them.

ETHICAL DECISION MAKING

A professional nurse in the twenty-first century will be deemed competent only if he or she can provide the scientific and technologic aspects of care and has the ability to deal effectively with the ethical problems encountered in patient care. A competent nurse is an ethically sensitive nurse (Weaver et al, 2008) who can deal with the human dimensions of care that include a search for what is good and right and for what is accurate and efficient. The previously listed "how should" questions are just as important as the how-to questions surrounding day-to-day decision making in the emergency department or the care of the 80-year-old patient introduced previously. As the nurse seeks to understand the how-to aspects of nurse management and patient care, such as how to best staff a busy emergency department at a time of nursing shortage and how to provide comfort measures for dyspnea and pharmacologic care against the threat of organ dysfunction, he or she also must seek to understand more.

Answering Difficult Questions

Care combining human dimensions with scientific and technical dimensions forces some basic questions:
- What is safe care?
  - What effect might a patient's cultural preferences have on safe care?
- When staffing is inadequate, what care should be accepted or refused?
  - What are other barriers to ethical practice brought about by the workplace environment?
- What does it mean to be ill or well?
- What is the proper balance between science and technology and the good of humans?
- Where do we find balance when science will allow us to experiment with the basic origins of life?
- What happens when the proper balance is in tension?

No tension in balance is created in the effort to save the life of a dying healthy adolescent or set the broken leg of a healthy older adult. Science and the human good are not in conflict here. No conflict exists when there is a competent nursing staff, sufficient in number to provide quality care. However, what is the answer when modern medicine can save or prolong the life of an 8-year-old child but the child's parents refuse treatment based on religious reasons? Or what is the answer when modern medicine has life to offer a 30-year-old mother in need of a transplanted organ but the woman is without the financial means to cover the cost of the treatment? What is the answer when an Asian family refuses to allow the physician to share news of a terminal illness with their grandmother? What is the answer when new discoveries allow some would-be parents to choose biologic characteristics of children not yet conceived? What is the answer when the emergency department is full of acutely ill patients and there are too few nurses expected for the next shift? At one end of the spectrum lies the obvious; at the other there is often only uncertainty. Health care professionals in everyday practice often find themselves somewhere between the two.

Balancing Science and Morality

If nursing care is to be competent, the right balance between science and morality must be sought and understood. Nurses must first attempt to understand not just what they are to do for their patients but who their patients are. They must examine life and its origins, in addition to its worth, usefulness, and importance. Nurses must determine their own values and seek to understand the values of others.

Health care decisions are seldom made independently of other people. Decisions are made with the patient, the family, other nurses, and other health care providers. Nurses must make a deliberate effort to recognize their own values and learn to consider and respect the values of others.

The nurse has an obligation to present himself or herself to the patient as competent. The dependent patient enters a mutual relationship with the nurse. This exchange places a patient who is vulnerable and wounded with a nurse who is educated, licensed, and knowledgeable. The patient expects nursing actions to be thorough because total caring is the defining characteristic of the patient-nurse relationship. The nurse promises to deliver holistic care to the best of his or her ability. The patient's expectations and the nurse's promises require a commitment to develop a reasoned thought process and sound judgment in all situations that take place within this important relationship. The more personal, subjective, and value-laden situations are deemed to be among the most difficult situations for which the nurse must prepare.

VALUES FORMATION AND MORAL DEVELOPMENT

A value is a personal belief about worth that acts as a standard to guide behavior; a value system is an entire framework on which actions are based and is the backbone to how one thinks, feels, and takes action. Perhaps many nursing students come to the educational setting with a strong backbone, an intact value system. No doubt anyone living in these times has faced many situations in which important choices had to be made. The challenges faced in this generation are too numerous to avoid difficult choices. Values have been applied to those decisions. Yet often people do not take time to seriously contemplate their value system, the forces that shaped those values, and the life and worldview decisions that have been made based on them.

Examining Value Systems

To become a competent professional in every dimension of nursing care, nurses must examine their own system of values and commit themselves to a virtuous value system. A clear understanding of what is right and wrong is a necessary first step to a process sometimes referred to as values clarification, a process by which people attempt to examine the values they hold and how each of those values functions as part of a whole. Nurses must acknowledge their own values by considering how they would act in a particular situation.

Diane Uustal was one of nursing's first leaders to describe the role of values clarification in the decision-making process of the nurse. A values clarification process (Uustal, 1992) is an important learning tool as nursing students prepare themselves to become competent professionals. The deliberate refinement of one's own value system leads to a clearer lens through which nurses can view ethical questions in the practice of their profession. A refined value system and worldview can serve professionals as they deal with the meaning of life and its many choices. A worldview provides a cohesive model for life; it encourages personal responsibility for the living of that life, and it prepares one for making ethical choices encountered throughout life. Tools to assist the reader in values clarification can be found online (http://evolve.elsevier.com/Cherry/).

Forming a worldview and a value system is an evolving, continuous, dynamic process that moves along a continuum of development often referred to as moral development. Just as there is an orderly sequence of physical and psychologic development, there is an orderly sequence of right and wrong conduct development. Consider an adult of strong physical prowess and strong moral character. With each biologic developmental milestone, there is a more mature, more expanded physical being; likewise with each life experience that has choices between right and wrong, there is a more mature, more virtuous person.

Learning Right and Wrong

The process of learning to distinguish right and wrong often is described in pediatric textbooks. Donna Wong describes such development in children (Hockenberry et al, 2007). Infants have no concept of right or wrong. Infants hold no beliefs and no convictions, although it is known that moral development begins in infancy. If the need for basic trust is met in infancy, children can begin to develop the foundation for secure moral thought. Toddlers begin to display behavior in response to the world around them. They will imitate behavior seen in others, even though they do not comprehend the meaning of the behavior that they are imitating. Furthermore even though toddlers may not know what they are doing or why they are doing it, they incorporate the values and beliefs of those around them into their own behavioral code.

By the time children reach school age, they have learned that behavior has consequences and that good behavior is associated with rewards and bad behavior with punishment. Through their experiences and social interactions with people outside their home or immediate surroundings, school-age children begin to make choices about how they will act based on an understanding of good and bad. Their conscience is developing, and it begins to govern the choices they make (Hockenberry et al, 2007).

The adolescent questions existing moral values and his or her relevance to society. Adolescents understand duty and obligation, but they sometimes seriously question the moral codes on which society operates as they become more aware of the contradictions they see in the value systems of adults.

Adults strive to make sense of the contradictions and learn to develop their own set of morals and values as autonomous people. They begin to make choices based on an internalized set of principles that provides them with the resources they need to evaluate situations in which they find themselves (Hockenberry et al, 2007).

Understanding Moral Development Theory

Perhaps the most widely accepted theory on moral development is the now classic theory developed by Lawrence Kohlberg (1971). Kohlberg theorizes a cognitive developmental process that is sequential in nature with progression through levels and stages that vary dramatically within society. At first morality is all about rules imposed by some source of authority. Moral decisions made at this level (preconventional) are simply in response to some threat of punishment. The good-bad, right-wrong labels have meaning, but are defined only in reference to a self-centered reward-and-punishment system. A person who is in the preconventional level has no concept of the underlying moral code informing the decision of good or bad or right or wrong.

At some point, people begin to internalize their view of themselves in response to something more meaningful and interpersonal (conventional level). A desire to be viewed as a good boy or nice girl develops when the person wants to find approval from others. He or she may want to please, help others, be dutiful, and show respect for authority. Conformity to expected social and religious mores and a sense of loyalty may emerge.

Not all people develop beyond the conventional level of moral development. A morally mature individual (postconventional level), one of the few to reach moral completeness, is an autonomous thinker who strives for a moral code beyond issues of authority and reverence.

The morally mature individual's actions are based on principles of justice and respect for the dignity of all humankind and not just on principles of responsibility, duty, or self-edification (Kohlberg, 1971).

Moving Toward Moral Maturity

The rightness or wrongness of the complex and confounding health care decisions that are being made today depends on the level of moral development of those professionals entrusted with the tough decisions. Moving toward the level of moral maturity required for sound ethical decision making is, for most, a learning endeavor that requires a strong commitment to the task. Nurses must commit themselves to such learning, to a process called ethics acculturation across the span of their career. The issues will only get more complex and confounding as new advances are introduced; the commitment to lifelong moral and ethical reasoning development is imperative. The desired outcomes as a result of ethics acculturation across the years are integrity, personal growth, practical wisdom, and effective problem solving on behalf of patients and their families (Weaver et al, 2008). These are the qualities that are characteristic of an ethically sensitive and morally mature person.

As a matter of the civil rights afforded to all members of United States society, health care professionals have been afforded rights of conscience to practice their own convictions about what is right and ethical care. Rights of conscience have been brought in to focus primarily over the debate on abortion and euthanasia. Historically there has been much liberty given professionals in choosing to participate in care they believe in, and to refuse to participate in care they may find ethically unsound. The current debate on health care reform has sparked discussion on threats to continued rights of conscience for practitioners as federal funding for abortion has been discussed. Professional nurses must be ready to take up the challenge of debating the matter of whether or not rights of conscience should continue to be a part of one's civil rights.

The development of values and value-based behavior is essential for professional nursing. The American Association of Colleges of Nursing (AACN) has delineated five essential values that are described in Table 9-1. The study and examination of these nursing values is a worthwhile endeavor for the nursing student. Students who seek to become morally mature health care providers will appraise the values of the nursing profession and strive to find a comfortable union of those values with their own. Furthermore the study of ethical theory and ethical principles can provide a basis for moving forward as a morally mature professional nurse.

ETHICAL THEORY

Ethical theory is a system of principles by which a person can determine what should and should not be done. Although there are others, utilitarianism and deontology are Western world theories that many health care professionals studying bioethics have embraced as a guide for answering the question regarding what is right to do in a given ethical dilemma (Tong, 2007).

Utilitarianism

Utilitarianism is an approach that is rooted in the assumption that an action or practice is right if it leads to the greatest possible balance of good consequences or to the least possible balance of bad consequences. For instance the utilitarian approach would be at work if a decision is made by the government to forgo Medicare funding treatment for patients 90 years old and older who have a diagnosis of Alzheimer's disease, redistributing Medicare funding to other

TABLE **9-1**

Essential Nursing Values and Behaviors

ESSENTIAL VALUES	ATTITUDES AND PERSONAL QUALITIES	PROFESSIONAL BEHAVIORS
Altruism—concern for the welfare of others	Caring, commitment, compassion, generosity, perseverance	Gives full attention to the client when giving care; assists other personnel in providing care when they are unable to do so Expresses concern about social trends and issues that have implications for health care
Autonomy—right to self-determination	Respectfulness, trust, objectivity	Provides nursing care based on respect of patients' rights to make decisions about their health care Honors individual's right to refuse treatment
Human dignity—respect for inherent worth and unique-ness of individuals and populations	Consideration, empathy, humaneness, kindness, respectfulness	Values and respects all patients and colleagues, regardless of background
Integrity—acting in accor-dance with an appropriate code of ethics	Moral, ethical, and legal professional behavior	The nurse is honest and provides care based on an ethical framework that is accepted in the profession
Social justice—acting in accordance with fair treat-ment regardless of economic status, race, ethnicity, age, citizenship, disability, or sexual orientation	Courage, integrity, morality, objectivity	Acts as a health care advocate Allocates resources fairly Reports incompetent, unethical, and illegal practices objectively and factually

From American Association of Colleges of Nursing: *Essentials of baccalaureate education for professional nursing*, Washington, DC, 2008, American Association of Colleges of Nursing.

Medicare-eligible individuals who have a greater likelihood of benefit to longevity or quality of life. Utilitarian ethics are noted to be the strongest approach used in bioethical decision making. An attempt is made to determine which actions will lead to the greatest ratio of benefit to harm for all persons involved in the dilemma.

Deontology

Deontology is an approach that is rooted in the assumption that humans are rational and act out of principles that are consistent and objective and compel them to do what is right. Ethics are based on a sense of a universal principle to consistently act one way. For instance, the deon-tological approach would be at work if a decision is made to resuscitate and provide mechanical ventilation to a 23-week, otherwise viable fetus, despite ability to pay for care and availability of newborn intensive care beds. In bioethical decision making, moral rightness is the act that is determined not by the consequences it produces, but by the moral qualities intrinsic to the act itself. Deontological theory claims that a decision is right only if it conforms to an overriding moral duty and wrong only if it violates that moral duty. All decisions must be made in such a way that the decision could become universal law. Persons are to be treated as ends in them-selves and never as means to the ends of others.

ETHICAL PRINCIPLES

Perhaps the most useful tool for the morally mature professional nurse is a set of principles, standards, or truths on which to base ethical actions. Common ground must be established between the nurse and the patient and the family, between fellow nurses, between the nurse and other health care providers, and between the nurse and other members of society. Such common ground can be established by adhering to a set of principles that can move everyone involved toward understanding and agreement.

The practice of ethics involves applying principles to the two ethical theories described—utilitarianism and deontology—or to other theories that are described elsewhere. Principles can permit people to take a consistent position on specific or related issues. If the principles, when applied to a particular act, make the act right or wrong in one situation, it seems reasonable to assume that the same principle, when applied to a new situation, can share similar features.

Three principles have proven to be highly relevant in bioethics: (1) autonomy, (2) beneficence, nonmaleficence, and (3) veracity. These principles are not related in such a way that they jointly form a complete moral framework. One may be relevant to a situation, whereas the others are not. Yet these principles are sufficiently comprehensive to provide an analytic framework by which moral problems can be evaluated.

Autonomy

Autonomy, the principle of respect for a person, is sometimes labeled as the primary moral principle. The umbrella concept says that humans have incalculable worth or moral dignity not possessed by other objects or creatures. There is unconditional intrinsic value for everyone. People are free to form their own judgments and whatever actions they choose. They are self-determining agents, entitled to determine their own destiny.

If an autonomous person's actions do not infringe on the autonomous actions of others, that person should be free to decide whatever he or she wishes. This freedom should be applied even if the decision creates risk to his or her health and even if the decision seems unwise to others. Concepts of freedom and informed consent are grounded in the principle of autonomy.

Although the principle of autonomy may seem basic and universal, there are times when this principle may be in conflict. For instance in some male-dominated or patriarchal cultures, the family leader's rights may override the individual and autonomous rights of a family member. In this situation, action based on the moral principle of autonomy may perpetuate conflict.

Beneficence, Nonmaleficence

In general terms, to be beneficent is to promote goodness, kindness, and charity. A different yet related principle is nonmaleficence, a principle that implies a duty not to inflict harm. In ethical terms nonmaleficence is to abstain from injuring others and to help others further their own well-being by removing harm and eliminating threats, whereas beneficence is to provide benefits to others by promoting their good. The beneficence-nonmaleficence principle is largely a balance of risk and benefit. At times the risk for harm must be weighed against possible benefits. The risk should never be greater than the importance of the problem to be solved.

Although it may seem natural to promote good at all times, the most common bioethical conflicts result from an imbalance between the demands of beneficence and those acts and decisions within the health care delivery system that might pose threats. For instance, it is not always clearly evident what is good and what is harmful. Is the resuscitation effort of the 80-year-old woman good or harmful to her overall sense of well-being? How much beneficence is there in supporting someone toward a peaceful death? What is the balance between beneficence and nonmaleficence in an understaffed emergency department? Is it better to do as much good as you can with the limited resources you have or to refuse to assume care in an effort to prevent harm that can come from being understaffed?

Veracity

Most contemporary professionals believe that telling the truth in personal communication is a moral and ethical requirement. If there is the belief in health care that truth telling is always right, then the principle of veracity can itself pose some interesting challenges.

In the past, truth telling was sometimes viewed as inconvenient, distressing, or even harmful to patients and families. In fact the first American Medical Association Code of Ethics in 1847 contained such a message:

> The life of a sick person can be shortened not only by the acts, but also by the words or the manner of a physician. It is, therefore, a sacred duty to guard himself carefully in this respect, and to avoid all things that have a tendency to discourage the patient and to depress his spirits.

The belief that the truth could at times be harmful was held for many years. Only recently with the shift from a provider-driven system to a consumer-driven system has the history of silence begun to break. With this shift have come interesting questions. Is the provider-patient relationship generally understood by both parties to include the right of the provider to control the truth by withholding some or all of the relevant information until an appropriate time for disclosure? How much deception with patients is morally acceptable in the communication of a poor or terminal prognosis?

Difficult questions surface, but at the heart of the principle of veracity is trust. Health care consumers today expect accurate and precise information that is revealed in an honest and respectful manner. A few generations ago the trust factor may have been such that it was acceptable for providers to share parts of truth or to distort the truth in the name of beneficence. Today, however, for trust to develop between providers and patients there must be truthful interaction and meaningful communication. The moral conflict that results from being less than truthful to patients is too troublesome for today's practitioner. The deontological theory of the health care provider having a duty to tell the patient the truth has taken precedence over the fear of harm that might result if the truth is revealed.

The challenge today is to mesh the need for truthful communication with the need to protect. Health care providers must lay aside fears that the truth will be harmful to patients and come to the realization that more often than not, the truth can alleviate anxiety, increase pain tolerance, facilitate recovery, and enhance cooperation with treatment. With a pledge toward human decency, health care providers must commit themselves to truth telling in all interactions and relationships.

ETHICAL DECISION-MAKING MODEL

Theories provide a cognitive plan for considering ethical issues; principles offer guiding truths on which to base ethical decisions. Using these theories and principles, it seems appropriate to consider a system for moving beyond a specific ethical dilemma toward a morally mature and reasoned ethical action.

Many ethical decision-making models exist for the purpose of defining a process by which a nurse or another health care provider actually can move through an ethical dilemma toward an informed decision. Box 9-3 depicts one ethical decision-making model.

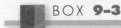

BOX **9-3**

Situation Assessment Procedure

1. Identify the ethical issues and problems.
2. Identify and analyze available alternatives for action.
3. Select one alternative.
4. Justify the selection.

From Wright RA: *The practice of ethics: human values in health care,* New York, 1987, McGraw-Hill.

Situation Assessment Procedure

Identify the ethical issues and problems. In the first step of assessment, there is an attempt to find out the technical and scientific facts and the human dimension of the situation—the feelings, emotions, attitudes, and opinions. A nurse must make an attempt to understand what values are inherent in the situation. Finally the nurse must deliberately state the nature of the ethical dilemma. This first step is important because the issues and problems to be addressed are often complex. Trying to understand the full picture of a situation is time consuming and requires examination from many different perspectives, but it is worth the time and effort to understand an issue fully before moving forward in the assessment procedure. Wright (1987) poses some important questions that must be addressed in this first step:

◆ What is the issue here?
◆ What are the hidden issues?
◆ What exactly are the complexities of this situation?
◆ Is anything being overlooked?

Identify and Analyze Available Alternatives for Action. In the second step, a set of alternatives for action is established. The second step is an important step to follow. Because actions are based most commonly on a nurse's personal value system, it is important to list all possible actions for a given situation, even actions that seem highly unlikely. Without deliberately listing possible alternatives, it is doubtful that the full consideration of all possible actions will take place. Wright's (1987) questions for the second step are these:

◆ What are the reasonable possibilities for action, and how do the different affected parties (patient, family, physician, nurse) want to resolve the problem?
◆ What ethical principles are required for each alternative?
◆ What assumptions are required for each alternative, and what are their implications for future action?
◆ What if any are the additional ethical problems that the alternatives raise?

Select One Alternative. Multiple factors come together in the third step. After identifying the issues and analyzing all possible alternatives, the skillful decision maker steps back to consider the situation again. There is an attempt to reflect on ethical theory and to mesh that thinking with the identified ethical principles for each alternative. The decision maker's value system is applied, along with an appraisal of the profession's values for the care of others. A reasoned and purposeful decision results from the blending of each of these factors.

Justify the Selection. The rational discourse on which the decision is based must be shared in an effort to justify the decision. The decision maker must be prepared to communicate his or her thoughts through an explanation of the reasoning process used. According to Wright (1987), the justification for a resolution to an ethical issue is an argument wherein relevant and sufficient reasons for the correctness of that resolution are presented. Defending an argument is not an easy task, but it is a necessary step to communicate the reasons or premises on which the decision is based. A systematic and logical argument will show why the particular resolution chosen is the correct one. This final step is important to advance ethical thought and to express sound judgment. Wright's formula for the justification process is as follows:

1. Specify reasons for the action.
2. Clearly present the ethical basis for these reasons.
3. Understand the shortcomings of the justification.
4. Anticipate objections to the justification.

Usefulness and Application of the Situation Assessment Procedure

A procedure or model for ethical decision making is useful for individuals and groups alike. The more subtle and tenuous issues that arise in health care often are resolved within the context of the patient-provider relationship that exists between two people. Dilemmas resulting from questions about truth telling, acknowledging uncertainty, paternalism, privacy, and fidelity are examples of issues that may be resolved between as few as two people.

Questions that are more encompassing often are addressed in group settings. Institutional ethics committees now are common within health care agencies. The purpose of the committee is to provide ethics education, aid in ethical policy development, and serve as a consultative body when resolution of an ethical dilemma cannot be reached otherwise. Although institutional ethics committees do not make legal decisions that are the province of the patient, the family, or the health care provider, a model such as the situation assessment procedure can be a useful procedure to guide the thinking of a group that has been asked to provide counsel.

More and more nurses are finding themselves facing ethical dilemmas as members of hospital administration teams or policymaking bodies within professional organizations or governmental bodies. Nurses contribute a highly relevant perspective to discussions and decisions about safe and effective care in these times of change. The situation assessment procedure can be applied to the decision-making process when procedures and policies are being developed to address conflicting variables.

Thus application of the situation assessment procedure can occur on two levels. The procedure is applicable to the daily practice level of ethical decision making as patients and providers make choices between right and wrong actions. The procedure is equally applicable to the policymaking level where professionals come together to consider right and wrong choices that affect society as a whole. Professional organizations including the American Nurses Association (ANA) have established committees, such as the ethics and human rights committee, that allow nurses to meet to set policy for the practice of nursing. Inherent in the policy formation are questions that affect patient care. The situation assessment procedure can be applied to difficult questions that arise in any setting in which the nurse is responsible for or contributes to ethical decision making.

BIOETHICAL DILEMMAS: LIFE, DEATH, AND DILEMMAS IN BETWEEN

Bioethical dilemmas are situations that pose a choice between perplexing alternatives in the delivery of health care because of the lack of a clear sense of right or wrong. It is imperative that every nursing student consider the potential dilemmas that might arise in a given practice setting. Concepts of life and death are central to nursing's body of knowledge, but a discussion of these concepts is incomplete unless the threats of conflict also are explored. A nursing student must not assume that conflict is rare or that it is to be dealt with primarily by other professionals on the health care team. Conflict must be addressed as the concepts of life and its origins, birth, death, and dying are addressed. However, conflict must also be addressed in the many varied situations that come up day after day in the practice of professional nursing.

Life

Entire textbooks are written to address the potential conflict that surrounds questions about the beginning of life. The most significant conflict that will be recorded in the historical accounts of the twentieth century will be the debate about when life begins. The abortion conflict became central in 1973 when the *Roe v. Wade* decision was made. Although the legal aspects of abortion have been resolved in courtrooms in the United States, the bioethical concerns continue to be debated 35 years later. The bioethical abortion conflict has been debated using ethical theories, ethical principles, value systems, rights issues, choice questions, and so on. Answers acceptable to society as a whole have not materialized; thus the right or wrong of abortion continues to rest with each person. Despite clear, generalizable answers to the abortion question, nurses serving in health settings for women and children must be prepared to face this morally laden issue.

Closely akin to the abortion question are newer questions about reproduction. Genetic screening, genetic engineering, stem cell therapy, and cloning are newer, highly advanced, and sophisticated techniques that bring with them the most ethically entangled questions ever encountered; the entire Human Genome Project with its rapidly developing advances represents the greatest challenge to date. Definitions of family, surrogacy, and other related issues also bring ethically entangled questions. Moving beyond the question about when life begins, health care providers must now address their patients' questions about the right or wrong of designing life itself through the manipulation and engineering of DNA or the right and wrong of new parenting models. Twenty-first-century life has created a whole new dimension of bioethics.

Death

The second most debated conflict in health care involves the issue of death and dying. Since the development of lifesaving procedures and mechanical ventilation, questions about quality of life and the definition of death have escalated. With the advances in health care, it has become unclear what is usual care and what is heroic care. The purpose and quality of life of a person in a vegetative state continue to be debated and even legislated, as seen in the nationally broadcasted court action in Florida in 2003. Health care providers regularly contend with questions of cerebral versus biologic death in their dealings with patients and families. The "dying with dignity" and "toward a peaceful death" concepts are examined in light of ever-evolving advances in life-prolonging care. Euthanasia and assisted suicide present the newest ethical questions surrounding the dying process. Because death is universal and part of human existence, every health care provider serving in every delivery setting must address the difficult end-of-life questions.

Dilemmas in Between

Life and death dilemmas receive the most attention in the written word through the media and in real-life drama played out in the news and on television and theater screens. However, a host of other questions make up most ethical decision-making activities for the professional nurse in the practice of today's health care. Between questions of life and death are questions of existence, reality, individual rights, responsibility, informed consent, cultural competence, equality, justice, ability to pay, and fairness. Added to these are an unlimited number of other questions that arise from the human dimension of caring.

It is in these ordinary day-to-day situations of caring that many professionals find the most important and troublesome questions. Basic notions of individual and social justice are viewed in terms of fairness and what is deserved. A person has been treated justly when he or she has been given what is due or owed. Any denial of something to which a person has a right or entitlement is an act of injustice.

The Right to Health Care. Handling injustice has been a part of nursing since the days of Florence Nightingale, but as health care delivery has shifted to a managed care system, new questions of injustices have surfaced. The system has become more selective in the amount and type of treatment offered. A full range of diagnostic testing may not be available to every person seeking answers for perplexing illnesses. The particular benefit package offered through one insurance company may be more limited in scope of services than the benefit package offered through another company. Two families living side by side in a typical suburban neighborhood may be entitled to different health care services based on where they are employed. Perhaps one family has access to health care, and the other does not.

What right to health care do people have? Is each person entitled to the same health care package? Should ability to pay affect the specific level of entitlement? How ethical is the reality of gatekeeping in the managed care system? Are employers and insurance groups removing patient autonomy by choosing the least costly insurance plans (Lee and Estes, 2003)? Resolutions to such questions have been based largely on the doctrine of justice, which states that like cases should be treated alike and equals ought to be treated equally. Such issues grip at the core of nursing practice wherein access to health care and a respect for human dignity are paramount. Justice becomes a bioethical issue at the point that it affects whether, when, where, and how a patient will receive health care.

Allocation of Scarce Resources. The issues of organ transplantation and the allocation of scarce resources flow from the doctrine of justice. The problem of scarce medical resources is becoming more common. Which people in need of transplantation should receive organs when available organs are in shorter supply than the number of people who could benefit from them? The justice question is applicable to this situation. The utilitarian view argues that the allocation decision should be framed so as to serve the greatest good for the greatest number of people affected. Should the selected recipient be the man with the largest, most loving family who does the greatest work for society? Or should a more universal law be applied? Should the people in need of organ transplantation be placed on a first-come, first-served list? Or should they be entered into a lottery? Distributive justice, or taking into consideration the needs, interests, and wishes of each patient, cannot alone answer allocation dilemmas. Who has the more meaningful life? Who has the best prognosis? Who can pay? As unjust as it may seem to some, these are the kinds of questions responsible parties must answer regarding the allocation of scarce resources. And what about the fact that nurses themselves are scarce resources? What about the challenge of the nurse's autonomous right to refuse to work in understaffed settings? Whose rights come first?

ETHICAL CHALLENGES

What about the doctrines of justice and freedom and the need for human experimentation and biomedical research? What about animal experimentation? It is accepted that human and animal experimentation is necessary for the progression of health care knowledge, but what about the risk for harm and the moral imperative that providers should, above all, do no harm? What about specifically problematic aspects of research, such as the use of institutionalized or imprisoned research subjects or the practice of research on a viable fetus? Memories of harmful medical research and human experimentation, such as the Nazi atrocities and the Tuskegee incident, have resulted in governmental regulations involving the use of human subjects in medical research. The Nuremberg Code is a set of provisions for research that must be followed for the federal government to approve research. Institutional review boards are established within research institutions for the purpose of overseeing that the degree of risk to the subject is minimized, if not eliminated. Human experimentation tests the principles of autonomy and respect for personhood.

The Challenge of Veracity

Everyday issues that test the principle of veracity are the concepts of alternative treatment and acknowledging uncertainty. It is the nature of health science that new knowledge must come forth to abolish less effective dogma. However, new ignorance comes along with these new discoveries. Which treatment among two or more is best for a patient in a specific situation? Which of the new drugs should be used? Should every patient be subjected to every possible form of diagnostic evaluation? Should this patient be treated with surgery, medication, or both? How do the economics of treatment costs factor in to the decision? And most important, should the patient be made aware of all these questions and various options for his or her care? Can patients comprehend medicine's esoteric knowledge, in general, and its accompanying certainties and uncertainties, in particular? Is disclosure of uncertainty ultimately beneficial or detrimental?

Acknowledging uncertainty is difficult for today's health care provider. As never before, it seems that providers need to present themselves as confident, knowledgeable, and sensitive to their patients, who may see them as arrogant, dogmatic, and insensitive. Acknowledging uncertainty may be worth the effort. For the diagnostician, it may lighten the burden by absolving him or her of the responsibility for implicitly making decisions for which there may be conflicting answers. For the patient, knowing about the uncertainty may give him or her a greater voice in decision making and, in the event of treatment failure, may leave him or her better informed and more trustful of the caregiver. It seems that disclosure of uncertainty is ultimately beneficial to both parties. In fact it seems that full disclosure and open communication through a commitment to veracity could prevent many everyday ethical situations. Optimal health care results from an exchange between patient and provider with open communication about the patient's wants and needs and the provider's judgment and advice. All too often time is not taken for open communication, and the exchange becomes one in which the patient listens to what the all-knowing and wise provider says about his or her needs. In this scenario it is easy for the provider to assume a paternalistic attitude in the delivery of health care.

The Challenge of Paternalism

Paternalism is an action and an attitude wherein the provider tries to act on behalf of the patient and believes that his or her actions are justified because of a commitment to act in the best interest of the patient. Paternalism is a reflection of the "father knows best" way of thinking. The phenomenon of paternalism presumes, in the name of beneficence, to overlook the patient's right to autonomy. Thus in the process of attempting to act in the best interest of the patient, paternalism involves actions not based on the patient's choices, wishes, and desires. Paternalism interferes with a patient's right to self-determination and occurs when the provider believes that he or she can make a better decision than the patient.

Whereas it must be recognized that some cultures are highly paternalistic, the most common belief and value system in North America views paternalism as a threat to the patient-provider relationship. Every provider must guard against actions and attitudes that are paternalistic. Perhaps in the past, paternalism was associated with the white-coat image of the physician as a sovereign god. Today paternalistic actions and attitudes can be found among nurses, pharmacists, physical therapists, occupational therapists, social workers, clergy, or anyone who assumes the image of the all knowing in the delivery of care. A current threat to a healthy patient-provider relationship is the emergence of entrepreneurship in medicine in which health care providers are more and more called on to be business managers. The bottom line financial realities can be threats to safe care.

The healthy patient-provider relationship is based on the open communication described previously, wherein patient choice and respect for personhood are deemed just as important as scientific knowledge and sound health care advice. The provider-patient relationship is built on trust when the right to confidentiality and privacy become ethical and legal obligations.

The Challenge of Autonomy

The provider-patient relationship makes way for the crucial legal concept of informed consent, which stipulates that the patient has the right to know and make decisions about his or her health. These decisions take the form of consent or refusal of treatment. Based on the principle of autonomy, the consent process must be voluntary and without coercion; the fully informed patient must clearly understand the choices being offered.

Informed consent dilemmas evolve from questions about whether patients are competent to make informed decisions and whether there are family members or surrogates to make those decisions by proxy. Difficult questions are posed for health care providers by the need for informed consent from minors, confused older adults, persons in emergency situations, and persons who are mentally compromised, imprisoned, inebriated, or unconscious. The burden of informed consent lies with the physician in most circumstances, although the nurse frequently is responsible for aspects of informing and obtaining consent.

In the latter part of the twentieth century, another crucial concept of consent was introduced. Advances in technology and the potential to keep people alive for extended periods have brought about legislation aimed at giving people choices about end-of-life decisions while they are still healthy and well enough to make informed decisions. The opportunity for people to make advance directives is now common and is even a requirement for admission to hospitals and other health care agencies that receive federal dollars. People are not required to decide, but must be given an opportunity to do so. Ideally the health care community will provide such an opportunity while the patient is well, perhaps in a community setting, such as a public library or community center. Health care professionals, such as nurses and other health care educators, have an ethical obligation to educate the public about the use of advance directives. These opportunities can serve as excellent means of educating patients not only about advance directives but also about their rights in general, changes in health care delivery and managed care, and the role of the various health care providers. These are excellent opportunities to educate the public about the scope of practice of today's professional nurse.

The Challenge of Accountability

A host of specific ethical issues exists within the practice of nursing itself. Professional nursing is a complex profession that is unlike most others. The accountability factor in the practice of nursing is such that a keen sense of responsibility and personal integrity are necessary qualities for every practicing nurse. It is the nurse's ethical obligation to uphold the highest standards of practice and care, assume full personal and professional responsibility for every action, and commit to maintaining quality in the skill and knowledge base of the profession. Failure to meet such obligations places the patient-nurse relationship at risk.

Failure to be accountable for one's own actions places a tremendous burden on the relationship with the patient and poses ethical dilemmas for fellow nurse professionals. In health professions in which the safety and health of society are at stake, the obligation of professionals to police the practice of their colleagues is important.

There are public and legal official policing bodies, such as the state board of nursing, for matters of public record and formal conviction. However, there are countless situations in which the official policing body will never be involved, and the obligation to denounce a harmful action or potentially threatening situation falls to a fellow member of the profession. Sometimes known as "whistle blowing," the obligation to denounce is based on the fact that to remain silent is to consent to the action or threatening situation. Whether denouncing a chemical impairment, negligence, abusiveness, incompetence, or cruelty, the obligation is a moral one based at least in part on the principle of beneficence.

Every person bearing the title of nurse must aspire to maintain himself or herself as a professional of integrity who is willing to blow the whistle on those whose actions are irresponsible and harmful. If this is not the case, the wrong will continue, and the harm to others will escalate. In the end, the profession as a whole will suffer, and the well-being of society will be diminished.

SUMMARY

Professional nurses must be prepared to face any number of potential ethical conflicts in the day-to-day practice of their profession. They must realize that each situation is different and that recognizing this uniqueness demands that responsible parties seek a loving and humane solution to every situation that poses an ethical dilemma. When the answer remains clouded, the decision maker must choose the most appropriate action, given the situation, based on a variety of potentially applicable principles.

To think that dilemmas, such as the ones described here, are unlikely or far removed is to think that the surgery patient will not be troubled by pain or the trauma patient by anxiety or the cancer patient by fear. Ethical conflict is inherent in the practice of nursing and is played out in every practice setting every day. The challenge is not to escape the conflict but to meet it with expectancy and preparedness.

The profession of nursing is often described as a discipline of human caring. Relationships are the foundation of safe practice, including ethical practice. Those seeking a career in nursing must realize the multifaceted aspects of the profession. They also should appreciate the rich and diverse opportunities that will be afforded them. Braced with scientific knowledge and the resources for critical examination of health and illness, the professional nurse is provided access to life's most intimate and precious encounters. Perhaps more than any other health care provider, a sensitive and caring nurse is invited to join patients who are experiencing the most intense moments of their lives. Nurses are given the opportunity to embrace patients in their joy over the birth of a child or the good news of a successful surgery or chemotherapy treatment for cancer. They also are privileged to support patients and their families during the trials of waiting for the outcome of a tragic head injury or the last breath in a life devastated by terminal illness. To all of this, nurses are invited.

With such privilege comes responsibility. The purpose of this chapter has been to introduce nursing students to the idea that ethical conflict in health care abounds and to increase students'

SUMMARY—cont'd

awareness of their role in resolving conflict. It is important for professional nurses to have a basic knowledge of the ethical thinking enterprise that is described in this chapter and realize that there are other resources for committed professionals to draw on in an effort to stay abreast of the issues they are likely to face in their practice. Some journals, such as The Hastings Center Report and Ethics in Medicine, come from centers and institutes, such as the Center for Health and Human Dignity; the Institute of Society, Ethics, and the Life Sciences; the Kennedy Institute Center for Bioethics; and the ANA Committee on Ethics and Human Rights. These groups prepare position statements and white papers on specific ethical dilemmas arising from today's health care practice. Learning centers, libraries, and websites generally provide access to these resources, although individual membership and subscriptions are available. Box 9-4 presents online resources available to learn more about ethics, bioethics, and the issues nurses are likely to face in their practice.

Bioethics and ethical decision making are philosophic enterprises, a thinking activity. Many activities in nursing practice require an actual skill that involves training, practice, and technique development. For example, nursing students are introduced to the principles of intravenous line insertion while in a campus laboratory setting. They may have an opportunity to practice starting an intravenous line in a simulated setting before actually assuming the responsibility for starting one on a "real" patient. The first few times that students insert an intravenous line, their effort is based on a deliberate thinking through of each step and each principle of asepsis, circulation and blood flow, and positioning. In time the principles of starting an intravenous line become a well-developed technique and skill activity.

The same process can be used when developing one's capacity for a critical thinking activity. This chapter has presented a vignette describing a nursing management situation laden with potential for ethical conflict within patient care. As nursing students move through their educational experience, they will be assigned to care for many patients. Every nursing management and patient care situation has the potential of presenting an ethical dilemma. As students are faced with ethical decisions, they refine their decision-making skills. Each time they reflect on ethical theories or consider ethical principles, they develop critical thinking ability. In time the professional nurse is able to incorporate what he or she has learned into a morally mature personal code of ethics. At that point, there is a liberating joy that comes from knowing that competence in professional nursing practice goes beyond technique and skill to include the ability to reason life's most difficult and challenging questions and all for the benefit of another human being. Although it is not as easy as it may sound, it is well worth the effort.

Girded with truth, nurses must commit themselves to take a bold stance for what is right and against what is wrong. Nurses should feel empowered through their roles as primary patient advocates to voice their morality in the face of a new century that promises sweeping changes in health care delivery. Nurses must speak in support of patient choice and self-determination in the era of managed care. They must speak against the moral wrong of understaffed practice trends wherein patient safety is jeopardized. Nurses must monitor legislation that affects health care and study current issues, such as assisted suicide and cloning. Professional nursing embodies a commitment, not just to think and act wisely in the administration of therapeutic nursing interventions, but also to think and act in accordance with specified values and basic principles of right and wrong. Nursing is making a commitment to all of the above.

ⓔvolve   Additional resources are available online at: http://evolve.elsevier.com/Cherry/

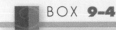

BOX **9-4**

Helpful Websites

ANA Center for Ethics and Human Rights
   www.nursingworld.org/ethics
Veterans Health Administration National Center for Ethics
   www.va.gov/VHAETHICS/index.cfm
Center for Bioethics and Human Dignity
   www.cbhd.org
The Nurse Friendly (nursing ethics and ethical issues; direct patient care)
   www.nursefriendly.com/nursing/directpatientcare/ethics.htm

REFERENCES

Hockenberry MJ, et al: *Wong's nursing care of infants and children*, ed 8, St Louis, 2007, Mosby.

Kohlberg L: Stages of moral development as a basis for moral development. In Beck CM, Crittenden BS, Sullivan EV, editors: *Moral interdisciplinary approaches*, Paramus, NJ, 1971, Newman.

Lee PA, Estes CL: *The nation's health*, ed 7, Boston, 2003, Jones and Bartlett.

Tong R: *New perspectives in healthcare ethics — an interdisciplinary and crosscultural approach*, Upper Saddle River, NJ, 2007, Pearson Prentice-Hall.

Uustal D: *Values and ethics in nursing: from theory to practice*, ed 4, Greenwich, RI, 1992, Educational Resources in Nursing and Holistic Health.

Weaver K, Morse J, Mitcham C: Ethical sensitivity in professional practice: concept analysis, *J Adv Nurs* 62(5):607–618, 2008.

Wright RA: *The practice of ethics: human values in health care*, New York, 1987, McGraw-Hill.

Cultural Competency and Social Issues in Nursing and Health Care

Susan R. Jacob, PhD, MSN, RN

evolve   Additional resources are available online at: http://evolve.elsevier.com/Cherry/

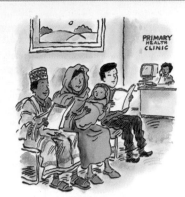

Clients deserve culturally competent care.

VIGNETTE

When my instructor taught the session on cultural differences, she stressed the high alcoholism rates of American Indians. I began to fear that my instructor and fellow classmates would stereotype me because of my American Indian background. However, no one in my family drinks alcohol because we belong to the Mormon church, where drinking is not accepted. I wish the instructor had stressed the importance of not stereotyping.

■ QUESTIONS TO CONSIDER WHILE READING THIS CHAPTER:

1 What preconceived ideas do you have about the following cultural groups: Hispanic, Appalachian, Moroccan, African-American, South African, and Chinese?

2 What strategies can you implement to overcome prejudice?

3 How can nurses provide effective care to different cultural groups who each have a unique set of beliefs about illness?

4 How can nursing research affect the attitudes and beliefs of health professionals in regard to minority and marginalized populations?

KEY TERMS

Acculturation The process of becoming adapted to a new or different culture.

Assimilation The cultural absorption of a minority group into the main cultural body.

Biculturalism Combining two distinct cultures in a single region.

Culture Shared values, beliefs, and practices of a particular group of people that are transmitted from one generation to the next and are identified as patterns that guide thinking and action.

Cultural humility Incorporates a lifelong commitment to self-evaluation and self-critique, to redressing the power imbalances in the patient-clinician dynamic and to developing mutually beneficial and advocacy partnerships with communities on behalf of individuals and defined populations (Tervalon and Murray-Garcia, 1998).

Cultural sensitivity Experienced when neutral language, both verbal and nonverbal, is used in a way that reflects sensitivity and appreciation for the diversity of another (American Academy of Nursing Expert Panel on Cultural Competence, 2007).

Enculturation Adaptation to the prevailing cultural patterns in society.

Ethnicity Affiliation resulting from shared linguistic, racial, or cultural background.

KEY TERMS—cont'd

Ethnocentrism Believing that one's own ethnic group, culture, or nation is best.

Marginalized population A subgroup of the population that tends to be hidden, overlooked, or on the outer edge.

Minority An ethnic group smaller than the majority group.

Prejudice Preconceived, deeply held, usually negative, judgment formed about other groups.

Stereotyping Assigning certain beliefs and behaviors to groups without recognizing individuality.

Transculturalism Being grounded in one's own culture, but having the skills to be able to work in a multicultural environment.

Worldview Perspective shared by a cultural group of general views of relationships within the universe. These broad views influence health and illness beliefs.

LEARNING OUTCOMES

After studying this chapter, the reader will be able to:

1 Integrate knowledge of demographic and sociocultural variations into culturally competent professional nursing care.

2 Provide culturally competent care to diverse client groups that incorporates variations in biologic characteristics, social organization, environmental control, communication, and other phenomena.

3 Critique education, practice, and research issues that influence culturally competent care.

4 Integrate respect for differences in beliefs and values of others as a critical component of nursing practice.

CHAPTER OVERVIEW

The United States has always been represented by a culturally diverse society. However, the volume of cultural groups entering our country is increasing rapidly. Professional nurses must provide care to persons of various cultures who have different values, beliefs, and perceptions of health and illness. This chapter explores cultural phenomena, including environmental control, biologic variations, social organization, communication, space, and time in relation to major cultural groups. It also examines different views toward health, illness, and cure. Federally defined minority groups, which include African-Americans, Asians, Hispanics, and American Indians, are emphasized, although the needs of marginalized populations, such as the homeless, refugees, and older adults also are addressed. The need for diversity in the health care force is explored, and strategies for recruiting and retaining minorities in health care are suggested. Strategies that nurses can use to increase their own cultural competence also are given.

POPULATION TRENDS

The demographic and ethnic composition of the U.S. population has experienced marked change in the past 100 years. The United States always has been a multicultural society, although changes in immigration laws have increased the number of cultural groups entering the United States (Stanhope and Lancaster, 2008). Minority groups have grown faster than the population as a whole. If migration trends continue, by the mid–twenty-first century minority populations will outnumber the white population. Approximately one in every three Americans will be an ethnic minority. In some U.S. cities the number of persons from diverse cultural groups is increasing at such a rapid pace that minorities constitute more than half the population. The nation will be more racially and ethnically diverse, as well as much older, by midcentury, according to 2008 projections released by the U.S. Census Bureau.

Minorities, now roughly one third of the U.S. population, are expected to become the majority in 2042, with the nation projected to be 54% minority in 2050. By 2023, minorities will comprise more than half of all children.

In 2030, when all of the baby-boomers will be 65 and older, nearly one in five U.S. residents is expected to be 65 and older. This age group is projected to increase to 88.5 million in 2050, more than doubling the number in 2008 (38.7 million). The aging population includes an increasing number of older adults whose age exceeds 85 years (U.S. Department of Commerce, Bureau of the Census, 2008).

This demographic change introduces many interrelated social, economic, political, educational, and health problems. The fact that people are living longer allows more opportunity for the development of chronic illness. Social isolation and depression that result from losses of friends and family will present a challenge for mental health care providers. Primary care providers will be faced with identifying risks to independence and health for the aging population (U.S. Department of Health and Human Services [USDHHS], 2000).

Federally Defined Minority Groups

Federally defined minority groups are African-Americans, Hispanics, American Indians, and Asians or Pacific Islanders. Although tremendous strides have been made in improving health and longevity in the United States, statistical trends show a disparity in key health indicators among certain subgroups of the population. There is a racial gap between African-Americans and whites of 5.6 years, with average life expectancy of 78 years for whites and 72.7 years for African-Americans. The infant death rate for African-Americans is twice that of whites (Nies and McEwen, 2007). Although the ranking of health problems according to excess deaths differs for minority groups, the six causes of death that are a priority are:
1. Cancer
2. Cardiovascular disease and stroke
3. Chemical dependency as measured by deaths caused by cirrhosis of the liver
4. Diabetes
5. Homicides and accidents
6. Infant mortality (Nies and McEwen, 2007)

Marginalized Populations

Not only should the concern for culturally competent care focus on ethnic minorities and populations that have a different heritage than Euro-Americans, but the needs of marginalized populations (Hall, Stevens, and Meleis, 1994), which are those populations that live on the periphery or in between, should be considered. Examples of such populations include gays and lesbians, older adults, recently arrived immigrants (e.g., from Russia, Afghanistan, and Rwanda), and groups that have been in this country for some time (e.g., from South America and the Middle East) who are less visible than the federally defined minorities (Lenburg et al, 1995). Their lives and health care needs often are kept secret and are understood only by them. Marginalized populations usually have extreme insights about their health care needs, although they often seem voiceless. This is in part a result of the different ways in which they both communicate and are silenced. It also may be because they feel even more peripheral or shut out from mainstream society when they are ill or experiencing a crisis.

ECONOMIC AND SOCIAL CHANGES

Changing world economics have had profound consequences, such as increased joblessness, homelessness, poverty, and limited access to health insurance and health care. Anxiety, hopelessness, depression, and despair commonly affect the individuals in our society who find themselves suddenly without a job and sometimes even without a home as a result of downsizing. These conditions often are associated with increased stress-related symptoms, substance abuse, violence, and crime (Lenburg et al, 1995). Dramatic changes in technology and specialization in the health care field have made health care costs skyrocket. Therefore not everyone can afford health care services. More minorities lack health insurance than the general population (Nies and McEwen, 2007). Higher costs and lower wages for minority groups make it difficult to rise out of poverty (Stanhope and Lancaster, 2008).

Poverty

Most families with racially or ethnically diverse backgrounds have a lower socioeconomic status than does the population at large. African-Americans, Hispanics, and American Indians have much higher rates of poverty than non-Hispanic whites and Asians. The median family income of Asians is slightly higher than that of non-Hispanic whites and is consistent with Asians' high levels of education and the higher percentage of families with two wage earners (Council of Economic Advisers, 1999). However, opportunities for education, occupation, income earning, and property ownership that are available to upper- and middle-class Americans often are not available to members of minority groups (Stanhope and Lancaster, 2008).

The poor also suffer more than the population as a whole for nearly every measure of health. Substantial disparities remain in health insurance coverage for certain populations. Among the nonelderly population, approximately 32.1% of Hispanic persons as well as American Indian and Alaska Native persons lacked health insurance coverage in 2007. For African-Americans, the percentage of uninsured in 2007 was 19.5. Lack of health care coverage has major implications for health (USDHHS, 2008).

Minority members of society often live in poverty. This social stratification leads to social inequality. For instance it is widely known that school systems and recreational facilities vary significantly between the inner city and the suburbs (Nies and McEwen, 2007). Residential segregation, substandard housing, unemployment, poor physical and mental health, and poor self-image are part of the cycle of poverty. This inequality is especially disturbing as it relates to health care. The United States has a history of providing the highest quality health care to those with the highest socioeconomic status and the worst health care to those with low socioeconomic status. Social, economic, and health problems have led to heated debates about the philosophy, scope and costs, and sources of funding for health care and insurance programs.

Violence

Changing economic and social conditions have contributed to the increasing level of violence in our society. Statistics indicate that homicide is the second leading cause of death among Americans ages 10 to 24 years and the leading cause of death among African-American males ages 15 to 34 years (Nies and McEwen, 2007). Businesses, schools, restaurants, playgrounds, and churches have become common settings for random acts of violence (Lenburg et al, 1995). Unemployment is associated with violence because it is an expectation in our society that people should be productive and gainfully employed. The inability to secure or hold a job may lead to feelings of inadequacy, guilt, and frustration, which in turn can precipitate acts of violence.

Although the increasing incidence of violence affects all segments of society, women, children, older adults, and culturally vulnerable groups are especially at risk. Unemployment rates among young minority men the United States are consistently low (Stanhope and Lancaster, 2008). This group also has the highest rate of violence, with homicide being a major problem for young African-American males. The differing rates of violence among races are more likely a result of poverty than race (Stanhope and Lancaster, 2008).

Societal changes have increased the tension between the empowered culturally dominant groups and the less visible vulnerable groups. This tension and behavioral response to tension has major implications for health care delivery and the education of nurses and other health care professionals (Lenburg et al, 1995).

ATTITUDES TOWARD CULTURALLY DIVERSE GROUPS

The range of attitudes toward culturally diverse groups can be viewed along a continuum of intensity, as illustrated in Figure 10-1 (Lenburg et al, 1995).

The extreme negative manifestation of prejudice is hate in its many violent and nonviolent forms. Contempt is somewhat less intense, but is problematic because it is so widespread and undermines many aspects of society. Tolerance reflects a more neutral attitude that accepts differences without attempting to convert them; it is the minimal-level attitude essential in democratic societies. Respect for diversity is manifested in behaviors that integrate differences into positive interactions and relationships. Respect is a demonstration of the inherent worth of the individual, regardless of differences. The most positive attitude is portrayed as a celebration (or affirmation) of the positive merits of cultural differences (i.e., of the value added to life experiences by multiple perspectives, traditions, rituals, foods, and art forms). The combination of ignorance of other cultures and arrogance about one's own culture fosters disrespect and hate. The deliberate attempt to discover and apply the positive benefits of cultural variation promotes respect and a celebration of the value of diversity, whereas perpetuating prejudice fosters narrow-mindedness and contempt. By integrating these perspectives as part of professional role behavior, educators can help students prepare for culturally competent practice in communities of diversity.

DIVERSITY IN THE HEALTH CARE WORKFORCE
Need for Diversity in the Health Care Workforce

Members of some cultural groups are demanding culturally relevant health care that incorporates their beliefs and practices (Nies and McEwen, 2007). Consumers are becoming much more aware of what constitutes culturally sensitive and competent care and are less willing to accept incompetent care (Meleis et al, 1995). There is a lack of diversity and ethnic representation of health care professionals, and there is limited knowledge about values, beliefs, experiences, and health care needs of certain populations, such as immigrants, the elderly, and gays and lesbians. Each of these groups has a unique set of responses to health and illness.

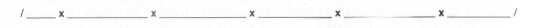

| Hate | Contempt | Tolerance | Respect | Celebration |

Figure 10-1 *A continuum of intensity of the range of attitudes toward culturally diverse groups. (From American Academy of Nursing:* Promoting cultural competence in and through nursing education: a critical review and comprehensive plan for action, *1995, Washington, DC, American Academy of Nursing.)*

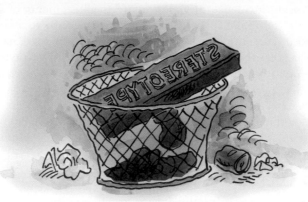

Stereotypes should be trashed.

Nurses make up the largest segment of the workforce in health care delivery. Therefore they have an opportunity to be proactive in changing health care inequities and access to health care (Meleis et al, 1995). The changing health care system must reflect the community and as health care moves into the community, it is vital that partnerships be formed between health care providers and the community. For these partnerships to become a reality, minority representation in all health professions is vital. Factors inhibiting minority members from attaining a career in nursing include inadequate academic preparation, especially in the sciences; financial costs; inadequate career counseling; and better recruitment efforts by other disciplines (Sullivan, 2004).

Current Status of Diversity in the Health Care Workforce

Although most nurses are white women, an increasing proportion of minority students is graduating from nursing programs. In a survey conducted by the American Association of Colleges of Nursing (AACN) in 2008, minority representation in baccalaureate programs was highest among those identified as black or African-American (11%) and lowest among American Indian/Alaska Natives (0.7%). Graduates from Hispanic or Latino groups totaled 6.1%, and Asian, Native Hawaiian, or other Pacific Islanders were 0.8% of the undergraduate students who responded to the survey. These totals lag behind the 74% reported white enrollment.

The number of men who graduate from basic registered nurse (RN) programs is also increasing. In the AACN survey conducted in 2008, 10.4% of the undergraduate respondents were men. Men continue to represent a minority in nursing, although recruitment efforts have focused more on men and minorities. Ad campaigns have highlighted men who were formerly firefighters, emergency responders, and law enforcement officers who have made the decision to pursue nursing as a career.

Of the nurses who indicated their racial or ethnic background in 2004, 88.4% were white, non-Hispanic; 4.6% were black or African-American, non-Hispanic; 3.3% were Asian or Pacific Islander, non-Hispanic; 1.8% were Hispanic; and 0.4% or 9453 were American Indian or Alaska Native (HRSA, 2005) (Figure 10-2). These figures are staggering in light of the demographics of our society. Although the number of minority nurses is increasing, the numbers have failed to keep up with our increasingly diverse population.

Men constituted 5.8% of the RN population in 2004. The initial nursing preparation for more male RNs was an associate's degree. The percentages of male and female RNs completing

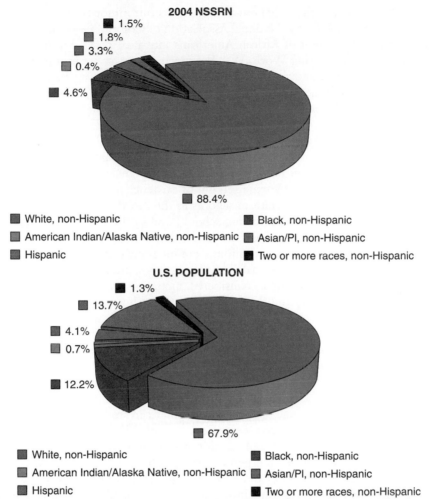

Figure 10-2 *Distribution of registered nurses and the U.S. population by racial/ethnic background, 2004, U.S. Census Bureau. (From Chart 5, HRSA 2005—Preliminary findings; Table 3: Annual estimates of the population by sex, race and Hispanic or Latino origin for the United States, 2004, U.S. Department of Health and Human Services, Health Resources Services Administration.)*

a baccalaureate or higher degree initial nursing program were similar, 32.7% and 31.5%, respectively (HRSA, 2005).

Recruitment and Retention of Minorities in Nursing

It is clear that we have been slow in preparing nurses to be reflective of our population, just as we have been unaware of the need for culturally sensitive patient care and sometimes less than welcoming to students different from the preponderant population (Sullivan, 1998). Recruitment and retention of students from minority populations must not be separated. In other words, recruitment programs must have retention as their primary focus because there is no point in recruiting minorities into nursing programs and then not helping them succeed.

Before World War II the only known effort to recruit minority students into nursing on a national scale was made by the National Association of Colored Graduate Nurses (NACGN), which had had recruitment of African-Americans into nursing as one of its objectives since its inception in 1908. During World War II a mechanism was set into motion by the federal government to produce additional nursing personnel by financing basic nursing education. This was done through the Cadet Nurse Corps. The corps had a number of recruiters, two of whom were African-Americans. These two African-American nurses confined their recruiting to 82 African-American colleges and universities. By the end of the war 21 African-American nursing schools had participated in the corps, and more than 2000 African-American nurses had acquired their basic nursing education through this mechanism.

After the war, recruitment efforts for African-Americans at the national level reverted to NACGN, an organization that voted itself out of existence in 1949 and was dissolved in 1951. However, individual African-American schools in the North and South continued to recruit. In the South, law segregated the nursing schools, and in the North they were segregated by custom. In 1954 the unanimous Supreme Court decision—*Brown v. the Board of Education*—asserted that "separate educational facilities were inherently unequal," making racial segregation in public schools unconstitutional. This decision was interpreted to mean that all kinds of educational discrimination would be considered, including nursing.

It was around the time of the Brown decision that schools of nursing were being accredited by national standards, and many schools, both African-American and white, just did not measure up to the standards. As a result, many schools closed. With integration permitting African-American students to be admitted to formerly all-white schools, quality African-American schools had difficulty attracting enough students, and many of the schools closed. However, the white schools that began admitting African-American students did not admit the number that would have been admitted by the African-American schools. For example, many white schools admitted only one or two African-American students per class.

In the late 1960s, many efforts were made to help the economically disadvantaged in this country. Although not all people of minority groups are economically disadvantaged, the vast majority of disadvantaged people are members of ethnic minority groups. Nursing too became concerned about the disadvantaged and began concerted efforts to recruit more members of minority groups into nursing schools. The Sealantic Fund, one of the Rockefeller Brothers funds, was one of the first foundations that helped minorities enter nursing school. Sealantic funded projects in 10 universities in different parts of the country to recruit students from minority groups and help them achieve success. The best example of an ongoing project, funded by the division of nursing since 1971, is the National Student Nurses Association's breakthrough in nursing to accelerate the recruitment of minorities, including men.

In 1997 the American Nurses Foundation published a report of a project it had funded titled Strategies for Recruitment, Retention and Graduation of Minority Nurses in Colleges of Nursing. Through survey and interview analysis, Bessent and a cadre of knowledgeable leaders investigated the most effective approach to increase the nursing profession's representation of minority nurses (Bessent, 1997). Members of Chi Eta Phi, a national African-American nursing society with chapters throughout the country, serve as mentors to minority nursing students. As mentors sorority members provide intellectual and inspirational stimulation along with counseling.

In 1997 AACN published a position statement stating that diversity and inclusion had emerged as central issues for organizations and institutions. AACN encouraged leadership in nursing to respond to these issues by finding ways to accelerate the inclusion of groups, cultures, and ideas that traditionally had been underrepresented in higher education.

As the demographics of the population rapidly changed in the twenty-first century there were numerous strategies to recruit and retain minority nursing faculty, students, and practicing nurses in the profession to better reflect the population demographics. Just as contributions of diverse cultural groups were increasingly valued, the profession began to value the need for diversity in their students and faculty and view this diversity as strength.

Strategies for Recruitment and Retention of Minorities in the Health Care Workforce

Recommendations of the American Academy of Nursing (AAN) expert panel on cultural competence (Meleis et al, 1995) include recruitment and retention of diversity in the workforce, raising consciousness, mentoring, and consultation. There also is a need to increase the number of nurse educators and researchers who are from diverse, marginalized, and vulnerable populations. Raising consciousness involves increasing the level of awareness of nurses and other health care professionals about the issues surrounding diversity. This can be accomplished by encouraging participation in forums related to different aspects of various cultural phenomena, such as environmental control, communication, and health beliefs. Such forums might be offered by state and local professional nurses' organizations and health care facilities.

Another successful strategy for recruiting and retaining minorities in education and clinical practice is matched mentoring, which involves matching same-culture mentors either in the same institution or different institutions. A different mentoring strategy involves teaching and modeling by nurses who have been trained in crosscultural care. Crosscultural nursing consultants in the care of specific groups are available to agencies, professional groups, licensing bodies, and individual nurses. (Organizations should contact the Transcultural Nursing Society at www.tcns.org to obtain the names of consultants in the field of transcultural nursing.)

Audiovisual media should be used to teach the importance of human health conditions cross-culturally. Video conferencing can provide international links for students and faculty who cannot travel. Students from various cultures can share their clinical experiences. One of the greatest benefits is the discovery that thinking, values, and decision making differ in various cultures. Collaborative arrangements should be encouraged between colleges and universities so that exchange programs can be offered to students. Such exchanges can provide firsthand in-depth experience with a culture that is different from their own. Interactive media could be used to gain a clearer perspective than can be obtained through the print medium on particular cultures.

Strategies such as mentoring by the same-culture professional are effective in recruiting and retaining minorities in nursing. In addition, the value of workshops, continuing education programs, and the use of consultants to promote culturally competent care should not be overlooked.

CULTURAL COMPETENCE

Health professionals, educators, and health care systems must all respond to the consequences of increasing cultural diversity for the future well-being of all populations. There is a shared responsibility to work collaboratively to achieve competence in nursing practice in order to deliver patient-centered care. It is evident that professional competence must incorporate cultural competence and the skillful use of knowledge and interpersonal and technical abilities

(Lenburg et al, 1995). Evaluation of cultural competence in students, faculty, and staff is essential. The authors suggest that it is essential that nurses take responsibility to:

◆ Be sensitive to and show respect for the differences in beliefs and values of others.

◆ Take responsibility to inquire, learn about, and integrate beliefs and values of others in professional encounters.

◆ Take responsibility to try to change negative and prejudicial behaviors in themselves and others.

In light of societal changes, responsible persons at all levels in education and health care delivery systems acknowledge the need to reassess the influence of culture on achieving expected health outcomes. There is an imperative need for nurse educators, administrators, students, and others to promote sensitivity to, acceptance of, and respect for the rights and mores of all individuals within the context of their cultural orientation and society as a whole. Nurses must be culturally competent because:

◆ The nurse's culture often is different from the client's culture.

◆ Care that is not culturally competent may be more costly.

◆ Care that is not culturally competent may be ineffective.

◆ Specific objectives for persons in different cultures need to be met as outlined in *Healthy People 2000*.

◆ Racial and minority groups experience profound disparities in health and health care.

◆ Nursing is committed to social justice, providing safe quality care to all.

◆ Nurses are expected to respond to global infectious disease epidemics.

◆ Achieving cultural competence should be our goal, although it may take most of us a lifetime to attain. However, we can all aspire to achieve cultural humility, which incorporates a lifelong commitment to self-evaluation and self-critique, to redressing the power imbalances in the patient-clinician dynamic, and to developing mutually beneficial and advocacy partnerships with communities on behalf of individuals and defined populations (Tervalon and Murray-Garcia, 1998). If we acquire cultural humility we should also demonstrate cultural sensitivity that shows appreciation of the diversity of others.

Cultural Competence in Nursing Education

Since the 1960s, there has been a united effort to include concepts sensitive to cultural diversity in nursing education. The National League for Nursing (NLN) and the American Association of Colleges of Nursing (AACN) have made this requirement mandatory for accreditation. In 2008 the AACN developed five end-of-program competencies for graduates of baccalaureate nursing programs as well as a faculty toolkit for integrating these competencies into undergraduate education. *The Essentials of Baccalaureate Education for Professional Nursing Practice* (2008) mandates the inclusion of culturally diverse nursing care concepts in the curriculum with attention to cultural, spiritual, ethnic, gender, and sexual orientation diversity. The following five competencies serve as a framework for integrating cultural content into existing curricula:

1. Apply knowledge of social and cultural factors that affect nursing and health care across multiple contexts.

2. Use relevant data sources and best evidence in providing culturally competent care.

3. Promote achievement of safe and quality outcomes of care for diverse populations.

4. Advocate for social justice, including commitment to the health of vulnerable populations and the elimination of health disparities.

5. Participate in continuous cultural competence development.

CULTURAL BELIEF SYSTEMS

A value is a standard that people use to assess themselves and others. It is a belief about what is worthwhile or important for well-being. There is a tendency for people to be "culture bound" (i.e., to assume that their values are superior, sensible, or right). Crosscultural health promotion requires the nurse to work with clients without making judgments as to the superiority of one set of values over another. Box 10-1 provides a comparison of Anglo-American values and those of more tradition-bound countries.

Each culture has a value system that dictates behavior directly or indirectly by setting norms and teaching that those norms are right. Health beliefs and practices tend to reflect a culture's value system. Nurses must understand the patient's value system to foster health promotion.

CULTURAL PHENOMENA

Giger and Davidhizar (2004) have identified six cultural phenomena that vary among cultural groups and affect health care. These phenomena are environmental control, biologic variations, social organization, communication, space, and time orientation.

Environmental Control

Environmental control is the ability of members of a particular culture to control nature or environmental factors. Some groups perceive humans as having mastery over nature; others perceive humans to be dominated by nature, and still other groups see humans as having a harmonious relationship with nature (Spector, 2008). People who perceive that they have mastery over nature believe that they can overcome the natural forces of nature. Such individuals would expect positive results from medications, surgery, and other treatment modalities. Persons who believe that they are subject to the forces of nature or that they have little control over what happens to them may not be compliant with treatments because they believe that whatever happens to them is part of their destiny. African-Americans and Mexican-Americans are most likely to subscribe to this view. Persons who hold the harmony with nature view, such as Asians and American Indians, believe that illness represents a disharmony with nature. These clients

BOX **10-1**

Anglo-American and Other Cultural Values

Anglo-American	Other Cultural Values
Personal control over the environment	Fate
Change	Tradition
Time dominates	Human interaction dominates
Human equality	Hierarchy, rank, status
Individualism, privacy	Group welfare
Self-help	Birthright inheritance
Competition	Cooperation
Future orientation	Past orientation
"Action-goal," work orientation	"Being" orientation
Informality	Formality
Directness, openness, honesty	Indirectness, ritual, "face"
Practicality, efficiency	Idealism, theory
Materialism	Spiritualism, detachment

may see medication as relieving only the symptoms and not curing the disease. Therefore, they are more likely to rely on naturalistic remedies, such as herbs or hot and cold treatments, to effect a cure (Stanhope and Lancaster, 2008). Included in this concept are the traditional health and illness beliefs, the practice of folk medicine, and the use of traditional and nontraditional healers. Environmental control plays an important role in the way clients respond to health-related experiences and use health resources (Spector, 2008).

Biologic Variations

Biologic variations, such as body build and structure, genetic variations, skin characteristics, susceptibility to disease, and nutritional variations, exist among different cultures. For example, babies who are born in Western culture weigh more than non-Western babies. Other common variations include skin color, eye shape, hair texture, adipose tissue deposits, shape of earlobes, and body configuration (Stanhope and Lancaster, 2008). For example, African-Americans have denser bones than whites, which may account for the low incidence of osteoporosis in the African-American population. The size of teeth varies among cultures, with whites having the smallest, followed by African-Americans, Asians, and American Indians. Larger teeth can cause protruding jaws, a condition common in African-Americans, which does not represent an orthodontic problem (Nies and McEwen, 2007).

Laboratory values for some tests also vary among cultural groups. For example, serum cholesterol levels essentially are the same for African-Americans and whites at birth. During childhood the levels are higher in African-Americans, but they are lower than in whites in adulthood. This finding is interesting because of the high morbidity and mortality from cardiovascular disease in African-Americans (Nies and McEwen, 2007). The maternal mortality rate of African-Americans is three times that of whites; occurrence of stomach cancer is twice as high among African-American men as white men; and occurrence of esophageal cancer is three times more common among African-Americans than the general population. Japanese-Americans have a lower incidence of cardiovascular and renal disease than the general population, but a higher incidence of stress-related diseases, such as ulcers, colitis, psoriasis, and depression. American Indians have a higher incidence of streptococcal sore throat and gastroenteritis than the general population (Medcom, 1997). American Indian women have the highest incidence of diabetes (Nies and McEwen, 2007).

Mexican-Americans have higher rates of obesity and diabetes than the general population, although they have lower rates of cardiovascular disease. The Mexican-American population has a pattern of less use of preventive services, including prenatal care, immunizations for children, and vision, hearing, and dental care (Nies and McEwen, 2007).

Social Organization

Social organization refers to the family unit (nuclear, single parent, or extended family) and the religious or ethnic groups with which families identify. Family is defined differently across cultures. For instance in the African-American culture, family often includes people who are unrelated or distantly related. Families depend on the extended family for emotional and financial support in times of crisis. Mothers and grandmothers play important roles in African-American families and are involved in decision making, especially as it relates to health (Stanhope and Lancaster, 2008).

Communication

Communication differences include language differences, verbal and nonverbal behaviors, and silence. Language can be the greatest obstacle to providing multicultural care. If the client does not speak the same language as the nurse, a skilled interpreter is mandatory (Giger and

Davidhizar, 2004). Comfort with direct eye contact during communication is an area that varies among cultures. Although some cultures, such as the Euro-American, value direct eye contact as a sign of attention, other cultures, such as African-American or American Indian, may view direct eye contact as rude behavior.

In the Asian culture it is considered important behavior to agree with those in authority. This aspect of the Asian culture has important implications for the nurse who is involved in patient education. The patient may seem compliant and nod his or her head as in agreement with the nurse's instruction even when the instruction is not clear or when the patient has no intention of carrying out the instruction (Stanhope and Lancaster, 2008).

Anglo-Americans tend to be informal in their style of communication, whereas other cultures may prefer a more formal style. Health professionals should not assume that a first-name basis is appropriate for client relationships. With any client, terms of endearment, such as "honey" or "dear" are unacceptable and can be interpreted as disrespectful, derogatory, or condescending. The best solution to the challenge of different communication styles and preferences is always to ask the client how he or she prefers to be addressed.

If the nurse and the client do not speak the same language, an interpreter should be consulted. An interpreter can help the nurse establish rapport with the client and explain concepts to the patient that are foreign to the nurse. When interpreters are needed, they should be selected carefully. Adult family members or friends are possible choices, as are bilingual staff and community volunteers. Nurses should be aware that some ethnic groups consider it a breach of confidentiality to have a stranger interpret, whereas certain individuals may not want other family members or friends to know the specifics of their medical condition.

The nurse also should be careful to consider the different dialects spoken in the same country and the culture's view of women and children. Children should not be used as interpreters because of the subject matter and because of certain cultural views of authority. Many cultures view adults as having more authority than children. In many cultures, women would not be acceptable interpreters because of the cultural view of women.

Nurses should be aware of the possibilities for interpreter services. A language line can be accessed 24 hours a day, 7 days a week by dialing 1-800-528-5888 and asking for the language you want. A live translator comes on the line to serve you in any one of 77 languages. You can conference call, use two phones on the same line, or simply pass the phone back and forth to the person with whom you wish to converse. For more information, see www.languageline.com.

Health care facilities may get a reasonable subscription rate for these services that is less costly than the individual rate.

Space

Space refers to people's attitudes and comfort level regarding the personal space around them. There are vast cultural differences in the comfort level associated with the distance between persons. Anglo-American nurses tend to feel comfortable with an intimate zone of 0 to 18 inches. This usually is the distance between the nurse and the patient when the nurse performs certain parts of a physical assessment, such as an eye or ear examination. Entering this zone could be uncomfortable for clients and nurses who have not had time to establish a trusting relationship. This discomfort would be increased for persons whose culture is not comfortable at all with such a limited space. For instance Asians frequently believe that touching strangers is inappropriate; therefore, they have a tendency to prefer more distance between themselves and others, particularly health professionals whom they have not previously known.

On the other hand, Mexican-Americans tend to be comfortable with less space because they like to touch persons with whom they are talking (Stanhope and Lancaster, 2008).

Time

Time orientation is the view of time in the present, past, or future. Present-oriented persons enjoy what they are experiencing at the moment and only move on to the next event or activity "when the time is right." Punctuality and "watching the clock" are definitely part of Western culture, but many cultural groups, such as American Indians, do not view time in the same way. This difference in time orientation can have implications for the present-oriented professional in the work setting, who may always be late for work without thinking it is an important issue. In addition, there are implications for health teaching. For example, when teaching medication schedules to a patient, it would be important to consider how that individual views time.

Clients who view the past as more important than the present or the future may focus on memories of the past. For instance the Vietnamese may take actions that they believe are consistent with the views of their ancestors and look to their ancestors for guidance (Giger and Davidhizar, 2004). In the Asian culture time is viewed as being more flexible than in the Western culture, and being on time or late for appointments is not a priority (Stanhope and Lancaster, 2008).

People who are future oriented are concerned with long-range goals and health care measures that can be taken in the present to prevent illness in the future. These persons plan ahead in scheduling appointments and organizing activities. They may be seen as having "distant" or "cold" personalities because they are not always engaged in communication at the moment because they may be thinking about their plans for the future. Persons who are oriented more to the present may be late for appointments because they are less concerned with planning ahead (Table 10-1).

PRACTICE ISSUES RELATED TO CULTURAL COMPETENCE
Health Information and Education

According to the task force on black and minority health, minority populations are less knowledgeable about specific health problems than are whites. African-Americans and Hispanics receive less information about cancer and heart disease than do nonminority groups. African-Americans tend to underestimate the prevalence of cancer, give less credence to the warning signs, obtain fewer screening tests, and are diagnosed at later stages of cancer than are whites. Hispanic women receive less information about breast cancer than do white women. Hispanic women are less aware that family history is a risk for breast cancer, and only 29% have heard of breast self-examination. Successful programs to increase public awareness about health problems are being offered to minority groups, but efforts must be continued to reach more of the population. Families, churches, employers, and community organizations need to be involved in facilitating behavior changes that will result in healthier lifestyles. Education programs have the greatest effect on diseases that are affected by lifestyle, such as hypertension, obesity, and diabetes. For example, if patients with diabetes could improve their self-management skills, 70% of complications could be prevented, saving human suffering and health care dollars (Nies and McEwen, 2007).

Education and Certification

Increasingly more universities and colleges offer graduate programs in transcultural, crosscultural, and international nursing. Many nurses have not been exposed to transcultural nursing in their basic education program. Therefore, the availability of graduate study in this area often is an unrecognized possibility.

TABLE **10-1**

Variations Among Selected Cultural Groups

	AFRICAN-AMERICANS	ASIANS	HISPANICS	AMERICAN INDIANS
Verbal communication	Asking personal questions of someone met for the first time is seen as improper and intrusive	High respect for others, especially those in positions of authority	Expression of negative feelings is considered impolite	Speaks in a low tone of voice and expects that the listener will be attentive
Nonverbal communication	Direct eye contact in conversation often is considered rude	Direct eye contact among superiors may be considered disrespectful	Avoidance of eye contact usually is a sign of attentiveness and respect	Direct eye contact often is considered disrespectful
Touch	Touching another's hair often is considered offensive	It is not customary to shake hands with persons of the opposite sex	Touching often is observed between two persons in conversation	A light touch of the person's hand instead of a firm handshake often is used when greeting a person
Family organization	Usually have close, extended family networks; women play key roles in health care decisions	Usually have close, extended family ties; emphasis may be on family needs rather than individual needs	Usually have close, extended family ties; all members of the family may be involved in health care decisions	Usually have close, extended family ties; emphasis tends to be on family rather than on individual needs
Time	Often present oriented	Often present oriented	Often present oriented	Often present oriented
Alternative healers	"Granny," "root doctor," voodoo priest, spiritualist	Acupuncturist, acupressurist, herbalist	Curandero, espiritualista, yerbo	Medicine man, shaman
Self-care practices	Poultices, herbs, oils, roots	Hot and cold foods, herbs, teas, soups, cupping, burning, rubbing, pinching	Hot and cold foods, herbs	Herbs, corn meal, medicine bundle
Biologic variations	Sickle cell anemia, mongolian spots, keloid formation, inverted T waves, lactose intolerance, skin color	Thalassemia, drug interactions, mongolian spots, lactose intolerance, skin color	Mongolian spots, lactose intolerance, skin color	Cleft uvula, lactose intolerance, skin color

Data from Giger JN, Davidhizar RE: *Transcultural nursing*, ed 4, St Louis, 2004, Mosby; Spector RE: *Cultural diversity in health and illness*, ed 5, Upper Saddle River, NJ, 2000, Prentice-Hall; Payne KT: Culturally valid testing: a proactive approach. In Taylor OL, editor: *Nature of communication disorders in culturally and linguistically diverse populations*, San Diego, 1986, College Hill Press.

Transcultural nursing is the study of differences and similarities of various cultural health values and beliefs among different ethnic and minority groups (Medcom, 1997). The Transcultural Nursing Society has been certifying nurses in transcultural nursing since 1988. Certification as a certified transcultural nurse is based on oral and written examinations and evaluation of the nurse's educational and experiential background. Certification has increased recognition of transcultural nursing as a legitimate nursing specialty. Transcultural nurses are interested in finding a universal care for clients that will improve, maintain, and restore health and improve client satisfaction.

International Marketplace

Nurses trained in the United States work, teach, and consult in hundreds of foreign countries on every continent. They often are recognized as international pacesetters and are viewed as "commodities for import" by both the more developed countries and the less developed third- or fourth-world nations. Nurses can make a difference in the health outcomes of people all over the world. Technology has enhanced global communication and facilitated travel. As nurses help solve emerging health problems in countries throughout the world, they are the most valuable assets of the health care system. They will be called on to design, implement, and evaluate international projects, educational endeavors, and research with an intercultural focus. Therefore, it is important that nurses understand the intercultural issues related to our global society (Nies and McEwen, 2007).

Nursing Literature

The number of journal articles about culturally diverse clients, transcultural nursing research, international nursing, and the inclusion of transcultural concepts in nursing curricula has increased considerably since the 1950s. The *Journal of Transcultural Nursing* is a refereed journal that was first published in 1989. This journal was created to advance transcultural nursing knowledge and practices. The *Journal of Transcultural Nursing* focuses on theory, research, and practice dimensions of transcultural nursing and provides a forum for researchers. Other journals that address cultural issues include the *Western Journal of Medicine: Cross Cultural Issues*, the *Journal of Cultural Diversity*, the *Journal of Multicultural Nursing*, the *International Journal of Nursing Studies*, the *International Nursing Review*, and the *Journal of Holistic Nursing*. Nurse authors also need to be encouraged to publish articles related to clients' cultural views and health care needs in nursing specialty and practice journals that are more widely read by nurses who actually are providing care on a daily basis to clients from diverse cultures.

Although research articles on transcultural issues are becoming a common feature in health care journals, there is a need for additional research that examines individual behavioral responses to normal life processes, such as pregnancy, birth, death, and human growth and development. There also is a need for well-designed studies that explore the biologic, psychologic, sociologic, and spiritual differences within, between, and among cultural groups (Purnell and Paulanka, 2003). Dr. Madeline Leininger created the theory of culture care diversity and universality to guide transcultural research. Even though numerous research studies have been conducted on cultural diversity issues, a significant time gap often exists between the identification of findings and publication of results. The limited dissemination of research findings inhibits widespread acceptance of new interventions that could improve health care practices of culturally diverse populations. Computer information technology and online networks help narrow this gap and distribute research findings in a timely manner (Purnell and Paulanka, 2003).

Responsibility of Health Care Facilities for Cultural Care

Nursing policies should reflect openness to including extended family members and folk healers in the nursing care plan, provided their presence is not harmful to the client's well-being. For example, Hispanic clients may want the support of a curandero, espiritualista (spiritualist), yerbo (herbalist), or sabador (equal to a chiropractor). African-Americans may turn to a hougan (voodoo priest or priestess) or "old lady." American Indians may seek assistance from a shaman or medicine man. Clients of Asian descent may want the services of an acupuncturist or bonesetter. In some religions, spiritual healers may be found among the ranks of the ordained and may be called priest, bishop, elder, deacon, rabbi, brother, or sister (Nies and McEwen, 2007). Most hospital chaplaincy programs have access to religious representatives available for patients of various religions.

Clients may need to consult with their support persons and folk healers before making medical decisions. Nurses must respect the client's right to privacy and allow time for the client to interact with his or her spiritual or cultural healers. Nurses must respect unconventional beliefs and health practices and work with clients to develop a plan of care that builds on their beliefs and incorporates nontraditional health practices that are not harmful. These nontraditional healers should be received with respect and provided privacy to enable the healers to interact with their patients (Nies and McEwen, 2007).

Health care facilities should provide resources for nurses and other health care professionals to assist with culture-specific needs of clients. Health care facilities should have a list of interpreters fluent in the major languages spoken by persons typically using the organization. Translators who have knowledge of health-related terminology are more effective than those who do not. Gender, birth origin, and socioeconomic class need to be considered when selecting a translator. Gender is an important consideration because many cultures prohibit discussion of intimate matters between women and men. Birth origin of the client and translator should be determined because often there are many dialects spoken within the same country, depending on the particular region (Stanhope and Lancaster, 2008). Differences in socioeconomic class between client and interpreter can lead to problems of interpretation.

Clinical nurse specialists (CNSs) in transcultural nursing should be added to the staff of institutions serving large numbers of culturally diverse individuals. The transcultural CNS could be a role model to the staff in delivery of culturally sensitive and competent care, provide in-service education to staff related to cultural differences, and conduct research related to cultural and social issues. In addition, consultants should be used to deal with specific cultural issues.

Continuing education programs for nurses should be offered by health care institutions. Programs should focus on promoting awareness of the nurses' own culturally based values, beliefs and attitudes, cultural assessment, biologic variations of cultural groups, crosscultural communication, and culture-specific beliefs and practices related to childbearing and childrearing, death and dying, issues of mental health, and cultural aspects of aging.

Recommended Standards for Culturally and Linguistically Appropriate Services (CLAS)

Culture and language have a considerable effect on how patients access and respond to health care services. To ensure equal access to quality health care by diverse populations, the Office of Minority Health in the Department of Health and Human Services developed guidelines for health care organizations. In their report *Assessing Cultural Competence in Health Care: Recommendations for National Standards and an Outcomes Focused Research Agenda*, the following standards are recommended:

- ◆ Promote and support the attitudes, behaviors, knowledge, and skills necessary for staff to work respectfully and effectively with patients and each other in a culturally diverse work environment.

◆ Have a comprehensive management strategy to address culturally and linguistically appropriate services, including strategic goals, plans, policies, procedures, and designated staff responsible for implementation.

◆ Utilize formal mechanisms for community and consumer involvement in the design and execution of service delivery, including planning, policymaking, operations, evaluation, training and, as appropriate, treatment planning.

◆ Develop and implement a strategy to recruit, retain, and promote qualified, diverse, and culturally competent administrative, clinical, and support staff members that are trained and qualified to address the needs of the racial and ethnic communities being served.

◆ Require and arrange for ongoing education and training for administrative, clinical, and support staff in culturally and linguistically competent service delivery.

◆ Provide all clients with limited English proficiency (LEP) access to bilingual staff or interpretation services.

◆ Provide oral and written notices, including translated signage at key points of contact, to clients in their primary language informing them of their right to receive interpreter services free of charge.

◆ Translate and make available signage and commonly used written patient educational material and other materials for members of the dominant language groups in service areas.

◆ Ensure that interpreters and bilingual staff can demonstrate bilingual proficiency and receive training that includes the skills and ethics of interpreting as well as knowledge in both languages of the terms and concepts relevant to clinical or nonclinical encounters. Family or friends are not considered adequate substitutes because they usually lack these abilities.

◆ Ensure that the clients' primary spoken language and self-identified race or ethnicity are included in the health care organization's management information system as well as any patient records used by provider staff.

◆ Utilize a variety of methods to collect and use accurate demographic, cultural, epidemiologic, and clinical outcome data for racial and ethnic groups in the service area. Become informed about the ethnic and cultural needs, resources, and assets of the surrounding community.

◆ Undertake ongoing organizational self-assessments of cultural and linguistic competence; integrate measures of access, satisfaction, quality, and outcomes for CLAS into other organizational internal audits and performance-improvement programs.

◆ Develop structures and procedures to address crosscultural ethical and legal conflicts in health care delivery and complaints or grievances by patients and staff about unfair, culturally insensitive, or discriminatory treatment; difficulty in accessing services; or denial of services.

◆ Prepare an annual progress report documenting the organizations' progress with implementing CLAS standards, including information on programs, staffing, and resources.

CULTURAL ASSESSMENT
Cultural Self-Assessment

The first step to becoming a culturally sensitive and competent health care provider is to conduct a cultural self-assessment. The nurse should engage in a cultural self-assessment to identify individual culturally based attitudes about clients who are from a different culture. Cultural self-assessment requires self-honesty and sincerity and reflection on attitudes of

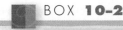

BOX **10-2**

Cultural Self-Assessment

- How do your parents, grandparents, other family members, and close friends view people from racially diverse groups?
- What is the cultural stereotype of African-Americans?
- Does the cultural stereotype allow for socioeconomic differences?
- Have your interactions with African-Americans been positive? Negative? Neutral?
- How do you feel about going into a predominantly African-American neighborhood or into the home of an African-American family? Are you afraid, anxious, curious, or ambivalent?
- What stereotypes do you have about African-American men, women, and children?
- What culturally based health beliefs and practices do you think characterize African-Americans? How are these different from your own culturally based health beliefs and practices?

From Swanson J, Nies M: *Community health nursing: promoting the health of aggregates,* ed 2, Philadelphia, 1997, Saunders.

parents, grandparents, and close friends in terms of their attitudes toward different cultures. Through identification of health-related attitudes, values, beliefs, and practices the nurse can better understand the cultural aspects of health care from the client's perspective. Everyone has ethnocentric tendencies that must be brought to a level of consciousness so that efforts can be made to temper the feeling that one's own culture is best. Box 10-2 shows a cultural self-assessment guide adapted from Swanson and Nies (1997) for the nurse who is not African-American, but is caring for an African-American client.

Cultural Client Assessment

After the nurse performs a cultural self-assessment, he or she should obtain a cultural assessment for the client. Nursing assessments in institutional and community settings should include the gathering of data pertinent to cultural beliefs and practices. Cultural assessments lead to culturally relevant nursing diagnoses and give direction to effective nursing intervention. Basic cultural data include ethnic affiliation, religious preference, family patterns, food patterns, and ethnic health care practices. Cultural assessments should be used as an adjunct to other patient assessments. These data will give the nurse sufficient information to determine if a more in-depth assessment of cultural factors is needed. A major reason that cultural assessments are performed is to identify patterns that may assist or interfere with a nursing intervention or treatment regimen (Giger and Davidhizar, 2004).

The nurse needs to find out if the client's beliefs, customs, values, and self-care practices are adaptive (beneficial), neutral, or maladaptive (harmful) in relation to nursing interventions. For example, if a Mexican-American client who is diagnosed with hypertension insists on taking garlic instead of an antihypertensive, this could be harmful. If the client agrees to take the garlic in addition to the antihypertensive, this would be a neutral practice. An adaptive or beneficial practice would include daily exercise in addition to the garlic and antihypertensive.

In the case of Southeast Asians, dermal practices, such as cupping, pinching, rubbing, and burning, are a common part of self-care. The dermal methods are perceived as ways to relieve headaches, muscle pains, sinusitis, colds, sore throats, diarrhea, or fever. Cupping involves placing a heated cup on the skin; as it cools, it contracts, drawing what is believed to be toxicity into the cup. A circular ecchymosis is left on the skin. Pinching may be at the base of the nose or between the eyes. Bruises or welts are left at the site of treatment. Rubbing or "coining" involves rubbing lubricated skin with a spoon or a coin to bring toxic "wind" to the body surface. A similar practice is burning, which involves touching a burning cigarette or piece of cotton to the skin, usually the abdomen, to compensate for "heat" lost through diarrhea (Nies and McEwen, 2007). These practices nurture the client's sense of well-being and security in being able to do something to correct disturbing symptoms. In most cases, the practice would be considered adaptive (beneficial) or neutral. However, if the client had a clotting disorder, the practices would pose a threat to physical integrity and therefore be considered maladaptive (harmful) (Nies and McEwen, 2007).

Cultural Client Nutrition Assessment

A cultural nutrition assessment should be obtained for clients who are minorities. It is necessary to assess the client's cultural definition of food. For example, certain Latin American groups do not consider greens to be food. Therefore, when asked to keep a food diary, these individuals would not list greens, which are an important source of vitamins and iron. Frequency and number of meals, amount and types of food eaten, and regularity of food consumption are other important factors that should be considered.

Among Asian-Americans dietary intake of calcium may appear inadequate because this group usually has a low rate of consumption of dairy products. However, they commonly consume pork bone and shells, thus taking in adequate quantities of calcium to meet minimum daily requirements. In cultures in which obesity is a problem, it is helpful for the nurse to have an idea of food preferences to help the client select low-calorie, low-fat foods. Asians tend to prefer spicy foods that may lead to the high incidence of stomach cancer, ulcers, and gastrointestinal bleeding (Purnell and Paulanka, 2003).

Nurses should avoid cultural stereotyping as it relates to food because all Italians do not necessarily like spaghetti, nor do all Chinese like rice. However, knowing the clients' food preferences makes it possible to develop therapeutic interventions that do not conflict with their cultural food practices (Stanhope and Lancaster, 2008). Food preferences of aggregate groups are described in Table 10-2.

Cultural Beliefs About Sickness and Cures

It also is important for the nurse to consider the nontraditional beliefs of sickness and cure of various cultures. For example, there are diseases that are not classified as Western culture diseases. For different cultural groups, they are real diseases for which the group has medicines and treatments. Examples of such diseases include mal ojo, susto, bilis, and empacho.

Mal ojo ("evil eye") is thought to be caused by persons giving admiration. "For example, Hispanic clients may beleiv in ma ojo (evil eye), in which an individual becomes ill as a result of excessive admiration by another" (Nies and McEwen, 2007, p. 221). For example, a stranger who lovingly admires a Mexican-American baby by looking into the baby's face actually can cause mal ojo. An infant who has mal ojo sleeps restlessly, has fever and diarrhea, and may ultimately die. Treatment consists of rubbing the body with an egg for three consecutive nights. The egg is broken and left under the bed overnight. In the morning, if the egg appears to be cooked, then mal ojo was definitely the cause of the illness. For protection, mothers often adorn their children with red yarn around their wrists or amulets that usually are a deer's eyes (Nies and McEwen, 2007).

TABLE **10-2**

Selected Food Preferences and Associated Risk Factors Among Selected Cultural Groups

CULTURAL GROUP	FOOD PREFERENCES	NUTRITIONAL EXCESS	RISK FACTORS
African-Americans	Fried foods, greens, bread, lard, pork, and rice	Cholesterol, fat, sodium carbohydrates, and calories	Coronary heart disease and obesity
Asians	Soy sauce, rice, pickled dishes, and raw fish	Cholesterol, fat, sodium, carbohydrates, and calories	Coronary heart disease, liver disease, cancer of the stomach, and ulcers
Hispanics	Fried foods, beans and rice, chili, carbonated beverages	Cholesterol, fat, sodium, carbohydrates, and calories	Coronary heart disease and obesity
American Indians	Blue cornmeal, fruits, game, and fish	Carbohydrates and calories	Diabetes, malnutrition, tuberculosis, infant and maternal mortality

Data from Andrews M, Boyle J: *Transcultural concepts in nursing,* ed 3, Philadelphia, 1998, Lippincott; Giger JN, Davidhizar RE: *Transcultural nursing,* ed 4, St Louis, 2004, Mosby; Jackson MY, Broussard BA: Cultural challenges in nutrition education among American Indians, *Diabetes Educ* 13(11):47-50, 1987.

Susto, or fright sickness, is an emotion-based illness that is common among Mexicans. An unexpected fall, a barking dog, or a car accident could cause susto. Symptoms include colic, diarrhea, high temperature, and vomiting. Treatment involves brushing the body with "ruda" for nine consecutive nights. The brushing is performed to allow the spirit that has been removed by the disease to return to the body. The treatment often is accompanied by burning candles and prayers in home or church (Nies and McEwen, 2007).

Bilis is a disease brought on by anger. It primarily affects adults and commonly occurs a day or two after a fit of rage. If untreated, bilis can cause acute nervous tension and chronic fatigue, although herbal remedies usually are effective (Giger and Davidhizar, 2004).

Empacho is a disease that can affect children or adults and is caused by food particles becoming lodged in the intestinal tract, causing sharp pains. To manage this illness the afflicted person lies face down on the bed with his or her back bared. The curer pinches a piece of skin at the waist, listening for a snap from the abdominal region. This is repeated several times in hope of dislodging the material. Empacho usually is not a serious disease (Nies and McEwen, 2007).

It is important to determine how culturally diverse clients define health and illness and whether their health beliefs and practices differ from the norm in the Western health care delivery system (Spector, 2008). For example, the Chinese often find many aspects of Western medicine distasteful. They cannot understand why so many diagnostic tests are necessary and tend to believe that a "good" physician has the ability to diagnose by thoroughly examining the client's body. Chinese clients dislike painful procedures, such as the practice of drawing blood. In their culture, blood is seen as the source of life for the entire body, and the Chinese believe that it is not regenerated. They have a deep respect for their bodies and prefer to die with their bodies intact. Therefore it is not uncommon for the Chinese to refuse surgery that would be mutilating to the body (Spector, 2008). Health represents a balance within the body, mind, and spirit. It is strongly affected by the family and community. Spector (2008) suggests a model for assessing health traditions (Box 10-3).

Spector (2008) also has developed a guide that can be used to assess clients' personal methods for maintaining health, protecting (preventing) illness, and restoring health (Table 10-3).

BOX **10-3**

Health Traditions Assessment Model

MAINTAINING HEALTH

Physical	Are there special clothes one must wear; foods one must eat or not eat, or combinations to avoid; exercises one must do?
Mental	Are there special sources of entertainment; games or other ways of concentrating; traditional "rules of behavior"?
Spiritual	Are there special religious customs; prayers; meditations?

PROTECTING HEALTH AND PREVENTING ILLNESS

Physical	Are there special foods that must be eaten after certain life events, such as childbirth; dietary taboos that must be adhered to; symbolic clothes that must be worn?
Mental	Are there special people who must be avoided, rituals for self-protection, familial roles?
Spiritual	Are there special religious customs, superstitions, amulets, oils, or waters?

RESTORING HEALTH

Physical	Are there special folk remedies; liniments; procedures, such as cupping, acupuncture, and moxibustion?
Mental	Are there special healers, such as curanderos, rituals, folk medicines?
Spiritual	Are there special rituals and prayers, meditations, healers?

From Spector RE: *Cultural diversity in health and illness,* ed 6, Upper Saddle River, NJ, 2008, Prentice-Hall.

SUMMARY

In a society as diverse as the United States, health care cannot come in one form to fit the needs of everyone. Culture has a powerful influence on one's interpretation of health and illness and response to health care. All clients have the right to be understood and respected, despite their differences. They have the right to expect health care providers to acknowledge that their perspectives on and interpretations of health are legitimate. Health care professionals must make a commitment to increase their knowledge, sensitivity, and competence in cultural concepts and care. Perhaps no other group in the health profession has recognized the effect of cultural diversity on outcomes of health care more than nursing. Nurses always have supported the concept of holistic care. By understanding the client's perspective, the nurse can be a better advocate for the client. With increased knowledge, sensitivity, respect, and understanding, therapeutic interventions can be maximized to promote the highest quality of health for clients in our multicultural society. Additional information can be found in the websites listed in Box 10-4.

evolve Additional resources are available online at: http://evolve.elsevier.com/Cherry/

TABLE **10-3**

Assessment Guide for Personal Methods to Maintain, Protect (Prevent Illness), and Restore Health

	PHYSICAL	MENTAL	SPIRITUAL
Maintain health	Are there special clothes you must wear at certain times of the day, week, year? Are there special foods you must eat at certain times? Do you have any dietary restrictions? Are there any foods that you cannot eat?	What do you do for activities, such as reading, sports, games? Do you have hobbies? Do you visit family often? Do you visit friends often?	Do you practice your religion and attend church or other communal activities? Do you pray or meditate? Do you observe religious customs? Do you belong to fraternal organizations?
Protect health or prevent illness	Are there foods that you cannot eat together? Are there special foods that you must eat? Are there any types of clothing that you are not allowed to wear?	Are there people or situations that you have been taught to avoid? Do you take extraordinary precautions under certain circumstances? Do you take time for yourself?	Do you observe religious customs? Do you wear any amulets or hang them in your house? Do you have any practices, such as always opening the window when you sleep? Do you have any other practices to protect yourself from "harm"?
Restore health	What kinds of medicines do you take before you see a doctor or nurse? Are there herbs that you take? Are there special treatments that you use?	Do you know of any specific practices your mother or grandmother may use to relax? Do you know how big problems can be cared for in your community? Do you drink special teas to help you unwind or relax?	Do you know any healers? Do you know of any religious rituals that help to restore health? Do you meditate? Do you ever go to a healing service? Do you know about exorcism?

From Spector RE: *Cultural diversity in health and illness,* ed 6, Upper Saddle River, NJ, 2008, Prentice-Hall.

 BOX **10-4**

Helpful Websites

CultureMed
   http://culturemed.sunyit.edu
The Office of Minority Health U.S. Department of Health and Human Services. Culturally Competent Nursing Modules
   www.thinkculturalhealth.org
Healthy People 2010
   www.health.gov/healthy people
Resources in Cultural Competence Education for Health Care Professionals
   www.calendow.org/uploadedFiles/resources_in_cultural_competence.pdf
National Collaborative of Ethnic Minority Nurse Organizations
   www.ncemna.org

Transcultural Nursing Society
   www.tcns.org
U.S. Census Bureau: *Money income in the United States, 1999*
   www.census.gov/hhes/www/income.html
American Cancer Society: *Cancer facts and figures—1997: racial and ethnic patterns*
   www.cancer.org/statistics
U.S. Census Bureau: *Poverty 1998: poverty by selected characteristics, 1999*
   www.census.gov/hhes/www/-poverty/povert.html

REFERENCES

American Association of Colleges of Nursing (AACN): *Enrollment and graduations in baccalaureate and graduate programs in nursing*, Washington DC, 2008-09, AACN.

American Association of Colleges of Nursing (AACN): *The Essentials of Baccalaureate Education for Professional Nursing Practice*, Washington DC, 2008, AACN.

American Academy of Nursing Expert Panel on Cultural Competence: *American Academy of Nursing Standards of Cultural Competence*, Washington DC, 2007, American Academy of Nursing.

AAN Expert Panel on Culturally Competent Health Care: Culturally competent health care, *Nurs Outlook* 40(6):277–283, 1992.

Bessent H: *Strategies for recruitment, retention and graduation of minority nurses in colleges of nursing*, Washington, DC, 1997, American Nurses Foundation.

Council of Economic Advisers for the President's Initiative on Race: *Changing America: indicators of social and economic well-being by race and Hispanic origin*, Washington, DC, 1999, US Government Printing Office.

Giger JN, Davidhizar RE: *Transcultural nursing: assessment and intervention*, ed 4, St Louis, 2004, Mosby.

Hall J, Stevens P, Meleis A: Marginalization: a guiding concept for valuing diversity in nursing knowledge development, *Adv Nurs Sci* 16(4):23–24, 1994.

Health Resources Service Administration Preliminary Findings: *2004 national sample survey of registered nurses*, Washington DC, 2005, US Department of Health and Human Services.

Lenburg C, et al: *Promoting cultural competence in and through nursing education; a critical review and comprehensive plan for action*, Washington, DC, 1995, American Academy of Nursing.

Medcom: *Cultural assessment (film)*, Cypress, CA, 1997, Medcom.

Meleis A, et al: *Diversity, marginalization, and culturally competent healthcare issues in knowledge development*, Washington, DC, 1995, American Academy of Nursing.

Nies M, McEwen M: *Community/public health nursing*, ed 4, Philadelphia, 2007, Saunders.

Purnell L, Paulanka B: *Transcultural health care*, ed 2, Philadelphia, 2003, FA Davis.

Spector R: *Culture care: guide to heritage assessment and health traditions*, ed 7, Upper Saddle River, NJ, 2008, Prentice-Hall.

Spector R: Cultural diversity in health and illness/culture care: guide to heritage assessment health. In Spector R, editor: *Cultural diversity in health and illness*, ed 7, Upper Saddle River, NJ, 2008, Prentice-Hall.

Stanhope M, Lancaster J: *Public health nursing: population-centered health care in the community*, ed 7, St Louis, 2008, Mosby.

Sullivan EJ: *Differences: reflections, second quarter*, Indianapolis, 1998, Sigma Theta Tau.

Sullivan LW: *Missing persons: minorities in the health professions, a report of the Sullivan commission on diversity in the healthcare workforce*, Washington, DC, 2004, The Sullivan Commission.

Swanson J, Nies M: *Community health nursing: promoting the health of aggregates*, ed 2, Philadelphia, 1997, Saunders.

Tervalon M, Murray-Garcia J: Cultural humility versus cultural competence: a critical distinction in defining physician training outcomes in multicultural education, *J Health Care Poor Underserved* 9(2):117, 1998.

U.S. Census Bureau News: *An older and more diverse nation by midcentury*. Accessed August 2009 from: www.census.gov/Press-Release/www/releases/archives/population/012496.html

U.S. Department of Commerce, Bureau of the Census, 2008. Washington DC, U.S. Government Printing Office.

U.S. Department of Health and Human Services: *Public Health Service: Healthy People 2000*, Washington, DC, 1990, U.S. Government Printing Office.

U.S. Department of Health and Human Services: *Healthy People 2010: national health promotion and disease prevention objectives—public health service*, Washington, DC, 2000, U.S. Government Printing Office.

U.S. Department of Health and Human Services: *The 2008 HHS Poverty Guidelines*, Washington, DC, 2008, U.S. Government Printing Office.

ADDITIONAL RESOURCES

American Academy of Nursing: Expert Panel on Culturally Competent Health Care: Culturally competent health care, *Nurs Outlook* 40(6):277–283, 1992.

American Association of Colleges of Nursing (AACN): *Cultural competency in baccalaureate nursing education*, Washington, DC, 2008, AACN. www.aacn.nche.edu/Education/cultural.htm.

Andrews M, Boyle J: *Transcultural concepts in nursing care*, ed 3, Philadelphia, 1999, Lippincott.

Baum F: Cracking the nut of health equity: top down and bottom up pressure for action on the social determinants of health, *Promot Educ* 14(2):90–95, 2007.

Campbell MK, et al: Church-based health promotion interventions: evidence and lessons learned, *Ann Rev Pub Health* 28:213–234, 2007.

Giger HJ: Health disparities: what do we know? What do we need to know? What should we do? In Schiulz AJ, Mullings L, editors: *Gender, race, class, health: intersectional approaches*, San Francisco, 2006, Jossey Bass, pp. 261–288.

Institute of Medicine (IOM): *Unequal treatment: confronting racial and ethnic disparities in healthcare. (Reports)*, Fairfax VA, March 2002, The Institute of Medicine.

Kawachi I, Daniels N, Robinson D: Disparities by race and class: why both matter, *Health Aff* 24:343–351, 2005.

Lipson J, Dibble S: *Culture and clinical care*, ed 2, San Francisco, 2005, University of California School of Nursing.

Complementary and Alternative Healing

Charlotte Eliopoulos, PhD, RN, MPH, ND

*e*volve   Additional resources are available online at: http://evolve.elsevier.com/Cherry/

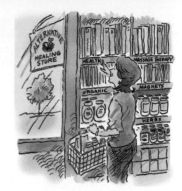

Consumers are seeking natural remedies; nurses have a responsibility to be aware of the potential effects.

VIGNETTE

Ruth Jeffers is a registered nurse (RN) who works in a rehabilitation unit of a community hospital. Many of the clients on this unit suffer from chronic musculoskeletal pain. Ms. Jeffers has noted that a growing number of clients have a history of independently using acupuncture, nutritional supplements, and other alternative and complementary healing therapies to improve their symptoms. Although they report beneficial results, most do not tell their physicians that they are using these therapies.

Last year Ms. Jeffers completed a course in the use of therapeutic touch and has used this therapy to promote relaxation and pain control with friends and family with considerable success. She is aware of many positive reports on the benefits of these unconventional approaches. She believes therapeutic touch and some other complementary healing therapies could benefit clients on the rehabilitation unit and informally introduces the topic to the team with whom she works. With the exception of one nurse who states that she believes these therapies are associated with the occult and wants no part of them, the nursing staff is enthusiastic and eager to implement complementary therapies. The physical and occupational therapists believe that complementary therapies could prove helpful to clients but that only therapists within their departments, not nursing, should provide these. The physician on the team opposes the use of all alternative and complementary therapies, claiming he "isn't about to put his license on the line for these unproven ideas."

■ QUESTIONS TO CONSIDER WHILE READING THIS CHAPTER:

1 What is the best course of action for Ruth Jeffers, RN, if she really believes that complementary and alternative therapies could benefit clients on the unit?

2 What would a hospital need to do to prepare for the inclusion of complementary and alternative therapies in its existing services?

3 What are some of the potential obstacles to introducing complementary and alternative therapies into a conventional setting?

4 What discipline(s) should be responsible for providing and/or coordinating or supervising the practitioners who provide complementary and alternative therapies in the hospital?

KEY TERMS

Alternative medical systems Acupuncture, anthroposophic Ayurvedic medicine, community-based health care practices (e.g., Native American, shamans), environmental medicine, homeopathy, naturopathy, traditional Oriental medicine.

Biologically based treatments Herbal therapies, individual and orthomolecular biologic therapies, special diets.

Complementary and alternative medicine (CAM) Healing philosophies, practices, and products that are outside of what Western society considers mainstream medicine and are not typically taught in the educational programs of physicians, nurses, and other health professionals.

Conventional medicine Western style of medicine practiced in the United States; also called allopathic.

Energy therapies Qi gong, Reiki, therapeutic touch, healing touch, bioelectromagnetic-based therapies.

Manipulative and body-based methods Chiropractic, massage, and related techniques (e.g., manual lymph drainage, Alexander technique, Feldenkrais method, pressure point therapies, Trager psychophysical integration), osteopathy.

Mind-body interventions Aromatherapy, art therapy, biofeedback, dance therapy, hypnosis, imagery, meditation, music therapy, prayer, relaxation, self-help support groups, tai chi, yoga.

LEARNING OUTCOMES

After studying this chapter, the reader will be able to:

1 Describe various complementary and alternative healing practices.

2 Identify how to effectively incorporate pertinent complementary and alternative therapies into patient care.

3 Provide patient education regarding uses, limitations, and precautions associated with selected complementary and alternative healing practices and products.

CHAPTER OVERVIEW

This chapter presents an overview of complementary and alternative medicine (CAM) therapies and products, which have gained popularity in Western society and are being integrated into health care. As increasing numbers of consumers and clinical settings become interested in and actually use CAM therapies, nurses must become knowledgeable about the uses, limitations, and precautions associated with these new practices and products. Professional nurses have an obligation to understand such practices and products to advise patients and effectively incorporate pertinent therapies into patients' care. Nurses who have knowledge and skills in this area are in key positions to empower patients for self-care that complements conventional medicine.

USE OF COMPLEMENTARY AND ALTERNATIVE HEALING METHODS

CAM includes healing philosophies, practices, and products that fall outside what Western society considers mainstream (conventional) medicine and that are not typically taught in the educational programs of physicians, nurses, pharmacists, and other health professionals.

The past few decades have seen CAM progress from a fringe movement to highly popular, widely used therapies that are being integrated into conventional care. According to a nationwide government survey, approximately 38% of U.S. adults ages 18 years and older and approximately 12% of children use some form of CAM, and most are paying for these services out of their own pockets (National Center for Complementary and Alternative Medicine [NCCAM], 2009a).

Rather than emerging from the leadership of health care professionals, the growing popularity of CAM has been consumer driven. Several factors contribute to consumers' desire for CAM:

- *Dissatisfaction with the conventional health care system:* The impersonal nature of health care has grown with costs. Shorter hospital stays, several months' waiting periods to see a physician, hurried staff that barely have time to provide basic care, and horror stories of the adverse effects of medications are causing consumers to look for alternative approaches that are safer, less costly, and more responsive and personalized than conventional health care.
- *Unwillingness to "grin and bear" the effects of diseases:* Today's consumers are less willing than their parents to live with symptoms that alter their lifestyles or to passively accept a terminal diagnosis and wait to die. They want options and to be empowered to do everything conceivable to promote the best possible quality and quantity of their lives, and they are willing to look to alternative healing measures to do so.
- *Shrinking world:* The rapid pace and ease of information sharing have enabled individuals to learn about diverse practices of cultures throughout the world.
- *Growing evidence of effectiveness:* The body of research supporting the effectiveness of alternative therapies increases almost daily. People hear testimonials from friends and family about the way they have been helped by acupuncture, herbs, and other forms of CAM. In addition, the media regularly report these findings, contributing to consumers' awareness of the body of evidence.

CAM practices and products are consistent with the values, beliefs, and philosophic orientations toward health held by many people (NCCAM, 2009a). With rare exceptions, consumers prefer natural approaches that afford them an active role in their care over high-tech interventions that relegate them to a passive, obedient role. They want to connect with their health care providers, have their individuality recognized, and gain education and skills to effectively make decisions and direct their care. Increasingly, consumers are seeking measures to enhance not just their bodies, but also their minds and spirits. The quality of their lives is equally, if not more, important to the quantity of years they live. Consumers often discover that CAM promotes many principles of holistic care that they value, such as individual empowerment, self-care, and a high quality of life.

PRINCIPLES UNDERLYING ALTERNATIVE HEALING

A wide range of healing therapies are encompassed in CAM, yet most share some common principles:

- *The body has the ability to heal itself.* Most conventional medicine works from the premise that the elimination of sickness requires an intervention "done to" the body (e.g., giving medications, surgery). In CAM there is the assumption that the body heals itself. Complementary and alternative healing therapies enhance the body's ability to self-heal.
- *Health and healing are related to a harmony of mind, body, and spirit.* The mind, body, and spirit are inseparable; what affects one affects all. Healing and the improvement of health demand that all of the facets of a person be addressed, not merely a single symptom or system.
- *Basic, positive health practices build the foundation for healing.* Good nutrition, exercise, rest, stress management, and avoidance of harmful habits (e.g., smoking) are essential ingredients to health maintenance and the improvement of health conditions. Practitioners of healing therapies are more likely than conventional practitioners to look at total lifestyle practices rather than the diseased body part.

◆ *Approaches to healing are individualized.* The unique composition and dynamics of each person are recognized in CAM. Practitioners of healing therapies explore the underlying cause of a problem and customize approaches accordingly. It is rare in CAM to find a standing protocol that treats everyone with similar conditions similarly.

◆ *Individuals are responsible for their own healing.* People can use a wide range of therapies, from conventional prescription drugs to herbal remedies, to treat illness. However, it is the responsibility of competent adults to seek health advice, make informed choices, gain necessary knowledge and skills for self-care, engage in practices that promote health and healing, and seek help when needed. Clients are responsible for getting their minds, bodies, and spirits in optimal condition to heal rather than look externally for a physician or nurse to heal them.

A holistic philosophy, promotion of positive health habits, and the client's responsibility for facilitating his or her own health and healing are common threads among healing therapies.

OVERVIEW OF POPULAR CAM HEALING THERAPIES

Hundreds of healing therapies are practiced throughout the world, with varying degrees of evidence to support their effectiveness. As the use of these therapies grew in the United States, the National Institutes of Health (NIH) established the Office of Alternative Medicine in 1992 to evaluate these complementary and alternative practices and products. In 1998 the Office of Alternative Medicine became a freestanding center within NIH and was named the National Center for Complementary and Alternative Medicine (NCCAM). NCCAM has categorized CAM into five fields of practice (Box 11-1); the center supports research and serves as a clearinghouse for information on alternative practices and products.

Consumers' growing use and the increased integration of CAM therapies into conventional care place a demand on nurses to become familiar with these therapies. Some of the frequently used CAM therapies are discussed in the following sections.

Acupuncture

Practiced in China for more than 2000 years, acupuncture is a major therapy within traditional Chinese medicine. It is based on the belief that there are invisible channels throughout the body called meridians, through which energy flows. This energy is called qi (pronounced chee)

 BOX **11-1**

Categories and Examples of Alternative and Complementary Therapies

Alternative medical systems Acupuncture, anthroposophic, Ayurvedic medicine, community-based health care practices (e.g., Native American, shamans), environmental medicine, homeopathy, naturopathy, traditional Oriental medicine

Mind-body interventions Aromatherapy, art therapy, biofeedback, dance therapy, hypnosis, imagery, meditation, music therapy, prayer, relaxation, self-help support groups, tai chi, yoga

Biologically based treatments Herbal therapies, individual and orthomolecular biologic therapies, special diets

Manipulative and body-based methods Chiropractic, massage, and related techniques (e.g., manual lymph drainage, Alexander technique, Feldenkrais method, pressure point therapies, Trager psychophysical integration), osteopathy

Energy therapies Qi gong, Reiki, therapeutic touch, bioelectromagnetic-based therapies

and is considered the vital life force. It is believed that illness and symptoms develop when the flow of energy becomes blocked or imbalanced. Health is restored when the energy becomes unblocked; this is achieved by stimulating acupuncture points on the meridian(s) affected (Figure 11-1).

The acupuncturist typically begins the treatment by taking a history, examining the tongue, and evaluating pulses. Based on where the acupuncturist assesses the energy imbalance to be, he or she places needles at specific points. The placement of the needles may have no obvious relationship to the area of the body that is symptomatic. Sometimes the acupuncturist applies heat to the acupoints by burning a dried herb on the top of the needle or skin; this procedure is known as moxibustion. Electroacupuncture, a process in which a small current of electricity is applied to the tip of the needle, is another means of stimulating acupoints.

Pain relief is the most common reason people seek acupuncture treatment, and research supports its effectiveness for this problem (Ahadian, Braun, and Schulteis, 2006; Cherkin and Sherman, 2005; Haigh, 2009; Last and Hulbert, 2009; Wang et al, 2009). The use of acupuncture for dental pain and chemotherapy-induced nausea and vomiting also has been supported by research. There is some evidence that acupuncture can be of help for nicotine withdrawal, asthma, stroke rehabilitation, carpal tunnel syndrome, and a growing list of other conditions.

Insurance companies vary in their coverage of acupuncture, so it is best for clients to call their individual insurer for determination of benefits. State health departments can be consulted for licensing requirements for acupuncturists in a given state.

Ayurveda

Although it recently has gained popularity because of the writings and lectures of Deepak Chopra, Ayurveda has existed in India for more than 5000 years. Ayurveda means "the science of life" and is a system of care that promotes spiritual, mental, and physical balance. Noninvasive approaches are used to achieve balance and include yoga, massage, diet, purification regimens, breathing exercises, meditation, and herbs.

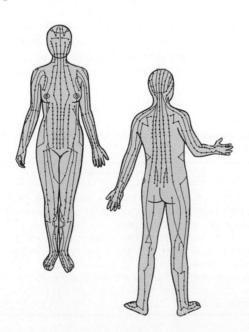

Figure 11-1 Acupuncture meridians. (From Eliopoulos C: Integrating alternative and conventional therapies, St Louis, 1999, Mosby.)

Individuals are believed to have distinct metabolic body types called doshas, which are vata, pitta, and kapha (Table 11-1). Signs of illness occur when the delicate balance of the doshas is disturbed.

The treatment to restore balance is influenced by the body type a client possesses and could include:

- ◆ Cleansing and detoxification
- ◆ Palliation
- ◆ Rejuvenation through special herbs and minerals
- ◆ Mental hygiene and spiritual healing

Currently there is no process for licensing or certifying Ayurvedic practitioners. Because some of the treatments have the potential to cause complications (e.g., dehydration from cleansing enemas, herb-drug interactions), finding a reputable trained practitioner is important. The Ayurveda websites listed in Box 11-2 can assist in locating qualified practitioners.

Biofeedback

Biofeedback is a technique in which the client is taught to alter specific bodily functions (e.g., heart rate, blood pressure, muscle tension). The client uses various relaxation and imagery exercises to affect desired responses. Machinery, such as electroencephalograms, electromyelograms, and thermistors, are used to measure and offer feedback about the function that the client is trying to alter. As the client becomes familiar with ways to successfully alter bodily responses, the equipment may no longer be necessary.

There are many conditions for which biofeedback can offer benefit, including urinary incontinence, anxiety, stress, irritable bowel syndrome, neck and back pain, and cardiac arrhythmias.

Chiropractic Medicine

Chiropractic medicine is a popular and widely accepted CAM therapy in the United States perhaps because it was developed here and has been practiced for more than a century. Chiropractors are licensed in every state, and most insurance companies will pay for chiropractic treatments.

Chiropractic medicine is based on the belief that misalignments of the spine, called subluxations, put pressure on the nerves, leading to pain and disruptions in normal bodily function. The misalignment is treated by manipulation and adjustment of the spine. Typically the chiropractor's hands do the alignment, although chiropractors increasingly are using heat, electrical stimulation, and other treatments.

TABLE **11-1**

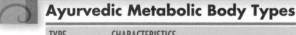

Ayurvedic Metabolic Body Types

TYPE	CHARACTERISTICS
Vata	Unpredictable, moody, vivacious, hyperactive, imaginative, intuitive, impulsive, fluctuating energy levels, slender, prominent features and joints, eats and sleeps at varying times throughout day, prone to insomnia, PMS, cramps, and constipation
Pitta	Predictable, orderly, efficient, perfectionist, intense, passionate, short-tempered, medium build, follows routine schedule, warm skin, prone to heavy perspiration, thirst, acne, ulcers, hemorrhoids, and stomach problems
Kapha	Relaxed; graceful; tendency toward procrastination; affectionate; forgiving; compassionate; sleeps long and deeply; cool, pale, and oily skin; eats slowly; prone to high cholesterol, obesity, allergies, sinusitis

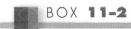

BOX **11-2**

Helpful Websites

GENERAL INFORMATION
NCCAM Clearinghouse
  www.nccam.nih.gov

ALTERNATIVE SYSTEMS OF MEDICAL PRACTICE
Acupuncture
Acupuncture and Oriental Medicine Alliance
  www.AOMalliance.org
American Academy of Medical Acupuncture
  www.medicalacupuncture.org
American Association of Acupuncture and
Oriental Medicine
  www.aaom.org

Ayurvedic Medicine
Ayurvedic Institute
  www.ayurveda.com

Homeopathy
National Center for Homeopathy
  www.homeopathic.org
North American Society of Homeopathy
  www.homeopathy.org

Naturopathy
American Association of Naturopathic Physicians
  www.naturopathic.org

BODYWORK—MOVEMENT THERAPY
The Alexander Therapy
www.alexandertech.com

The Feldenkrais Method
Feldenkrais Guild of North America
  www.feldenkrais.com

The Trager Approach
Trager International
  www.trager.com

MANUAL HEALING METHODS
Chiropractic
American Chiropractic Association
  www.amerchiro.org
World Chiropractic Alliance
  www.worldchiropracticalliance.org

Craniosacral Therapy
www.upledger.com

Energy Medicine/Healing
American Holistic Nurses Association
  www.ahna.org
Colorado Center for Healing Touch
  www.healingtouch.net

Nurse Healers Professional Associates
  www.therapeutic-touch.org
International Center for Reiki Training
  www.reiki.org

Massage Therapy
American Massage Therapy Association
  www.amtamassage.org
Associated Bodywork and Massage Professionals
  www.abmp.com
Massage Bodywork Resource Center
  www.massageresource.com

MIND-BODY THERAPIES
Biofeedback
Association of Applied Psychophysiology and
Biofeedback and Biofeedback Certification
Institute
  www.aapb.org

Guided Imagery
Academy for Guided Imagery
  www.interactiveimagery.com
Nurse Certificate Program in Imagery
  www.imageryrn.com

Hypnotherapy
American Board of Hypnotherapy
  www.hypnosis.com
American Society of Clinical Hypnosis
  www.asch.net

Meditation/Relaxation
American Meditation Institute
  www.americanmeditation.org
The Stress Reduction Clinic
Department of Medicine
University of Massachusetts Medical Center
  www.umassmed.edu/behavmed/clinical.cfm
The Center for Mind-Body Medicine
  www.cmbm.org

Tai Chi
Classic Tai Chi
  www.classictaichi.com

Yoga
American Yoga Association
  www.americanyogaassociation.org
Yoga Alliance
  www.yogaalliance.org
Yoga Science Research Foundation
  www.yogasite.com

Continued

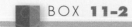

BOX **11-2**

Helpful Websites—cont'd

PHARMACOLOGIC AND BIOLOGIC TREATMENTS
Aromatherapy
Institute of Aromatherapy
Aromatherapy Consultant Program
 www.instituteofaromatherapy.com
National Association for Holistic Aromatherapy
(NAHA)
 www.naha.org
The Institute of Integrative Aromatherapy
 www.Aroma-RN.com

Herbal Medicine
Herb Research Foundation
 www.herbs.org
American Botanical Council
 www.herbalgram.org
American Herbalists Guild
 www.americanherbalistsguild.com

Dietary Supplements

The past advice that vitamin and mineral supplements are unnecessary if one is eating well has been replaced with the recommendation that everyone should take a daily vitamin and mineral supplement. This shift in thinking has resulted from the realization that many people do not consume the proper nutrients through their diets. Pollutants, stress, and other factors that are more common today than in previous generations heighten the body's need for added protection. Also unlike our ancestors, who consumed produce that was picked the same day, we tend to eat more processed foods and produce that may have been in transit for several days before reaching us; therefore, the foods we consume contain fewer vitamins and minerals. Given these factors, the National Research Council of the National Academy of Sciences is reevaluating the need to increase the recommended dietary allowances (RDAs).

Specific dietary supplements are believed to be beneficial for specific health conditions. However, too much of a good thing could prove harmful, and high doses of vitamins and minerals can lead to serious complications (Huang et al, 2006; Whitworth, 2006). For example, high doses of folic acid can mask a vitamin B_{12} deficiency (a cause of dementia), and calcium in excess of 2500 mg/day can cause kidney stones and impair the body's ability to absorb other minerals. In addition, because new research may disprove earlier claims about supplements, nurses need to keep abreast of new findings so that they can use supplements wisely and educate consumers to do the same.

Herbs

Plants have been used for medicinal purposes for nearly as long as humans have inhabited the earth. It is estimated that as many as 70,000 plant species have been used at one time or another by various cultures for medicinal purposes (Thomson Healthcare, 2007). Botanical medicine was a mainstream practice in the United States until the early nineteenth century, when medicine's shift toward a more scientific approach caused drugs to be viewed more favorably than herbs. But in the 1960s when the movement toward natural health began to grow, interest in herbal products increased. The use and sales of herbal remedies have grown significantly since.

In reality herbs are not that foreign to conventional medicine. Many modern drugs are derived from plants, including:

◆ Atropine from *Atropa belladonna*
◆ Digoxin from *Digitalis purpurea*

BOX **11-3**

Facts About Commonly Used Herbs

CHAMOMILE
Uses: Sedative effect, calming upset digestive tract
Cautions: Because it contains coumarin, it could affect coagulation, although clinical studies have not proven this to date; if client is using an anticoagulant and chamomile, monitor.

ECHINACEA
Uses: Antimicrobial; stimulates immune system
Cautions: Some persons with ragweed and other environmental allergies may have sensitivity; although immunosuppressive effects with long-term use are inconclusive at present, best to limit to short-term use. Should not be used in people with autoimmune diseases.

FEVERFEW
Use: Relief of migraines
Cautions: Contraindicated for clients with allergies to ragweed and other members of the *Compositae* family; can affect coagulation so contraindicated in persons on anticoagulant therapy.

GARLIC
Uses: Lowers blood pressure; reduces "bad" cholesterol; stimulates immune system; heart tonic; antioxidant
Cautions: Close monitoring necessary if taken by person using anticoagulant because it can prolong bleeding time; can potentiate action of hypoglycemic drugs.

GINGER
Use: Antiemetic
Caution: Regular use can prolong bleeding time; monitor if used with an anticoagulant.

GINKGO BILOBA
Use: Increases circulation to brain, which may improve cognitive performance in persons with dementia
Cautions: Close monitoring necessary if taken by person using anticoagulant because it can prolong bleeding time; can reduce effectiveness of anticonvulsants. Should not be used by people who have fragile blood vessels and a tendency to easily bleed.

GINSENG
Uses: Improves resistance to stress, immune stimulant; general stimulant
Cautions: Raises blood pressure; close monitoring necessary if taken by person using anticoagulant because it can prolong bleeding time; may increase digoxin levels; contraindicated when other stimulants are used; can cause insomnia, headache, epistaxis, vomiting. Can cause breast tenderness in some menstruating women.

SAW PALMETTO
Uses: Improves symptoms with benign prostatic hypertrophy; diuretic; urinary antiseptic
Caution: Do not take with hormonal therapies. Can increase risk of bleeding when taken with other drugs that increase risk of bleeding.

ST. JOHN'S WORT
Uses: Antianxiety; mild depression
Cautions: Can cause photosensitivity, particularly in fair-skinned individuals; contraindicated when other antidepressants are used. Causes dry mouth, dizziness, nausea in some individuals.

VALERIAN
Use: Sedative
Caution: Do not use with barbiturates.

◆ Ipecac from *Cephaelis ipecacuanha*
◆ Reserpine from *Rauwolfia serpentina*

With more than 20,000 herbs and related products on the market, staying current of uses, dosage, interactions, and adverse effects is a near impossibility. However, nurses would be wise to become familiar with some of the most commonly used herbs (Box 11-3) and know where to obtain information on other herbs when needed (see Box 11-2). Because of consumers' widespread use of herbs, questions regarding use of all supplements and education to ensure safe use are significant nursing responsibilities.

Homeopathy

Homeopathy is a branch of medicine developed in the late eighteenth century by Samuel Hahnemann. It was widely practiced in the United States until the early 1900s, when modern (i.e., conventional) medicine discredited it as being unscientific and ineffective. Homeopathy remained popular in other parts of the world, however, and recently has regained popularity in our country.

The origin of the word *homeopathy* helps in understanding this therapy. In Greek the word *homos* means "similar," and *pathos* means "suffering." The foundation of homeopathy are the laws of *similars*, the *minimum dose*, and *cure* Box 11-4.

Although the reason for their effectiveness is not fully understood, homeopathic remedies have been shown to be effective for a variety of conditions. People use homeopathy for a range of health concerns, from wellness promotion and disease prevention to the treatment of diseases and conditions such as allergies, asthma, chronic fatigue syndrome, depression, digestive disorders, ear infections, headaches, and skin rashes (NCCAM, 2009b).

The ideal way to use homeopathic remedies is to have a homeopath prescribe a customized remedy based on individual characteristics and symptoms. However, homeopathic practitioners are not plentiful, so the next best thing is to buy over-the-counter preparations that are labeled for their intended purpose (e.g., arthritis, headache, hay fever, cold).

Hypnotherapy

Although the use of trance states for healing purposes dates back to primitive cultures, hypnotherapy was not approved as a valid medical treatment until the 1950s. This mind-body therapy is now widely and successfully used for a wide range of conditions, including chronic pain, migraines, asthma, smoking cessation, and irritable bowel syndrome.

The process of hypnosis begins by the therapist guiding the client into a relaxed state and then creating an image that focuses attention to the specific symptom or problem that needs to

---

 BOX **11-4**

Principles Underlying Homeopathy

Law of similars: This law builds on the idea of prescribing remedies that produce symptoms similar to those of the illness being treated. This is the same principle on which vaccines are based. In homeopathy a dilute preparation is made from a plant or other biologic material; the more dilute the preparation, the higher its potency. The solution typically is added to a sugar tablet or powder for oral use or to a lotion or ointment for external use.

Law of minimum dose: This law, also known as the principle of dilutions, states that the lower the dosage of the substance, the greater its effectiveness. In preparing homeopathic remedies, substances are diluted and shaken vigorously; a portion of that substance is then diluted and shaken. This procedure is repeated to the point that the final substance is so dilute that no molecules of the original plant or substance remain. This process, referred to as potentization, is believed to transmit some form of information or energy from the original substance to the final diluted remedy. It is believed that the substance has left its imprint or "essence," which stimulates the body to heal itself (this theory is called the "memory of water").

Law of cure: This is the principle used to evaluate the effectiveness of a remedy. If the treatment is successful, symptoms should travel from vital to less vital organs of the body, move from within the body outward, and disappear in reverse order of appearance. If symptoms do not follow this sequence, a new or additional treatment is used. In homeopathic medicine, a worsening of symptoms after a remedy is given is considered a positive sign that healing is taking place.

be improved. The client must be in a state of deep relaxation to be receptive to a posthypnotic suggestion. Most people are capable of being hypnotized if they are willing.

Imagery

Imagery is the process of creating a "picture" (image) in the mind that can cause a specific bodily response. Although hypnosis uses imagery, in hypnosis an image and suggestion are presented to the person, whereas in imagery the person creates an image on his or her own. The process of imagery begins by the client establishing a desired outcome (e.g., to relieve stress, enhance circulation, reduce blood pressure). The nurse or other practitioner assists the client in creating an image that helps to achieve the outcome (e.g., the nurse may describe how the blood circulates through the body, help the client develop an image of how cancer cells can be eliminated, or suggest that the client think of a peaceful place where cares can "melt away") and guides the client in reaching a relaxed state. As an alternative to having someone guide him or her through an imagery exercise, a client can learn the process from books or use commercially prepared audiotapes.

Imagery is not a difficult mind-body healing therapy to master and can be easily implemented in virtually every practice setting.

Magnet Therapy

Although a mainstream therapy in Germany and Japan, the use of magnets has only recently become popular in the United States. The most common uses of magnet therapy are for pain and wound healing.

The mechanism by which magnets work is not completely understood and is being investigated. It is believed that magnets relieve pain by creating a slight electrical current that stimulates the nervous system and consequently blocks nerve sensations. Magnets are hypothesized to speed wound healing by dilating vessels and increasing circulation to an area. Distributors of magnet products make additional claims about the health benefits of magnets, ranging from improving attention deficit disorder to boosting the immune system, although these benefits are yet to be proven.

Magnets come in a variety of forms, strengths, and prices. There are magnet disks that can be strapped to limbs, magnet mattresses that one can sleep on, and magnet jewelry. To be effective for therapeutic purposes, the magnet should have a strength of at least 500 gauss (which is about eight times stronger than the magnets used for attaching things to your refrigerator door).

Persons with pacemakers should not use magnets, and, because the effects of magnets on fetal growth are not fully understood, they should not be applied to the abdomen of a pregnant woman.

Massage, Bodywork, and Energy Therapies

Massage for healing purposes has been used for thousands of years to maintain health. Many people today receive regular massages as an important component of their self-care to aid in stress management. In addition to promoting relaxation, massage can be beneficial for reducing edema, promoting circulation and respirations, and relieving pain, anxiety, and depression.

Massage is the manipulation of soft tissue by rubbing, kneading, rolling, pressing, slapping, and tapping movements. The term "bodywork" is applied to the combination of massage with deep tissue manipulation, movement awareness, and energy balancing. Touch therapies include techniques in which the hands of the nurse or therapist are near the body, in the client's energy field. Examples of various types of massage, bodywork, and touch therapies are described in Box 11-5.

Because therapeutic touch (TT) is a popular alternative healing therapy among nurses, it deserves some discussion. TT became popular in nursing in the 1970s with the work and research of Delores Krieger (Krieger, 1979; Nurse Healers Professional Association, 2009). Krieger advanced the theory that people are energy fields and that obstructed energy could be responsible for unhealthy states. She proposed that the nurse could draw on the universal field of energy and transfer this energy to the client. This incoming energy could help the client mobilize his or her own inner resources for healing and help unblock the client's obstructed energy.

In TT there is little direct physical contact between the practitioner and the individual being treated. Rather TT is an energy-based therapy; the nurse enters the client's energy field to assess and treat energy imbalances.

In the first step of TT, the nurse centers herself or himself and focuses on the intent to heal (this is sometimes referred to as healing meditation). During this phase the nurse quiets the mind and prepares physically and psychologically to connect with the client. This is considered a crucial step in the process to enable the nurse to be fully present in the moment with the client. This is followed by the nurse passing his or her hands over the client's body to assess the energy field and mobilizing areas in which energy is blocked or sluggish by directing energies to that area. TT is used to reduce anxiety, relieve pain, and enhance immune function.

Healing touch (HT) is an energy therapy that is an offshoot of TT. It combines additional healing approaches to the basic ones of TT to open energy blockages, seal energy leaks, and rebalance the energy field. There is a six-level educational program for HT. (The Healing Touch International website offers a full description of their program, in addition to a bibliography of recent research related to this therapy.)

 BOX **11-5**

Types of Massage, Bodywork, and Touch Therapies

ALEXANDER TECHNIQUE
Teaches improved balanced, posture, and coordination by using gentle hands-on guidance and verbal instruction

FELDENKRAIS METHOD
Teaches movement reeducation by using gentle manipulations to heighten awareness of the body; believes each person has an individualized optimal style of movement

HEALING TOUCH
A multilevel energy healing program that incorporates aspects of therapeutic touch with other healing measures

REFLEXOLOGY
Application of pressure to pressure points on the hands and feet that correspond to various parts of the body

REIKI
A therapy that uses techniques to direct universal life energy to specific sites

ROLFING (STRUCTURAL INTEGRATION)
Use of manual manipulation and stretching of body's fascial tissues to establish balance and symmetry

SWEDISH MASSAGE
Most prevalent form of massage that uses long strokes, friction, and kneading of muscles

TRAGER APPROACH
Use of gentle, rhythmic rocking and touch to promote relaxation and energy flow

Reiki is a practice in which the Reiki practitioner (of which there are several levels) channels energy to others using a series of hand positions. It is believed that healing energy flows through the hands without the need for any special skills. Like other forms of energy work, Reiki is believed to be useful for pain management, wound healing, stroke rehabilitation, and general relaxation (Ringdahl and Halcon, 2006).

Meditation and Progressive Relaxation

Meditation, the act of focusing on the present moment, has been used for centuries throughout the world. This practice gained considerable attention in the United States in the 1970s when Harvard Medical School cardiologist Herbert Benson published research on the relaxation response (Benson and Beary, 1974). Benson reported that after 20 minutes of meditation, participants' heart rate, respirations, blood pressure, oxygen consumption, carbon dioxide production, and serum lactic acid levels decreased. This led to meditation being used for a variety of conditions, including stress, anxiety, pain, and high blood pressure.

Progressive relaxation is another exercise that shares some of the same benefits as meditation. Typically a person learns to guide himself or herself through a series of exercises that relax the body, such as tightening and relaxing various muscle groups. Many audiotapes are available in bookstores and health food stores that offer scripts to guide meditation and progressive relaxation exercises.

Naturopathy

An intense interest in natural cures in Europe during the nineteenth century led to the development of spas that offered natural treatments to promote health and healing. Soon the movement spread to the United States, and in 1896 the American School of Naturopathy was founded. Naturopathic physicians and treatment facilities using natural cures became popular in the early part of the twentieth century. For example, John Kellogg ran such a facility in Battle Creek in which he subsequently became famous for the natural breakfast cereals that he used. As time progressed, medications and high-tech interventions caused naturopathy to pale by comparison; however, as consumers seek approaches that are more natural, this form of alternative medicine is making a comeback.

Naturopathy is based on the principle that the body has inherent healing abilities that can be stimulated to treat disease. Naturopathic physicians assess and treat the cause of the disease rather than merely alleviate symptoms. They help clients identify unhealthy practices, encourage healthy lifestyle habits, and guide them in managing health problems using natural approaches, such as herbs, homeopathic remedies, diet modifications, dietary supplements, and exercise.

There are a limited number of accredited schools of naturopathic medicine (e.g., Bastyr University, Southwest College of Naturopathic Medicine and Health Sciences, and National College of Naturopathic Medicine). A handful of states license naturopaths and require that they must have graduated from an accredited program. However, there are many individuals practicing as naturopaths who have obtained their education and experience through other means or who practice in states that do not require licensure; thus learning about the credentials of a naturopath before receiving services is beneficial for clients.

Prayer and Faith

Many people consider their faith to be an integral part of their total being rather than a therapy, but now there is scientific evidence supporting the therapeutic benefits of faith and prayer in health and healing. Hundreds of well-conducted studies have revealed that people who profess a faith, pray, and attend religious services are generally healthier, live longer, have lower rates of disability, recover faster, have lower rates of emotional disorders, and otherwise enjoy better health states than those who do not (Barnum, 2006; O'Brien, 2007). Not only do the faith and religious practices of individuals themselves affect health and healing, but research also supports the benefit of intercessory prayer.

Nurses need to appreciate that many people believe in the healing power of prayer and may expect their health care providers to join them in prayer if requested. This does not suggest that nurses or other health professionals should be forced into prayer if it is contrary to their beliefs; rather if there is no objection from either party, prayer by the client and health care provider can be used as a valuable healing measure.

Tai Chi

Tai chi is another practice from traditional Chinese medicine used to stimulate the flow of qi, the life energy. It is a combination of exercise and energy work that looks like a slow, graceful dance using continuous, controlled movements of the arms and legs. There is a specific sequence of steps to follow in doing tai chi, but fortunately there are many inexpensive videos that can be used, in addition to classes that are offered to aid people in learning this practice.

Tai chi has some proven benefits, including reduction of falls, improved coordination in older adults, and improved function in persons with arthritis (Adler and Roberts, 2006). Many people find that tai chi helps to reduce stress and promotes a general sense of well-being.

Yoga

Yoga has changed from a mystical form of Hindu worship practiced more than 5000 years ago to what is now known as a system of exercises involving various postures, meditation, and deep breathing. The word *yoga* means "union"; the union of body, mind, and spirit is achieved through yoga. Research suggests that yoga has many beneficial effects, such as to reduce stress, improve mood and sense of well-being, decrease heart rate and blood pressure, increase lung capacity, improve flexibility, and promote relaxation (NCCAM, 2009c).Yoga can be adapted to any level and capability so that it can be easily used.

There are many other alternative healing modalities, and new ones are appearing regularly. Some may be safe and effective, but lack sufficient experience or clinical research to support their claims; others may be worthless and merely an attempt to sell a product or service. Discretion is crucial. (Assistance in gaining objective information regarding CAM therapies can be obtained from NCCAM 1-888-644-6226; www. nccam.nih.gov.)

NURSING AND COMPLEMENTARY AND ALTERNATIVE MEDICINE THERAPIES
A Holistic Approach

The use of natural or "alternative" healing measures is hardly new to nursing. From Florence Nightingale (1860), who wrote about the importance of creating an environment in which natural healing could occur, through contemporary nurse theorists who discuss human and environmental energy fields (Meleis, 2006; Rogers, 1975), nurses have long realized that healing quite effectively occurs in ways not encompassed within the conventional biomedical system. Nursing also has promoted many of the same principles evident in CAM, particularly care of the body, mind, and spirit. In fact, this is the essence of holistic nursing (Box 11-6). Nurses must ensure that the integration of CAM into their practice is done within a holistic

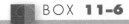

BOX **11-6**

Beliefs Guiding Holistic Nursing Practice

- The uniqueness of each individual is honored.
- Health is a harmonious balance of body, mind, and spirit.
- The needs of individuals' bodies, minds, and spirits are assessed and addressed in the caregiving process.
- Health and disease are natural parts of the human experience.
- Disease is an opportunity for increased awareness of the interconnectiveness of body, mind, and spirit.
- Individuals have the capacity for self-healing; the nurse facilitates this process.
- Nurses empower individuals for self-care.
- Individuals' cultural values, beliefs, and practices are honored and incorporated into the caregiving process.
- Individuals have a dynamic relationship with their environment; the environment is part of the healing process.
- Nurses, through their presence and being, are tools of the healing process.
- Nurses engage in self-care and an ongoing process of unfolding inner wisdom.
- Nurses can learn about holistic nursing and network with holistic nurses through involvement in the American Holistic Nurses' Association; learn more by visiting the AHNA website (www.ahna.org).

paradigm to truly make them healing therapies and not merely disconnected procedures within an already fragmented health care system.

Facilitating Use of Complementary and Alternative Medicine

Nurses need to integrate CAM into their nursing practice. This begins during the assessment process by exploring clients' use of CAM practices and products. Because it is not unusual for clients to use these without the knowledge of their physicians, nurses may be the first health professional with whom clients have discussed this issue. Factors to assess include:

- ◆ CAM practices and products being used and their sources
- ◆ Appropriateness of use of CAM practices and products
- ◆ Side effects and risks associated with use of CAM
- ◆ Conditions for which CAM currently is not used that could benefit by its use

Through the assessment process, nurses may identify the need to educate clients about the appropriateness of the CAM products and practices they are using. For example, a client with a pacemaker who uses magnets needs to be advised against continuing this practice; likewise a client drinking ginseng tea at bedtime requires an explanation that his insomnia may be the result of the stimulant effects of the herb. There may be situations in which nurses identify that specific conditions could benefit from the use of CAM therapies. As client advocates, nurses could bring this to the attention of the physician and other members of the health care team and make recommendations accordingly.

Nurses traditionally have been responsible for the coordination of client care. As CAM therapies are integrated into conventional care, nurses are the logical professionals to oversee the various parts and ensure that they are working in harmony for the client's benefit.

Nurses can learn to use many alternative healing measures to enhance nursing care. Among these are acupressure, aromatherapy, biofeedback, imagery, massage, and therapeutic touch. Nurses should seek whatever additional education and training are required to gain competency in these therapies and ensure compliance with state licensing laws.

Integrating Complementary and Alternative Medicine into Conventional Settings

Nurses can demonstrate leadership in helping conventional clinical settings integrate CAM therapies. In fact, nursing's holistic orientation and traditional coordination responsibilities make nurses logical for this role. Let us look at the way in which one nurse accomplished this.

CASE STUDY

Becky Blake, RN, recently joined the nursing staff in a combined coronary care and step-down unit. It did not take her long to note the expert technical skill of her colleagues, who could read monitors in a flash and respond to emergencies without missing a beat. The skill, efficiency, and organization of the nursing staff were evidenced by the lack of medication errors, infections, and pressure ulcers, coupled with the lowest length of stays of comparable hospital units in the area.

Yet there seemed to be something missing. Clients and their families often showed signs of anxiety and fear that were not addressed. Familiar faces reappeared as some clients were readmitted because they failed to alter lifestyle habits that contributed to their conditions. The same nursing staff who cared for people with hearts damaged by the effects of smoking, poor diet, and stress were guilty of the same unhealthy practices themselves.

It came to a head for Ms. Blake one morning when she was at a bedside changing an intravenous bag and checking equipment. The client, a man in his 50s, pulled at her arm, looked Ms. Blake in the eyes, and tearfully said, "How do you think I'm going to do? I've been awake all night wondering if I'll be able to do my job, take care of my wife, see my grandkids grow up, do the things I like to do." For the first time, Ms. Blake saw beyond the body in the bed to a human being experiencing considerable emotional distress—distress that was hardly beneficial to his condition. "We have managed to get this man's heart repaired," she thought, "but we have not begun to help him heal the emotional and spiritual pain that this illness created." This began a journey for Ms. Blake of discovering measures to help clients that went beyond the conventional treatments that were regularly prescribed.

Ms. Blake found a local network of holistic nurses and began attending their meetings. Through this group she learned of the difference between healing and curing and the importance of addressing the needs of body, mind, and spirit. She also heard nurses discussing their own need to be nurtured and committed to positive self-care practices. She met nurses who shared how they were using alternative healing practices and who led her to resources from which she could learn more.

In the months that followed, Ms. Blake attended several workshops and learned how progressive relaxation, meditation, therapeutic touch, and aromatherapy could be used to benefit the clients on her unit. As her understanding of holism grew, she recognized that stress reduction and improved health habits for her coworkers were sorely needed.

After planting seeds through informal discussions and sharing of articles, Ms. Blake requested a formal meeting with the interdisciplinary team on the unit. In this meeting, she described her areas of concern, which included the need to:

- Address clients' emotional and spiritual needs more effectively.
- Promote improved health habits of the staff.
- Develop practices that would reduce stress for clients, their families, and staff.

The staff concurred with these needs and expressed a desire to take actions to address them. Ms. Blake offered some suggestions:

- Coordinate with the staff development instructor to have classes offered on progressive relaxation, imagery, meditation, therapeutic touch, and stress reduction.
- Form an ad hoc committee to develop guidelines, policies, and procedures on how these healing therapies could be safely and legally implemented.
- Begin to include healing therapies into the care plans.
- Arrange for the nutritionist to offer classes to staff on healthy eating.
- Add healthy snacks to the break room.

CASE STUDY—cont'd

- Coordinate with the housekeeping and maintenance departments to introduce aromatherapy diffusers, plants, and piped-in music in the unit.
- Develop a system to remind staff to use stress reduction measures throughout their shift.
- Collaborate with the nutritionist, social worker, spiritual care counselor, and nursing clinical resources to provide group sessions for clients and their families on topics, such as coping with illness, stress management, and promoting healthy lifestyle habits.
- Request the quality improvement coordinator to monitor and evaluate the effect of these interventions.

It did not take long for the effects of these new approaches to be realized. Clients requested fewer sedatives and analgesics. Surveys of clients and families revealed higher levels of satisfaction. Staff sick days were reduced, and there seemed to be a greater sense of team spirit and cooperation. Soon staff in other parts of the hospital began requesting that similar interventions be implemented in their units.

Using Complementary and Alternative Medicine Competently

As increasing numbers of consumers and clinical settings are interested in or actually using CAM therapies, nurses are challenged to become knowledgeable about the uses, limitations, and precautions associated with these new practices and products. Maintaining a resource library and becoming familiar with websites to stay current are beneficial measures.

Nurses must become familiar with cultural factors that can influence acceptance and use of alternative healing practices. For instance some individuals may object to energy therapies (e.g., TT, HT) on the grounds that they associate these therapies with occult practices, or they may have anxiety about meditation because they believe evil spirits could invade their minds. As comforting as a massage can be, some people who come from cultures that believe it is inappropriate for someone to touch a person of the opposite sex could become distressed with this measure. Knowledge and sensitivity to personal and cultural preferences are essential.

Legal Considerations

The use of CAM could present some legal issues for which nurses need to be concerned. As growing numbers of practitioners of healing therapies advocate for recognition and separate licensure, some of the healing therapies once considered part of nursing care may require separate licensure. Such is the case with massage. In some states nurses may not provide a massage unless they are licensed as massage therapists. Acupressure and biofeedback are among the other areas in which the nurse could be challenged if not licensed. Nurses need to clarify the therapies that fall within the realm of nursing practice and take a proactive role in ensuring that other disciplines do not attempt to limit them.

Another legal concern for nurses in the growing arena of CAM is the question of to whom the nurse is responsible when practicing CAM therapies. New, nonconventional practice settings are developing. For example, a nurse may be employed in a setting in which there is an acupuncturist, hypnotherapist, and homeopath. Some questions that could arise include: Who supervises the nurse? Can these therapists delegate responsibilities to the nurse? How does the nurse ensure that in such a practice setting diagnoses are not being made or treatments being prescribed that are beyond the scope of the CAM practitioners? Nurses need to begin to consider the implications of new practice models and develop clear practice guidelines that ensure a legally sound practice.

SUMMARY

An opportunity exists for nursing to demonstrate leadership in the integration of CAM with conventional care. Representing the largest number of health care professionals, nurses can have a significant effect on implementing CAM throughout the health care system. Nurses' historical holistic orientation to care enables them to ensure that the integration of CAM and conventional services is done in a manner that addresses the client's body, mind, and spirit. Without such coordinated efforts, there is the risk that these new therapies will merely be additional ingredients in an already fragmented system of care. Nurses have proven that they can coordinate and promote comprehensive care like no other discipline. Therefore, nursing is the logical discipline to be the hub of the wheel of integrative services.

evolve   Additional resources are available online at: http://evolve.elsevier.com/Cherry/

REFERENCES

Adler PA, Roberts BL: The use of tai chi to improve health in older adults, *Orthop Nurs* 25(2):122–126, 2006.

Ahadian FM, Braun JC, Schulteis G: Quantitative assessment of acupuncture analgesia using a human experimental pain model: a randomized, crossover pilot study, *Med Acupunct* 17(3):12–15, 2006.

Barnum B: *Spirituality in nursing*, ed 2, New York, 2006, Springer.

Benson H, Beary JZ: The relaxation response, *Psychiatry* 37:37–46, 1974.

Cherkin DC, Sherman KJ: Acupuncture and knee osteoarthritis, *Ann Intern Med* 142(10):872–873, 2005.

Haigh C: Acupuncture reduced frequency and pain intensity of primary migraine or tension-type headaches, *Evid Based Nurs* 12(2):47, 2009.

Huang HY, Cabalerro B, Chang S, et al: The efficacy and safety of multivitamin and mineral supplement use to prevent cancer and chronic disease in adults: a systematic review for a National Institutes of Health State-of-the-Science Conference, *Ann Intern Med*, July 31, 2006.

Krieger D: *The therapeutic touch*, Englewood Cliffs, NJ, 1979, Prentice-Hall.

Last AR, Hulbert K: Chronic low back pain: evaluation and management, *Am Fam Physician* 79(12):1067–1074, 2009.

Meleis AI: *Theoretical nursing: development and progress*, ed 4, Philadelphia, 2006, Lippincott.

National Center for Complementary and Alternative Medicine: *Statistics on CAM use in the United states*. 2009a. Retrieved July 2009 from: http://nccam.nih.gov/news/camstats/2007/index.htm.

National Center for Complementary and Alternative Medicine: *Homeopathy: an introduction*. 2009b. Retrieved July 2009 from: http://nccam.nih.gov/health/homeopathy/homeopathy.pdf.

National Center for Complementary and Alternative Medicine: *Yoga for health*. 2009c. Retrieved August 2009 from: http://nccam.nih.gov/health/yoga/introduction.htm.

Nightingale F: *Notes on nursing*, London, 1860, Harrison.

Nurse Healers Professional Association: *TT facts*. Retrieved July 2009 from: www.therapeutic-touch.org/newsarticle.php?newsID=1.

O'Brien ME: *Spirituality in nursing: standing on holy ground*, ed 3, Sudbury, MA, 2007, Jones and Bartlett.

Ringdahl D, Halcon LL: Reiki. In Snyder M, Lindquist R, editors: *Complementary/alternative therapies in nursing*, New York, 2006, Springer, pp 243–253.

Rogers M: *An introduction to the theoretical basis for nursing*, ed 3, Philadelphia, 1975, FA Davis.

Thomson Healthcare: *PDR for herbal medicines*, ed 4, Montvale, NJ, 2007, Thomson Reuters.

Wang SM, et al: Auricular acupuncture as a treatment for pregnant women who have low back and posterior pelvic pain: a pilot study, *Am J Obstet Gynecol* 200(6):589, 2009.

Whitworth A: Micronutrients: to supplement, or not to supplement? *J Natl Cancer Inst* 98(4):230–232, 2006.

ADDITIONAL RESOURCES

Bauer R: *Mayo Clinic guide to alternative medicine*, New York, 2007, Time Inc.

Caspi O, Baranovitch O: When science meets medical tradition: what is needed for a dialogue on integrative medicine? *J Altern Complement Med* 15(5):579–583, 2009.

Conners MS, Altshuler L: *The everything guide to herbal remedies*, Avon, MA, 2009, Adams Media.

Eliopoulos C, editor: *Invitation to holistic health: a guide to living a balanced life*, ed 2, Boston, 2010, Jones and Bartlett.

Furlan A, et al: Acupuncture and dry-needling for low back pain, *Cochrane Database Syst Rev* (1):CD001351, 2005.

Kabat-Zinn J: *Coming to our senses: healing ourselves and the world through mindfulness*, New York, 2006, Hyperion.

Kalauokalani D, Cherkin DC, Sherman KJ: A comparison of physician and nonphysician acupuncture treatment for chronic low back pain, *Clin J Pain* 21(5):406–411, 2005.

Kawas CW: Medications and diet: protective factors for AD? *Alzheimer Dis Assoc Disord* 20(Suppl 2):S89–S96, 2006.

Lind BK, et al: Chiropractic use by urban and rural residents with insurance coverage, *J Rural Health* 25(3):253–258, 2009.

Mantle F, Tiran D: *A-Z of complementary and alternative medicine: a guide for health professionals*, New York, 2009, Churchill Livingstone.

National Center for Complementary and Alternative Medicine: *Herbs at a glance*. Retrieved July 2009 from: http://nccam.nih.gov/health/herbsataglance.htm.

Selin R: *Medicine across cultures*, Boston, 2003, Kluwer Academic Publishers.

Snyder M, Lindquist R, editors: *Complementary/alternative therapies in nursing*, New York, 2006, Springer.

Workforce Advocacy and the Nursing Shortage

Debra D. Hatmaker, PhD, RN-BC, SANE-A

evolve Additional resources are available online at: http://evolve.elsevier.com/Cherry/

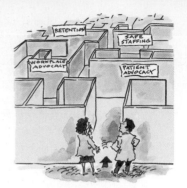

A changing workplace and the nursing shortage require nurses to embrace workforce advocacy to ensure quality health care delivery.

VIGNETTE

As a new graduate, 26-year-old Elena Gonzalez is searching for her first position as a registered nurse (RN) in a large metropolitan city. As part of her education she learns about the importance of a nurse's role in advocating for a workplace conducive to delivering safe and effective quality health care. She also understands that the workplace is filled with complex issues—nursing shortages, staffing issues, potential exposure to bloodborne diseases—affecting the nurse, the patient, the organization, and the profession. As a result of the nursing shortage, Elena receives offers from various organizations. However, she wisely chooses not to accept a job on its "face value" and decides to investigate her opportunities more thoroughly. Using the Internet, she searches the websites of hospitals in her target area. She is looking for the answers to questions, such as:

- *Have any organizations within my area received Magnet hospital status?*
- *Which organizations have shared governance models?*
- *Are nurses encouraged to participate in shared governance?*
- *What is the content and length of orientation for new nurses?*
- *What is the organization's philosophy regarding staff mix designations?*
- *Does the organization have a conflict resolution process?*
- *What is the organization's turnover rate and what is the average time that nurses are employed in the organization?*

Answers to these questions can be found on health care organizations' websites or from their nurse recruiters or nurse educators. Armed with answers to these and other questions, Elena decides to accept a position with a large tertiary care center that she believes has created an environment most supportive of ensuring the delivery of quality patient care. However, she knows that with the acceptance of this position, her role as a workforce and patient advocate has not ended; rather it has only just begun.

■ QUESTIONS TO CONSIDER WHILE READING THIS CHAPTER:

1 What workforce advocacy strategies can Elena use to promote quality patient care and a safe work environment?

2 What is the value of shared governance to Elena's individual nursing practice?

3 If Elena becomes concerned about floating assignments, what questions can help guide her decision about accepting such assignments?

4 What online resources are available to help Elena learn more about important workplace issues and workforce advocacy?

5 How can Elena gain increased marketability of her nursing expertise?

KEY TERMS

Patient advocacy The nurse and the nursing profession's powerful voice at the local, state, and national levels in supporting policies that protect consumers and enhance accountability for quality by promoting safer health care systems. Patient advocacy is a cornerstone of the nursing profession, and patients depend on nurses to ensure that they receive quality care. Workforce advocacy is a component of patient advocacy.

Workforce advocacy An array of services and tools designed to help nurses promote an optimal professional work environment and support their professional and personal development. Elements of workforce advocacy include staffing, workflow design, personal and social factors, physical environment, and organizational factors (Center for American Nurses, 2009).

Workplace issues An array of complex issues nurses face in the workplace on a daily basis. These complex issues affect the nurse, the patient, the organization, and the profession. Examples include the nursing shortage, adequate staffing levels, errors in health care delivery, and violence in the workplace.

LEARNING OUTCOMES

After studying this chapter, the reader will be able to:

1 Describe workforce advocacy as a means of improving the quality of health care delivery.

2 Identify issues that affect the practice of professional nursing in the health care workplace.

3 Identify available resources to assist in improving the workplace environment.

4 Define the role of nurses in advocating for safe and effective workplace environments.

5 Describe internal and external workforce strategies that support efficient and effective quality patient care.

6 Identify unique opportunities within the organization to improve the work environment for nurses.

CHAPTER OVERVIEW

In today's modern health care system nurses are faced with many workplace issues. These complex issues affect not only the nurse but also the patient, the organization, and the profession. This chapter attempts to identify a few select critical issues facing nurses and the nursing profession, including the nursing shortage, appropriate staffing, patient safety and advocacy, and workplace rights and safety. Workforce advocacy is defined, and its specific strategies are highlighted. To be a successful and accountable professional, nurses must recognize current issues and know where to seek support for workforce advocacy.

PROMOTING WORKFORCE ADVOCACY AND A PROFESSIONAL PRACTICE ENVIRONMENT

Professional nurses are seeing the dawn of an era of involvement and control in the work environment that was unheard of a decade ago. Important research is validating the contribution and value of RNs in the following areas:

- ◆ Improved patient outcomes (Kane et al, 2007)
- ◆ Prevention of premature mortality (Cho, Hwang, and Kim, 2008)
- ◆ Increased hospital profitability (Needleman et al, 2006; Unruh, 2008)

BOX **12-1**

Examples of Workforce Advocacy

- Promoting and protecting the occupational safety and health of nurses
- Using nurse practice acts and other legislative and regulatory protections
- Using the political process to influence legislative and regulatory agencies for the protection of nurses and patients
- Providing education regarding employment rights and responsibilities
- Developing skills related to public relations, media presentations, and conflict resolution
- Building coalitions and support groups to enable nurses to speak and advocate for their professional practices
- Participating in committee structures of the health care organization to ensure a nursing voice in safety and workplace issues

Adapted from American Nurses Association: *Definition of professional practice advocacy adopted by House of Delegates (internal document)*, Washington, DC, 1999, ANA.

Within this context of the important contributions that nurses make to patients, hospitals, and health care in general, we find nurses challenged to deliver care against all kinds of barriers and with dwindling resources. Nurses' strong concern and commitment to patient care and their role as patient advocates often place them in direct conflict with those who have more control, such as physicians and health care administrators. How a nurse reacts to such conflicts within the workplace and continues to advocate to improve patient care are a new focus for the profession—a focus called "workforce advocacy."

As we visit Elena Gonzalez 6 months after she assumed her new position, we find that she has become involved in advocating for a safe work environment. Elena and the other nurses working on the medical unit are concerned because there is a limited amount of safe patient handling equipment available on their unit. The patients on the medical unit often have mobility issues, and the nurses are worried about suffering musculoskeletal injuries when transferring and repositioning patients. Where will they find information about ergonomic safety and other workplace safety issues? Are there regulations that require hospitals to implement safety measures to protect their staff against debilitating musculoskeletal injuries? What legal rights do nurses have to demand safe patient handling equipment? Is there an avenue to work with hospital administrators to decrease the costs associated with unsafe practices and to move toward a user-friendly work environment? All of these questions are related to workforce advocacy. Examples of workforce advocacy are included in Box 12-1.

In 2003 the American Nurses Association's (ANA) commitment to workforce advocacy was advanced with creation of the Center for American Nurses (CAN). The CAN (http://centerfor americannurses.org) addresses the needs of individual nurses who are not represented by collective bargaining in their employment setting by offering services and tools designated to help nurses self-advocate in their professional and personal development. The CAN's focus is on the individual nurse rather than the nurse's workplace and addresses key elements of the nursing workforce: staffing, workflow design, personal and social factors, physical environment, and organizational factors (CAN, 2009). The CAN model and definitions of its elements are included in Box 12-2.

The CAN's vision is to be recognized as the voice of workforce advocacy for professional nurses, contributing to the creation of healthy workplaces that value and respect the contributions of nurses. Through research, continuing education, and knowledge sharing among today's nursing community, the CAN offers powerful resources to nurses seeking to overcome

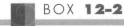

BOX **12-2**

Workforce Advocacy Ecosystem Model

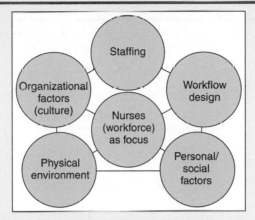

- **Staffing:** Refers to job assignments including the volume of work assigned to individuals, the professional skills required for particular job assignments, the duration of experience in a particular job category, and work schedules.
- **Workflow design:** Pertains to on-the-job activities of health care workers, including interactions among workers and the nature and scope of the work.
- **Personal and social factors:** Refer to individual and group factors, such as stress, job satisfaction, and professionalism, in addition to skills that may be underdeveloped in the nursing population, such as financial literacy.
- **Physical environment:** Includes aspects of the workplace, such as light, aesthetics, and sound. These elements will be crucial as the CAN explores the needs of a maturing workforce and offers solutions to health care employers.
- **Organizational factors:** Structural and process aspects of the organization as a whole, such as the use of teams, divisions of labor, shared beliefs, and an increasing leadership capacity among nurses.

Adapted from Hickam DH et al: *The effect of health care working conditions on patient safety.* Evidence report/technology assessment number 74. Prepared by Oregon Health & Science University under Contract No 290-97-0018. AHRQ Publication No 03-E031, Rockville, MD, Agency for Healthcare Research and Quality, April 2003; www.ahrq.gov. Available online at www.centerforamericannurses.org (Resources/Workforce Ecosystem).

workforce challenges and realize opportunities. Five opportunities and challenges for workforce advocacy programs are highlighted in Box 12-3. Other examples of workforce and patient advocacy are discussed, along with specific workplace issues, in the following sections.

THE NURSING SHORTAGE

The nursing profession has a long history of cyclic shortages, which have been documented since World War II (Minnick, 2000). The acute cyclic shortage affecting the nation during the late 1990s and the early 2000s was a direct result of the struggle to implement managed care as a means of controlling the escalating cost of health care. The nursing shortage has attracted significant attention from key groups including state and federal policymakers and leaders in education, health care, and manufacturing. Interventions by these groups have positively affected the shortage, resulting in growth in RN employment and nursing school enrollment.

As the result of an aging population and an aging nursing workforce, the nursing shortage will remain an important issue for health care providers for years to come (Buerhaus, Staiger,

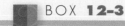

BOX **12-3**

Five Opportunities and Challenges for Workforce Advocacy Programs

1. Identify mechanisms within health care systems that provide opportunities for RNs to affect institutional policies.
   - Shared governance
   - Participatory management models
   - Magnet hospital recognition
   - Statewide staffing regulations
2. Develop conflict resolution models for use within organizations that address RNs' concerns about patient care and delivery issues.
   - Identification of the reporting loop
   - Appointment of a final arbiter in disputes
3. Seek legislative solutions for workplace problems by reviewing issues of concern to nurses in employment settings and introducing appropriate legislation, such as:
   - Whistle-blower protection
   - "Safe harbor" peer review
   - Support for rules outlining strong nursing practice standards
4. Develop legal centers for nurses that could provide legal support and decision-making advice as a last recourse to resolve workplace issues.
   - Provide fast and efficient legal assistance to nurses
   - Earmark precedent-setting cases that could affect case law and health care policy
5. Provide RNs with self-advocacy and patient advocacy information, such as:
   - Laws and regulations governing practice
   - Use of applicable nursing practice standards
   - Conflict resolution and negotiation techniques
   - Identify state and national reporting mechanisms that allow RNs to report concerns about health care organizations and/or professionals

Center for American Nurses: *Five opportunities/challenges for workforce advocacy programs.* Adapted from the Texas Nurses Association: Workplace advocacy program. Available at: www.centerforamericannurses.org (Resources/Workforce Advocacy).

and Auerbach, 2009). The downturn in the U.S. economy in 2009 led to an easing of the nursing shortage in some parts of the country (Thrall, 2009). This was largely due to many retired nurses reentering the workforce due to economic pressures, nurses who had planned to retire who are holding on to their positions, some nurses working part-time who have taken full-time positions, and hospitals treating fewer patients because many people are delaying procedures or not seeking care due to loss of insurance (American Hospital Association, 2008; Buerhaus, 2008). Despite this positive sign of stabilization, workforce analysts caution nurse educators, policymakers, employers, and other stakeholders that this will likely not result in a long-term resolution of the nursing shortage. It is projected that the number of nurses in the U.S. workforce will plateau in 2015, and by 2025 the nursing shortage could be nearly 500,000 with a 40% RN vacancy rate nationwide (Buerhaus et al, 2009).

Professional nursing is the largest U.S. health care occupation according to the Bureau of Labor Statistics (U.S. Department of Labor, 2009). In fact RNs are projected to create more than half a million new jobs over the 2006-2016 period, one of the largest numbers among all occupations. Thousands of job openings will result from:

- ◆ The need to replace experienced nurses who leave the occupation, especially as the median age of RNs continues to rise (Health Resources and Services Administration [HRSA], 2006)

+ Technologic advances in patient care that result in more patients accessing the health care system and needing more specialized care
+ Increasing emphasis on preventive care
+ The rapid growth in the older population, who are much more likely than younger people to need nursing care

Despite increases in graduation rates of new nurses over the past 8 years, the demand for nurses will continue to outpace the supply (Buerhaus et al, 2009). Planning for an adequate workforce will remain one of the most critical challenges of the new century. Although the current nursing shortage is related to supply and demand issues, a closer look at several confounding variables provides an insight into the complexity of the shortage and the need for an array of actions.

Health Care Is No Longer a Favored Employer

In examining the shortage of nurses, which is also accompanied by a shortage of other health care workers, the attractiveness of careers in health care, especially hospital care, declined in the 1980s and 1990s (Buerhaus et al, 2009). The women's movement sparked greater opportunities beyond female-dominated professions. This occurred at the same time the applicant pool for nursing (predominantly young women between the ages of 18 and 40) declined.

In a comparison of three national random sample surveys of RNs in 2002, 2004, and 2006, certain areas of the workplace environment continue to negatively affect nursing satisfaction as a preferred career choice: opportunities to influence decisions about workplace organization, recognition of accomplishments and work well done, opportunities for professional development, opportunities for professional advancement, and opportunities to influence decisions about patient care (Buerhaus et al, 2007). The identification and recognition of these workplace issues charge health care systems with the unavoidable requirement to redesign work and workplace environments so that they are able to attract, retain, and develop the best RN workforce.

Nursing School Enrollments and Recruitment

One contribution to a decline in nursing school enrollments during the 1990s was the younger birth cohorts (i.e., those born after 1955) that were smaller in population size and significantly less likely to choose nursing as a career (Buerhaus et al, 2009). Because many young nurses are attracted to the excitement of a critical care setting, acute care settings in particular have been hit hard by this decline in younger nurses entering the workforce. A second factor contributing to the shrinking shortage is the expanded career opportunities for women outside of nursing. Women make up 90% of the professional nursing workforce (U.S. Department of Labor, 2009). The first factor of an overall smaller number of individuals available to enter the workforce is beyond the control of the profession; however, we are challenged to make our profession attractive to young men and women as a viable career alternative.

Numerous efforts were undertaken over the past decade to recruit more students into nursing—efforts that have been largely successful. Professional nursing associations and health care companies educated the public regarding the shortage and the benefits of a nursing career. The Johnson & Johnson Campaign for Nursing's Future, a multiyear $30-million national initiative, was designed to enhance the image of the nursing profession, recruit new nurses and nurse faculty, and help retain nurses currently in the profession (Johnson & Johnson, 2009). Unfortunately, even when attempts to recruit more people into nursing have been successful, most schools and universities find themselves unable to expand their nursing programs to accept the qualified applicants because they are faced with a serious shortage of nursing faculty.

National and statewide efforts have resulted in increases in nursing school enrollments for 8 consecutive years (2001 to 2008), yet these increases continue to fall below the projected need to reverse the nursing shortage (American Association of Colleges of Nursing [AACN], 2009).

Along with the need to recruit into the profession, nursing must continue to examine the ways in which new nurses are introduced into the nursing work culture. Adequate orientation, mentoring, and preceptor programs are essential to introduce and retain new nurses.

Educational Preparation

During past shortages, employers have hired RNs regardless of their degree preparation. The current and projected demands for RNs require not simply more RNs, but more RNs of the right type and right educational and skill mix to handle increasingly complex care demands. Demand has intensified for more baccalaureate-prepared nurses with critical thinking, leadership, quality improvement, case management, and health promotion skills who are capable of delivering care across a variety of health care settings. Demand has also increased for experienced RNs; for nurses in key clinical specialties, such as critical care, emergency department (ED), operating room, and neonatal intensive care; and for master's- and doctoral-prepared RNs in advanced clinical specialties, teaching, and research.

In 2005 the American Organization of Nurse Executives (AONE), which is composed of chief nursing officers of U.S. hospitals, issued a position paper that supported the need for baccalaureate-prepared nurses as the minimal requirement for employment in today's complex health care environments (AONE, 2005). The National Quality Forum (2006) recognized the important contribution of nursing to quality care and the potential for emerging science to show evidence that nurses who are prepared with a bachelor of science in nursing or higher degree positively affect patient outcomes in acute care settings.

Faculty Shortage

One of the most critical problems facing nursing and nursing workforce planning is the aging of nursing faculty (Yordy, 2006). According to the AACN (2009) the mean age of nursing faculty has steadily increased to 59.1, 56.1, and 51.7 for doctoral faculty at the ranks of professor, associate professor, and assistant professor, respectively. For master's-prepared faculty the average ages for professors, associate professors, and assistant professors were 58.9, 55.2, and 50.1 years, respectively. Unfortunately the shortage of faculty is contributing to the current nursing shortage by limiting the number of students admitted to nursing programs. In 2008 an AACN survey determined that 49,948 qualified applications to nursing baccalaureate programs were not accepted, and an insufficient number of faculty were cited by schools as a reason for not accepting all qualified applicants (AACN, 2009). The National League for Nursing (NLN) reported that 99,000 qualified applicants were turned away from their member schools, which are primarily associate degree programs (NLN, 2009). Faculty salaries continue to be a major contributor to the faculty shortage. According to Yordy (2006), academic institutions, especially those faced with budget cuts, generally cannot compete with nonacademic employers.

Nurse Retention

Past nursing shortages have proven that the retention of professional nurses is a key to any organization's success. The ability of an organization to retain nurses primarily depends on the creation of an environment conducive to professional autonomy. Nurses want to work in an environment that supports decision making and effective nurse-physician relationships, which are critically important to patient safety. Although some progress has been achieved, RNs' perceptions of the hospital workplace environment as measured across three national surveys, demonstrate there is much need for improvement (Buerhaus et al, 2009).

In the national surveys many areas of work-related quality of life were rated poorly by RNs employed in hospitals, with fewer than one in four RNs rating them "excellent" or "very good" (Buerhaus et al, 2009). When asked to rate the quality of their relationships with others in the workplace, RNs assigned their highest overall ratings to their relationships with other RNs, followed next by their relationships with physicians and nurse practitioners, and then frontline nurse managers. RNs ranked their relationships with administration and management the lowest. In contrast to these perceptions, RNs in the surveys were generally satisfied with their jobs, and satisfaction had increased over time. The increase in job satisfaction was predicted by several factors: organizations who emphasized the quality of patient care, management recognized the importance of their personal and family lives, satisfaction with salary and benefits, high job security, and positive relationships with other nurses and with management. Decreases in job satisfaction were predicted by feeling stressed to the point of burnout, feeling burdened by too many non-nursing tasks, experiencing an increase in the number of patients assigned, and having a general negative overall view of the healthcare system.

Magnet Hospitals. One of the most successful retention models focuses on promoting standards for professional nursing practice and recognizing quality, excellence, and service. In 1980 recognizing a critical and widespread national shortage of nurses, the American Academy of Nurses undertook a study to identify a national sample of what are referred to as Magnet hospitals (i.e., those that attract and retain professional nurses in their employment) and to identify the factors that seem to be associated with their success in doing so (McClure et al, 1983). This landmark study, titled "Magnet Hospitals: Attraction and Retention of Professional Nurses," identified workplace factors, such as management style, nursing autonomy, quality of leadership, organizational structure, professional practice, career development, and quality of patient care as influencing nurse job satisfaction and low turnover rates in the acute care setting. Out of 163 hospitals initially participating, only 41 were deemed Magnet hospitals for their ability to support nurse autonomy and decision making in the workplace.

As a result, ANA's credentialing arm, the American Nurses Credentialing Center (ANCC), began a program recognizing hospitals with excellent nursing recruitment and high retention rates. As the Magnet Recognition Program evolved, it sought to combine the strengths of the original study with quality indicators identified by ANA and the standards of nursing practice as defined in ANA's *Scope and Standards for Nurse Administrators* so that both quantitative and qualitative factors of nursing services were measured. The qualitative factors in nursing, referred to as the 14 "Forces of Magnetism," provided the conceptual framework for the appraisal process. In 2007, ANCC commissioned a statistical analysis of Magnet appraisal team scores from evaluations conducted using the *2005 Magnet Recognition Program Application Manual.* This analysis clustered the sources of evidence into more than 30 groups, yielding an empirical model for the Magnet Recognition Program. The new, simpler model reflects a greater focus on measuring outcomes and allows for more streamlined documentation, while retaining the 14 Forces as foundational to the program (Box 12-4).

With its link between quality patient care and nursing excellence, the Magnet Recognition Program has reached a coveted level of prestige within the nursing community and among acute care facilities (Aiken, 2005). Research has consistently shown that Magnet hospital nurses have higher levels of autonomy, more control over the practice setting, and better relationships with physicians (Aiken et al, 2008; Aiken et al, 2009; Aiken, Havens, and Sloane, 2000;

BOX **12-4**

The Magnet Model and 14 Forces of Magnetism

Model Components	Forces of Magnetism
Transformational Leadership	• Quality of Nursing Leadership (Force 1)
	• Management Style (Force 3)
Structural Empowerment	• Organizational Structure (Force 2)
	• Personnel Policies and Programs (Force 4)
	• Community and the Healthcare Organization (Force 10)
	• Image of Nursing (Force 12)
	• Professional Development (Force 14)
Exemplary Professional Practice	• Professional Models of Care (Force 5)
	• Quality of Care: Ethics, Patient Safety, and Quality Infrastructure (Force 6)
	• Quality Improvement (Force 7)
	• Consultation and Resources (Force 8)
	• Autonomy (Force 9)
	• Nurses as Teachers (Force 11)
	• Interdisciplinary Relationships (Force 13)
New Knowledge, Innovations, and Improvements	• Quality of Care: Research and Evidence-Based Practice (Force 6)
	• Quality Improvement (Force 7)
Empirical Quality Outcomes	• Quality of Care (Force 6)

Reprinted with permission of the American Nurses Credentialing Center: *Application manual Magnet Recognition Program,* Silver Spring, MD, 2008, ANA.

Armstrong, Laschinger, and Wong, 2009; Wade et al, 2008). Magnet status is now seen as the single most effective mechanism for providing consumers and nurses with comparative information, the gold standard for quality nursing care. Nurses advocating for a strong workplace should advocate for their hospital to achieve Magnet status.

Pathway to Excellence Hospitals. In 2003 the Texas Nurses Association (TNA) began work to positively affect nurse retention by improving the workplace for nurses and established the Texas Nurse-Friendly Program for Small/Rural Hospitals. The program was partially funded with a 5-year grant from the HRSA. The goal of this program was to improve both the quality of patient care and professional satisfaction of nurses working in small and rural hospitals in Texas. To be responsive to a national market for this program, TNA sold the rights to the Nurse-Friendly Program to the ANCC in 2006, and it has undergone revision to meet national criteria. The Pathway to Excellence recognition is earned by health care organizations that create work environments where nurses can flourish. The award substantiates the professional satisfaction of nurses and identifies best places to work. As this program matures, research focused on nursing and patient outcomes will demonstrate the value of an improved work environment.

Aging Workforce and Retention

As the nation works to increase the supply of professional nurses through education, strategies must be developed to retain the older, expert professional nurse within the nursing workforce. The following statistics detail the extent of the aging workforce issue (HRSA, 2006):
   ♦ In 2004 the national average age of professional nurses was 46.8 years.
   ♦ In 2004 RNs younger than 30 years of age represented only 8% of the total nurse population.
   ♦ Professional nurses older than the age of 40 represent nearly 60% of the workforce with 25% older than 54 years.

There has been little research to test the effectiveness of recruitment and retention strategies with older nurses. A review of the existing literature (Hatcher et al, 2006) identified four key themes that contribute to older nurses' decisions about continuing to work: health status, financial status, attitude toward retirement, and current job satisfaction. The study's authors also interviewed seasoned nurses to determine what changes are needed to make nursing attractive to and supportive of older nurses. Findings included (Hatcher et al, 2006):

◆ Revised employment policies with greater flexibility in scheduling, innovative new nursing positions, such as mentor, research assistant, or safety officer, and smoother transitions into management.

◆ Better ergonomics and health care design to decrease the time nurses spend walking and reduce the physical demands of their work with aids such as mechanical lifts, decentralized supply storage, and better lighting at the bedside.

◆ Improved introduction to technology with adequate training and input of experienced nurses in the choice of technology purchases and outfitting equipment with features, such as larger fonts.

◆ Changes in organizational culture as nurses seek greater autonomy and participation in decision making. "Nurses are tired of doing a difficult job under stressful conditions and of not having their contributions acknowledged," the report states.

◆ Commitment to training and education for older nurses who view ongoing learning as especially critical to retain senior nurses promoted to managerial or other innovative positions that require new skills.

Although many organizations have added on-site day and sick care for children of younger nurses, organizations may need to consider adding adult daycare to assist older nurses who are caring for aging parents. Creative staffing plans with shorter shifts and identified respite periods may help extend the work life of aging nurses. Technology has provided many workplace accessories that reduce the physical demands on nurses that can result in injury or stress, especially to aging nurses. ANA's Handle With Care campaign aims at eliminating lifting in the hospital environment by using technology and assistive devices to do the heavy work (ANA, 2009a). Ergonomic issues are important for staff of any age, but additional attention is needed as the workforce ages. Organizations that strategically plan for an aging workforce will be best positioned to deliver quality health care to their customers.

Emerging Workforce Recruitment and Retention

In addition to planning for retention of an aging workforce, health care is challenged to become the employer of choice for the younger emerging workforce. The younger generation, born between 1969 and 1985, presents unique problems for the health care environment. Tulgan (2007) has written extensively about the work and management expectations of today's young worker who expects balance and perspective in the workplace. Elena, the young nurse described at the beginning of the chapter, will be searching for opportunities to gain advanced training, education, and certification as she seeks to make herself more marketable in her professional nursing role. She expects feedback on her performance to help refine her skills and build her confidence. She also expects her manager to take a personal interest in her, to know her name, and to help her build a competitive portfolio. Many managers are unaware of these expectations in emerging workforce employees and contribute to their hastened exit from the workplace by not attending to their personal and career needs.

Foreign Nurse Recruitment

For several decades the United States has regularly imported nurses to ease its nurse shortages. From 2002 to 2006, the number of full time equivalent (FTE) positions filled by foreign-born RNs working in the United States increased rapidly, growing by 93,000 (Buerhaus et al, 2009). In 1994 foreign-born RNs comprised 9% of the U.S. FTE RN workforce and grew to 15% of the FTE workforce by 2006. The Philippines has dominated the nurse migration pipeline to the United States and to other recruiting countries. In 2007 the top-five countries from which foreign-educated nurses came to the United States were: Philippines 57.2%, India 20.9%, South Korea 17%, Canada 3.6%, and the United Kingdom 1.3% (Commission for Graduates of Foreign Nursing Schools, 2008).

Relying on the recruitment of foreign nurse graduates as a method of resolving the U.S. nursing shortage is particularly problematic for two reasons. First, the current shortage is worldwide; therefore, recruitment of foreign nurses results in an intensified shortage in the country from which the nurses were recruited. As more industrialized countries rely on the importation of foreign nurses to meet their health care needs, those resources are being depleted in underdeveloped countries. Second, foreign nurse recruitment is open to abuse because of rules surrounding the granting of visas and the foreign nurses' vulnerable status, limited social support, and language challenges. Any indication that foreign nurses are being deprived of their rights or unfairly treated in compensation or work requirements should be reported to the state nurses association. Monitoring of foreign nurses' employment falls under the authority of the U.S. Department of Labor.

In fall 2008, a collaborative of nursing organizations, health care organizations, educational and licensure bodies, and recruiters endorsed a *Code of Ethical Conduct for the Recruitment of Foreign Educated Nurses* (ANA, 2008a). The Code provides voluntary guidelines that aim to ensure the growing practice of recruiting foreign-educated nurses is done in a responsible and transparent manner throughout the process of recruitment. It also provides guidance to health care organizations and recruiters on ways to ensure recruitment is not harmful to source countries. This announcement was highlighted by an example of foreign nurse abuse that occurred earlier that year when ANA filed an amicus brief in New York supporting a motion to drop criminal charges against a group of Filipino RNs charged with patient endangerment after resigning their positions. The "Sentosa nurses," as they had come to be known, had been recruited by the Sentosa Recruitment Agency to work at specific nursing home facilities on Long Island. When they arrived in the United States, they discovered they actually were working for a staffing agency, and over a period of months, the nurses said the agency refused to pay them according to the terms of their contracts. They also said they were not properly trained for their new jobs and were required to care for more patients than they believed were safe. In January 2009, after a 3-year legal battle supported by ANA and the New York State Nurses Association, the New York Supreme Court Appellate Division ruled that the nurses could not be prosecuted for resigning their positions.

Nursing Salaries

Buerhaus and colleagues (2009) found that during the 1980s, professional nursing hourly wages increased by approximately 3% each year. Unfortunately during the 1990s nursing salaries remained flat—low compensation levels definitely contributed to the current nursing shortage. Salary compression has long plagued the nursing profession, with little opportunity for extended growth of salary as nurses gain more experience.

In the early 2000s, health care agencies moved to offer relocation bonuses and other financial and fringe benefits to attract nurses. Health care employers used sign-on bonuses of up to $30,000, increased recruitment of foreign nurses, offered new concessions in flexible scheduling, and developed a growing reliance on "traveling nurses" (May, Bazzoli, and Gerland, 2006). All of these mechanisms resulted in considerable expenditures by health care organizations. Many believed that these recruitment-related costs could be better spent by increasing basic compensation levels of professional nurses. As past shortages have abated, so has the offering of financial bonuses and differential pay scales.

A sharp increase in RN wages occurred in 2002 and 2003. This increase reflects the acceleration in the demand for RNs that occurred from 2001 to 2004, along with increasing collective bargaining activity and several labor strikes. In 2004 and 2005 the growth in real RN wages stopped, hospital RN employment subsequently decreased by more than 50,000 FTE RNs, and the RN vacancy rate increased to 8.5% (Buerhaus et al, 2009). In 2006 hospitals raised real RN wages slightly and vacancy rates dropped back to 8.1%, but hospitals still reported that 116,000 RN positions remained unfilled.

The hospital RN shortages of the 1960s, 1970s, 1980s, and early 1990s were transitory until wage increases brought the demand and supply of RNs into equilibrium; however, the current shortage began in hospital specialty units in 1998 and continues through today (Buerhaus et al, 2009). Workforce analysts believe that further wage increases will be needed to bring about a new equilibrium in the hospital RN labor market. However, the current nursing shortage is unique, and concerted additional efforts must be made to rectify the problem.

Work Environment

A number of studies in the late 1990s focused on the work environment as a significant contributor to the difficulty in recruiting and retaining RNs (Mercer, 1999; Nolan, Lundh, and Brown, 1999). One of the primary factors for the increasing nurse turnover rate was identified as workload and staffing patterns. Other issues identified as affecting the shortage and turnover were insufficient supply of qualified managers and experienced staff, increased market demand, and inappropriate staffing. The importance of addressing issues related to the work environment were clear—efforts at increasing the overall supply of nurses were unlikely to be successful if retention strategies were not developed. Health care employers have begun to direct their attention to improving the workplace. Nursing school enrollments are at capacity, and it is vitally important to retain nurses in an effort to boost overall supply. Although work environment issues persist, employers have begun to implement strategies to improve nurse retention.

Several national initiatives have been undertaken to promote positive and safe work environments for nurses. The Nursing Organizations Alliance, a coalition of more than 65 national nursing organizations, developed and presented its *Principles and Elements of a Healthful Practice/Work Environment* (Nursing Organizations Alliance, 2004) (Box 12-5), which provides a framework for organizations to improve nurses' work environments. The Center for American Nurses (2009) adopted a position statement on restructuring and redesigning nurses' work environments. The statement cites a number of recommendations for improving the environment including additional research related to technology solutions for safe patient handling, nurses as full partners in work redesign, and education regarding evidence-based practice of ergonomics. It has been noted "if the staffing levels and work environments are not safe for the nurses, they will not be safe for the patients" (Joint Commission on Accreditation of Healthcare Organizations, 2002, p.12). Improving the design of the individual nurse's work can increase satisfaction with the professional role, in addition to improving patient outcomes and cost of care (Stichler and Ecoff, 2009).

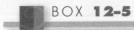

BOX **12-5**

Principles and Elements of a Healthful Practice/Work Environment

The Nursing Organizations Alliance believes that a healthful practice and work environment is supported by the presence of the following elements:

1. Collaborative practice culture
   - Respectful collegial communication and behavior
   - Team orientation
   - Presence of trust
   - Respect for diversity
2. Communication-rich culture
   - Clear and respectful
   - Open and trusting
3. A culture of accountability
   - Role expectations are clearly defined
   - Everyone is accountable
4. The presence of adequate numbers of qualified nurses
   - Ability to provide quality care to meet client's or patient's needs
   - Work and home life balance
5. The presence of expert, competent, credible, visible leadership
   - Serves as an advocate for nursing practice
   - Supports shared decision making
   - Allocates resources to support nursing

6. Shared decision making at all levels
   - Nurses participate in system, organizational, and process decisions
   - Formal structure exists to support shared decision making
   - Nurses have control over their practice
7. The encouragement of professional practice and continued growth and development
   - Continuing education and certification are supported and encouraged
   - Participation in professional association is encouraged
   - An information-rich environment is supported
8. Recognition of the value of nursing's contributions
   - Reward and pay for performance
   - Career mobility and expansion
9. Recognition by nurses for their meaningful contribution to practice

These nine elements will be fostered and promoted, as best fits, into the work of individual member organizations of the alliance, 2004.

Nursing Organizations Alliance: *Principles and elements of a healthful practice work/environment*, 2004. Available at: www.nursing-alliance.org.

APPROPRIATE STAFFING AND MANDATORY OVERTIME

Inappropriate staffing levels and use of mandatory overtime are two major contributing factors to dissatisfaction within the workplace. A landmark study by Aiken and colleagues (2002) found that in hospitals with fewer nurses per patient, surgical patients were more likely to experience higher death rates from failure to rescue (insufficient nursing care) and death from complications. The same study also found that nurses working in institutions plagued by insufficient staffing and workforce shortages were more likely to experience emotional exhaustion and greater job dissatisfaction. Subsequent research has reinforced the importance of appropriate nurse staffing and positive patient outcomes. However, many questions still exist about how to quantify appropriate staffing and how to appropriately use unlicensed personnel to assist in the delivery of care to patient populations who are more acutely ill, who require high-tech care, and whose lengths of stay are being reduced to keep costs in check.

Floating and Mandatory Overtime

By the late 1990s an emerging shortage of professional nurses further complicated staffing levels. The shortage resulted in (1) professional nurses being required to "float" to other patient care units for which they had little or no orientation, experience, or support and (2) the implementation of mandatory overtime and/or mandatory on-call requirements by some employers. The practice of requiring nurses to work mandatory overtime spread across the United States

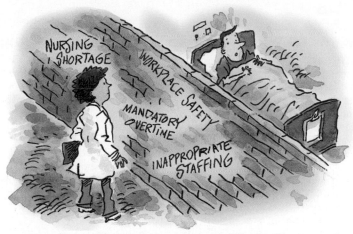

Professional nurses are struggling to deliver patient care against all kinds of barriers and with dwindling resources.

in the year 2000. In studies of mandatory overtime in other industries, the U.S. Department of Labor found that increasing scheduled work time increased time lost to absenteeism and increased injuries, and it usually required 3 hours of work to produce an additional 2 hours of productivity. In the health care sector, in-hospital deaths declined when the schedules of medical residents in teaching hospitals were reduced in the face of public outcry related to care from exhausted residents (Osterweil, 2007).

Nurses believe that employers' ability to mandate last-minute overtime or to use peer pressure as a negative motivator relieves the employers' sense of urgency to find safer and more appropriate staffing. Although nurses are fully cognizant and concerned about inadequate staffing, they are also resentful that they bear the personal, professional, and legal burden for this problem that is in large part a direct result of earlier changes in skill mix and care delivery models made acceptable by national imperatives to work swiftly to reduce the cost of health care (ANA, 2009b; Robert Wood Johnson Foundation [RWJF], 2007). By the late 1990s many nurses began to unite to push mandatory overtime and inadequate staffing issues to the forefront through workforce advocacy mechanisms. RN surveys suggest that these efforts are yielding results: from 2002 to 2006 the percentage of RNs who perceived that overtime was strictly voluntary increased significantly from 46% in 2002 to 55% in 2006, whereas significantly fewer RNs perceived that overtime was required in the hospitals where they worked—21% in 2002 and 14% in 2006 (Buerhaus et al, 2009).

Advocating for Safe Staffing

Many nurses across the country are concerned about the inadequacies of staffing to meet patient care needs. Before accepting a position with an organization, professional nurses should ask the questions identified in Box 12-6 regarding safe staffing. Resources to help professional nurse decision making relative to adequate staffing and mandatory overtime are included in Box 12-7.

The immediate concern for most nurses in a staffing conflict is whether to accept an assignment. Often this comes down to a disagreement between the nurse manager making the assignment and the staff nurse asked to accept the assignment. Box 12-8 identifies questions to help the staff nurse in making a decision to accept an assignment. These questions are designed to

BOX **12-6**

Questions to Ask About Safe Staffing Before Accepting Employment

1. Who is the chief nursing officer, to whom does she or he report, and does she or he have authority over staffing?
2. Who controls the staffing budget?
3. Is the level of staffing an active and ongoing discussion in the organization, and do staff nurses have input?
4. Does the organization have a shared governance model?
5. When, where, and how is staffing input obtained from staff nurses?
6. How do ratios in the organization compare with recommendations of national and regional organizations, such as the American Organization of Nurse Executives and the American Association of Critical-Care Nurses?
7. What is the content and length of orientation for new nurses?
8. What is the philosophy regarding staff mix designations?
9. What is the frequency of floating to other nursing units?
10. What are the criteria used by the organization in determining competency of cross-trained staff?
11. What resources does the organization use to supplement staff during peak census?
12. If concerns arise about the adequacy of staffing, where and to whom is it appropriate to voice those concerns?
13. How are overtime, on-call time, and cancellation of regularly scheduled shifts handled?
14. Does the organization mandate overtime? If so can the staff nurse refuse to participate without repercussions?
15. What is the turnover rate, and what is the average longevity of staff nurses?
16. What opportunities for advancement exist in the organization, such as clinical ladders or other systems of recognition?
17. Where does the organization expect discussions about staffing or practice issues to take place?
18. Is there a conflict resolution process in place?

Center for American Nurses: Questions to ask about safe staffing before accepting employment. Adapted from the Texas Nurses Association: *Nurse staffing task force document.* Available at www.centerforamericannurses.org (Resources/Workforce Advocacy).

BOX **12-7**

Resources for Decision Making Related to Adequacy of Staffing and Mandatory Overtime

GUIDEBOOKS
- *Utilization Guide for the ANA Principles for Nurse Staffing*—This guidebook will direct RNs on how to determine the level of nurse staffing for any setting. It focuses on patient acuity systems, the basics of workload measurement, patient classification, unlicensed assistive personnel, the role of professional judgment, and the development of principles.
- *Principles for Delegation*—This guidebook provides the principles and guidelines for delegation of tasks to others. Its purpose is to define relevant principles and provide RNs with practice strategies when delegating patient care to nursing assistive personnel. It also covers needed definitions and the essentials of care provision and related nurse education.
- *Principles for Documentation*—This guidebook focuses on managing the increasingly complex requirements of documenting patient care activities in both paper and electronic formats.

These three documents are available as a Principles for Practice set at www.nursesbooks.org.

BOX **12-7**

Resources for Decision Making Related to Adequacy of Staffing and Mandatory Overtime—cont'd

OTHER RESOURCES
ANA's Safe Staffing Saves Lives campaign
  www.safestaffingsaveslives.org
ANA's Position Statements Regarding Workplace Advocacy
  http://nursingworld.org/MainMenuCategories/HealthcareandPolicyIssues/ANAPositionStatements/
  workplac.aspx
Nursing Quality Indicators: Definitions and Implications
  www.nursesbooks.org
  http://nursingworld.org/quality
State Nurses Association
ANA's Constituent Member Associations
  www.nursingworld.org

BOX **12-8**

Questions to Ask in Making the Decision to Accept a Staffing Assignment

1. *What is the assignment?*
   Clarify the assignment. Do not assume. Be certain that what you believe is the assignment is indeed correct.
2. *What are the characteristics of the patients being assigned?*
   Do not just respond to the number of patients; make a critical assessment of the needs of each patient, his or her age, condition, other factors that contribute to special needs, and the resources available to meet those needs. Who else is on the unit or within the facility that might be a resource for the assignment? Do nurses on the unit have access to those resources? How stable are the patients, and how long have they been stable? Do any patients have communication and/or physical limitations that will require accommodation and extra supervision during the shift? Will there be discharges to offset the load? If there are discharges, will there be admissions, which require extra time and energy?
3. *Do I have the expertise to care for the patients?*
   Am I familiar with caring for the types of patients assigned? If this is a float assignment, am I cross-trained to care for these patients? Is there a buddy system in place with staff who are familiar with the unit? If there is no cross-training or buddy system, has the patient load been modified accordingly?
4. *Do I have the experience and knowledge to manage the patients for whom I am being assigned care?*
   If the answer to this question is no, you have an obligation to articulate limitations. Limitations in experience and knowledge may not require refusal of the assignment but rather an agreement regarding supervision or a modification of the assignment to ensure patient safety. If no accommodation for limitations is considered, the nurse has an obligation to refuse an assignment for which she or he lacks education or experience.
5. *What is the geography of the assignment?*
   Am I being asked to care for patients who are in proximity for efficient management, or are the patients at opposite ends of the hall or on different units? If there are geographic difficulties, what resources are available to manage the situation? If my patients are on more than one unit and I must go to another unit to provide care, who will monitor patients out of my immediate attention?

Continued

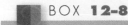

BOX **12-8**

Questions to Ask in Making the Decision to Accept a Staffing Assignment—cont'd

6. *Is this a temporary assignment?*

    When other staff are located to assist, will I be relieved? If the assignment is temporary it may be possible to accept a difficult assignment, knowing that there will soon be reinforcements. Is there a pattern of short staffing, or is this truly an emergency?

7. *Is this a crisis or an ongoing staffing pattern?*

    If the assignment is being made because of an immediate need on the unit, a crisis, the decision to accept the assignment may be based on that immediate need. However, if the staffing pattern is an ongoing problem, the nurse has the obligation to identify unmet standards of care that are occurring as a result of ongoing staffing inadequacies. This may result in a request for "safe harbor" and/or peer review.

8. *Can I take the assignment in good faith? (If not you will need to get the assignment modified or refuse the assignment.)*

    Consult your individual state's nurse practice act regarding clarification of accepting an assignment in good faith. In understanding good faith it is sometimes easier to identify what would constitute bad faith. For example, if you had not taken care of pediatric patients since nursing school and you were asked to take charge of a pediatric unit, unless this were an extreme emergency, such as a disaster (in which case you would need to let people know your limitations, but you might still be the best person, given all factors for the assignment), it would be bad faith to take the assignment. It is always your responsibility to articulate your limitations and to get an adjustment to the assignment that acknowledges the limitations you have articulated. Good faith acceptance of the assignment means that you are concerned about the situation and believe that a different pattern of care or policy should be considered. However, you acknowledge the difference of opinion on the subject between you and your supervisor and are willing to take the assignment and await the judgment of other peers and supervisors.

Center for American Nurses: *Questions to ask in making the decision to accept a staffing assignment.* Adapted from the Texas Nurses Association: Workplace advocacy program. Available at: www.centerforamericannurses.org (Resources/Workforce Advocacy).

help the staff nurse think critically about the assignment so that if there is a problem, the nurse can be clear in telling the manager what makes her or him uncomfortable with the assignment.

Mandatory overtime and adequate staffing levels have become a legislative issue at the national and state levels of government (ANA, 2009b). As of 2009, 15 states placed restrictions on the use of mandatory overtime for nurses: 13 states enacted legislation (CT, IL, MD, MN, NJ, NH, NY, OR, PA, RI, TX, WA, WV), and 2 states have provisions in regulations (CA, MO) (ANA, 2009b). A variety of federal legislation also has been proposed to prohibit the requirement that a nurse work more than 12 hours in a 24-hour period and 80 hours in a consecutive 14-day period, except under certain circumstances.

Federal regulations require hospitals to "have adequate numbers of licensed registered nurses, licensed practical [vocational] nurses, and other personnel to provide nursing care to all patients as needed" (Department of Health and Human Services, 2009, p. 517). With such nebulous language, it has been left to the states to ensure that staffing is appropriate to meet patients' needs safely. Three models of staffing are informing policymakers in the current environment: fixed minimum ratios, patient classification systems, and pay-for-performance (RWJF, 2007). In 1999 California became the first state to enact fixed minimum ratios legislation requiring hospitals to meet minimal staffing standards, limiting the numbers of patients that RNs and licensed vocational nurses (LVNs—known in most other states as licensed practical nurses, or LPNs) may care for at any one time. Under the California rules initiated in 2005 and fully implemented in 2008, one nurse will not care for more than five patients in medical-surgical units, in addition to one nurse per four patients in specialty care and telemetry units and one nurse per three patients in step-down units. Years after California's nurse staffing law was signed, there is no clear picture of the policy's effectiveness because no provision was included for evaluation (RWJF, 2007). Results from a 2009 study showed that although the legislation increased the use of RNs, the ratios had no clear effect on nursing-sensitive quality measures that affect quality patient care (California Healthcare Foundation, 2009).

Other states have implemented strategies focused on patient classification systems or nurse staffing plans to address patients' and nurses' concerns about safe staffing. Nurse staffing plans require direct-care nurses have input into a plan to ensure safe nurse-to-patient ratios based on patient need and other influencing criteria (e.g., nursing skill mix, ancillary support staff). ANA endorses this approach through its *Principles for Nurse Staffing*, which provides recommendations on appropriate staffing and require nurses to be an integral part of the nurse staffing plan development and decision-making process (ANA, 2009c). Texas, Oregon, and Washington focused on improving the work environment by incorporating the ANA staffing principles into state rules and regulations. These unique collaborative initiatives used the political and regulatory arenas to bring together historically competing groups (nurses and hospital administrators) to work toward a mutually acceptable policy initiative that actually increased nurses' ability to influence staffing in hospitals.

Another approach being debated in some state legislatures is that of requiring facilities to disclose staffing levels to the public and/or a regulatory body. Disclosure of staffing plans without evaluation and recourse for those that represent inadequate levels for safe, quality care would seem to be futile. It will be imperative for evaluation to occur as these new statues for nurse staffing plans are implemented. As of 2009, 13 states have enacted some type of legislation focused on nurse staffing plans.

A pay-for-performance (P4P) model has been proposed in recent years (RWJF, 2007). With the P4P concept, insurance companies and government health care programs would provide greater payments to hospitals that meet or exceed certain quality standards. Payments would be linked to outcomes, thus providing an incentive to boost staffing. Questions still surround the P4P model; however, it is receiving a good deal of attention in the health care policy arena.

Shared Governance as a Method of Advocating for Excellence in Nursing Practice

Introduced in the 1970s, shared governance has been identified by RNs as a key indicator of excellence in nursing practice (ANCC, 2008; Porter-O'Grady, 1987, 1991, 2003; Steinbinder, 2005). The concept of professional practice models, such as shared governance, has attracted the attention of nursing over the past 15 years in response to maintaining nursing job satisfaction, quality care, and fiscal viability. During the past two decades there has been proliferation of such models to redesign care delivery roles and systems and restructure the governance of professional nursing.

The importance of shared governance is that such models provide an organizational framework for nurses in direct care to become committed to nursing practice within their organizations. The implementation of such models allows nurses to have an active role in decision making by providing maximal participation and accountability for the outcomes of those decisions. Shared governance models render a structure and an environment that empowers staff

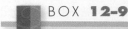

BOX **12-9**

Three Developmental Phases of Shared Governance

PHASE 1
- Staff nurse representatives—members of clinical forums, have authority for designated practice issues and some authority for determining roles, functions, and processes.
- Managers—members of management forums, responsible for facilitation of practice through resource management and allocation.
- Executive committee—administrative and staff membership, often in disproportionate numbers, accept recommendations from staff nurses and managers.
- Chief nurse executive—retains final decision-making authority.

PHASE 2
- Staff nurse representatives—members of nursing committees that are designated for specific management and/or clinical functions.
- Managers—serve on same committees with staff nurses.
- Committee chairs—appointed by chief nurse executive.
- Nursing cabinet—composed of multiple committee chairs that make final decisions on recommendations from the committees.

PHASE 3
- Staff nurse representatives—belong to councils with authority for specific functions.
- Council chairs—make up management committee charged with making all final operational decisions.

Adapted from Texas Nurses Association: *Workplace advocacy program,* Austin, 2001, TNA. Available online at www.texasnurses.org.

to make care decisions. Shared governance results in more than job satisfaction for nurses; it includes as equally important increased efficiency and better patient outcomes.

Shared governance of nursing services often develops in phases that offer organizations the opportunity to adjust to the changing roles and decision-making authority of nurses. Each phase provides greater autonomy to practicing nurses in determining practice policy. However, the structure allows nursing delivery decisions to be integrated with other policy needs of the organization. Box 12-9 provides an overview of potential developmental phases for shared governance. As a shared governance model is developed in the health care organization, it is important that it does not become isolated from other organizational problem-solving and policymaking bodies, such as quality improvement, ethics, and risk management.

Not all health care organizations place quality patient care at the top of their agenda; rather they focus more on bottom-line profits. In these situations, nurses may find themselves challenged to provide quality care. Therefore, it is important that nurses have access and input to the various organizational structures where decisions that affect the nurse and patient are made. Nurses need to be integral members of such organizational structures as quality improvement and ethics committees. Staff nurses need to know who their representatives are and how to access such committees. Box 12-10 identifies questions that should be asked about shared governance or participatory management models when nurses are trying to identify the organization that would be most conducive to the delivery of quality nursing care.

Nurses working under shared governance models should have access to conflict resolution procedures that define the processes they should follow if they are in disagreement with the organization. However, organizations without shared governance models may also have systems in place that could be of assistance. Examples of these are open-door policies, ombudsman programs, or dispute-resolution processes. When seeking dispute resolution, the nurse may

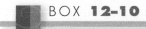

BOX **12-10**

Questions to Ask About Shared Governance Models

- Are nurses encouraged to participate in shared governance?
- How do nurses become involved in the shared governance process?
- What is the ratio of staff nurses to managers involved in shared governance within the organization?
- Is adequate work time allowed to participate in governance councils?
- How does the organization communicate shared governance decisions with staff nurses?
- How did shared governance improve nursing care delivery in the organization?
- Do nurses feel shared governance within their organization is beneficial to their practice?
- Does the organization have outcomes data related to shared governance?
- If so how have those data affected changes in nursing practice?

Adapted from Texas Nurses Association: *Workplace advocacy program*, Austin, 2001, TNA. Available online at www.texasnurses.org.

---

use a third party or resources internal to the organization to assist in the resolution. Some states have processes that can assist in resolving patient care or professional issues. These processes include peer review, safe harbor, and mandatory reporting.

PATIENT ADVOCACY AND SAFETY

Patient advocacy is a cornerstone of the nursing profession, and patients depend on nurses to ensure that they receive proper care. Although nurses have always advocated for their patients, it has only been during the past 30 years that the recognized role of the nurse as patient advocate has begun to clearly emerge. Today's health care systems have created an environment in which errors and adverse events are attributed to complex systems and complicated uses of technology. This complex environment demands that the nursing profession assert its powerful voice in the role of patient advocate by supporting public policies that protect consumers and enhance accountability for quality by promoting safer health care systems.

Patient Safety

The IOM's report, *To Err Is Human* (Kohn, Corrigan, and Donaldson, 2000), focused a great deal of attention on the issue of patient safety when it reported that between 44,000 and 98,000 patients die in U.S. hospitals each year from preventable medical errors. Subsequently, the IOM released its report, *Keeping Patients Safe: Transforming the Work Environment of Nurses* (Page, 2004), which examined patient safety from the perspective of the work environment in which nurses provide patient care. The report provided evidence of the critical role nurses have in the health care system and found that the typical work environment of nurses is characterized by many serious threats to patient safety. These threats were found in all four of the basic components of all organizations, including:

- **Leadership and management:** Frequent failure to follow management practices necessary for safety, leading to a loss of trust in administration by nurses, along with the reduction of clinical nursing leadership at multiple levels leading to a diminished voice for nurses
- **Workforce:** Unsafe workforce deployment as evidenced by a wide variation in nurse staffing levels across hospitals and nursing homes and a need for all health care professionals (nurses and physicians alike) to have better training and active involvement in interdisciplinary collaboration and teamwork

♦ **Work processes:** Unsafe work and workspace design including long work hours, insufficient technology to support tasks, such as medication administration, and undue time commitment to document patient information and care processes resulting in insufficient time for patient care

♦ **Organizational culture:** Punitive cultures that hinder the reporting and prevention of errors

The 2004 IOM report recommended that no single action can, by itself, keep patients safe from health care errors. It recommended defenses be created in all four of the above organizational components.

ANA's National Center for Nursing Quality (NCNQ) was created to address patient safety and quality in nursing care and nurses' work lives (ANA, 2009d). NCNQ advocates for nursing quality through quality measurement, novel research, and collaborative learning. The National Database for Nursing Quality Indicators (NDNQI), a program of NCNQ, is the only database containing data collected at the nursing unit level and allows for empirical linkages between nursing care and patient outcomes. Indicators such as patient falls, physical restraints, nosocomial infections, nursing care hours provided per patient day, and RN satisfaction surveys are used for quality improvement, reporting requirements (e.g., The Joint Commission [TJC], Magnet Recognition Program), staff retention efforts, budget allocation, and research.

An initiative called Transforming Care at the Bedside (TCAB) was begun in 2003 as a joint effort between the Robert Wood Johnson Foundation (RWJF) and the Institute for Healthcare Improvement (IHI) to create a framework for change on hospital medical/surgical units by engaging front-line nurses and leaders to (RWJF, 2008):

♦ Improve the quality and safety of patient care
♦ Increase the vitality and retention of nurses
♦ Engage and improve the patient's and family members' experience of care
♦ Improve the effectiveness of the entire care team

After an initial pilot project, the TCAB initiative is being implemented in scores of hospitals across the country to test new concepts, develop exemplary care models, and demonstrate institutional commitment and resources to support and sustain these innovations. Ideas for transforming the way care is delivered come from the nurses and other health care team members who are engaged in direct patient care. These teams identify where change is needed, suggest and test potential solutions, and decide whether those innovations should be implemented.

Another issue that contributes to patient safety is interaction among health professionals. In an alert posted in 2008, TJC warned that rude interactions among health care professionals threaten patient safety. The alert stated: "Intimidating and disruptive behaviors can foster medical errors, contribute to poor patient satisfaction and to preventable adverse outcomes, increase the cost of care, and cause qualified clinicians, administrators and managers to seek new positions in more professional environments. Safety and quality of patient care is dependent on teamwork, communication, and a collaborative work environment. To ensure quality and to promote a culture of safety, health care organizations must address the problem of behaviors that threaten the performance of the health care team" (TJC, 2008, para. 1).

Although efforts to address and improve patient safety are significant, there is still much work to be done. In early 2009 Secretary of Health and Human Services Kathleen Sebelius reported that some safety measures have worsened with a substantial number of Americans not receiving recommended care (Agency for Healthcare Research and Quality [AHRQ], 2009). Secretary Sebelius noted that patient safety has declined in part because of the rise in health care–associated infections (HAIs), infections that patients acquire during the course of their stay in a health care setting such as a nursing home or a hospital. HAIs are among the top 10 leading causes of death in the United States, and drive up the cost of health care by up to $20 billion per year.

Whistle-Blower Protection

Nurses want the assurance that if they are acting within the scope of their practice, they will be able to speak up for their patients through appropriate channels without fear of retaliation. Whistle-blower legislation has been advocated for at the federal level and has actually passed in some states (ANA, 2009b). Whistle-blower protection basically prohibits health care organizations from retaliating against nurses when the professional nurse in good faith discloses information or participates in agency investigations. Specifically, whistle-blower protection protects nurses who speak out about unsafe situations from being fired or subjected to other disciplinary actions by their employers.

An example of how whistle-blower protection promotes workplace advocacy is illustrated by a case in Texas. A Texas jury awarded a nurse formerly employed by a large health science center $810,000 in her lawsuit filed under the Texas Whistle-Blower Act. She witnessed patients, who in her assessment were not in imminent danger of death, having their rights to informed consent disregarded. Patients refusing treatment were treated despite their protests to physicians. This nurse sought counsel from her state nurses association and, based on their recommendations, documented her concerns about these incidents according to the hospital's policies and tried to work within the system to stop what she believed to be serious patient rights violations. The nurse further protected herself by documenting her interactions with those who were retaliating against her for speaking out and reported the situation to the state board of nurse examiners, the Texas Department of Health, and the local police department. She was eventually terminated by the employing hospital. However, the jury found that she acted in accordance with the state nurse practice act in reporting her concerns about patient care practices and upheld her suit for defamation and wrongful termination. Box 12-11 provides an overview of things to know about whistle-blowing. Nurses should check with their state nurses association to assess the status of whistle-blower protection in their state.

WORKPLACE SAFETY

Nurses are battling to provide safe, quality care for patients in an environment that is becoming increasingly dangerous. The occupational safety and health of nurses continue to be ongoing concerns for individual nurses as well as professional nursing associations. Workplace injuries for all industries cost Americans annually $175.3 billion, with 4689 workplace fatalities caused by unintentional injuries and 3.5 million disabling injuries (National Safety Council, 2007). Rates of occupational injury to health care workers have risen over the past decade. By contrast two of the most hazardous industries, agriculture and construction, are safer today than they were a decade ago (National Institute for Occupational Safety and Health [NIOSH], 2008). Box 12-12 describes categories of health hazards in the health care workplace.

Exposure to Bloodborne Pathogens

Nurses and other health care professionals are at major risk for exposure to bloodborne diseases including hepatitis B, hepatitis C, and human immunodeficiency virus–acquired immunodeficiency syndrome (HIV-AIDS). In 1991 the Occupational Safety and Health Administration (OSHA, 2009) issued the bloodborne pathogens standard to protect health care workers from this risk. In 2000 the Needlestick Safety and Prevention Act passed at the federal level

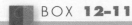

BOX **12-11**

Things to Know About Whistle-Blowing

- If you identify an illegal or unethical practice, reserve judgment until you have adequate documentation to establish wrongdoing.
- Do not expect those that are engaged in unethical or illegal conduct to welcome your questions or concerns about this practice.
- Seek the counsel of someone you trust outside of the situation to provide you with an objective perspective.
- Consult with your state nurses association or legal counsel if possible before taking action to determine how best to document your concerns.
- Remember that you are not protected in a whistle-blower situation from retaliation by your employer until you blow the whistle.
- Blowing the whistle means that you report your concern to the national and/or state agency responsible for regulation of the organization for which you work or, in the case of criminal activity, to law enforcement agencies as well.
- Private groups, such as The Joint Commission or the National Committee for Quality Assurance, do not confer protection. You must report to a state or national regulator.
- Although it is not required by every regulatory agency, it is a good rule of thumb to put your complaint in writing.
- Document all interactions related to the whistle-blowing situation and keep copies for your personal file.
- Keep documentation and interactions objective.
- Remain calm and do not lose your temper, even if those who learn of your actions attempt to provoke you.
- Remember that blowing the whistle is a very serious matter. Do not blow the whistle frivolously. Make sure you have the facts straight before taking action.

Center for American Nurses: Things to know about whistle-blowing. Adapted from Tabone S: 2000 Update: foreign nurse recruitment, *Texas Nurs* 74(8):9, 15, 2000. Available at www.centerforamericannurses.org (Resources/Workforce Advocacy).

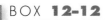

BOX **12-12**

Categories of Health Hazards in the Health Care Workplace

BIOLOGIC HAZARDS
Bacteria, viruses, fungi, or parasites that may be transmitted by contact with infected patients or contaminated body secretions or fluids (e.g., human immunodeficiency virus, hepatitis B and C, tuberculosis, and varicella)

CHEMICAL HAZARDS
Medications, solutions, gases (such as ethylene oxide, formaldehyde, glutaraldehyde, waste anesthetic and laser gases), cytotoxic agents, pentamidine, latex, PVC plastics, di(2-ethylhexyl) phthalate (DEHP), mercury

ERGONOMIC HAZARDS
Musculoskeletal injury to the back and extremities resulting from lifting, standing for long periods, and repeated hand motions

PSYCHOLOGIC HAZARDS
Stress, shiftwork, mandatory overtime, verbal abuse by patients and other health care providers

PHYSICAL HAZARDS
Radiation, lasers, noise, electricity, violence

Adapted from National Institute for Occupational Safety and Health, Centers for Disease Control and Prevention: *NIOSH safety and health topic: health care workers.* 2007. Available at: www.cdc.gov/niosh/topics/healthcare.

to require the use of safer needle devices to protect from sharps injuries (ANA, 2009e). The law requires employers to solicit the input of nonmanagerial employees responsible for direct patient care who are potentially exposed to sharps injuries in the identification, evaluation, and selection of effective engineering and work-practice controls. This law also requires employers to maintain a sharps injury log to contain, at a minimum, the brand of device involved in the incident, the department or work area where the exposure incident occurred, and an explanation of how the incident occurred. A 2008 study of nurses views on workplace safety and needlestick injuries (ANA, 2008b) revealed that needlestick injuries and bloodborne infections remain major concerns for nearly two thirds (64%) of nurses. The research also highlighted that safety concerns influence the decisions made by the vast majority of nurses (87%) about the type of nursing they do and that nearly two thirds of nurses (64%) have been accidentally stuck by a needle while working.

Ergonomic Injuries

Although nurses have suffered from back and other musculoskeletal disorders (MSDs) for decades, it is only during the past few years that these injuries are directly attributed to the workplace. Strong data demonstrate the problem of overexertion injuries in hospitals, nursing homes, and home care settings over the past decade. Nursing is ranked second after industrial work for physical workload intensity. Nurse aides, orderlies, and attendants reported the highest incidence of MSDs requiring days away from work in 2006 (ANA, 2009a). This group was ranked second in overall MSDs requiring days away from work, with RNs ranked fifth. The extent of MSDs among the U.S. nursing workforce is distressing when considered in light of the current nursing shortage. It is estimated that 12% of nurses leave the profession annually due to back injuries and greater than 52% complain of chronic back pain. Two decades of research have demonstrated that use of a single approach (i.e., engineering controls, administrative changes, or worker training) to reduce the incidence of MSDs has been ineffective. There has been a shift toward evidence-based practices such as a program within a facility that creates no-lift policies, secures appropriate patient handling equipment and lifts, and trains staff on usage, with a comprehensive tracking system of MSD injuries that includes ongoing evaluation of the program. ANA's Handle With Care campaign (2009a) supports safer practices with regards to patient handling. A number of states have enacted legislation to support the development of safe patient handling and movement programs. The campaign also seeks to reshape nursing education and federal and state ergonomics policies by highlighting the ways technology-oriented safe-patient handling benefits patients and the nursing workforce.

Many nurses find themselves suffering from workplace injuries, which they are reluctant to report because of perceived potential negative consequences to their employment status. Reporting a work-related injury or illness is not always easy. In past surveys nurses and other employees have indicated they did not report injuries that occurred on the job due to fear of repercussions such as disciplinary action, stigmatization as a complainer, harassment, denial of opportunities for promotion, and even termination of employment (U.S. House of Representatives, 2008).

Every organization should have specific policies concerning reporting of workplace injuries and illness. The ANA provides a number of resources and information concerning nurses' health and safety rights. The U.S. Department of Labor—OSHA's record keeping standard—requires employers to keep a log of workplace injuries and to keep the OSHA 300 Log available to employees and their representatives. The OSHA standard also prevents discrimination against employees who report a work-related injury, illness, or fatality.

Workplace Violence

Workplace violence has become a major societal issue. Its most extreme form, homicide, is the fourth-leading cause of fatal occupational injury in the United States with 564 workplace homicides in 2005 out of a total of 5702 fatal work injuries (OSHA, 2007). Among all American workers, health care workers have the highest rates of nonfatal assault injuries in the workplace (ANA, 2006). In the first national study of ED nurses and perceptions of workplace violence, investigators determined that violence against ED nurses is prevalent. More than 25% of nurses who responded to the survey reported experiencing physical violence more than 20 times in the past 3 years and almost 20% reported experiencing verbal abuse more than 200 times during the same period (Gacki-Smith et al, 2009).

Nurses in all settings must proactively advocate for safe workplaces. Workplace violence prevention programs should create a zero tolerance for workplace violence, verbal and nonverbal threats, and related actions; ensure that no employee who reports or experiences workplace violence faces reprisals; have detailed record keeping to assess risk and measure progress; develop a comprehensive plan for maintaining security in the workplace; and demonstrate management commitment and employee training. Nursing safety is imperative and includes adequate staffing levels, adequate staff training, and environmental safeguards.

Advocating for a Safer Workplace

The ANA has emerged as a leader in health care worker health and safety, working in collaboration with other nursing organizations, including the Center for American Nurses, American Association of Occupational Health Nurses, Association of periOperative Registered Nurses, the Emergency Nurses Association, and labor unions representing health care workers. These organizations advocate for administrative controls, such as adequate staffing, health and safety committees; engineering controls, such as ventilation and safer needlestick devices; and personal protective equipment, such as respirators and synthetic gloves that will prevent exposure to hazardous substances and/or prevent illness or injury from unavoidable exposure. Although the health care industry can be a dangerous place to work, many of the risks are avoidable and dangerous exposures preventable. Box 12-13 identifies resources available to improve the safety of the workplace for nurses as well as patients.

BOX **12-13**

Helpful Websites and Online Resources

American Nurses Association—Occupational Health and Safety
www.nursingworld.org/MainMenuCategories/OccupationalandEnvironmental/occupationalhealth.aspx
American Nurses Association—ANA's Principles of Environmental Health for Nursing Practice with Implementation Strategies
www.nursesbooks.org or 1-800-637-0323 to request publication 9781558102545
American Nurses Association—Safe Needles Save Lives Campaign
www.needlestick.org
American Nurses Association—Safe Staffing Saves Lives Campaign
www.safestaffingsaveslives.org
Center for American Nurses
www.centerforamericannurses.org

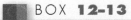

BOX **12-13**

Helpful Websites and Online Resources—cont'd

Citizens Advocacy Center—unique support program for public members who serve on health care regulatory boards and governing bodies as representatives of consumer interest
   www.cacenter.org
FDA MedWatch Program—report reactions to latex products and other chemical exposures
   www.fda.gov/medwatch/ or 1-888-INFO-FDA
Health Care Without Harm—publications list
   www.noharm.org (for educational brochures, click on library)
Hospitals for a Healthy Environment (H2E)—now a part of Practice GreenHealth, resources to facilitate sustainable/eco-friendly practices
   www.h2e-online.org
   www.practicegreenhealth.org
Information on mercury
   www.epa.gov/mercury
   www.nwf.org/mercury/housetour.cfm
Institute for Healthcare Improvement
   www.ihi.org
Johnson & Johnson Campaign for Nursing's Future
   www.discovernursing.com/
National Academy of Sciences—IOM reports
   www.nap.edu
National Institute for Occupational Safety and Health—databases/information resources
   www.cdc.gov/niosh/database.html
Nightingale Institute for Health and the Environment
   www.nihe.org
Nursing Organizations Alliance
   www.nursing-alliance.org/
U.S. Department of Labor, Occupational Safety and Health Administration   How to report a workplace injury or illness
   www.osha.gov/

SUMMARY

This chapter has covered a variety of significant workplace issues and identified workforce advocacy strategies for a nurse to use to improve the workplace environment and quality of patient care. A rapidly changing health care environment, significantly affected by an aging workforce and a nursing shortage, creates a challenge for all nurses. Nurses must be aware of the issues facing the profession and know where to seek assistance, information, and resources to address workplace issues. Working together with the resources of such organizations as the ANA, nurses can create a workplace that promotes career satisfaction and quality patient care.

ℯvolve Additional resources are available online at: http://evolve.elsevier.com/Cherry/

REFERENCES

Agency for Healthcare Research and Quality (AHRQ): *Secretary Sebelius highlights two new reports on health care quality, says improving quality is key component of health reform*. Retrieved May 2009 from: www.ahrq.gov/news/press/pr2009/qrdr08pr.htm.

Aiken L: Journey to excellence, *Reflect Nurs Leader* 31(1):16–19, 2005.

Aiken L, et al: Hospital nurse staffing and patient mortality, nurse burnout, and job dissatisfaction, *JAMA* 288(16):1987–1993, 2002.

Aiken L, et al: Effects of hospital care environment on patient mortality and nurse outcomes, *JONA* 39 (7/8 Suppl):S5–S14, 2009.

Aiken L, Havens D, Sloane D: The Magnet Nursing Services Recognition Program: a comparison of two groups of magnet hospitals, *Am J Nurs* 100(3):26–34, 2000.

Aiken L, et al: Transformative impact of Magnet designation: England case study, *J Clin Nurs* 17(24):3330–3337, 2008.

American Association of Colleges of Nursing (AACN): *Nursing faculty shortage fact sheet*, Washington, DC, 2009, AACN.

American Hospital Association (AHA): *New report details impact of economic downturn on patients and hospitals*, 2008. Retrieved May 2009 from: www.aha.org/aha/press-release/2008/081119-pr-econcrisis.html.

American Nurses Association (ANA): *Preventing workplace violence*, 2006. Retrieved May 2009 from: http://nursingworld.org/MainMenuCategories/Occupationaland Environmental/occupationalhealth/workplaceviolence/ANAResources/PreventingWorkplaceViolence.aspx.

American Nurses Association (ANA): *The American Nurses Association advances the prevention of unethical recruitment of foreign-educated nurses*, 2008a. Retrieved May 2009 from: www.nursingworld.org/FunctionalMenu Categories/MediaResources/PressReleases/2008PR/ANAAdvancesthePreventionofUnethicalRecruitmentofForeigneducatedNurses.aspx.

American Nurses Association (ANA): *Study of nurses' views on workplace safety and needlestick injuries*, 2008b. Retrieved May 2009 from: www.nursingworld.org/MainMenuCategories/OccupationalandEnvironmental/occupationalhealth/SafeNeedles/2008InviroStudy.aspx.

American Nurses Association (ANA): *Safe patient handling and movement*. 2009a. Retrieved May 2009 from: www.nursingworld.org/MainMenuCategories/ANAPolitical Power/State/StateLegislativeAgenda/SPHM.aspx.

American Nurses Association (ANA): *State governmental affairs program*, 2009b. Retrieved May 2009 from: www.nursingworld.org/gova.

American Nurses Association (ANA): *Nurse staffing plans and ratios*, 2009c. Retrieved May 2009 from: http://nursingworld.org/mainmenucategories/ANAPolitical Power/State/StateLegislativeAgenda/StaffingPlansand Ratios_1.aspx.

American Nurses Association (ANA): *Patient safety and nursing quality*, 2009d. Retrieved May 2009 from: www.nursingworld.org/MainMenuCategories/ThePracticeof ProfessionalNursing/PatientSafetyQuality.aspx.

American Nurses Association (ANA): *Safe needles save lives*, 2009e. Retrieved May 2009 from: http://nursingworld.org/MainMenuCategories/OccupationalandEnvironmental/occupationalhealth/SafeNeedles.aspx.

American Nurses Credentialing Center (ANCC): *Application manual for Magnet Recognition Program*, Silver Spring, MD, 2008, ANCC.

American Organization of Nurse Executives (AONE): *Practiceeducation partnerships for the future*, 2005. Retrieved May 2009 from: www.aone.org/aone/pdf/PracticeEducationPartnership0405.pdf.

Armstrong K, Laschinger H, Wong C: Workplace empowerment and Magnet hospital characteristics as predictors of patient safety climate, *J Nurs Care Qual* 24(1):55–62, 2009.

Buerhaus P: Current and future state of the US nursing workforce, *JAMA* 300(20):2422–2424, 2008.

Buerhaus P, Staiger D, Auerbach D: *The future of the nursing workforce in the United States: data, trends, and implications*, Sudbury, MA, 2009, Jones and Bartlett.

Buerhaus, et al: Trends in the experiences of hospital-employed registered nurses: results from three national surveys, *Nurs Econ* 25(2):55, 69–79, 80, 2007.

California Healthcare Foundation (CHF): *Assessing the impact of California's nurse staffing ratios on hospitals and patient care*, 2009. Retrieved May 2099 from: www.chcf.org/documents/hospitals/AssessingCANurse StaffingRatios.pdf.

Center for American Nurses: *Workforce advocacy resources*, 2009. Retrieved May 2009 from: www.can.affiniscape.com/displaycommon.cfm?an=1&subarticlenbr=257.

Cho SH, Hwang JH, Kim J: Nurse staffing and patient mortality in intensive care units, *Nurs Res* 57(5):322–330, 2008.

Commission for Graduates of Foreign Nursing Schools: *2007 Annual Report*, 2008. Retrieved May 2009 from: www.cgfns.org/files/pdf/annualreport/2007%20CGFNS%20Annual%20Report.pdf.

Gacki-Smith J, et al: Violence against nurses working in U.S. emergency departments, *JONA* 39(7/8):340–348, 2009.

Hatcher B, et al: *Wisdom at work: the importance of the older and experienced nurse in the workplace*, Princeton, NJ, 2006, Robert Wood Johnson Foundation, Retrieved May 2009 from: www.rwjf.org/files/publications/other/wisdomatwork.pdf.

Health Resources and Services Administration (HRSA): *Department of Health and Human Services: Preliminary findings: 2004 national sample survey of registered nurses*, 2006. Retrieved May 2009 from: http://bhpr.hrsa.gov/healthworkforce/rnsurvey04.

Johnson & Johnson: *Campaign for nursing's future*, 2009. Available at: www.jnj.com/community/contributions/programs/support.htm.

Kane RL, et al: The association of registered nurse staffing levels and patient outcomes: systematic review and meta-analysis, *Med Care* 45(12):1195–1204, 2007.

Kohn L, Corrigan J, Donaldson M: *To err is human: building a safer health system*, Institute of Medicine, Washington, DC, 2000, National Academy Press.

May UJ, Bazzoli G, Gerland A: Hospitals' responses to nurse staffing shortages, *Health Aff* 25(4):316–323, 2006.

McClure M, et al: *Magnet® hospitals: attraction and retention of professional nurses: American Academy of Nursing Task Force on Nursing Practice in Hospitals*, Kansas City, MO, 1983, American Nurses Association.

Mercer W: *Attracting and retaining registered nurses—survey results*, Chicago, 1999, William M Mercer.

Minnick A: Retirement, the nursing workforce, and the year 2005, *Nurs Outlook* 48:211–217, 2000.

National Institute for Occupational Safety and Health, Centers for Disease Control and Prevention: *NIOSH safety and health topic: health care workers*, 2008. Retrieved May 2009 from: www.cdc.gov/niosh/topics/healthcare.

National League for Nursing: *Demand for spots in nursing programs continues to dramatically outstrip supply*, 2009. Available at: www.nln.org/newsreleases/annual_survery_031609.htm.

National Quality Forum: *Nurses educational preparation and patient outcomes in acute care: a case for quality*, July, 2006. Retrieved September 2009 from: http://qualityforum.org/pdf/nursing-quality/FinalNursesEdPreparation.pdf.

National Safety Council: *Report on injuries in America*, 2007. Retrieved May 2009 from: www.nsc.org/lrs/injuriesinamerica08.aspx.

Needleman J, et al: Nurse staffing in hospitals: is there a business case for quality? *Health Aff* 25(1):71–79, 2006.

Nolan M, Lundh U, Brown J: Changing aspects of nurses' work environment: a comparison of perceptions in two hospitals in Sweden and the UK and implications for recruitment and retention of staff, *J Nurs Res* 4(3):221–233, 1999.

Nursing Organizations Alliance: *Principles and elements of a healthful practice work/environment*. 2004. Retrieved May 2009 from: www.nursing-alliance.org/about.cfm.

Occupational Safety and Health Administration: *Workplace violence*, 2007. Retrieved May 2009 from: www.osha.gov/SLTC/workplaceviolence/index.html.

Occupational Safety and Health Administration: *Bloodborne pathogens and needlestick prevention*, 2009. Retrieved May 2009 from: www.osha.gov/SLTC/bloodbornepathogens/index.html.

Osterweil N: Patients don't get short shrift from shorter shifts for residents, *MedPage Today*, June 12, 2007. Retrieved May 2009 from: www.medpagetoday.com/PublicHealthPolicy/HealthPolicy/5915.

Page A, editor: *Keeping patients safe: transforming the work environment of nurses*, Washington, DC, 2004, Institute of Medicine, National Academy Press.

Porter-O'Grady T: Shared governance and new organizational models, *Nurs Econ* 5(6):281–286, 1987.

Porter-O'Grady T: Shared governance for nursing, part II: putting the organization into action, *AORN J* 53(3):694–703, 1991.

Porter-O'Grady T: Researching shared governance: a futility of focus, *JONA* 33(4):251–252, 2003.

Robert Wood Johnson Foundation (RWJF): *Charting nursing's future*, 2007. Retrieved May 2009 from: www.rwjf.org/files/research/nursingissue5revfinal.pdf.

Robert Wood Johnson Foundation (RWJF): *Transforming care at thebeside (TCAB)*, 2008. Retrieved May 2009 from: www.rwjf.org/pr/product.jsp?id=30053.

Steinbinder A: The Magnet process: one appraiser's perspective, *Nurs Adm Q* 29(3):268–274, 2005.

Stichler JF, Ecoff L: Joint optimization: merging a new culture with a new physical environment, *J Nurs Adm* 39(4):156–159, 2009.

The Joint Commission: *Behaviors that undermine a culture of safety*, 2008. Retrieved May 2009 from: www.jointcommission.org/SentinelEvents/SentinelEventAlert/sea_40.htm.

The Joint Commission on Accreditation of Healthcare Organizations: *Health care at the crossroads: strategies for addressing the evolving nursing crisis*, Oakbrook Terrace, IL, 2002, JCAHO.

Thrall TH: The return of the RNs, *Hosp Health Netw* 83(4):22–24, 2009.

Tulgan B: *Managing the generation mix*, 2007. Retrieved May 2009 from: www.rainmakerthinking.com/pdf%20files/mix2007.pdf.

Unruh L: Nurse staffing and patient, nurse, and financial outcomes, *Am J Nurs* 108(1):67–71, 72, 2008.

U.S. Department of Health and Human Services, Centers for Medicare and Medicaid Services: *§482.23 Condition of participation: nursing services*. Retrieved May 2009. from: http://edocket.access.gpo.gov/cfr_2007/octqtr/pdf/42cfr482.23.pdf.

U.S. Department of Labor, Bureau of Labor Statistics: *Occupational outlook handbook*, 2008-2009. Retrieved May 2009 from: www.bls.gov/oco/ocos083.htm.

U.S. House of Representatives: *Hidden tragedy: underreporting of workplace injuries and illnesses*, 2008. Retrieved May 2009 from: http://edlabor.house.gov/publications/20080619WorkplaceInjuriesReport.pdf.

Wade G, et al: Influence of organizational characteristics and caring attributes of managers on nurses' job enjoyment, *J Adv Nurs* 64(4):344–353, 2008.

Yordy K: *Factors affecting the health workforce compendium: the nursing faculty shortage: a crisis for health care*, 2006. Retrieved May 2009 from: www.rwjf.org/files/publications/other/NursingFacultyShortage071006.pdf.

Collective Bargaining and Unions in Today's Workplace

Carolyn Roe, MSM, BSN
Barbara Cherry, DNSc, MBA, RN, NEA-BC

*e*volve   Additional resources are available online at: http://evolve.elsevier.com/Cherry/

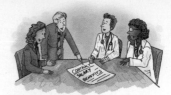

Collective bargaining is a method for achieving power-sharing in the workplace.

VIGNETTE

Addison Mitchell graduated in June from nursing school. She passed the NCLEX® examination and can now call herself a registered nurse (RN). As she drives to the hospital on the first day of her new job, she is feeling a sense of pride and joy, mixed with sheer fright, as she realizes that this is the world-class place she has chosen for her first job. She had always dreamed of working at this hospital. It was the hospital she always heard about from her family and the one that the press always headed to when a local comment on health care events was needed as background for a news story. She would now have a chance to become a seasoned nurse at one of the finest hospitals in the country.

Addison is realistic enough to know that her feelings of joy may not last, but she is unaware that she is on the verge of walking into a battleground. As she enters the drive leading to the hospital parking area, there are picketers shouting about unfair working conditions and patient deaths. Signs tell of cruelty to nurses. As Addison walks to the building, with her new name tag that reads "Registered Nurse," she is approached by a person asking her to sign a card. Addison states, "I'm sorry. I'm new here. I need to get my feet on the ground, then I will be happy to talk to you about the card." Addison begins to feel very anxious because she does not have a good understanding of union organizing efforts or the issues the nurses at the hospital are facing.

Addison does not yet know that she will be approached many times in the coming days by coworkers who will tell her how she should feel and what she should do. She has much to consider before making a decision between two alternatives that she does not fully understand.

■ QUESTIONS TO CONSIDER WHILE READING THIS CHAPTER:

1 What questions should the nurse ask about collective bargaining and labor relations?

2 What does signing a card mean and what questions should Addison ask before signing?

3 How can Addison establish good relationships with both nurse managers and staff nurses in an atmosphere in which collective bargaining has put these two groups in adversarial positions?

4 What skills and information will Addison need to navigate and make effective decisions in this hospital?

5 What provisions in a union contract are in a patient's best interest as well as a nurse's?

6 What resources are available to Addison to help her learn more about labor and management issues occurring in the hospital?

We thank Corinne Grimes, DNSc, RN for her contribution to this chapter in the first edition.

KEY TERMS

Arbitration The process of negotiation sanctioned in the United States by the National Labor Relations Board. It is the method used for formal talks between management and labor within modern business, industry, or service organizations. Binding arbitration means that all parties must obey the arbitrator's recommendations.

Collective bargaining The process whereby workers organize under the representation of a union in order to share a degree of power with management to determine selected aspects of the conditions of employment.

Grievance A term associated with a negative workplace event that results in an allegation by an employee that he or she has not been treated fairly and equitably. Grievances can occur in union and nonunion settings. In a union setting, a grievance generally arises when two parties, such as an employee and a manager, interpret contract provisions differently. Grievances often involve job security or safety, which is a union priority, or job performance or discipline, which is a management priority.

Industrial unionism Occurs when there is a single union for all workers in a corporation. For example, all people who work in an automobile manufacturing company may be grouped together under the United Auto Workers (UAW). It is possible that the industrial union, with its massive numbers of union members, is the strongest possible collective group.

Labor A group composed of those who work for others to receive a salary.

Management The group of people within a business or company who plan, organize, lead, or control the activities of employees who have agreed to work to receive a salary.

Mediation A form of settling disputes that involves a trained person who listens to all parties and makes recommendations. Such mediation is generally not legally binding.

Occupational unionism Each occupation within a given company has separate unions; these occupational groups might join others of like work across boundaries and across the country. White-collar workers coming from a background of higher education and some measure of job security tend to prefer occupational unionism and organizing with like-minded professionals. In general, nurses prefer occupational unionism.

Picketing A form of protest in which people (called picketers) congregate outside a place of work or location where an event is taking place. Often this is done in an attempt to dissuade others from going in ("crossing the picket line"), but it can also be done to draw public attention to a cause.

Right-to-work laws Statutes enforced in 22 U.S. states, mostly in the southern and western United States, allowed under provisions of the Taft-Hartley Act, which prohibit agreements between unions and employers making membership or payment of union dues or "fees" a condition of employment, either before or after hiring.

Secret ballot elections To establish a union in a workplace, a majority of employees must express support for the union. The employees prove majority through a secret ballot election conducted by the National Labor Relations Board.

Strike A work stoppage caused by the refusal of a large portion of employees to perform work; usually takes place to enforce demands relating to employment conditions on their employer or to protest unfair labor practices. Sympathy strike occurs when a union stops work to support the strike of another union.

Unfair labor practices Actions that interfere with the rights of employees or employers as identified under the National Labor Relations Act. An unfair labor practice can be something as simple as suspicion by an employee that he or she was assigned to an unpopular task unfairly, or it can be as complex as the identification of a pattern of many employees receiving discriminatory treatment in the workplace because of being union supporters. Unfair labor practices are a frequent source of either strikes or the initiation of union activity within a setting.

Union A group of workers who band together to accomplish goals related to conditions of employment.

Union shop Refers to a worksite that requires all new employees in a specific work group to join the union. Dues will be deducted automatically from employees' paychecks as defined in the facility's contract.

LEARNING OUTCOMES

After studying this chapter, the reader will be able to:

1 Use terms associated with collective bargaining correctly in written and oral communications.

2 Examine key events in the historical development of collective bargaining and unions.

3 Recognize questionable labor or management practices in the workplace.

4 Analyze collective bargaining as a method for achieving power sharing in the workplace.

5 Evaluate current conflicts and controversies associated with collective bargaining by professional nurses.

CHAPTER OVERVIEW

Collective bargaining is a very complex and often an emotionally charged issue. Because the future of nursing may be influenced by our collective and individual efforts to be fairly represented and to have a voice in the conditions of our work, it is important to understand the costs and benefits of collective action, as well as the motives of those who would represent nursing. This chapter attempts to present a balanced view of collective bargaining in the hope that students, staff nurses, and nurses in managerial positions will use the information to make effective decisions when confronted with collective bargaining issues.

DEVELOPMENT OF COLLECTIVE BARGAINING IN AMERICA
Early Activities

During the late nineteenth century, when the Industrial Revolution was a force throughout North America, a cadre of thinkers arose who believed that to protect workers from circumstances such as long work hours, child labor, and unhealthy factory conditions, there needed to be collectivization of workers. These early groups sought such basic conditions as safety in work situations, adequate pay for hours worked, and the right not to be arbitrarily dismissed. This banding together of workers to accomplish goals was termed trade unionism. This technique was successful in many instances and remains with us today.

Federal Legislation

As a result of these early efforts at unionization, Congress passed the National Labor Relations Act (NLRA) in 1935. Under the terms of the NLRA, employees were given the right to self-organize, to form labor unions, and to bargain collectively. As part of the 1935 NLRA, the National Labor Relations Board (NLRB) was established to implement provisions of the NLRA. The NLRB continues to play a vital role in labor-management relations and, working through 52 regional and field offices in major U.S. cities, they conduct union elections and prosecute unfair labor practices.

With employees' rights protected by federal legislation, collective bargaining now could occur in companies across the country. Employees could organize themselves into units recognized under terms of the NLRA without fear of being fired for belonging to the union or for participating in union activities, such as collective bargaining. Typical goals in collective bargaining activities were to establish reasonable working conditions and formal agreements between employees and management for wages and health and retirement benefits.

However, exemptions to the NLRA were established for nonprofit companies. This meant that employees of nonprofit hospitals such as nurses were not protected under the NLRA and therefore were not legally protected for participation in collective bargaining activities. Hospitals' employees may have been excluded from protection by the NLRA because it was believed that services provided were so essential that organizing activities would be contrary to the public's interest. Eventually in 1974 legislation allowed for the inclusion of nonprofit hospitals in coverage under provisions of the NLRA. Nurses could form collective bargaining units. The 1974 amendments also included the requirement for a 10-day written notice of the intent to picket or to strike. This notice would allow the health care facility time to prepare and would protect the relative health and safety of the public.

Development of Collective Bargaining in Nursing

Formal unionization in nursing began in 1946 when the American Nurses Association (ANA) endorsed collective bargaining as a way to gain economic security and influence other employment issues. Its efforts were dealt a serious blow, however, when Congress passed the 1947 Taft-Hartley Act, exempting charitable institutions, including nonprofit hospitals, from the 1935 NLRA Act. The ANA immediately began efforts to get the Taft-Hartley provisions related to charitable institutions repealed. As noted, legislation enacted in 1974 finally allowed for the inclusion of nonprofit hospitals in coverage under the NLRA.

While ANA worked to pave the way for collective bargaining for nurses, it also struggled with its role in representing nurses who were part of unions as well as nurses from right-to-work states who did not support unionization. Finally in 1999, a national nurses union, the United American Nurses (UAN), was established as an ANA affiliate to create an independent voice for union nurses. UAN is also affiliated with the American Federation of Labor and Congress of Industrial Organizations (AFL-CIO), which is the largest federation of unions in the United States. The mission of UAN is to "shape the future of all staff nurses and the health care system for the better by improving the economic and general welfare of nurses, providing a quality work environment, protecting nurse and patient safety and influencing nursing practice standards" (UAN, 2009, p. 1). Today, UAN represents a significant number of the estimated 200,000 unionized nurses, but virtually all major unions now represent nurses at some level.

THE COLLECTIVE BARGAINING PROCESS

Collective bargaining is a method of equalizing power. As such, it involves negotiation and administrative agreements between employees and employers. Because the individual employee, or even a small group of employees, has limited power to bargain with the employer, the idea of banding together in a union enhances the position of employees in situations calling for negotiation. The goals of collective bargaining are achieved by imposing rules regarding how employers must treat employees represented by a union. The union movement in the United States is involved with strengthening a worker's position in the relationship between management and labor.

Nurses and nurse managers need to understand the steps involved in the union organizing and election process, as well as what are considered appropriate or inappropriate management responses and labor responses. Since union organizing involves power sharing and sometimes a temporary sense of distrust between bedside nurses and management, it can become a nerve-racking and emotional process. Knowing allowable patterns for the process of union organizing can help alleviate unnecessary distress.

The following discussion of steps in the union organizing process is based on information taken from the *Basic Guide to the National Labor Relations Act* (NLRB, 1997). The reader will see that careful attention is given to ensuring fairness for employer, employees, and the unions that may be involved in an election to determine if employees agree to unionize.

The Preformal Period in Union Organizing

The goal of collective bargaining is the equalization of power between labor and management. To initiate collective bargaining activities, an organizing drive is instituted by union forces who attempt to create an official NLRB-sanctioned bargaining unit in a particular institution.

The bargaining unit is either accepted or rejected through an election process in which non-management employees vote. If accepted, the bargaining unit will be made up of union members who are workers at the unionized facility and will be designed to protect the workers against arbitrary treatment and unfair labor practices.

A union organizing drive may be initiated when nurses in a particular health care facility contact a union because they feel a need for help in negotiating with their employer. The stimulus for this initial contact is usually not frivolous. There is typically a pervasive feeling among the nurses on a particular unit or in the health care facility as a whole that working conditions are unsatisfactory and that there is no possibility of making improvements under conventional existing circumstances.

It is helpful at this point to examine what is to be gained by those petitioning the NLRB for an election for union representation. For a group of workers, a newly formed union will:

◆ Have the power to make certain demands of the employer
◆ Provide some degree of political power on a local level

For the union organization, a newly formed union will:

◆ Give the union additional power by adding more bargaining units, especially if the union is part of a larger national union.
◆ Increase monetary support for the union through dues paid by employees. The additional money can be used to pay union officials' salaries, organize other bargaining units, or contribute to political causes or candidates.

Once a union has been contacted by nurses and told that there is some interest in establishing a collective bargaining unit, union forces try to determine whether efforts to organize the majority of nurses in the facility will be successful. This determination is made through a process of "signing cards." Union authorization cards help the union organizer, a professional who works for the union, to decide whether there is enough interest in unionization on the part of nurses employed in the facility. Such cards are simply index cards that help union organizers keep track of the numbers of workers who are interested in information about the union or in joining or otherwise supporting the union (Box 13-1 lists more information about union authorization cards and questions to ask before signing a card).

BOX **13-1**

Union Authorization Cards

The single-purpose authorization card:
• Requests a signature, date, name and address of the person signing, and a brief description of the person's job (department, shift, and type of work).
• Does not indicate that the person is requesting union membership or asking for a union election.
• Only requests information to assist union forces with identifying total numbers of employed nurses and whether their status would permit them to take part in union-organizing efforts.
• Allows accurate counting and updating of information about potential union members.

The dual-purpose authorization card:
• Calls for the same background information as the single-purpose authorization card.
• Also contains a statement that when signed by a nurse indicates a request for an election and that the person is applying for union membership.

Questions to ask before signing a card:
• Is the card merely asking for information about the nurse's employment status?
• Does signing the card indicate the nurse is applying for actual union membership?

If 30% of employed nurses sign cards, signaling an interest in representation by the union, the employer and NLRB are officially notified, and the employer must refrain from antilabor action such as firing those favoring the union (NLRB, 1997). If 50% plus one of nurses who are eligible (non-management nurses) to vote respond in the affirmative to accept union representation, then nurses in the facility become represented by the union and are unionized.

To follow the process effectively, a nurse should be aware of details of what is and is not allowed and what is and is not likely to occur during union organizing efforts. When a specific union, such as the Teamsters, UAN, or the Service Employees International Union, initiates organizing activities in a particular facility, an organizer goes to the facility. The organizer, who may also be called a business agent or field representative, is then responsible for developing and implementing plans to ensure success of the unionizing effort.

To form a core support group in the facility, the organizer locates respected leaders in the workplace. Meetings are then held at nonwork settings such as homes or restaurants to gain initial information about grievances and workplace inequities. These later are used as a basis for campaign literature. To gain additional supporters, discussion and card-signing take place in areas in the actual facility: locker rooms, bathrooms, lunch areas, lounges, and less visible work areas.

As the union drive surfaces to gain management's attention, organizers begin to distribute cards more openly. At this point the union organizer sends a registered letter to the employer with the names of employees on the organizing committee. Management will probably have already become aware of organizing activities through clues such as employee behavior changes during this period. There will be times when individuals seem distracted or when there is an increase in the number or aggressive quality of complaints about workplace conditions. Conversely, there may be a feeling of distancing between labor and management and an air of unnatural silence among employees.

Although peaceful strikes and picketing may occur for the purpose of publicity or seeking recognition, the NLRB prohibits certain behaviors during the pre-election period. The union may not:

◆ Inflame racial prejudices
◆ Lie about loss of jobs if the union loses the election
◆ Forge documents or signatures
◆ Meet or distribute literature in work areas during work times
◆ Hold meetings within 24 hours of an election

During the pre-election period, management may not:

◆ Solicit spying
◆ Photograph employees engaged in union activities
◆ Visit employees in their homes
◆ Lie about what will happen if the union is the victor in an election
◆ Question employees about their preferences regarding union activity

The Election Process

There are several steps in the election process. Either the union or the employer must petition the NLRB for an election. Once this petition is made, the request is passed along to the regional NLRB director. Within 48 hours the union must submit proof of its claim that 30% of eligible nurses are interested in forming a collective bargaining unit. Eligible nurses are generally considered to be those nurses who are engaged in patient care and are not in management positions. Normally, for a 10-day period literature will be mailed to eligible employees.

The union and the employer may circulate literature; however, both sides must cease activities within 24 hours of the election.

On the day actually designated for the election, the three parties (NLRB, union representatives, and employer representatives) meet to review the list of those eligible to vote. The three parties then count ballots and, in case of a true tie, a victory for the employer is declared. However, any votes in dispute will be set aside for a later recount. Objections must be made within 5 working days after the election and may be made on the grounds of problems with the conduct of the election or unfair labor practices.

Post Election

After the election, in the case of a union victory, federal law guarantees workers the right to collectively bargain and strike. Nurses may subsequently change a bargaining agent or remove the union representation by having 30% of nurses sign cards. An election would follow, requiring a vote of 50% plus one in favor of the change (NLRB, 1997).

The NLRA mandates that under the rules of collective bargaining, meetings between management and labor will be held at reasonable times for the purpose of conferring in good faith. Mandatory topics include wages; the establishment of rules about the use of labor (such as hours of work and worker safety); individual workers' rights; resolution of grievances; and methods of enforcement, interpretation, and administration of the union agreement. Negotiations between union and management occur in cycles following the initial year of collective bargaining. Negotiations are held before a contract is ratified (approved) by both union and management and again just before the contract expires.

Principles to Guide Fairness During Union Organizing

In an unprecedented collaboration between a major U.S. health care employer and unions, a set of guiding principles have been established to ensure a fair process for union organizing efforts. The principles, which can serve as a guide for employers and unions across the country, will help ensure that health care employees are able to make informed decisions regarding unionization without undue influence or pressure from either side. Based on the seven principles, employers as well as unions should agree in writing how they will (Catholic Healthcare Association of America, 2009):

- ◆ Demonstrate respect for each other's organization and mission
- ◆ Provide workers with equal access to information from both sides
- ◆ Adhere to standards for truthfulness and balance in their communications
- ◆ Create a pressure-free environment
- ◆ Allow workers to vote through a fair and expeditious process
- ◆ Honor employees' decision regardless of the outcome
- ◆ Create a system for enforcing these principles during the course of an organizing drive

UNIONS AND PROFESSIONAL NURSING
Professionalism vs. Unionization

Nurses in the workplace are buffeted by cost cutting, nursing shortages, shuffled duties, concerns about patient safety and quality care, and hospital reorganizations that bring job insecurity and uncertainty. Despite these difficult working conditions, it is often problematic for nurses to come to grips with their feelings related to the emotionally charged issues associated with unionization. Many nurses may be reluctant to become involved with what they view as trouble-making groups who exaggerate the issues just to win the contest against the adversary, which is management. It is difficult to reconcile feelings of professionalism and service with the perceived union connotations of strife and discord.

In addition, when nurses try to update their thoughts about unionization through reading, it becomes difficult to find objective reading material. Few experienced authorities on collective bargaining can remain neutral or objective. It is difficult to read about unionization without encountering biased language and the attempt to paint one side or the other in extremely unflattering terms. This doesn't help in clearing away the fog of conflict surrounding unionization decisions for nurses.

Questions to Answer

Four major questions need to be answered as nurses consider collective bargaining and unionization.

1. Are there relevant gains to be made for the nursing profession and for improved patient care through collective bargaining—or is this a myth?
2. Should nurses, who frequently are called on to supervise the work of others, be classified for collective bargaining purposes as management or labor? The answer to this question will determine the ultimate success of collective bargaining efforts for nurses.
3. Will nurses be too reluctant to strike, which is one of the most powerful tools that a union has at its disposal? There is concern that strikes by nurses could destroy the public's image of nursing. More importantly, the strike is contrary to nursing ethics and licensure to do no harm and avoid patient abandonment.
4. How will unionization of the nursing department affect functions of the interprofessional team, which is essential for quality patient care (e.g., physical therapy, dietary, pharmacy, housekeeping)? Will the nursing collective bargaining contract create inequities for other departments?

These questions are addressed in more detail in the following sections.

Gains for the Nursing Profession and Patient Care?

When considering collective bargaining and unionization, nurses need to seriously reflect on issues that affect the practice of professional nursing and on the patient care environment beyond what unions typically address during negotiations (wages and benefits, work hours, worker safety, and resolution of grievances). The primary triggers that spark interest in joining a union often are forgotten in the challenges confronted by nurses during the union organization process. Consider the following issues that may trigger a group of nurses to seek union representation:

◆ Physicians not seeing critical patients in a timely manner, putting patients at risk
◆ Lack of administrative support for collegial, professional relationships among nurses, physicians, and other interprofessional team members
◆ Inadequate medical and nursing hand-off procedures causing errors, frustration, interdepartmental conflicts, and delay in care
◆ Nursing staff continuing education and unit specific competencies not adequately addressed
◆ Self-scheduling designed around staff needs, not patient and unit needs

Nurses are cautioned that gains in wages and benefits may be achieved through unionization, but the nursing practice environment may suffer. A survey of more than 3500 RNs in Minnesota found that nurses who were members of collective bargaining units had higher satisfaction regarding wages but they had overall lower job satisfaction than their nonmember counterparts; nonmembers had significantly higher satisfaction regarding professional relationships, work setting, supervision, patient care, and overall job satisfaction (Pittman, 2007). When faced with union organizing efforts, nurses need to carefully consider all factors including the professional practice environment. Box 13-2 presents a list of questions the nurse should ask when confronted by a union organizing effort.

Regardless of whether the nurse works in a union environment, there are several strategies he or she can use to develop and encourage sound relationships between management and labor and promote a positive work environment:

- ◆ Assess your knowledge of the labor laws and practices in your area and seek to understand the unique culture of the facility; seek help before union activity begins or grievances are filed.
- ◆ Identify and be proactive in situations where the nurse, peers, or leaders, disrespect others, ignore serious staff concerns, or neglect appropriate communication and follow-up.
- ◆ Participate in education and training that will improve your labor relations skills in union and nonunion environments.
- ◆ Be proactive in solving issues that compromise patient care; embrace your role in achieving timely outcomes that truly improve care.

Management or Staff?

One of the difficult issues for nursing in relation to collective bargaining is that in the eyes of the NLRB certain nurses are singled out as management or supervisory personnel and are not allowed NLRA protection, which applies only to nonmanagement employees. Charge nurses and shift supervisors have traditionally been considered part of management rather than labor. But what about nurses who routinely supervise others who act merely as extenders of care, such as in nursing homes? Are these nurses acting exclusively on behalf of the company that employs them or are they routinely carrying out their responsibilities as a professional nurse?

The definition of manager or supervisor is problematic even in non–health care settings. In nursing things become even more complicated. Most experienced RNs are involved in some type of supervisory or management work. For example, most staff nurses who ordinarily

 BOX **13-2**

Questions to Ask When Confronted by a Union Organizer

- What measures has the union successfully used to improve quality of care and promote the national patient safety goals?
- Will the union guarantee in writing that it will be getting employees a specified wage increase and better benefits or be liable to employees if it doesn't?
- How much are union dues? What portion of union dues goes to paying union salaries?
- Are there special union assessments and, if so, how much are they and how often will they be imposed?
- Are dues used to help organize other union groups?
- What are the consequences if employees violate the union constitution and/or bylaws?
- Will the union guarantee in writing that employees will not be permanently replaced during an economic strike?
- Will the union pay wages to employees if they are called on to strike?
- Will union members be expected to picket at other unionized facilities in the event of a strike or an informational picket?

provide bedside care have been called on to be in charge of a particular nursing unit for a particular working shift. Does this mean that the nurse should no longer be considered non-management?

Another trend that has an effect on decisions about supervisory status is the increasing use of unlicensed personnel in health care workplaces. More nurses could now be classified as supervisory because they direct the activities of unlicensed workers. In 1994 in *NLRB v. the Health Care and Retirement Corporation*, the Supreme Court ruled that nurses do indeed direct the work of others and therefore are not eligible for protection under the NLRA. This case was important to the nursing profession because had the ruling been upheld, it would have dramatically lowered the numbers of nurses who could act as "laborers" and engage in collective bargaining. However, in 1997 the decision of the U.S. Court of Appeals for the Ninth Circuit helped clarify this point. The court ruled that RNs who performed charge nurse duties were not management and therefore were eligible for collective bargaining protection. In another case, *Providence Alaska Medical Center v. NLRB*, the ruling recognized that the judgment used by RNs in assigning patients and coordinating patient care was part of their professional role rather than part of any statutory supervision as defined by the NLRA.

And beyond the issue of recognizing who is management and who is staff, there is the uncomfortable prospect of pitting nurse managers against their colleagues in the workplace. A definite schism occurs when managers and staff are placed on opposite sides of the table. Bad feelings arise. For example, a supervisor nurse represents management but is not insulated in an executive office. In addition, the supervisor nurse or nurse manager must often assume duties routinely performed by staff nurses in the event of a strike. This can lead to lingering negative feelings even after the strike is resolved.

Techniques frequently used by nurse managers to maintain smooth and efficient job performance in their work settings may be relatively ineffective when unionization or collective bargaining initiatives occur. For example, the nurse supervisor who believes that open communication in both upward and downward directions is useful for problem solving may become frustrated during unionization initiatives. Union tactics may involve coaching nurses at staff levels to use the "silent treatment" and not cooperate with nurse managers' attempts to communicate.

To Strike or Not?

Strikes can have very powerful effects. The economic effect of a strike can best be understood by noting that hospitals become concerned over lost revenues when the average daily census drops only a few percentage points. Hospitals could possibly have to turn away patients because of a strike and could lose that market share permanently, resulting in long-term losses to the hospital. Thus strikes or the threat of a strike can be effective in gaining concessions (i.e., salary increases, better benefits) from management in an effort to avoid the strike completely or to end it as soon as possible. However, it is important to note that in some states, collective bargaining contracts may contain "no strike" clauses prohibiting the collective bargaining unit from having the power of the strike.

Nursing is a trusted profession, and for many nurses, the strike is a symbol of negative behavior. To safeguard nursing's image and allow for hospitals to react effectively in safeguarding patient care, a 10-day notice of intent to strike is required. On receipt of such notice, the NLRB attempts to mediate, and the hospital is encouraged to decrease census and halt elective admissions. Schedules are developed for covering the emergency department, operating room, and intensive care areas.

BOX **13-3**

Helpful Websites and Online Resources

United American Nurses
  www.uannurse.org
Respecting the Just Rights of Workers: Guidance and Options for Catholic Health Care and Unions
  www.usccb.org/sdwp/national/respecting_the_just_rights_of_workers.pdf
ANA Publication: *A Seat at the Table: 50 Years of Progress*
  www.uannurse.org/who/historyBook/A%20Seat%20at%20the%20Table-%2050%20years.pdf
Basic Guide to the National Labor Relations Act
  www.nlrb.gov/nlrb/shared_files/brochures/basicguide.pdf
Online Article: Roe, C. (2009). Navigating the muddy waters of labor relations. *Business of Caring*, May, 2009. Available online at *www.hfma.org/NR/exeres/EE62DCA0-CC42-40B2-91F0-DEB603B48511.htm*

As nurses are confronted with making decisions about unionization, it is important to consider the many issues that will affect their personal economic welfare, their practice environment, and the quality of patient care they are able to provide. There are no easy answers as the issues and challenges vary depending on each organization's unique set of circumstances. To successfully negotiate unionization initiatives and make good decisions, nurses are encouraged to learn more about collective bargaining and unions. Box 13-3 provides online resources regarding collective bargaining and unions.

SUMMARY

This chapter has provided a history and overview of the collective bargaining process and addressed some important issues for nurses to consider as they face questions regarding unionization. These important issues include the role of unionization in addressing the professional practice environment and quality care, the questions surrounding management versus labor in collective bargaining, and the controversy of the strike as a strategy to gain concessions from the employer. The role of unions in the future of health care may hinge on cooperation versus conflict, on relative productivity gains in union versus nonunion facilities, and on success of human relations practices in union as well as nonunion workplaces. Nurses live in a new era in health care and will need to continue to grow in their knowledge regarding unions and collective bargaining

 evolve Additional resources are available online at: http://evolve.elsevier.com/Cherry/

REFERENCES

Catholic Healthcare Association of America: *Respecting the just rights of workers: guidance and options for Catholic health care and unions.* 2009. Available at: www.usccb.org/sdwp/national/respecting_the_just_rights_of_workers.pdf.

National Labor Relations Board: *Basic guide to the National Labor Relations Act*, Washington, DC, 1997, U.S. Government Printing Office.

Pittman J: Registered nurse job satisfaction and collective bargaining unit membership status, *J Nurs Adm* 37(10):471–476, 2007.

United American Nurses: *Our mission for patients and nurses.* 2009. Available at: www.uannurse.org/who/index.html.

Information Technology in the Clinical Setting

Cynthia K. Russell, PhD, APN

*e*volve Additional resources are available online at: http://evolve.elsevier.com/Cherry/

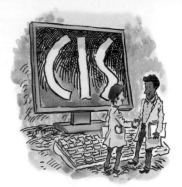

Information systems offer nurses and other team members information when, where, and how they need it.

VIGNETTE

Jerry White is a recent graduate who is employed in the intensive care unit (ICU) of a large, multisite hospital organization. In his professional entry program he had the opportunity to have a clinical rotation at a local veterans affairs medical center, where he saw an integrated clinical information system that supported computerized provider order entry, reporting of diagnostic tests, and clinical alerts and reminders. During his educational program he heard about the president's 2004 initiative to make electronic health records available to most Americans within the next 10 years. His employer currently uses the CERNER system for ordering and reviewing diagnostic tests. He is told that this system will be discontinued, and a new computerized system will be phased in over a period of 2 years, with his unit expected to be the last for implementation.

Jerry wonders precisely how a system such as this can be phased in. How will it affect health care providers who practice in different parts of the institution, and how will nurses and other health care providers be educated about the new system? He is interested in whether the new system will actually help increase efficiency and promote patient safety as has been promised. He realizes that this is a time of rapid change in the technologies being used in the care environment and is unsure how everyone will adapt to the changes, especially given the variability that he has witnessed in terms of the information technology and computer literacy competencies of his fellow nurses and other health care providers.

■ QUESTIONS TO CONSIDER WHILE READING THIS CHAPTER:

1 What are the various components of a clinical information system (CIS)?

2 What are the potential benefits of a CIS to nurses, other health care providers, and patients?

3 How can technologically savvy nurses help fellow nurses and other health care providers adjust to a new CIS?

4 What are some of the advantages of telehealth interventions in the home health setting?

5 How does the information literacy of nurses affect patient outcomes?

We thank Leslie H. Nicoll, PhD, MBA, RN for her contribution to this chapter in the 1st, 2nd and 3rd editions.

KEY TERMS

Clinical information system (CIS) The software and associated hardware that supports the entry, retrieval, update, and analysis of patient care information and associated clinical information related to patient care.

Computer literacy The knowledge and understanding of computers combined with the ability to use them effectively.

Decision support systems Software programs that process data to produce or recommend decisions by linking with an electronic knowledge base controlled by established rules for combining data elements; the knowledge base and rules mimic the knowledge and reasoning an expert clinician would apply to data and information to solve a problem.

Dock Connecting a device through cable or other connector so that data can be transferred, by either uploading the device's information to a CIS or downloading information from a CIS to the device.

Hardware The physical computer and its components, such as the central processing unit (CPU), the monitor, and the printer.

Information literacy The ability to identify when information is needed combined with the ability to locate, evaluate, and use the information.

Information technology The hardware and software that enable information to be stored, retrieved, communicated, and managed.

Point of care technology (POCT) Initially, POCT referred to technologies that allowed for decentralized tests done on patients by non-laboratory staff. Current definitions of POCT include technologies that allow for real-time data retrieval, documentation, and decision support at the bedside or where direct care is provided.

Software Programs that run the computer (programs that perform different tasks, such as statistics or word processing, are known as applications).

URL Uniform resource locator; the system of addresses used on the Internet.

LEARNING OUTCOMES

After studying this chapter, the reader will be able to:

1 Describe the role of the CIS in patient care.

2 Explain the importance of security and confidentiality in the use of various CISs.

3 Predict future trends in computing as they relate to health care and nursing practice.

4 Conduct Internet searches for relevant health-related information.

5 Use established criteria to evaluate the content of health-related sites found on the Internet.

CHAPTER OVERVIEW

The clinical settings of today are undergoing an explosion in the types of technology used by all health care providers. Yesterday's clinical settings saw the use of telephones, fax and copy machines, and slow computers that primarily stored patients' contact and billing information. Today you are likely to see voice communication systems, handheld computers (HHCs), robots, and fast computers that contain patients' electronic health records and can display charts, graphs, and tables to help health care providers view important trends in a patient's progress. In this chapter you will explore the important role of CISs in today's clinical environment, review the evolution of computer technology, and learn about the importance of information literacy, information technology literacy, and computer literacy in the twenty-first century nursing environment.

CLINICAL INFORMATION SYSTEMS

CISs are changing the way that health care is delivered, whether in the hospital, the clinic, the provider's office, or the patient's home. With capabilities ranging from advanced instrumentation to high-level decision support, the CIS offers nurses and other clinicians information when, where, and how they need it. Increasingly, CIS applications function as the mechanisms for delivering patient-centered care and for supporting the move toward the electronic health record (EHR).

What exactly is a CIS? Definitions vary, often from organization to organization. A CIS facilitates reporting of results, management of orders, and documentation of clinical care (Knecht, Simpson, and Weaver, 2006). The CIS integrates with other systems to provide clinical information for patient care.

A CIS can be patient focused or departmental. In patient-focused systems, automation supports patient care processes. Typical applications found in a patient-focused system include order entry, results reporting, clinical documentation, care planning, and clinical pathways. As data are entered into the system, data repositories are established that can be accessed to look for trends in patient care. Departmental systems evolved to meet the operational needs of a particular department, such as the laboratory, radiology, pharmacy, medical records, or billing. Early systems often were stand-alone systems designed for an individual department. A major challenge facing CIS developers is to integrate these stand-alone systems to work with one another and with the newer patient-focused systems.

Electronic Health Records

A CIS is not the same as an EHR (electronic health record). Ideally the EHR includes all information about an individual's lifetime health status and health care maintained electronically. The EHR is a replacement for the paper medical record as the primary source of information for health care, meeting all clinical, legal, and administrative requirements. However, the EHR is more than today's medical record. Information technology permits much more data to be captured, processed, and integrated, which results in information that is broader than that found in a linear paper record.

It is important to note that a wide variety of terms are used in health care settings to refer to these types of electronic health information management systems. In addition to EHR, some of the more common terms are electronic medical record (EMR), electronic patient record (EPR), and computerized patient record (CPR). (For this chapter, we will use EHR.)

The EHR is not a record in the traditional sense of the term. "Record" connotes a repository with limitations of size, content, and location. The term traditionally has suggested that the sole purpose for maintaining health data is to document events. Although this is an important purpose, the EHR permits health information to be used to support the generation and communication of knowledge. Figures 14-1 and 14-2 illustrate selected screens from a patient's EHR.

The health care delivery system is dramatically changing, with a strong emphasis on improving outcomes of care and maintaining health. The EHR needs to be considered in a broader context and is not applicable only to patients (i.e., individuals with the presence of an illness or disease). Rather in the EHR the focus is on the individual's health, encompassing both wellness and illness.

As a result of this focus on the individual, the EHR is a virtual compilation of health data about the person across his or her lifetime, including facts, observations, interpretations, plans,

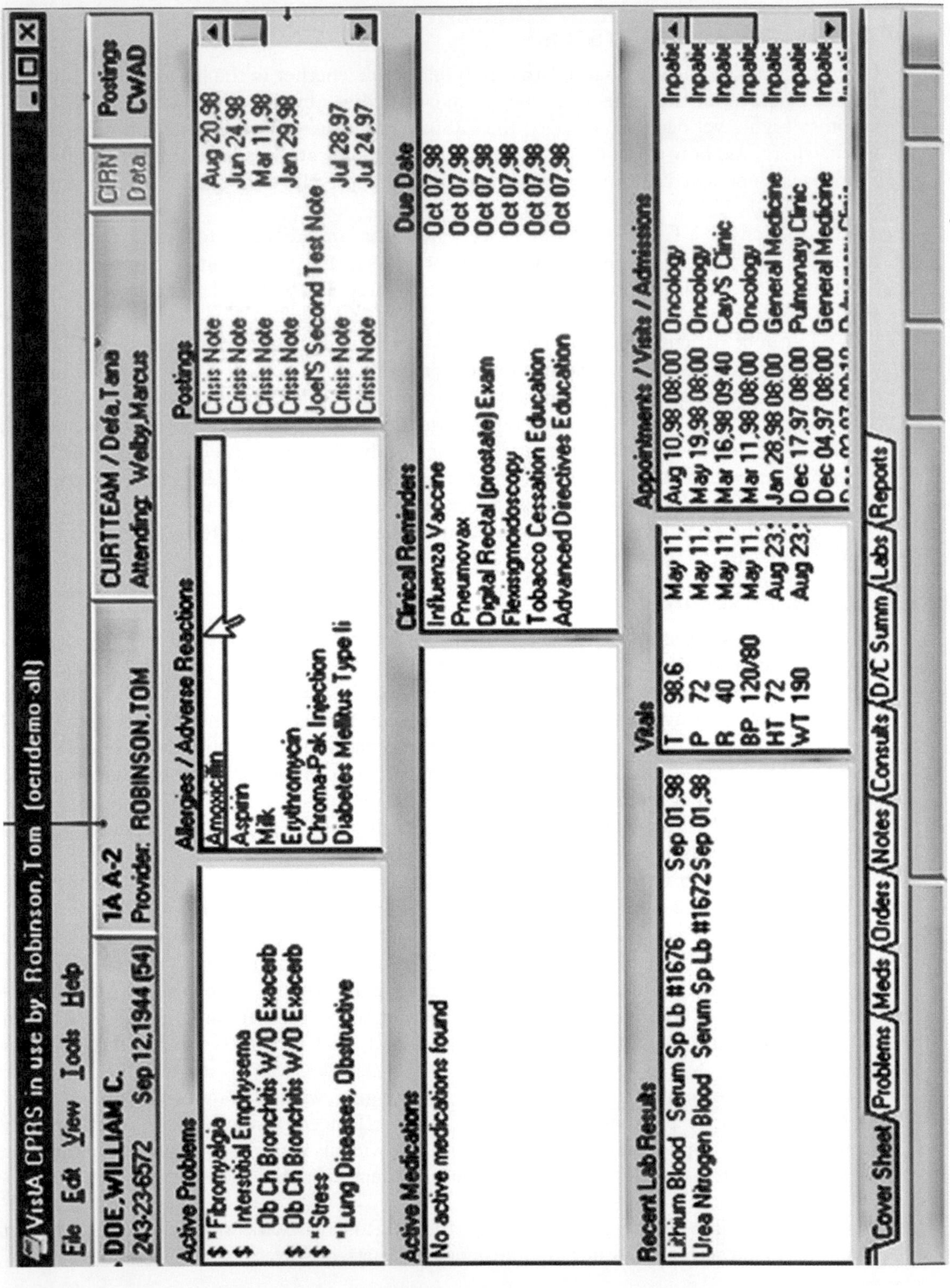

Figure 14-1 Selected screen from a patient's electronic health record (EHR). (Courtesy the Veterans Health Administration from its VisTA system.)

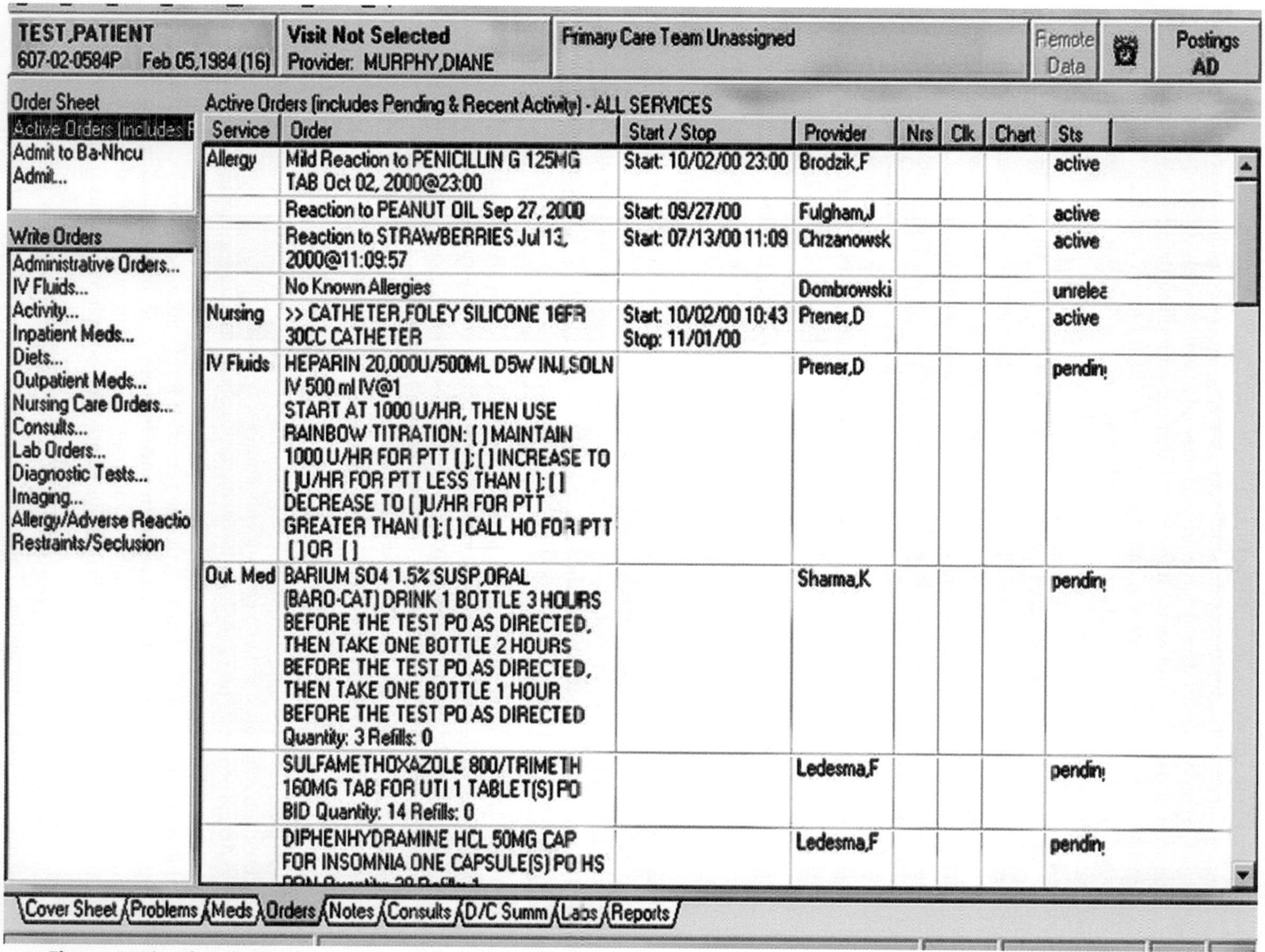

TEST,PATIENT	Visit Not Selected	Primary Care Team: Unassigned				Remote Data		Postings AD
607-02-0584P Feb 05,1984 (16)	Provider: MURPHY,DIANE							

Order Sheet

Active Orders (includes Pending & Recent Activity) - ALL SERVICES

Service	Order	Start / Stop	Provider	Nrs	Clk	Chart	Sts
Allergy	Mild Reaction to PENICILLIN G 125MG TAB Oct 02, 2000@23:00	Start: 10/02/00 23:00	Brodzik,F				active
	Reaction to PEANUT OIL Sep 27, 2000	Start: 09/27/00	Fulgham,J				active
	Reaction to STRAWBERRIES Jul 13, 2000@11:09:57	Start: 07/13/00 11:09	Chizanowsk				unrelec
	No Known Allergies		Dombrowski				unrelec
Nursing	>> CATHETER,FOLEY SILICONE 16FR 30CC CATHETER	Start: 10/02/00 10:43 Stop: 11/01/00	Prener,D				active
IV Fluids	HEPARIN 20,000U/500ML D5W INJ,SOLN IV 500 ml IV@1 START AT 1000 U/HR, THEN USE RAINBOw TITRATION: [ ] MAINTAIN 1000 U/HR FOR PTT [ ]; [ ] INCREASE TO [ ]U/HR FOR PTT LESS THAN [ ]; [ ] DECREASE TO [ ]U/HR FOR PTT GREATER THAN [ ]; [ ] CALL HO FOR PTT [ ] OR [ ]		Prener,D				pending
Out. Med	BARIUM SO4 1.5% SUSP,ORAL [BARO-CAT] DRINK 1 BOTTLE 3 HOURS BEFORE THE TEST PO AS DIRECTED, THEN TAKE ONE BOTTLE 2 HOURS BEFORE THE TEST PO AS DIRECTED, THEN TAKE ONE BOTTLE 1 HOUR BEFORE THE TEST PO AS DIRECTED Quantity: 3 Refills: 0		Sharma,K				pending
	SULFAMETHOXAZOLE 800/TRIMETH 160MG TAB FOR UTI 1 TABLET(S) PO BID Quantity: 14 Refills: 0		Ledesma,F				pending
	DIPHENHYDRAMINE HCL 50MG CAP FOR INSOMNIA ONE CAPSULE(S) PO HS		Ledesma,F				pending

Active Orders (includes

Admit to Ba-Nhcu
Admit ...

Write Orders

Administrative Orders...
IV Fluids...
Activity...
Inpatient Meds...
Diets...
Outpatient Meds...
Nursing Care Orders...
Consults...
Lab Orders...
Diagnostic Tests...
Imaging...
Allergy/Adverse Reactio
Restraints/Seclusion

Cover Sheet \ Problems \ Meds \ Orders \ Notes \ Consults \ D/C Summ \ Labs \ Reports

Figure 14-2 Selected screen from a patient's *electronic health record (EHR)*. (Courtesy the Veterans Health Administration from its VisTA system.)

actions, and outcomes. Health data include information on allergies, history of illness and injury, functional status, diagnostic studies, assessments, orders, consultation reports, and treatment records. Health data also include wellness information, such as immunization history, behavioral data, environmental information, demographics, health insurance, administrative data for care delivery processes, and legal data, such as informed consents. The who, what, when, and where of data capture are also identified. The structure of the data includes text, numbers, sounds, images, and full-motion video. These are thoroughly integrated so that any given view of health data may incorporate one or more structural elements.

Ideally, within an EHR, an individual's health data should be maintained and distributed over different systems in different locations, such as a hospital, clinic, physician's office, and pharmacy. Intelligent software agents with appropriate security measures are necessary to access data across these distributed systems. The nurse or other user who is retrieving these data must be able to assemble it in such a way as to provide a chronology of health information about the individual.

The EHR is maintained in a system that captures, processes, communicates, secures, and presents the data about the patient. This system may include the CIS. Other components of the EHR system include clinical rules, literature for patient education, expert opinions, and payer rules related to reimbursement. When these elements work together in an integrated fashion, the EHR becomes much more than a patient record—it becomes a knowledge tool. The system is able to integrate information from multiple sources and provide decision support; thus the EHR serves as the primary source of information for patient care.

A fully functional EHR is a complex system. Consider a single data element (datum), such as a person's weight. The system must be able to capture, or record, the weight, then store it, process it, communicate it to others, and present it in a different format, such as a bar graph or chart. All of this must be done in a secure environment that protects the patient's confidentiality and privacy. The complexity of these issues and the development of the necessary systems help explain why few fully functional EHR systems are in place today.

Data Capture. Data capture refers to the collection and entry of data into a computer system. The origin of the data may be local or remote from patient-monitoring devices, from telehealth applications, directly from the individual recipient of health care, and even from others who have information about the recipient's health or environment, such as relatives, friends, and public health agencies. Data may be captured by multiple means, including key entry, pattern recognition (voice, handwriting, or biologic characteristics), and medical device transmission.

Storage. Storage refers to the physical location of data. In EHR systems, health data need to be distributed across multiple systems at different sites. For this reason, common access protocols, retention schedules, and universal identification are necessary.

Access protocols permit only authorized users to obtain data for legitimate uses. The systems must have backup and recovery mechanisms in the event of failure. Retention schedules address the maintenance of the data in active and inactive form and the permanence of the storage medium. A person's identity can be determined by many types of data in addition to common identifiers, such as name and number. Universal identifiers or other methods are required for integrating health data of an individual distributed across multiple systems at different sites.

Information Processing. Application functions provide for effective retrieval and processing of data into useful information. These include decision support tools, such as alerts and alarms for drug interactions, allergies, and abnormal laboratory results. Reminders can be provided for appointments, critical path actions, medication administration, and other activities. The systems also may provide access to consensus- and evidence-driven diagnostic and treatment guidelines and protocols. The nurse could integrate a standard guideline, protocol, or critical path into a specific individual's EHR, modify it to meet unique circumstances, and use it as a basis for managing and documenting care. Outcome data communicated from various caregivers and health care recipients themselves also may be analyzed and used for continual improvement of the guidelines and protocols. Data may also be downloaded into statistical software programs for more sophisticated analysis for research purposes.

Information Communication. Information communication refers to the interoperability of systems and linkages for exchange of data across disparate systems. To integrate health data across multiple systems at different sites, identifier systems (unique numbers or other methodology) for health care recipients, caregivers, providers, payers, and sites are essential. Local, regional, and national health information infrastructures that tie all participants together using standard data communication protocols are key to the linkage function. There are hundreds of types of transactions or messages that must be defined and agreed to by the participating stakeholders. Vocabulary and code systems must permit the exchange and processing of data into meaningful information. EHR systems must provide access to point-of-care information databases and knowledge sources, such as pharmaceutical formularies, referral databases, and reference literature.

Security. Computer-based patient record systems provide better protection of confidential health information than paper-based systems because such systems incorporate controls designed to ensure that only authorized users with legitimate uses have access to health information. Security functions address the confidentiality of private health information and the integrity of the data. Security functions must be designed to ensure compliance with applicable laws, regulations, and standards. Security systems must ensure that access to data is provided only to those who are authorized and have a legitimate purpose for its use. Security functions also must provide a means to audit for inappropriate access. Three important terms must be clearly understood when discussing the issues surrounding access: privacy, confidentiality, and security.

- *Privacy* refers to the right of an individual to keep information about himself or herself from being disclosed to anyone else. If a patient has had an abortion and chooses not to tell a health care provider this fact, the patient would be keeping that information private.
- *Confidentiality* refers to the act of limiting disclosure of private matters. Once a patient has disclosed private information to a health care provider, that provider has a responsibility to maintain the confidentiality of that information and not reveal the information to others who do not have a legitimate need to know.
- *Security* refers to the means to control access and protect information from accidental or intentional disclosure to unauthorized persons and from alteration, destruction, or loss. When private information is placed in a confidential EHR, the system must have controls in place to maintain the security of the system and not allow unauthorized persons access to the data (Computer-Based Patient Record Institute [CPRI], 1995).

Information Presentation. The wealth of information available through EHR systems must be managed to ensure that authorized caregivers (including nurses) and others with legitimate uses have the information they need in their preferred presentation form. For example, a nurse may want to see data organized by source, caregiver, encounter, problem, or date. Data can be presented in detail or summary form. Tables, graphs, narrative, and other forms of information presentation must be accommodated. Some users may need only to know of the presence or absence of certain data, not the nature of the data itself. For example, blood donation centers draw blood for testing for human immunodeficiency virus, hepatitis, and other conditions. If a donor has a positive test result, the center may not be given the specific information regarding the test, but only general information that a test result was abnormal and that the donor should be referred to an appropriate health care provider.

Decision Support and Computerized Provider Order Entry

The Institute of Medicine (IOM) (2003) recommends that EHR systems offer the eight functionalities presented in Table 14-1. Two specific functionalities recommended by the IOM—clinical decision support and computerized provider order entry (CPOE)—are frequently mentioned in the literature as essential to improve the quality and safety of health care. Clinical decision support contributes to safety and quality by providing automatic reminders about preventive practices, such as immunizations, drug alerts for dosing and interactions, and electronic resources for data interpretation and clinical decision making (IOM, 2003; Smith, 2004).

CPOE is defined as the "process by which the physician or another health care provider, such as a nurse practitioner, physician's assistant, or physical or occupational therapist, directly enters orders for client care into a hospital information system" (Hebda and Czar, 2009, p. 23). CPOE contributes to safety and quality by eliminating lost orders and illegible handwriting; generating related orders automatically (e.g., lab test needed to monitor a specific medication); monitoring for duplicate or contradictory orders; and reducing time to fill orders (Hebda and

TABLE **14-1**

Core Functionalities for EHR Systems as Recommended by the IOM (2003)

Health information and data	Information to make sound clinical decisions, such as past medical history, laboratory tests, allergies, current medications, and consent forms
Results management	Electronic reports of laboratory results and radiology procedures with automated display of previous results; electronic consultation reports
Order entry and order management	Computerized provider order entry with or without decision support to eliminate lost orders and illegible handwriting, generate related orders automatically, monitor for duplicate or contradictory orders, and reduce time to fill orders
Decision support	Enhance clinical performance by providing reminders about preventive practices, such as immunizations, drug alerts for dosing and interactions, and clinical decision making
Electronic communication and connectivity	Electronic communication between heath care team members and other care partners, such as radiology and lab personnel, and connectivity to the patient record across multiple care settings
Patient support	Computer-based patient education and home monitoring where applicable
Administrative processes	Scheduling systems, billing and claims management, insurance eligibility, and inventory management
Reporting and population health management	Meet public and private sector reporting requirements at the federal, state and local level; address internal quality improvement initiatives

Czar, 2009; IOM, 2003). CPOE functions also contribute to medical error prevention through (1) improved communication; (2) more readily accessible knowledge; (3) requirement for key pieces of information (such as the dose of a drug); (4) assistance with calculations; (5) checks performed in real time; (6) assistance with monitoring; (7) decision support; and (8) rapid response to, and tracking of, adverse events (Bates and Gawande, 2003).

Point-of-Care Technology

Historically, POCT devices were used to test for occult blood, dipstick urinalysis, urine pregnancy, and blood glucose. Today these devices are being used at the point of care to test blood gas, clotting time, cardiac markers, rapid strep, bilirubin, breathalyzer, rapid influenza A and B, rapid human immunodeficiency virus (HIV), and salivary testing for drugs of abuse (Lewandrowski et al, 2005; Newbold, 2004; Nichols, 2004). One advantage to POCT is that the identification badge of the nurse can be scanned, thereby indicating who conducted the test, and in the case of repeated errors or problems, the nurse can be identified for additional training. The patient's identification badge can also be scanned, thereby allowing the test report to be uploaded directly to the patient's health care record. Once the test is done, the POCT device can be docked to a computer and the data uploaded to a central database for recording in a patient's electronic record, accessible by other nurses, physicians, and laboratory personnel.

Improving Patient Safety. Another advantage in using POCT devices is a reduction in errors and an increase in patient safety. The IOM's (2001) report about medical errors pointed to the important role of the STEEEP principles in providing health care that is safe, timely, effective, efficient, equitable, and patient centered. Garritty and Eman's (2006) systematic review of PDA usage surveys that were published between 2000 and 2005 showed an increase in health care providers' use of PDAs, with an adoption rate between 45% and 85%. Another systematic review of PDAs showed some evidence that PDA use in health care settings improves decision making, enhances learning of students and health care providers, and reduces the number of medical errors (Lindquist et al, 2008). Some of the most common sources of error in patient care environments include misinterpretation of physician orders, incorrect calculations, inaccurate charting, illegible writing, and inappropriate anticoagulation parameters. POCT, whether CPOE, EHRs, and/or HHCs, has the potential to help decrease these errors. Technology can help redesign processes to improve patient safety. Technology can capture and display data to show important trends and provide a mechanism to quickly screen. Bar-coded patient identification bracelets or identity cards can be scanned to confirm correct administration of medications. Being able to instantly receive lab test results that could alter medication dosing is another important feature (Ehrmeyer, Hausman, and Lebo, 2005; Savage et al, 2002).

Saving Time and Money. POCT devices are timesavers because of their portability and documentation features. They are small enough, whether an HHC or a tablet personal computer (PC), to be carried by health care providers. When health care providers have these devices with them, they are much more apt to use them at the time they need them—whether to look for information or to document. Immediate documentation of data eliminates the need to wait for that "down time" that never seems to come.

A 2003 survey of 900 physicians noted that for 20% of respondents, the PDA helped them see an additional three patients per day, whereas another 20% said the PDA helped them see an additional one or two patients per day (Versel, 2003). At St. Agnes Healthcare, the use of wireless voice communications saved more than 3000 person-hours annually (Breslin, Greskovich, and Turisco, 2004).

Enabling Evidence-Based Practice. POCT devices facilitate evidence-based decision making and quality of care. Promoting patient safety and enabling evidence-based practice are two cornerstones for ensuring health care quality. Improving access to evidence-based material is important in providing high-quality care. Access to this reliable, trustworthy information needs to be as close to the bedside as possible. In multiple studies, it has been noted that nurses are the health care providers that often lack access to evidence-based resources, whether in the institution's library or online. In many facilities, the library is used almost solely by physicians and is often locked. This could present a barrier to nurses who may not feel welcome to use the library. Also in many facilities, the Internet is inaccessible from patient care areas, in a belief that Internet access would be abused. This means that nurses must make special efforts to acquire material that ought to be readily available—via desktop or HHC.

It is important that nursing practice goes from practice that relies on memory to one that emphasizes continuous use of resources as they are needed. This means that nurses must transform from being technical experts to knowledge workers and rely on the ever-increasing and reliable computer memory versus the overburdened and fallible human memory. Computer-based alerts and reminders are helpful in detecting and preventing potential adverse drug events related to drug-drug interactions and abnormal lab values. Standardized protocols and clinical practice guidelines are other important materials that need to be more readily available than the oft-disappearing and outdated protocol and procedure books on shelves (Bakken, Cimino, and Hripcsak, 2004; Hoenich, Lindley, and Stoves, 2003; Thompson, 2005a).

Health Insurance Portability and Accountability Act

In the early 1990s, the President of the United States called together health care industry leaders for the purpose of determining how the administrative costs of health care could be decreased. The leaders determined that the use of electronic data interchange within the health care industry held the most promise for decreasing costs. Given the numerous electronic systems that were available, it was recommended that national standards for electronic data interchange and information privacy and security be established.

The Health Insurance Portability and Accountability Act (HIPAA) was signed into law in August 1996. HIPAA regulations focus on the privacy and security of patient data, including standard formats for transmitting electronic patient information. Civil and criminal penalties can result from noncompliance with HIPAA and from not protecting protected health information (PHI). By April 2005, health care institutions were required to be in compliance with federal HIPAA regulations.

HIPAA and Clinical Information Systems. All offices, organizations, and institutions that collect or store PHI are required to name an individual as a privacy officer. They must also develop policies and procedures to ensure that HIPAA regulations are followed. Each health care entity must provide privacy and security training for employees, in addition to information for patients. Controlling employee access to PHI so that only employees with a need to know specific information are able to access that information is another requirement of HIPAA. Individuals who knowingly use or disclose PHI in violation of HIPAA may be subject to criminal penalties and civil monetary penalties.

HIPAA and HHCs. HHCs include PDAs and laptops. Common patient information that may be on HHCs includes names, contact information, room numbers (if hospitalized), diagnoses, diagnostic tests, images, medications, and other treatments. Various institutional policies consider HHCs "at-risk devices" in terms of security issues important to HIPAA. The systems and security of institutional computers are typically managed by trained computer security personnel. In contrast HHCs are individually owned and, as such, the individual assumes responsibility for ensuring the security of the information contained on the device. Unregulated HHCs are being used by health care providers in increasing numbers each year.

Various measures required by institutions to protect PHI on HHCs include a password protecting the device with a programmed timeout, using biometric fingerprint identification, encrypting information, implementing data self-destruct mechanisms if security is breached, disabling the infrared transmission capabilities (beaming), avoiding wireless transmission of data, and installing virus protection and firewall protection software and/or hardware (Pancoast, Patrick, and Mitchell, 2003). Additionally, before an HHC is transferred to a new owner or otherwise disposed of, all PHI on the device must be destroyed unless the new owner has a right to access that PHI. Centralized registration of HHCs is recommended so that audits can be performed to ensure users' compliance with security measures, and access to institutional networks can be prevented if a device is reported lost or stolen.

Users of HHCs must be as cognizant of HIPAA guidelines as users of EHRs (Thompson, 2005b). Some HHCs have patient scheduling or other programs that enable entry of patients' laboratory, physical, and treatment data; all of which would be considered PHI. If PHI is stored on an HHC, additional care must be taken to password the device and/or use encryption if transmitting data wirelessly.

Telehealth

Telehealth is the use of telecommunications technology to assess, diagnose, and, in some cases, treat persons who are at a distance from the health care provider. Nurses, physicians, radiologists, psychiatrists, and others use this technology via telephones, computers, and interactive video or teleconferencing. In many instances, telehealth makes possible the delivery of health care services to populations, such as rural communities, older adults, or prisoners that may have difficulty accessing necessary services. Demonstrated benefits of telehealth include improved quality of care, enhanced continuity of care, increased availability of experts, improved access to care, improved decision making and time savings, and higher quality records related to the incorporation of digital information (Hebda and Czar, 2009). Telehealth interventions that have demonstrated cost-effectiveness include enhanced self-care management, early detection of health deterioration, and symptom management (Agency for Healthcare Research and Quality [AHRQ], 2006).

The home care arena is seeing significant changes as a result of telehealth. Telehome care devices used to be as simple as a blood pressure cuff and sphygmomanometer. Today, devices such as automated blood pressure monitors, glucose testing meters, peak flowmeters, pulse oximeters, weight scales, and two-way digital video transport systems are used. The devices offer data recording, audible alarms or reminders, and data uploading, in addition to reports on disease progression and trends. They are used for diverse patient populations, including persons with heart failure, hypertension, diabetes, asthma, chronic obstructive pulmonary disease (COPD), cystic fibrosis, depression, and bipolar disorder. Real-time data capture is particularly important in the management of numerous chronic diseases (Kerkenbush and Lasome, 2003).

Telehealth has brought to the forefront some significant practice issues. For instance telehealth has the potential to transcend state boundaries, which creates issues given that nurses and most health care providers are licensed in specific states. The scopes of practice and standards for practice vary from state to state, as do the laws and regulations that cover practice. Additionally, not all telehealth networks offer secure communications, which may limit the acceptability of this intervention for some persons. The process of referrals, a need for technical support personnel, and a lack of standards for interoperability of equipment are significant issues facing telehealth providers.

PAST, PRESENT, AND FUTURE COMPUTING TRENDS

Computers have moved from the realm of a "nice to know" luxury item to a "need to know" essential resource for professional practice. Nurses are knowledge workers who require accurate and up-to-date information for their professional work. The explosion in information—some estimate that all information is replaced every 9 to 12 months—requires nurses to be on the cutting edge of knowledge to practice ethically and safely. Trends in computing will affect the work of professional nurses in areas beyond the development of the CIS and EHR. Research advances, new devices, monitoring equipment, sensors, and "smart body parts" will all change the way that health care is conceptualized, practiced, and delivered.

Weiser and Brown (1996) have characterized the history and future of computing in three phases. The first phase is known as the "mainframe era," in which many people shared one computer. Computers during this phase were found behind closed doors and run by experts with specialized knowledge and skills. Although we have mostly moved beyond the mainframe era, it still exists in certain health care CIS settings (for instance in the departmental systems discussed earlier) and other industries that rely on large mainframe systems, such as banking, weather forecasting, and legacy systems in academic institutions.

Phase II in modern computing is the era of personal computers (PCs), which is characterized by one person (linked) to one computer. In this era, the computing relationship is personal and intimate. Similar to how consumers think of a car, perception of a computer is that of a special, relatively expensive item that requires attention, but provides a very valuable service in one's life.

Phase III has been dubbed the era of ubiquitous computing (UC), in which there will be many computers to each person. Weiser and Brown (1996) estimate that the crossover of the UC era with the PC era will occur between 2005 to 2020. In this phase, computers will be everywhere: in walls, chairs, clothing, light switches, cars, appliances, and so on. Computers will become so fundamental to our human experience that they will "disappear," and we will cease to be aware of them.

The Internet can also be considered an integral component of UC. Each time you connect to the Internet, you are connecting with millions of information resources and hundreds of information delivery systems. A person truly does become one person linked to hundreds of computers. Ironically the interface to the UC world of the Internet is still through a PC. However, this is changing. Wireless infrared connections have started to eliminate wires; handheld devices will eliminate the relatively bulky PC. Network wireless technologies are becoming more prevalent, are in continuous evolution, and enable the following:

- ◆ Instant access via HHCs to prescription writing, charge capture, research, patient education, daily schedules, memo writing, voice dictation, photography, drug calculations, and lab orders

+ Telehealth for sending and receiving data
+ Voice communication
+ Once we become wireless and mobile, UC will become a reality.

Voice Systems

Voice recognition (computer users talk to a computer) is becoming commonplace. Some institutions have found the accuracy of voice recognition to be sufficient for health care providers to use in dictating patient encounters. Individual users train their PCs to recognize their voices and are able to dictate documents and e-mails and direct their computers to perform specific activities on voice command.

Voice communication systems are being integrated into some clinical institutions. Unlike the overhead paging system or the digital pager that is worn on a belt, these sophisticated systems provide an efficient mechanism for communication among health care providers. Located in Baltimore, Maryland, St. Agnes Healthcare has been featured for its wireless technology using the Vocera communication system. Staff wear badges that weigh less than 2 ounces—think of the *Star Trek* communicator—that allow them to answer or initiate internal and external calls and designate the party to be called by name, title, function, or group, thereby eliminating the need to know phone numbers or who is on duty. As *Forbes* magazine rightly noted, "Communication in a hospital is often an amazingly inefficient affair. Nurses and doctors spend a lot of time playing phone and page tag" (Hesseldahl, 2004, p. 1). To understand the value of Vocera, St. Agnes's staff conducted a study of two units: one with Vocera deployed and the other operating in its normal fashion. In the Vocera-enabled unit, a total of 3477 annual labor hours were saved. There was reduction in overhead paging, more efficient workflow, support of quality care delivery, and time savings. More than half the nurses and three quarters of the unit secretaries believed they saved at least 30 minutes per shift. That is amazing (Breslin et al, 2004; Kuruzovich et al, 2006).

Robot Technology

Mobile robotic technology combined with wireless communications are in use in several institutions. The Remote Presence Robotic system, developed by InTouch Health in 2002, enables hospital intensivists and specialists to interview and examine patients—even when the health care providers are at their offices or homes. Robotic technology is being used to connect language translators, who are at home at night, with patients who need translation services in hospitals (Greenback, 2007). Robots also have been used to deliver additional sensorimotor activity to persons whose arms were paralyzed as a result of stroke, to distribute medications, and as couriers within institutional settings. Data indicate that (1) patients and health care providers are satisfied with the technology, (2) patient outcomes when using this technology are as good as or better than control groups, (3) medication dispensing and administration errors are decreased, and (4) efficiency may be improved (InTouch Health, 2006; Thacker, 2005; Van den Bent et al, 2009; Volpe et al, 1999).

Biometric Technology

Increasingly, biometric technology is being used for authentication and security. Biometric technologies use human characteristics, such as fingerprints, retinas, irises, voices, and facial patterns, to authenticate or grant access to data or information. More and more HHCs are including biometric options to provide an additional layer of security.

World Wide Web Advances

While the initial World Wide Web has been described as Web 1.0, there have been significant advances in Web 2.0 and the subsequent Web 3.0. Web 2.0 significantly changed the way people shared, collaborated, and connected with each other and with ideas and information. Specific Web 2.0 technologies include web logs (blogs), social bookmarking sites, wikis, podcasts, shared databases, and collaborative writing spaces.

The promises of Web 3.0 are portability and personalization. Intelligent portable devices, such as the iPhone and others, put capabilities and power in the palm of the hand that were recently only found in desktop or laptop computers. Opportunities to personalize web pages, using iGoogle and widgets for instance, shift the focus from a generic web space to one focused on an individual's preferences.

INFORMATION LITERACY AND INFORMATION TECHNOLOGY

The rapid growth in and turnover of information and the enormous changes in technologies that allow access to and storage of information make it imperative that nurses possess information literacy and fluency with information technology. Information literacy is defined as the ability to "recognize when information is needed and have the ability to locate, evaluate, and use effectively the needed information" (Association of College and Research Libraries [ACRL], 1998, par. 3).

Information technology is defined as the hardware and software that facilitate the storage, retrieval, communication, and management of information. According to the National Academy of Sciences report, "Being Fluent with Information Technology" (Computer Science and Telecommunications Board, 1999):

◆ Information technology has entered our lives over a relatively brief period of time with little warning and essentially no formal educational preparation for most people.

◆ Many people who currently use information technology have only a limited understanding of the tools they use and a (probably correct) belief that they are underutilizing them.

◆ Many people do not feel confident or in control when confronted by information technology, and they would like to be more certain of themselves.

Whereas not every nurse will need to be an informatics specialist, every nurse must be computer literate. Computer literacy is defined as the knowledge and understanding of computers, combined with the ability to use them effectively (Joos et al, 1996). Computer literacy may be interpreted as different levels of expertise for different people in various roles. On the least specialized level, computer literacy involves knowing how to turn on a computer, start and stop simple application programs, and save and print information. For health care professionals, computer literacy requires having an understanding of systems used in clinical practice, education, and research settings. For example, in clinical practice, electronic patient records and clinical information systems are becoming more widely used. The computer-literate nurse is able to use these systems effectively and can address issues discussed earlier, such as confidentiality, security, and privacy. At the same time, the nurse must be able to effectively use applications typically found on PCs, such as word processing software, spreadsheets, presentation graphics, and statistics for research. Finally the computer-literate nurse must know how to access information from a variety of electronic sources and how to evaluate the appropriateness of the information at the professional and patient levels alike.

Information Competencies in Clinical Practice

The need to stay current with clinical advances and new knowledge comes from patients, colleagues, third-party payers, and certifying boards. Even with the growth of information technology, the increase of health care information is exponential, and the task of reliably and quickly finding that needle in the haystack is daunting. Evidence-based nursing grew out of the general need to efficiently and effectively sift through the haystack to find the high-quality information needed to answer patient care questions (Mclnyk and Fineout-Overholt, 2004). Information technology and the ability to access reliable electronic resources are crucial to ensure that health care delivery is based on current knowledge and best practices (Alpay and Russell, 2002; IOM, 2001; Parker, 2005; Stein and Deese, 2004). The ability to access up-to-date evidence-based practice information results in (1) improved quality of patient care (California HealthCare Foundation, 2002), (2) improved patient safety (Sensmeier and Horowitz, 2003; Simpson, 2005), (3) increased confidence (Shorten, Wallace, and Crooks, 2001), and (4) improved nursing productivity and efficiency (Bartholomew and Curtis, 2004; Bower and McCullough, 2004; Sensmeier and Horowitz, 2003).

Unfortunately many, if not most, nurses do not possess adequate information technology, information literacy, and computer literacy (Gosling, Westbrook, and Spencer, 2004; Skiba, 2004). A national survey of 2000 randomly selected members of the American Organization of Nurse Executives (McCannon and O'Neal, 2003) found that using e-mail effectively, operating basic Windows applications, and searching databases were considered critical skills for new nurses entering the workforce. Of nurses who use the Internet to access health care information, many received no formal training (Estabrooks et al, 2002). In fact, studies indicate that nurses receive less education related to information technology, information literacy, and computer literacy than do most health care workers (Alpay and Russell, 2002). As a result of inadequate competencies, nurses are twice as likely to seek out general and less credible information instead of targeted information relevant to practice (Estabrooks et al, 2002).

There is evidence that most nurses are not using the knowledge base of their profession to answer clinical questions. In one study (Bostrom and Suer, 1993), only 21% of 1200 nurses used evidence in their practice. Like other health care providers, nurses have a low awareness of available Internet resources (Sigouin and Jkadad, 2002), in part at least because they are not prepared to use the health care information available on the Internet (Pravikoff, Tanner, and Pierce, 2005) and in part because Internet access and support for Internet resources are not widely available in the patient care setting (Retsas, 2000). Two important initiatives designed to address nursing students' and nurses' limited competencies in information technology, information literacy, and computer literacy are Technology Informatics Guiding Educational Reform (TIGER, 2009) and a Health Resources and Services Administration (HRSA)–funded Learning Information Seeking and Technology for Evidence-Based Nursing Practice (LISTEN) program (LISTENUPHEALTH, 2009). For more information on these two initiatives, visit www.tigersummit.com and http://listenuphealth.org.

Nursing Informatics

Although all nurses are involved with computers to some degree, some nurses have chosen to specialize in the area of nursing practice that relates to computers. This field is known as nursing informatics (NI), a relatively new specialty within the profession of nursing. Ozbolt and Saba (2008) provide a timeline of the brief history of nursing informatics in the United States. The early 1970s saw the emergence of computing applications in the nursing literature; in the

1980s nursing informatics was recognized as a distinct specialty in nursing, and in the 1990s the American Nurses Association (ANA) published the first Scope and Standards of Practice for the specialty. The American Nurses Credentialing Center has a certification examination for nurses who are involved in informatics. There is tremendous potential for nurses within this specialty to have a major effect on the way care is planned and delivered in the current complex health care environment.

Informatics is more than just computers—it includes all aspects of technology and science, from the theoretic to the applied. Health care informatics is an interprofessional arena. NI refers to that component of informatics designed for and relevant to nurses. Several definitions of NI have been developed, but the one that generally is accepted has been set forth by the ANA, which states,

> "Nursing informatics is a specialty that integrates nursing science, computer science, and information science to manage and communicate data, information, knowledge, and wisdom in nursing practice. Nursing informatics supports consumers, patients, nurses, and other providers in their decision-making in all roles and settings. This support is accomplished through the use of information structures, information processes, and information technology" (ANA, 2008, p. 1).

Embedded in this definition are the many components of NI: information processing, language development, applications of the system's life cycle, and human-computer interface issues.

Nurse informaticists are knowledge workers (IOM, 2004) that enact their roles in a variety of settings. Some nurse informaticists serve as liaisons to users of computer systems, through designing, implementing, and evaluating CISs. Other nurse informaticists are involved with quality improvement or administrative roles. Most nurse informaticists work in hospitals or health systems, with about one fifth employed by vendors (Sensmeier and Weaver, 2007). Future trends for nurse informaticists, as identified in a 2007 Healthcare Information and Management Systems Society (HIMSS) Nursing Informatics Survey, include (1) leadership in the development, selection, and implementation of health information technology; (2) an increasing focus on interoperability and integration of systems; (3) creating systems that support patient-centric care; (4) integrating informatics roles across all areas of nursing, including specialty areas; and (5) the need for more education and training to prevent a shortage of nurse informaticists (Sensmeier and Weaver, 2007).

Applied Information Literacy

Students entering nursing programs directly from high school are members of the net generation, those "digital natives" born after 1980 who have grown up with technology, including computers, video games, CDs, mobile phones, and the Internet (Caruso and Kvavik, 2005; Prensky, 2001a; Rodgers and Starrett, 2005). Net generation students favor multimedia and are known for their multitasking, multiprocessing, and connectivity to people and ideas (Oblinger and Oblinger, 2005; Rodgers and Starrett, 2005). As native speakers of the digital language of computers and video games (Jukes, 2005), they think and process information fundamentally differently than people who are older and spend less time on reflection and critical thinking (Prensky, 2001b).

In part because of their technology experiences to date, net generation students expect that they will instantaneously find answers to their questions on the Internet. They expect to find the right answer using free Internet resources and expect that the right answer will be somewhere within the first 10 items of a Google search (Livingstone, 2005a). Of concern is that although

BOX **14-1**

Illustration of Search Strategy Effectiveness

The term being explored is "never events," which are considered by Medicare to be preventable errors for which Medicare will no longer reimburse organizations if they occur.

Type of Search	Site	Results
Quick & Dirty	www.google.com	54,200—a majority of results are newspaper articles and general websites and articles that list the never events but do not provide useful information
Advanced	www.google.com/advanced_search	For .gov = 1830 For .org = 6520 For .edu = 406
Brute Force	Searched "www.neverevents.com"	Page returned that said "Page coming soon"
Link Searching	Using the .gov advanced search: • 1st result is the Centers for Medicare & Medicaid Services (CMS) • 2nd result is the Agency for Healthcare Research and Quality (AHRQ)	From 1st result—no links From 2nd result—many helpful links, including: • What's New in Never Events • Editor's Picks for Never Events including those from AHRQ, journal articles, books/reports, newspaper/magazine articles, tools/toolkits, and web resources

they may know how to get answers quickly, they are not able to evaluate the accuracy and integrity of their results (Rodgers and Starrett, 2005). Once in college, net generation students' dependence on Google and other search engines continues, at the expense of using library resources and databases (Lippincott, 2005). Students in a nationwide study reported using an electronic device (excluding cell phones) for 11 to 15 hours per week, but using a library resource to complete a course assignment less than 1 hour per week (Caruso and Kvavik, 2005).

Research has demonstrated that students (1) regularly overrate themselves on their ability to find information on the Internet, (2) recognize they struggle and waste time when attempting to find useful materials for class, (3) have not been taught how to evaluate if the information they locate is reliable and trustworthy, (4) do not understand how and when to use library databases for resources, and (5) enter their educational programs with varying degrees of experience and ability in computer skills and knowledge (Livingstone, 2005b; McEuen, 2001; Sinclair and Gardner, 1999).

Finding Information on the Internet

Effective and efficient searching is a must in today's information overloaded society. Purposeful use of a variety of strategies can improve search results (Box 14-1 lists an example of these search strategies).

- ◆ Quick and dirty searching can be useful if you're looking for information in an unfamiliar area. Type your search term into a search engine such as Google (www.google.com). Review your results to see which ones sound most promising.
- ◆ Advanced searching allows you to set specific limits on your searches. For instance, at Google's advanced search (www.google.com/advanced_search) you can limit

your searching to educational (.edu), organizational (.org), or governmental (.gov) domains, as well as by language, file type, and date. Another advanced search option is www.googlescholar.com, where you are more likely to find information related to research and evidence-based practice. Limiting your searches in this way can help ensure your results are more credible, authoritative, useful, and up-to-date.

♦ Brute force is a method of searching where you type in what you think might logically be a web address and see what happens. Sometimes you'll receive an error message, but sometimes you find precisely what you're looking for.

♦ Link searching can be helpful once you find a relevant website. Explore links from the site you find that connect to other relevant sites.

It is important to be persistent and purposeful in searching because no one search strategy or search engine will work for all purposes every time. The "deep web," that portion of the Internet that search engines do not access, is likely composed of as many pages as the public web. Although the number of pages and quality of search results have improved over time (Henzinger, 2007), it can still be a challenge to find what you need on the Internet. You can augment your searching by incorporating additional strategies.

First, you should target your search by conducting a "purpose-focus-approach" (PFA) assessment. To determine your purpose, ask yourself why you are doing the search and why you need the information. Consider questions, such as the following:

♦ Is the information for personal interest?
♦ Do you want to obtain information to share with coworkers or a client?
♦ Are you verifying information given to you by someone else?
♦ Are you preparing a report or writing a paper for a class or project?

Based on your purpose, your focus may be:

♦ Broad and general (basic information for yourself)
♦ Lay-oriented (to give information to a patient)
♦ Professionally oriented (for colleagues)
♦ Narrow and technical with a research orientation

Purpose combined with focus determines your approach. For example, information that is broad and general can be found using brute force methods or quick and dirty searching. Lay information can be quickly accessed at a few key sites, including MEDLINEplus and consumer health organizations. Similarly, professional associations and societies are a good starting point for professionally oriented information. Scientific and research information usually requires literature resources that can be found in scholarly databases, such as MEDLINE or the Cumulative Index to Nursing and Allied Health Literature (CINAHL).

Evaluating Information Found on the Internet

As you access information on the Internet, it is imperative that you perform a critical evaluation of what you have obtained. The Internet is open to anyone with access to a computer, and material that looks official may actually be posted by persons without formal education in an area. Some of the information you access may also contain inaccuracies. There are several forms that can assist you in your evaluation. Table 14-2 shows a website evaluation form from Kent State University that offers five criteria and examples of the types of evidence that should factor into your rating of a website. Following are the specific criteria that are useful in evaluating a website.

Authority with Regard to the Topic. For this criterion you are interested in the author of the site. It is important to review the author's credentials to ascertain whether the author's

TABLE **14-2**

Website Evaluation Form

WEBSITE EVALUATION							

Name:

Course:

Instructor:

Website title:

Web URL:

Date visited:

Brief description of the contents of the site:

CRITERIA AND TYPES OF EVIDENCE	HOW THE WEBSITE BEING EVALUATED MET THE CRITERION	(low) 1	2	RATING 3	4	(high) 5
1. Authority with regard to topic—who is responsible for the site? Author of site (individual or institutional affiliation, organization) Credentials, expertise, experience Contact information (name, e-mail, postal address) URL type suggests reputable affiliation						
2. Objectivity—is the purpose of the site clear, including any particular viewpoint? Statement of purpose and scope Intended audience Information presented as factual or opinion, primary or secondary in origin Criteria for inclusion of information Disclosure of sponsorship or underwriting						
3. Accuracy—is the information accurate? Facts documented or well researched Facts compare with related print or other online sources Links provided to quality web resources						
4. Currency—is the information current? Evidence of current content Pages date-stamped with latest update						
5. Usability—is the site well designed and stable? Site organization logical and easy to maneuver Content readable by intended audience Information presented is error free (spelling, punctuation) Readily identifiable link back to the institutional or organizational home page Site reliably accessible Pages loaded quickly Subtotal by rating of points awarded for each of the five criteria						

Continued

TABLE 14–2

Website Evaluation Form—cont'd

ASSESSMENT OF WEBSITE	
Rating based on the total number of points: 5-9 points: poor 10-14 points: fair 15-19 points: good 20-25 points: excellent	Your personal assessment—would you recommend this site? Why or why not?

Courtesy Kent State University Libraries and Media Services, Kent, OH; www.library.kent.edu/files/webevalform.pdf.

background prepares him or her to write on the subject of the website. The author's contact information should be provided. The affiliation of the website is important—*.edu* is an educational institution; *.org* is a nonprofit organization; *.com* is a commercial enterprise; *.net* is an Internet service provider; *.gov* is a governmental body; and *.mil* is military.

Objectivity. This criterion is concerned with whether the purpose of the website is clear, particularly whether a specific viewpoint is advanced at the expense of alternative views. Reviewing the site's statement of purpose and intended audience is important. Identifying whether information that is presented is factual or opinion and whether the information is primary or secondary in origin is also important. Some sites are sponsored or underwritten by other organizations. In assessing health care websites, it is particularly important to note whether a pharmaceutical company is sponsoring the information because that may influence the objectivity of the content.

Accuracy. Determine whether the information is accurate by looking for documentation and referencing. Compare information on the website with other sources. Review links that go from the website to other Internet resources. Ensure that the links are going to quality resources.

Currency. Review the website for evidence that the information it contains is current. Look for dates at the top and bottom of the page. Given the rapid changes in health care information, you should expect that the website is updated regularly. Compare the last update of the website with current literature. For example, if you review a website about diabetes, make sure that the information incorporates the latest practice standards and resources.

Usability. This criterion is concerned with whether the site is well designed and stable. The website should be accessible, logically organized, and easy for users to maneuver. The content should be error-free and readable by the intended audience.

Get in the habit of evaluating websites that you access to ensure that the information is authoritative, objective, accurate, current, and usable. Merely because a Web page is published and accessible on the Internet does not imply that it is a resource that would be useful to you, other professionals, or the lay public. Box 14-2 provides several credible websites where you can find good information related to health care technology and NI.

BOX **14-2**

Helpful Websites and Online Resources

CIS-HIT WEBSITES

Healthcare Information and Management Systems Society (HIMSS)
   www.himss.org/ASP/index.asp
   The HIMSS focuses on providing leadership for optimal use of health care information technology and management systems. A comprehensive site about various aspects of clinical information systems.

U.S. Department of Health and Human Services (DHHS) Health Information Technology (HIT) website
   http://healthit.hhs.gov
Official central governmental hub for all HIT-related items, including reports and standards.

NI WEBSITES

American Nursing Informatics Association
   www.ania.org
Nursing Informatics section of the HIMSS website
   www.himss.org/ASP/topics_nursingInformatics.asp

INFORMATION/COMPUTER LITERACY WEBSITES

Association of College and Research Libraries information literacy competency standards for higher education
   www.ala.org/ala/mgrps/divs/acrl/issues/infolit/index.cfm
   A comprehensive look at the information literacy competency standards that were proposed by the Association of College and Research Libraries to guide higher education.

Twenty-First-Century Information Fluency Project
   http://21cif.com/
   Comprehensive site for teaching and learning about information fluency. Free online documents and interactive games and exercises to help people learn to locate, evaluate, and use digital information resources more effectively, efficiently, and ethically.

HIPAA WEBSITES

Office for Civil Rights—HIPAA site
   www.hhs.gov/ocr/privacy
   The official central governmental hub for all HIPAA issues including rules, standards, and implementation guides.

   www.hipaa.org
   The law, identifiers, transactions, enforcement, security, privacy, code sets, industry discussion, collaboration, and other resources.

HANDHELD COMPUTING WEBSITES

University of Connecticut Health Center
   http://libdatabase.uchc.edu/temphome/pda/index.html
   In addition to background information about HHCs and considerations for purchasing an HHC, this site has numerous links to general and health care–related software for HHCs. Specific categories, noting palm or pocket PC operating system, include medical link resources, medical databases, medical calculators, drug guides, patient information, texts and journals, and evidence-based medicine.

Johns Hopkins University
   www.welch.jhu.edu/internet/mobile.html
   This site lists HHC software by subject area, such as anesthesiology, complementary and alternative medicine, and cardiology. Specific notations for cost are included.

TELEMEDICINE WEBSITES

Health Resources and Services Association
   www.hrsa.gov/telehealth
   Official governmental site for telehealth. Contains links to publications, funded telehealth projects, and links to relevant websites.

Telemedicine Information Exchange
   http://tie.telemed.org/default.asp
   This site claims to be "an unbiased and all-inclusive platform for information on telemedicine and telehealth." Established early on with the support of the federal government, it is now supported and maintained by the Association of Telehealth Service Providers.

SUMMARY

As a profession, nurses must understand and manage information technology, information literacy, and computer literacy. As the largest group of organized health care professionals in the United States, nurses have a responsibility to patients and society to continually improve and refine their competencies and knowledge base. Findings of multiple studies confirm that nurses in every role and at each level of education and practice exhibit large gaps in knowledge and competencies for information technology, information literacy, and computer literacy. The saying, "you don't know what you don't know" applies because nurses are often unaware that they need information.

Nurses have an important role in tracking, interpreting, and improving quality of care, in addition to translating research into practice. Technology continues to change and evolve at an ever-increasing pace. Be a lifelong learner. Take face-to-face or online classes. Arrange groups in your place of employment to learn more about technology and information literacy. Buddy up with someone who is a sophisticated user of technology. Get gadgets and software and start using them. Just do it.

 Additional resources are available online at: http://evolve.elsevier.com/Cherry/

REFERENCES

Agency for Healthcare Research and Quality (AHRQ): *Conference proceedings: creating a national telehealth nursing research agenda.* 2006. Retrieved October 2009 from: http://tie.telemed.org/articles/article.asp?path=articles &article=telehealthNursingAgenda_ca_tie06.xml.

Alpay L, Russell A: Information technology training in primary care: the nurses' voice, *Comput Inform Nurs* 20:136–142, 2002.

American Nurses Association: *Nursing informatics: Scope and standards of practice,* ed 3, Washington, DC, 2008, ANA.

Association of College and Research Libraries (ACRL): *A progress report on information literacy: an update on the American Library Association Presidential Committee on Information Literacy: final report.* 1998. Retrieved October 2009 from: www.ala.org/ala/mgrps/divs/acrl/publications/whitepapers/progressreport.cfm.

Bakken S, Cimino JJ, Hripcsak G: Promoting patient safety and enabling evidence-based practice through informatics, *Med Care* (Suppl 2):II-49–II-56, 2004.

Bartholomew K, Curtis K: High-tech, high-touch: why wait? *Nurs Manage* 35(9):48–54, 2004.

Bates D, Gawande AA: Improving safety with information technology, *N Engl J Med* 348(25):2526–2534, 2003.

Bostrom J, Suer WN: Research utilization: making the link to practice, *J Nurs Staff Dev* 9:28–34, 1993.

Bower FL, McCullough C: Nurse shortage or nursing shortage: have we missed the real problem? *Nurs Econ* 22:200–203, 2004.

Breslin S, Greskovich W, Turisco F: Wireless technology improves nursing workflow and communications, *Comput Inform Nurs* 22:275–281, 2004.

California HealthCare Foundation: *The nursing shortage: can technology help?* 2002. Retrieved October 2009 from: www.wha.org/workForce/pdf/nursingshortagetech.pdf.

Caruso JB, Kvavik RB: *ECAR study of students and information technology, 2005: convenience, connection, control, and learning,* Boulder, CO, 2005, EDUCAUSE Center for Applied Research. Retrieved October 2009 from: www.educause.edu/ECAR/ECARStudyofStudentsand Informat/158586.

Computer-Based Patient Record Institute: *Guidelines for establishing information security policies at organizations using computer-based patient records: work group on confidentiality, privacy, and security,* Schaumburg, IL, 1995, CPRI.

Computer Science and Telecommunications Board: *Being fluent with information technology,* Washington, DC, 1999, National Academies Press.

Ehrmeyer SS, Hausman P, Lebo R: Using technology to improve patient safety at point of care, *Point Care* 4:146–149, 2005.

Estabrooks CA, et al: The internet and access to evidence: how are nurses positioned? *J Adv Nurs* 42(1):73–81, 2002.

Garritty C, Eman KL: Who's using PDAs? Estimates of PDA use by health care providers: a systematic review of surveys, *J Med Internet Res* 8:e7, 2006.

Gosling AS, Westbrook JI, Spencer R: Nurses' use of online clinical evidence, *J Adv Nurs* 47:201–211, 2004.

Greenback L: Robot aids Johns Hopkins patients, *The Examiner,* January 9, 2007. Retrieved February 2007 from: www.examiner.com/articlePDF.cfm?articleID=498079~Robot_aids_Johns_Hopkins_patients.html.

Hebda T, Czar P: *Handbook of informatics for nurses & healthcare professionals*, ed 4, Upper Saddle River, NJ, 2009, Pearson-Prentice Hall.

Henzinger M: Search technologies for the internet, *Science* 317:468–471, 2007.

Hesseldahl A: *Your Trekkie communicator is ready*. 2004. Retrieved March 2006 from: www.forbes.com/technology/2004/03/16/cx_ah_0316chips.html.

Hoenich N, Lindley E, Stoves J: Technological advances in renal care, *J Med Eng Technol* 27.1–10, 2003.

Institute of Medicine: *Crossing the quality chasm: a new health care system for the 21st century*. 2001. Retrieved August 2005 from: www.iom.edu/Object.File/Master/27/184/0.pdf.

Institute of Medicine (IOM): *Key capabilities of an electronic health record system: letter report*. 2003. Washington, DC, Institute of Medicine of the National Academies.

Institute of Medicine (IOM): *Keeping patients safe: transforming the work environment of nurses*. 2004. Washington, DC. Retrieved June 2007 from: www.nap.edu/openbook.php?isbn=0309090679.

InTouch Health: InTouch technologies. Retrieved February 2006 from: www.intouch-health.com/index.html.

Joos I, et al: *Computers in small bytes: the computer workbook*, ed 2, New York, 1996, National League for Nursing Press.

Jukes I: *Understanding digital kids (DKs): teaching & learning in the new digital landscape*. 2005. Retrieved May 2005 from: http://thecommittedsardine.net/infosavvy/education/handouts/ndl.pdf.

Kerkenbush NL, Lasome CEM: The emerging role of electronic diaries in the management of diabetes mellitus, *AACN Clin Issues Adv Prac Acute Crit Care* 14:371–378, 2003.

Knecht K, Simpson RL, Weaver CA: Clinical transformation and nursing executive leadership. In Weaver CA, et al, editors: *Nursing and informatics for the 21st century: an international look at practice, trends, and the future*, Chicago, IL, 2006, Healthcare Information and Management Systems Society (pp. 57–85).

Kuruzovich J, et al: *Wireless communication role in patient response time: a study of Vocera integration with a nurse call system*. 2006. Retrieved March 2006 from: www.vocera.com/downloads/UofMD_St_Agnes2.pdf.

Lewandrowski K, et al: Evolution of point-of-care testing in a large academic teaching hospital: current applications and observations from the Massachusetts General Hospital, *Point Care* 4:128–132, 2005.

Lindquist AM, et al: The use of the personal digital assistant (PDA) among personnel and students in health care: a review, *J Med Internet Res* 10:e31, 2008.

Lippincott JK: *Net generation students and libraries*. 2005, EDUCAUSE Resources. Retrieved November 2005 from: www.educause.edu/Resources/EducatingtheNet Generation/NetGenerationStudentsandLibrar/6067.

LISTENUPHEALTH: 2009. Retrieved October 2009 from: http://listenuphealth.org.

Livingstone S: *UK children go online: end of Award report*. 2005a. Retrieved November 2005 from: www.lse.ac.uk/collections/children-go-online.

Livingstone S: *Internet literacy among children and young people: findings from the UK Children Go Online project*. 2005b. Retrieved November 2005 from: http://eprints.lse.ac.uk/397/1/UKCGOonlineLiteracy.pdf.

McCannon M, O'Neal PV: Results of a national survey indicating information technology skills needed by nurses at time of entry into the work force, *J Nurs Educ* 42:337–340, 2003.

McEuen SF: How fluent with information technology are our students? *Educause* 4:8–17, 2001.

Melnyk BM, Fineout-Overholt E: *Evidence-based practice in nursing & healthcare: a guide to best practice*, Philadelphia, 2004, Lippincott Williams & Wilkins.

Newbold SK: New uses for wireless technology, *Nurs Pract* 29(4):45–46, 2004.

Nichols JH: Point-of-care testing data management, *Point Care* 3:8–10, 2004.

Oblinger DG, Oblinger JL: *Educating the net generation*. 2005. Retrieved October 2009 from: www.educause.edu/educatingthenetgen.

Ozbolt JG, Saba VK: A brief history of nursing informatics in the United States of America, *Nurs Outlook* 56:199–205, 2008.

Pancoast PE, Patrick TB, Mitchell JA: Physician PDA use and the HIPAA privacy rule, *J Am Med Inform Assoc* 10:611–612, 2003.

Parker PJ: One nurse informatics specialist views the future: technology in the crystal ball, *Nurs Adm Q* 29:123–124, 2005.

Pravikoff DS, Tanner AB, Pierce ST: Readiness of US nurses for evidence-based practice, *AJN* 105(9):40–51, 2005.

Prensky M: Digital natives, digital immigrants, *On the Horizon* 9(5), October, 2001a. Retrieved May 2005 from: www.marcprensky.com/writing/.

Prensky M: Digital natives, digital immigrants, part II: Do they really *think* differently? *On the horizon* 9 2001b. Retrieved May 2005 from: www.marcprensky.com/writing/Prensky%20-%20Digital%20Natives,%20Digital%20Immigrants%20-%20Part2.pdf.

Retsas A: Barriers to using research evidence in nursing practice, *J Adv Nurs* 31(3):599–606, 2000.

Rodgers M, Starrett D: TECHPED: don't be left in the e-dust, *Natl Teach Learn Forum Newslett* 14(5), 2005. Retrieved November 2005 from: www.ntlf.com/html/ti/techped.htm.

Savage B, et al: Information technology and acute dialysis, *Curr Opin Crit Care* 8:544–548, 2002.

Sensmeier J, Horowitz JK: Advance care delivery through technology: align information technology initiatives with staff expectations regarding patient safety, *Nurs Manage* 34(10):2–6, 2003.

Sensmeier J, Weaver C: *HIMSS 2007 Nursing informatics survey.* 2007. Retrieved October 2009 from: www.himss.org/content/files/CBO/Meeting9/Nursing_Informatics_Survey.pdf.

Shorten A, Wallace MC, Crooks PA: Developing information literacy: a key to evidence-based nursing, *Int Nurs Rev* 48:86–92, 2001.

Sigouin C, Jkadad AR: Awareness of sources of peer-reviewed research evidence on the internet, *JAMA* 287:2867–2869, 2002.

Simpson RL: Patient and nurse safety: how information technology makes a difference, *Nurs Adm Q* 29:97–101, 2005.

Sinclair M, Gardner J: Planning for information technology key skills in nurse education, *J Adv Nurs* 30:1441–1450, 1999.

Skiba DJ: Informatics competencies, *Nurs Educ Perspect* 25:312, 2004.

Smith C: New technology continues to invade healthcare: what are the strategic implications/outcomes? *Nurs Adm Q* 28(2):92–98, 2004.

Stein M, Deese D: Information systems and technology: addressing the next decade of nursing challenges, *Nurs Econ* 22:273–279, 2004.

Technology Informatics Guiding Education Reform (TIGER): *The TIGER initiative: evidence and informatics transforming nursing: 3-year action steps toward a 10-year vision.* Retrieved October 2009 from: www.aacn.nche.edu/Education/pdf/TIGER.pdf.

Thacker PD: Physician-robot makes the rounds, *JAMA* 293:150, 2005.

Thompson BW: The transforming effect of handheld computers on nursing practice, *Nurs Adm Q* 29:308–314, 2005a.

Thompson BW: HIPAA guidelines for using PDAs, *Nursing* 35(11):24, 2005b.

Van den Bent PMLA, et al: Medication administration errors in nursing homes using an automated medication dispensing system, *J Am Med Inform Assoc* 16:486–492, 2009.

Versel N: PDAs greatly improve practice efficiency, *Modern Physician* 7(12):11, 2003.

Volpe BT, et al: Robot training enhanced motor outcome in patients with stroke maintained over 3 years, *Neurology* 53:1874–1876, 1999.

Weiser M, Brown JS: *The coming age of calm technology.* Retrieved October 1996 from: www.ubiq.com/hypertext/weiser/acmfuture2endnote.htm.

Emergency Preparedness and Response for Today's World

Linda D. Norman, DSN, RN, FAAN
Elizabeth E. Weiner, PhD, RN, BC, FAAN

evolve Additional resources are available online at: http://evolve.elsevier.com/Cherry/

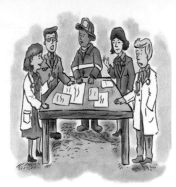

Partnering to respond to disaster.

VIGNETTE

Jane Wolverton works as a staff nurse on a medical-surgical unit at the Culverton General Hospital. She is in a patient's room giving an intravenous (IV) medication when the news program announces that there has been a major explosion at a chemical plant. The plant has 400 workers, including her husband.

■ QUESTIONS TO CONSIDER WHILE READING THIS CHAPTER:

1 How do we prepare for mass casualty events that will overwhelm the resources of our health facility?

2 How are response efforts coordinated so that the needs of the local area are met?

3 How do hospitals organize themselves to manage disaster situations while continuing to communicate with other external agencies?

4 How does the response differ when the hospital suffers damage and cannot function normally?

5 Where can I find current information about this ever-changing area?

KEY TERMS

All-hazards approach A process approach for all sectors to prepare for any emergency or disaster that may occur.

Biologic agents Microorganisms or toxins from living organisms with infectious or noninfectious properties that produce lethal or serious effects in plants and animals.

Chemical agents Solids, liquids, or gases with chemical properties that produce lethal or serious effects in plants and animals.

Comprehensive emergency management A broad style of emergency management, encompassing prevention, preparedness, response, and recovery.

Consequence management Measures to protect public health and safety, restore essential government services, and provide emergency relief to governments, businesses, and individuals affected by the consequences of terrorism.

Containment Limitation of an emergency situation within a well-defined area.

Credible threat Situation in which the Federal Bureau of Investigation (FBI) determines that a terrorist threat is credible and confirms the involvement of a weapon of mass destruction (WMD) in the developing terrorist incident.

Crisis management Measures to identify, acquire, and plan the use of resources needed to anticipate, prevent, and/or resolve a threat or act of terrorism.

Decontamination The physical process of removing harmful substances from personnel, equipment, and supplies.

Disaster condition A significant natural disaster or man-made event that overwhelms the affected state, necessitating both federal public health and medical care assistance.

Disaster medical assistance teams (DMATs) Regionally organized teams consisting of physicians, nurses, and other health care providers that can be sent into areas outside their own regions to assist in providing care for ill or injured victims at the location of a disaster or emergency. DMATs provide triage, medical or surgical stabilization, and continued monitoring and care of patients until they can be evacuated to locations where they will receive definitive medical care. Specialty DMATs can also be deployed to address, for example, mass burn injuries, pediatric care requirements, and chemical injury or contamination.

Emergency As defined in the Stafford Act, any occasion or instance for which, in the determination of the President, federal assistance is needed to supplement state and local efforts and capabilities to save lives and protect property, public health, and safety; includes emergencies other than natural disasters.

Emergency Management Assistance Compact (EMAC) An organization authorized by the U.S Congress through which a state impacted by a disaster can request and receive assistance from other member states quickly and efficiently (EMAC, 2009).

Incident command system (ICS) A multiagency operational structure that uses a model adopted by the fire and rescue community. ICS can be used in any size or type of disaster to control response personnel, facilities, and equipment. ICS principles include use of common terminology, modular organization, integrated communications, unified command structure, action planning, manageable span-of-control, predesignated facilities, and comprehensive resource management. The basic functional modules of ICS (e.g., operations, logistics) can be expanded or contracted to meet requirements as an event progresses.

Lead agency As defined by the FBI, the federal department or organization assigned primary responsibility to manage and coordinate a specific function—either crisis management or consequence management. Lead agencies are designated on the basis of their having the most authority, resources, capabilities, or expertise relative to accomplishment of the specific function. Lead agencies support the overall lead federal agency during all phases of the disaster response.

Major disaster As defined under the Stafford Act, any natural catastrophe (including any hurricane, tornado, storm, high water, wind-driven water, tidal wave, tsunami, earthquake, volcanic eruption, landslide, mudslide, snowstorm, or drought) or, regardless of cause, any fire, flood, or explosion in any part of the United States that in the determination of the President causes damage of sufficient severity and magnitude to warrant major disaster assistance under the Stafford Act to supplement the efforts and available resources of states, local governments, and disaster relief organizations in alleviating the damage, loss, hardship, or suffering caused thereby.

Mass casualty incident (MCI) A disaster situation that results in a large number of victims who need the response of multiple organizations.

Mitigation Those activities designed to alleviate the effects of a major disaster or emergency or long-term activities to minimize the potentially adverse effects of future disasters in affected areas.

National disaster medical system (NDMS) A nationwide medical mutual aid network between the federal and nonfederal sectors that includes medical response, patient evacuation, and definitive medical care. At the federal level it is a partnership among the U.S. Department of Health and Human Services (DHHS), the Department of Defense (DOD), the Department of Veterans Affairs (VA), and the Federal Emergency Management Agency (FEMA).

Nuclear weapons Weapons that release nuclear energy in an explosive manner as the result of nuclear chain reactions involving fission and/or fusion of atomic nuclei.

Personal protective equipment (PPE) Equipment designed to shield or isolate individuals from chemical, physical, and biologic hazards.

Preparedness Activities that build capability and capacity to address potential needs identified by the threat and vulnerability study.

Recovery Activities designed to return responders and the facility to full normal operational status and to restore fully the capability to respond to future emergencies and disasters; activities traditionally associated with providing federal supplemental disaster relief assistance under a presidential major disaster declaration. These activities usually begin within days after the event and continue after response activity ceases. Recovery includes individual and public assistance programs that provide temporary housing assistance, in addition to grants and loans to eligible individuals and government entities to recover from the effects of a disaster.

Response Activities to address the immediate and short-term effects of an emergency or disaster. Response includes immediate actions to save lives, protect property, and meet basic human needs. Based on the requirements of the situation, response assistance will be provided to an affected state under the federal response plan.

Scene assessment The act of reviewing the location of an event to look for information that might help to determine treatment options.

Technical operations Actions to identify, assess, dismantle, transfer, dispose of, or decontaminate personnel and property exposed to explosive ordnance or weapons of mass destruction (WMD).

Terrorist incident As defined by the FBI, a violent act or an act that is dangerous to human life, in violation of the criminal laws of the United States or of any state, and intended to intimidate or coerce a government, the civilian population, or any segment thereof in furtherance of political or social objectives.

Triage Process of prioritizing which patients are to be treated first; first action in any disaster response (Veenema, 2007).

Weapon of mass destruction (WMDs) As defined by Title 18, US Code 2332a, (1) any destructive device as defined in section 921 of this title, [which reads] any explosive, incendiary, or poison gas, bomb, grenade, rocket having a propellant charge of more than 4 ounces, missile having an explosive or incendiary charge of more than one quarter ounce, mine or device similar to the above; (2) poison gas; (3) any weapon involving a disease organism; or (4) any weapon designed to release radiation or radioactivity at a level dangerous to human life.

LEARNING OUTCOMES

After studying this chapter, the reader will be able to:

1 Describe the interaction between local, state, and federal emergency response systems.

2 Examine the roles of public and private agencies in preparing for and responding to a mass casualty event.

3 Compare and contrast chemical, biologic, radiologic, nuclear, and explosive agents and treatment protocols.

4 Access resources related to disaster preparedness on the Internet.

5 Communicate effectively (using correct emergency preparedness terminology) in regard to an MCI.

6 Describe the need for personal preparedness for individuals and households.

CHAPTER OVERVIEW

During the past decade we have seen many mass casualty events on U.S. property, some from natural disasters and some as a result of terrorist attacks. Examples of terrorist attacks include the New York World Trade Center bombing in 1993; the bombing of the Murrah Federal Building in Oklahoma City in 1995; the attacks on the U.S. embassies in Kenya and Tanzania in 1998; the attack in 2000 on the U.S.S. Cole, an American warship refueling in Yemen; and the anthrax scare in 2002 (Johns Hopkins Evidence-Based Practice Center, 2002). None of these events, however, had the same effect as the events of September 11, 2001, when the United States experienced devastating well-coordinated attacks in New York City and Washington, D.C., that led to the deaths of more than 3000 people.

Although a great deal of attention has been targeted to preparing for an MCI related to a terrorist attack, the United States has suffered major damage from natural disasters. Recent major natural catastrophic events have been the result of Hurricanes Katrina and Rita. Although the death toll from these events was not at the level of the destruction from the World Trade Center, the damage to the health care systems in the affected areas was substantial. It became evident very quickly that the response systems in place could not be effective in dealing with the destruction of the health care infrastructure, and, in fact, the health care agencies themselves were sites of mass casualty. The extensive need for immediate and long-term shelters for large numbers of victims also highlighted the need for nurses to have knowledge and skills in how to meet the needs of victims with psychologic and chronic diseases in a sheltered environment. Although the hurricanes took place in 2005, by their fourth anniversary it was clear that the area had not fully recovered from that event, and one of the area hospitals had not reopened.

Emergency management plans must address adequate response systems that can be used regardless of the cause of the MCI. A more reasonable approach has been the movement to plan and improve responses to a variety of hazards, called an all-hazards approach. Nurses have traditionally received disaster education as a part of community health content within nursing education programs as it related to natural disasters; however, the education has been focused on responding to a disaster site of victims when the health care system is still intact. In addition, they have not routinely received education related to biologic, chemical, nuclear, explosive, or radiologic hazards. It is imperative that all health care providers become knowledgeable about how to provide care for victims of all types of hazards and in situations where the health care system itself has been damaged, destroyed, or has no contact with the other parts of the community.

It is recognized by all federal agencies that the most serious knowledge deficit for health care providers is in the area of bioterrorism attacks and pandemic flu events. Unlike the other hazards, these situations place the health care providers in a different position of being first responders. Traditionally, first responders to emergencies have been the police, firefighters, and emergency medical technicians who respond with ambulances. In a biologic event (covert or natural transmission), however, victims will first appear in emergency departments, physicians' offices, nurse-managed clinics, or even in school health settings. Health care professionals need to be able to identify symptoms, patterns of similar events, and other irregularities. If they fail to recognize or report significant events, a biologic event could go unrecognized until it is of epidemic proportions. The same principles of responding to a bioterrorist event are pertinent for coping with a natural biologic outbreak, such as a pandemic flu event or severe acute respiratory syndrome (SARS). It is these types of diseases and exposures that are becoming the target of education for not only the health care community but also the general community at large to cooperate to prevent spread of a disease that would eventually become pandemic and a mass casualty event.

The purpose of this chapter is to describe the various components of our nation's local, state, and federal National Response Framework and how these components interrelate in the event of an MCI. The problems associated with natural or terrorist disasters when the health care system is damaged or rendered ineffective because of the event are reviewed. The kinds of agents that may be used in a terrorist attack are described along with the activities and response systems related to the preimpact and impact phase of a disaster. Readers will be particularly interested to note how standard triage and patient care priorities change when care is provided during an MCI. Additionally, readers are encouraged to closely review the list of key terms to understand and be able to use emergency preparedness terminology and explore the online resources about emergency preparedness and disaster management provided at the end of the chapter.

THE BASICS OF EMERGENCY PREPAREDNESS AND RESPONSE

Nurses have significant experience in dealing with natural disasters and are familiar with the work of the Red Cross in bringing disaster relief to affected areas. A disaster condition is defined as a significant natural disaster or man-made event that overwhelms the affected state and necessitates both federal public health and medical care assistance (Federal Emergency

Management Agency [FEMA], 2009a). The disaster condition must be declared of significant impact to warrant federal resources. It is important for nurses to understand the stages of a disaster to be able to determine the actions that are needed during each phase. In addition, understanding the responsibilities of the multiple agencies that respond to a disaster is imperative to be able to communicate with patients, families, and other health care providers.

In some situations the number of victims is so large that multiple organizations will be called to respond. A mass gathering is usually defined as a group of 1000 persons or more gathered together in a specific area for a specific purpose (Veenema, 2007). When casualties occur at this level, the event is termed an MCI. Although the situation may be unfamiliar for some nurses, it is important to remember that the nursing fundamentals practiced in other settings and during smaller crises are generally still applicable (Veenema, 2007). Traditionally, triage that is practiced in most health care agencies categorizes patients into low risk, intermediate care, and critically ill (those who need immediate care to save their lives). With such large numbers, however, there is a paradigm shift to change priorities into doing the greatest good for the greatest number of people. Care is given to those patients who have the greatest chance of survival. This type of triage typically places nurses in ethical situations in which they experience discomfort, particularly if patients are triaged and tagged to receive only pain management rather than typical extensive treatment that might be provided during normal health care conditions. Furthermore, the public responds to the visible tags placed on patients and can provide added stress when calling out to health care providers to provide further care. Nurses may also find themselves in positions in which there is a lack of necessary resources, and they will then have to come up with creative solutions. The literature has described the situations and triage decisions that health care providers, nurses, and physicians had to make to be able to provide care during the time of Hurricanes Katrina and Rita (Ginsberg, 2006; Johnson, 2006; Walsh and Orsega, 2006).

Terrorism has created the need for us to prepare against a variety of different agents. A standardized nomenclature has been developed for five categories using the acronym CBRNE, which stands for **c**hemical, **b**iologic, **r**adiologic, **n**uclear, and **e**xplosive. Table 15-1 describes the similarities and differences related to the CBRNE agents and provides information about treatment protocols for each agent.

STAGES OF DISASTER

Veenema (2007) describes three phases of the disaster continuum: preimpact, impact, and postimpact. In the preimpact phase, activities are focused on planning, preparedness, prevention, and warning. In the impact phase, all efforts are directed to responding to the disaster, initiating the emergency management system, and mitigating the effects of the hazard. During the postimpact phase, which usually begins 72 hours after the disaster and may continue for 2 to 3 years, a network of activities is designed to enhance recovery, rehabilitation, and reconstruction. Evaluation of the disaster preparedness and response plan is a major activity that needs to be included in the postimpact phase. The following sections describe components of the preimpact and impact phases of a disaster.

Preimpact Phase

Every disaster, regardless of the cause, begins as a local event. Each locale has the responsibility for responding to the emergencies within its community first. Thus the heaviest burden falls on the local community when a mass casualty occurs. Assistance from state and federal levels is appropriated when the local system is unable to provide the necessary level of care. It is

TABLE **15-1**

CBRNE Agents

AGENTS	ACTION	ADVANTAGES	DISADVANTAGES	TREATMENT
Chemical	Agents injure or kill through variety of means: vesicant, nerve, blood, respiratory	Spread easily through air; cause immediate effects; require decontamination	Less toxic than biologic agents; need to be used in large quantities; subject to dispersion by wind; terrorists need to protect themselves; require trained HAZMAT teams	Dependent on agent used; in some cases have agent-specific medications; require decontamination; require use of personal protective equipment by personnel
Biologic	Disease-causing organisms (bacteria, viruses, toxins)	Available; small quantities can have large effect; spread through large areas; can remain in air or on surfaces; difficult to prepare against	Delayed effects; production hazardous to terrorists; difficult to develop	Dependent on agent used; most cause flulike symptoms; plague and smallpox most contagious; timing of specific treatment critical; in some cases can have vaccinations
Radiologic	Ionizing radiation able to strip electrons from atoms, causing chemical changes in molecules; expression may be delayed; radiation depends on time, distance, shielding, and quantity of radioactive material	Available; psychologic effect likely to be substantial; often used in conjunction with explosive devices ("dirty bomb")	Delayed effects of radiation materials; difficult to shield against	Dirty bomb causes immediate effects (radiation burns, acute poisoning) and long-term effects (cancer, contamination of drinking water); decontamination must occur before patient care can be safely provided by the health care worker
Nuclear	Depends on yield of nuclear weapon, but consists of blast range effects, thermal radiation, nuclear radiation, and radioactive fallout	Requires decontamination; contamination can remain for many years; psychologic effect likely to be substantial	Large, heavy, and dangerous weapons; hazardous to terrorist; expensive and difficult to make weapons of this type	Symptomatic treatment of thermal burns, shrapnel injuries, and radioactive fallout; depends on distance from source and time of exposure
Explosive	Most common method for terrorists; capable of violent decomposition; pressure, temperature changes and propellants cause injury and/or death	Easy to find materials to construct explosive device; large devices can be placed in abandoned vehicles; smaller devices can be placed on bodies of persons willing to commit suicide by igniting the device	Volatile ingredients could cause premature explosion of device, thus creating danger for terrorists; government agencies have improved training and processes for identifying incendiary devices	Symptomatic; often requires treatment for burns

Linking Response Systems

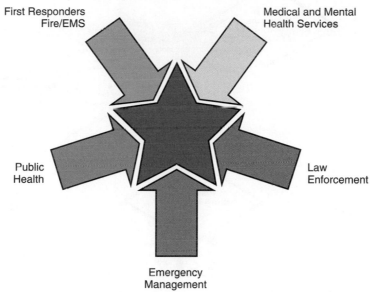

First Responders
Fire/EMS

Medical and Mental
Health Services

Public
Health

Law
Enforcement

Emergency
Management

Figure 15-1 *Agencies and services involved at the time of a disaster. (From http://emergency.cdc.gov/coca/ppt/ cdcopsdisasters_032806.ppt.)*

imperative then that communities plan for the services that will be needed in a time of disaster and train the providers within each agency about responding to all hazard types of mass casualty events. Efforts must be directed toward the interrelationship of roles and responsibilities of the agencies and services that will be needed at the time of a disaster (Figure 15-1).

The key elements of a community preparedness program should include the following:

- Assessing the community for risks and determining the types of events that may occur
- Planning the emergency activities to ensure a coordinated response effort
- Building the capabilities that are necessary to respond to the consequences of the events

There must be agreements between agencies within the community and between neighboring communities for such entities as emergency response units, hospitals, long-term care facilities, clinics, and health departments to be able to provide mutual aid and transfer of people and materials during a time of disaster. This part of the health care system was certainly stressed during the response to the Katrina and Rita hurricanes.

Agreements should be in place that address issues related to credentialing health care providers who may be shared among institutions. The Medical Reserve Corps (MRC) was initiated in 2002 to improve the health and safety of communities across the country by organizing and utilizing public health, nursing, medical, and other volunteers (Office of the Civilian Volunteer Medical Reserve Corps, 2009). Part of the requirements for membership in the MRC is to complete an emergency response curriculum. The MRC is the responsibility of the local area, with many states receiving funding to establish the network of volunteers. They function as a way to locally organize and utilize volunteers who want to donate their time and expertise to prepare for and respond to emergencies and promote healthy living throughout the year. MRC volunteers supplement existing emergency and public health resources. There are situations (such as Hurricane Katrina) that local units deployed outside of their region to respond to the

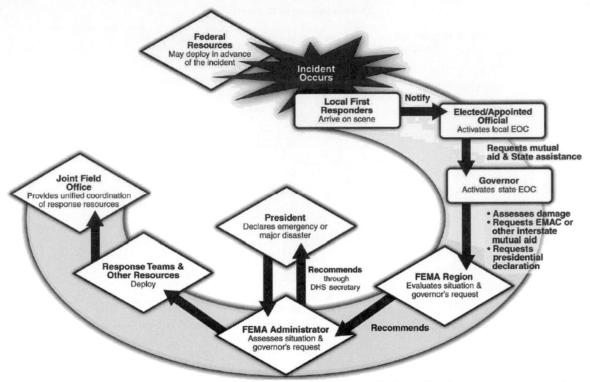

Figure 15-2 *Emergency response flows from the community to the state to the federal level. (From FEMA: National response framework. 2009. Available at: www.fema.gov/pdf/emergency/nrf/nrf-overview.pdf.)*

additional needs that were not being met. (See www.medicalreservecorps.gov/about/ for more information about how to volunteer to participate in the MRC system.)

Plans and contracts also need to be developed with school systems, YMCAs, or other large facilities to provide shelter for large numbers of victims. The interface with volunteer agencies, such as the Red Cross, also needs to be arranged. Each agency should have a well-developed emergency operating plan (EOP) that includes its responsibilities and capabilities for responding to a mass casualty event, an identified chain of command, and a plan for interaction with other community agencies. Agency personnel should be knowledgeable about their role in the EOP and receive education concerning the ways to respond to all types of hazards.

Several federal level programs are designed to assist communities in planning their emergency response to a mass casualty event and to provide assistance during a time of disaster. Agency and community EOPs should outline their relationship with the federal system. The National Response Framework (formerly known as the National Response Plan) is a guide to how the nation conducts an all-hazard response—from the smallest incident to the largest catastrophe—using a comprehensive, national, all-hazards approach to domestic incident response (FEMA, 2009b). Figure 15-2 illustrates the relationship among local, state, and federal response systems. Following is a description of the key components of the federal response system.

Metropolitan Medical Response System (MMRS). The MMRS builds a cadre of specialty trained responders and equipment. The system is coordinated with area and statewide planning systems and integrates the efforts of all of the emergency response teams. The MMRS includes plans for expanding hospital-based care, enhancing emergency medical transport and emergency department capabilities, locating specialized pharmaceuticals to respond to a mass casualty event, managing mass fatalities, and providing mental health care for the community, victims, and health care providers. Scenarios designed to test the effectiveness of the MMRS in the community in providing an integrated response to an MCI are conducted on a regular basis.

National Disaster Medical System (NDMS). NDMS is a federally coordinated system that augments the nation's medical response capability during times of major peacetime disasters and to provide support to the military and the Department of Veterans Affairs medical systems in caring for casualties evacuated back to the U.S. from overseas armed conventional conflicts (U.S. Dept. of Health and Human Services [USDHHS], 2009a). The National Response Framework utilizes the NDMS under Emergency Support Function #8, Health and Medical Services, to support the federal medical response to major emergencies and federally declared disasters including national disasters, major transportation accidents, technologic disasters, and acts of terrorism. Included in the NDMS are disaster medical assistance teams (DMATs), disaster mortuary operational response teams (DMORTs), national veterinary response teams (NVRTs), national nurse response teams (NNRTs), and national pharmacy response teams (NPRTs). (For more information about becoming involved in NDMS go to www.hhs.gov/aspr/opeo/ndms/join/index.html.)

Commissioned Corps. The Commissioned Corps emergency response teams are managed by the Office of the Surgeon General and are part of the U.S. Public Health Service. These teams are an additional asset capable of responding in times of extraordinary need when the public health needs exceed the ability of the local or state agencies. The Commissioned Corps is composed of more than 6000 health care professionals that can be deployed to respond to a disaster, either as a large group or in small numbers to support the DMAT effort. (For more information go to www.usphs.gov/AboutUs/emergencyresponse.aspx.)

Strategic National Stockpile (SNS). The Centers for Disease Control and Prevention (CDC) host an SNS that has large quantities of medicine and medical supplies to protect the American public if there is a public health emergency severe enough to cause local supplies to be depleted. The SNS has a national repository of antibiotics, chemical antidotes, antitoxins, IV administrations, airway supplies, and other medical-surgical items. A 12-hour "push-pack" of supplies can be deployed within 12 hours of the decision to activate the SNS. The community emergency plan should include procedures to receive the push package. Follow-up pharmaceutical or medical supplies can be shipped within 24 to 36 hours if required. This supply can be tailored to the specific needs of the event if the needs are known at that time (CDC, 2009).

Community emergency operating plans must include strategies for the community's interaction with these various state and federal response teams and systems to efficiently use the services and materials provided for mass casualty response. Hospital EOPs should include descriptions of the federal responses and how they will be incorporated into the emergency operations.

Though not formally part of emergency operations, individuals and households play an important role in the overall emergency management strategy. They can contribute by reducing hazards in and around their homes, preparing emergency supply kits and household emergency plans, and monitoring emergency communications carefully. The Ready government website provides additional disaster response information and can be found at www.ready.gov.

Impact Phase

Response Activities. Response activities are first initiated during the impact phase of disasters. These activities begin at the time of the event and are focused on providing the first emergency response to victims of the disaster, stabilizing the situation, and providing adequate treatment for the victims. This phase requires the interaction of emergency responders from fire and police departments, emergency medical services, hazardous materials teams, health care agencies, health departments, and other agencies to be able to triage and provide assistance to the victims and stabilize the scene. Usually the first unit responding establishes an incident command post from which to coordinate the activities. However, as other units arrive and as the cause of the incident becomes known, one of the law enforcement agencies may assume control if there is suspicion of a crime before the establishment of a community-based emergency operations center (EOC).

National Incident Management System (NIMS). Emergencies breed chaos, and it is essential to bring order to the situation for an effective response. The NIMS provides a systematic proactive approach to guide departments and agencies at all levels of government, nongovernmental organizations, and the private sector to work seamlessly during disaster situations (FEMA, 2009a). The system is designed to expand from one person or agency performing all roles to having hundreds of people involved in the process. An efficient NIMS requires a hierarchic chain of command led by the incident manager or commander. Job assignments are consistently followed by assigned personnel who refer to a specific job action sheet. An NIMS will be established at the scene of the disaster and include representatives of all agencies needed to provide the emergency services.

At the time of a mass casualty, each hospital system will initiate its emergency response plans. Structures may vary from hospital to hospital, but most are using the system called the hospital incident command system (HICS). The assumption is that in a time of crisis, communication will be improved if all disaster responders begin from a common structure. HICS defines responsibilities, reporting channels, and common terminology for hospitals, fire departments, local governments, and other agencies (California Emergency Medical Services Authority, 2009). The HICS can be customized for organizations of varying sizes. (The HICS chart can be downloaded online at no charge at www.emsa.ca.gov/HICS.)

Regardless of the structure of the NIMS, the ultimate aim is to coordinate the safe and effective response of emergency resources to an incident. In the HICS there is only one incident commander, supported by clearly identified levels in the command structure. The hierarchy of command is important so that there is no confusion as to who reports to whom or about who is managing the incident. The chain of command is established to allow for communication to flow from the top down or the bottom up. (FEMA provides online training modules about the incident command system for hospitals and health care providers at: www.training.fema.gov/emiweb/IS/is100HC.asp.)

It is important to understand that although a community event may trigger the establishment of an EOC using incident management, the local hospitals establish their own centers to manage the incident within that hospital. Careful attention is paid, however, to designate a liaison officer to coordinate the response between the community EOC and the hospital EOC. Successful use of incident command principles depends on a unified command structure with a clearly established chain of command, along with incident objectives and strategies. In the aftermath of Katrina and Rita, multiple hospitals reported that the HICS was one of the most important aspects of the disaster response that kept the system intact and functioning when the hospital lost power and flooded.

Personal Protection and Safety. Personal protection and safety are important regardless of the situational factors causing an MCI. What is important to note, however, is that situational factors dictate how to be personally protected and safe. Protecting the lives of emergency responders takes precedence over other incident issues because if emergency responders are exposed or injured, they will not be able to provide care to others.

Because of the varied routes of exposure from CBRNE agents, personal protective equipment (PPE) must be designed to impede the most vulnerable route(s), thereby blocking the agent from entering the body. Specially designed PPE is available in a variety of levels, each level designed to meet specific protection needs:

- *Level A* provides a totally encapsulated chemical resistant suit, including supplied air. As a result, maximum respiratory and skin protection is provided. In addition, this level of equipment is used to provide protection against liquid splashes or in situations in which agents are still unidentified.
- *Level B* provides a chemical splash–resistant suit with hood and self-contained breathing apparatus (SCBA). It provides maximum respiratory protection but less skin protection than level A equipment.
- *Level C* equipment is chemical-resistant clothing with a hood and an air-purifying respirator. The respirator can remove all anticipated contaminants and concentrations of chemical materials, thus providing adequate protection against airborne biologic agents and radiologic materials.
- *Level D* protection may consist of a uniform or scrubs and is appropriate when it has been determined that no respiratory or skin hazard is present.

Although each level provides some protection, it is important to understand the limitations of all PPE. Typically, first responders to community emergencies are firefighters, police, and emergency medical technicians. These professionals have traditionally been trained in the effective use of PPE and can be a good community resource. In addition, hospital infection control personnel can be an excellent resource for the use of PPE. As health care providers assume the care of patients who may have been contaminated, it is important to note whether they have been decontaminated and require no further protective equipment or what additional level of protection is required.

Communication Within the Health Care Facility. At the initial time of the event, when news stories are first breaking, staff, patients, and families may hear of the incident before the EOP and HICS have been initiated. In this case it is crucial for the facility information officer to take charge of communicating with the news media and for administrators to initiate a plan to communicate within the health care facility. Crisis intervention strategies to prevent group panic must be instituted immediately. Communication officers need to do the following:

- Determine the effects the crisis will have on the audience.
- Speak clearly and simply about the facts.
- Be direct, honest, and to the point.
- Reassure and calm the audience.

Regular updates of information (every 30 minutes) need to be planned and distributed to all hospital units as quickly as possible (Veenema, 2007). Patients and families need to be informed of measures that will be taken with the initiation of the EOP, such as early discharge or relocation of less ill patients to other areas of the hospital or to other facilities. Family members may not be able to leave the hospital to return home; arrangements will need to be made to care for them, including providing medications that they take regularly.

Lessons Learned from Mass Casualty Incidents

The most recent U.S. mass casualty incidents were Hurricanes Katrina and Rita. Lessons learned from these events have informed health care agencies of the extensive nature of disaster preparation that needs to occur. The Agency for Healthcare Research and Quality (AHRQ) provides several valuable guidelines to assist hospitals and communities with disaster preparedness including:

- *Community-Based Mass Prophylaxis: A Planning Guide for Public Health Preparedness*
- *Disaster Alternate Care Facilities: Selection and Operation*
- *Evaluation of Hospital Disaster Drills: A Module-Based Approach*
- *Mass Medical Care with Scarce Resources: A Community Planning Guide*

The AHRQ Guidelines are available online at www.ahrq.gov/prep/.

Although preparation for all types of causes of MCIs (natural or man-made) is necessary, nurses must understand the actions needed when the health care agency is damaged and how health care providers must function during those times. Issues related to use of personnel, rotation and resting of personnel, use of family or volunteers, methods of evacuation, and care of hospital staff and families must be included in emergency preparedness preparations and education. Alterations in the standard of care during an MCI need to be understood. The DHHS prepared a report that makes recommendations about the adjustments to standards of care to be able to serve the greatest number of people. This report is available online at www.ahrq.gov/research/altstand.

Hospitals are viewed by the community and employees as places of safe haven when a disaster strikes. Incoming staff will be limited, and decisions about how care will be provided must be made. Places to provide rest and measures to encourage staff to rest should be determined early in the MCI. Mechanisms for staff to contact their families or significant others should be initiated as soon as possible. Arrangements need to be made for the care of children, other dependents, and pets for those staff members who will be staying at the hospital for extended periods. In addition, measures need to be included to provide information to the staff for those who are not able to locate their family because of the disaster. The role of the information liaison office of HICS is most important for this function.

Staff need to be prepared to cope with power outages and damage to the institution. All hospitals are equipped with emergency generators, and most hospital staff members assume that these will be operational. Emergency plans and drills need to include scenarios of how to adapt care if the generators are not functioning. It is important that the staff delivering care have the skill set to know how they will function in these situations. Lessons learned from previous disasters emphasize the necessity to include the care delivery staff in this level of detail (Ginsberg, 2006). Some examples of decisions that had to be made were how to:

- Deliver medications when the usual pumps were not functioning.
- Decide what medications would be given when the medication supply was depleted.
- Provide for ventilation and suctioning without electricity.

Nurse managers and staff on the nursing units need to be prepared for these situations. Preparing unit-based scenarios for discussion can be helpful in preparing for an MCI.

Nurses need to understand the steps for evacuation of patients to other areas of the hospital or to other health care agencies. Research conducted in Japan recommends that nurses include planning for evacuation of the patients on a unit as a part of the shift report at least once a week. They suggest a 3-minute plan to decide which patients should be evacuated first, how each patient would be evacuated, what personnel would be needed, and to assess the evacuation route to ensure there are no impediments (Yamamoto, 2006). Evacuation of patients in a hospital is not included routinely in hospital drills; however, evacuation posed major problems for hospitals during Hurricane Katrina (Johnson, 2006; Walsh and Orsega, 2006).

BIOLOGIC CAUSES OF MASS CASUALTY: PANDEMIC INFLUENZA

Nurses also need to be prepared to respond to MCIs that result from biologic agents. Although terrorist dissemination of biologic agents was initially the focus of emergency preparedness efforts following the World Trade Center attack, the natural dissemination of biologic agents such as influenza has been the priority for disaster preparedness efforts for communities. The threat of pandemic flu has been heightened recently because of the H1N1 virus (swine flu) and H5N1 virus (avian flu) outbreaks. A pandemic influenza is a global outbreak that occurs when a new influenza virus emerges in the human population, causing serious illness and death as it spreads worldwide. The United States has had three previous pandemic flu experiences: 1918—50 million died worldwide and 675,000 in the United States; 1957—1 to 2 million worldwide and 70,000 in the United States; and 1968—700,000 worldwide and 34,000 died in the United States (DHHS, 2009b).

The world has been watching outbreaks of different types of flu over the last few years. Detection efforts were most recently directed toward people who had contracted flu in other countries such as H1N1 from Mexico and those who became infected in other countries as a result of coming into contact with infected birds (H5N1). Cambodia, China, Indonesia, Thailand, Iraq, Turkey, Vietnam, and Egypt reported human deaths from H5N1 virus after coming into contact with infected birds or contaminated food (World Health Organization [WHO], 2006) and in Mexico from H1N1 virus. The mortality rate for H5N1 virus was initially 50% to 70% for human cases. The infected birds moved from Asia to Europe and Africa. Although the CDC prepared for it only being a matter of time before the infected birds reach the United States, few cases were actually reported. However, the H1N1 virus rapidly spread to the United States and other countries. Initially it was predicted that the H1N1 virus would have a high fatality rate, but as of 2009, the virus has been less virulent than predicted, with few fatalities in the absence of chronic disease and other disabilities (WHO, 2009).

The advent of the H5N1 virus focused the world's attention on pandemic flu. The immediate concern of the H5N1 virus was whether it was capable of human-to-human transmission. The strain closely resembled the 1918 influenza strain but was capable of mutation so rapidly that producing vaccines would be like "shooting a moving target." However, a vaccine for the H1N1 virus was produced within months of its initial detection. The effectiveness of a vaccine might not be known until time to use it.

It needs to be emphasized that vaccines may not be available in the early stages of a pandemic. Antivirals might be helpful, but the current supply of antiviral medication is grossly inadequate to meet our projected needs. Depending on the type of virus or bacteria, it is estimated that new vaccines may not be available until 4 to 6 months after the pandemic actually starts as a result of production limitations. Regular flu shots are not designed for the specific strain of flu (H5N1 or H1N1) and thus will not provide immunity to the various types of flu.

Experts at the WHO have designated phases of pandemic alert, which includes decisions on when to move from one phase to another. Figure 15-3 provides the details related to the

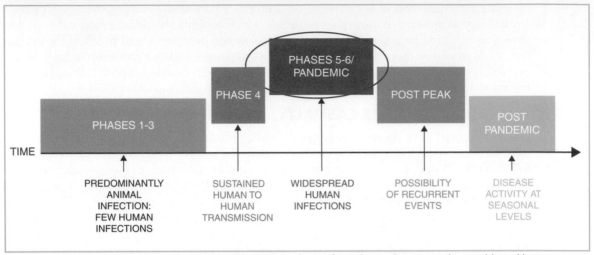

Figure 15-3 *Current World Health Organization (WHO) phase of pandemic alert. (From the World Health Organization. Retrieved August 2009 from: www.who.int/csr/disease/avian_influenza/phase/en.)*

six phases of alert with the alert phase in 2009 being at level 6. (The WHO global influenza preparedness plans can be found at: www.who.int/csr/disease/influenza/pipguidance2009/en.)

As with other mass casualty events, planning is aimed at saving the largest number of people. It is likely that flu varieties would strike nearly simultaneously in multiple geographic regions at nearly the same time and cause multiple waves of disease lasting 4 to 6 weeks in communities and 12 to 16 weeks nationally. Localities will need to make their plans self-sufficient because other areas will be dealing with the same problem. Control methods include isolation, quarantine, and restrictions. Limitations include suspension of large public gatherings, school closures, and social distancing. The term "social distancing" refers to the attempt to keep people as far apart as possible to limit the possibilities of spreading germs.

The most frequently recommended type of social distancing that has proved to be effective for H1N1 virus has been keeping people suspected of the illness at home until 24 hours after the fever has subsided. Health care providers are advised to treat patients symptomatically without encouraging them to come to offices or emergency departments. Many health care facilities set up separate screening facilities for those who have flulike symptoms.

Health care providers need to take the time to become familiar with their institutions' preparedness plan. Most will have a plan specific to the threat of pandemic flu. Know what your role is, how you would be notified, and where and how you would report if an emergency is declared. The U.S. government strategy will be to focus on saving lives: slow the spread, decrease illness and death, and buy time.

Being prepared means that you and your family need to be prepared as well. Practice good health hygiene and follow the general principles of sound public health. Teach family members how to cover their mouths when coughing, how to appropriately dispose of used tissues, and how and when to wash their hands. Develop contingency plans to address school and business closures, unavailability of public transportation, and disruption in social activities. Grocery stores and gas stations may not be open during their typical hours. That means that personal

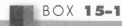

BOX **15-1**

Helpful Websites and Online Resources

Providing mass medical care with scarce resources: A community planning guide
   www.ahrq.gov/research/mce/
Centers for Disease Control and Prevention: Strategic national stockpile: emergency preparedness and response
   www.bt.cdc.gov/stockpile/index.asp
Federal Emergency Management Agency: National Response Framework, 2009
   www.fema.gov/emergency/nrf
Federal Emergency Management Agency: Online training about the incident command system for hospitals and health care providers
   www.training.fema.gov/emiweb/IS/is100HC.asp
Hospital Incident Command System (HICS)
   www.emsa.ca.gov/hics
Current information regarding the status of pandemic flu in the United States
   www.pandemicflu.gov
World Health Organization global influenza preparedness plans
   www.who.int/topics/influenza/en
How to volunteer for the Medical Reserve Corps
   www.medicalreservecorps.gov
Sigma Theta Tau: Disaster preparedness and response for nurses
   www.nursingknowledge.org/Portal/main.aspx?PageID=36&;SKU=91775
Vanderbilt University School of Nursing: Online modules for nurses in emergency preparedness
   www.nursing.vanderbilt.edu/incmce/modules.html

stockpiling of food and medications would help you and your family get through this event with minimal contact with others. Ideally the goal is to keep the number of people infected within range of existing medical capabilities.

For current information regarding the status of any pandemic flu, visit www.pandemicflu.gov for updates in the United States. Planning guides are available for federal, state, business, local, and individuals at this website. Global updates can be found at the website of the WHO (www.who.org, Pandemic influenza).

SUMMARY

Preparing for a mass casualty event requires a complex set of activities. All nurses need to be aware of the emergency response system at the local, state, and federal levels and how they should interface with the systems. They should be involved in developing and evaluating the emergency response plans for their health care agencies and communities. Consider Jane in the opening vignette. Her understanding of the resources available in the community's emergency response system will help her better cope with the disaster facing her family and the hospital where she works. Just as in Jane's situation, disaster can strike anytime and preparation for an effective emergency response is absolutely critical to ensure the very best outcome for everyone involved. Nurses are well positioned to serve in leadership roles within health care agencies during the time of a disaster because of their excellent skills in communication and collaboration. Box 15-1 provides a list of online resources for more information about emergency preparedness.

REFERENCES

California Emergency Medical Services Authority: *Disaster medical services: hospital incident command system (HICS)*. 2009. Available at: www.emsa.ca.gov/HICS.

Centers for Disease Control and Prevention: *Strategic national stockpile: emergency preparedness and response*. 2009. Available at: www.bt.cdc.gov/stockpile.

Emergency Management Assistance Compact. *EMAC* 2009. Available at: www.emacweb.org.

Federal Emergency Management Agency: *National incident management system*. 2009a. Available at: www.fema.gov/emergency/nims/AboutNIMS.shtm.

Federal Emergency Management Agency: *NRF resource center*. 2009b. Available at: www.fema.gov/emergency/nrf.

Ginsberg HG: Sweating it out in a level III regional NICU: disaster preparation and lessons learned at the Ochsner Foundation Hospital, *Pediatrics* 117(5 Pt 3):S375–S380, 2006.

Johns Hopkins Evidence-Based Practice Center: *Training of clinicians for public health events relevant to bioterrorism preparedness*, AHRQ Publication No. 02-E011, Rockville, MD, 2002, Agency for Healthcare Research and Quality.

Johnson C: *Emergency planning after hurricane Katrina: using task analysis with observational studies to simulate hospital evacuation*. 2006. Available at: www.dcs.gla.ac.uk/~johnson/papers/Katrina.pdf.

Office of the Civilian Volunteer Medical Reserve Corps: *Volunteers building strong, healthy, prepared communities*. 2009. Available at: www.medicalreservecorps.gov/HomePage.

U.S. Department of Health and Human Services (USDHHS): National disaster medical system (NDMS). 2009a. Available at: www.hhs.gov/aspr/opeo/ndms/index.html.

U.S. Department of Health and Human Services: Flu.gov. 2009b. Available at: www.pandemicflu.gov/general/index.html.

Veenema TG, editor: *Disaster nursing and emergency preparedness for chemical, biological, and radiological terrorism and other hazards*, New York, 2007, Springer.

Walsh T, Orsega S: Lessons from hurricane Rita: organizing to provide medical care during a natural disaster, *Ann Intern Med* 145:469–470, 2006.

World Health Organization: *Avian influenza in Egypt*. 2006. Retrieved January 2007 from: www.who.int/csr/don/2006_12_27a/en/index.html.

World Health Organization: *Current WHO phase of pandemic alert*. 2009. Retrieved September 2009 from: www.who.int/csr/disease/avian_influenza/phase/en.

Yamamoto A: Mid-term report on the project "disaster nursing in a ubiquitous society" in the academic years 2003 and 2004, *Japan J Nurs Sci* 3(1):65–69, 2006.

CHAPTER

16

Nursing Leadership and Management

Barbara Cherry, DNSc, MBA, RN, NEA-BC

evolve   Additional resources are available online at: http://evolve.elsevier.com/Cherry/

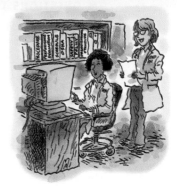

As a manager, the nurse will coordinate many aspects of care delivery.

VIGNETTE

Nancy Brown, a new registered nurse (RN), has accepted a position in a busy outpatient dialysis unit. During nursing school Nancy worked in the facility as a patient care technician, and she is confident in her clinical skills because of this experience. Mary, the nurse manager of the dialysis unit, has scheduled Nancy to attend the new-nurse orientation. Although Nancy thinks to herself, "I know what the RNs do around here; I'd like to jump right in without attending orientation," she readily accepts the assignment.

The nurse manager begins the orientation program with a discussion about the mission of the organization and the RN's responsibility to ensure that quality patient care is provided in a safe and cost-effective manner. As Nancy progresses through the orientation program, her confidence quickly fades. She becomes overwhelmed as she listens to a description of her new responsibilities as an RN. The RN's duties involve much more than the expected physical assessment, identifying nursing diagnoses, and developing and implementing care plans. Some of Nancy's many new responsibilities as a staff RN are to:

- *Supervise patient care technicians and manage assignments and supply use for a group of patients.*
- *Meet with the interprofessional team including the social worker, dietitian, nephrologist, nurse manager, and the patient and family to develop the patient's care plan and then follow up to coordinate and implement the plan.*
- *Serve on a task force charged with developing and implementing a new training and mentoring program for patient care technicians.*
- *Perform chart audits to review nursing documentation, identify problems, develop recommendations, and report to the quality management committee.*

As Nancy is trying to assimilate the information being presented, she almost fails to hear Mary say that within 6 months of employment all staff RNs are expected to begin orientation for the charge nurse position to provide backup coverage. At the end of the orientation, Nancy has a new perspective about professional nursing practice—it seems to be more about managing the delivery of patient care than actually giving the care!

■ QUESTIONS TO CONSIDER WHILE READING THIS CHAPTER:

1 What leadership and management skills will assist Nancy as she begins her new role as a staff RN responsible for supervising a group of patient care technicians, managing supply use, and serving on a task force to implement a new training program?

2 Why is it important for the nursing staff to understand the mission and values of the organization to provide direct patient care?

3 What type of team-building skills will help Nancy as she learns to work with the interprofessional team and coordinate the patient's plan of care with a diverse group of health professionals?

4 What resources are available to help Nancy learn and enhance her management and leadership skills?

KEY TERMS

Authority The legitimate right to direct others given to a person by the employer through an authorized position, such as manager or administrator.

External customers People in need of services from an organization who are not employed by the organization, including patients, family members, physicians, students, payers, discharge planners, and other groups that are a source of patient referrals.

Health care organization Any business, company, institution, or facility (e.g., hospital, home health agency, ambulatory care clinic, health insurance company, nursing home) engaged in providing health care services or products.

Internal customers People who are employed by the organization to provide services to various groups and individuals across the organization (e.g., nurses and other patient care staff, administrators, social workers, dietitians, therapists, housekeeping staff, and clerical support staff).

Leadership The act of guiding or influencing people to achieve desired outcomes; occurs any time a person attempts to influence the beliefs, opinions, or behaviors of an individual or group (Hersey and Blanchard, 1988).

Management Coordination of resources, such as time, people, and supplies, to achieve outcomes; involves problem-solving and decision-making processes.

Organizational chart A visual picture of the organization that identifies lines of communication and authority.

Productivity The amount of output or work produced (e.g., home visits made) by a specific amount of input or resources (e.g., nursing hours worked).

Resources Personnel, time, and supplies needed to accomplish the goals of the organization.

LEARNING OUTCOMES

After studying this chapter, the reader will be able to:

1 Relate leadership and management theory to nursing leadership and management activities.

2 Differentiate among the five functions of management and essential activities related to each function.

3 Integrate principles of patient-centered care and customer service in professional nursing practice.

4 Implement effective team-building skills as an essential component of nursing practice.

5 Implement the nursing process as a method of problem solving and planning.

6 Apply principles and strategies of change theory in the management role.

7 Discuss implications of leadership and management challenges of the twenty-first century.

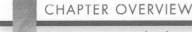

CHAPTER OVERVIEW

During nursing school students are often more concerned with developing clinical knowledge and skills and are less concerned with management and leadership skills. However, immediately after graduation the new nurse is placed in many situations that require leadership and management skills—managing a group of assigned patients, serving on a task force or committee, acting as team leader or charge nurse, or supervising unlicensed assistive personnel and licensed vocational or practical nurses. In addition to providing safe, evidence-based, high-quality clinical care, the challenges for RNs today are to manage nursing units that are constantly admitting and discharging higher-acuity patients, motivate and coordinate a variety of diverse health professionals and nonprofessionals, embrace change to develop work environments that are safer and more conducive to professional nursing practice, and manage limited resources and shrinking budgets.

Regardless of in which position or area the nurse is employed, the health care organization will expect the professional nurse to have leadership and management skills, including to:

- *Make good clinical decisions based on safety, quality, cost, legal, and ethical aspects of care.*
- *Promote evidence-based practice (see Chapter 6).*
- *Promote patient safety and quality improvement in the work environment.*
- *Coordinate patient care activities for the interprofessional team.*
- *Promote staff satisfaction, patient satisfaction, and overall unit productivity.*
- *Create and sustain trust between and among managers and staff.*
- *Actively manage the process of change through good communication, staff involvement, training, sustained attention, and measurement and feedback.*
- *Provide leadership to maintain compliance with governmental regulations and accreditation standards.*

As the reader can easily visualize, leadership and management activities are a primary responsibility for the RN. In fact professional nursing within the health care organization has as much to do with managing the delivery of care as it does with actually providing that care. This chapter presents key leadership and management concepts that will guide the nurse to grow and develop in this important aspect of the professional practice role.

Throughout this chapter "organization" is used to refer to the hospital, home health agency, post-acute care facility, long-term care facility, ambulatory clinic, managed care company, or any other area in which a nurse might be employed to practice professional nursing. Legal and ethical issues are a critical component of nursing management, although it is not within the scope of this chapter to discuss these issues. The reader is encouraged to review Chapter 8 regarding legal issues and Chapter 9 regarding ethical issues.

LEADERSHIP AND MANAGEMENT DEFINED AND DISTINGUISHED
Leadership Defined

Leadership occurs any time a person attempts to influence the beliefs, opinions, or behaviors of a person or group (Hersey and Blanchard, 1988). Leadership is a combination of intrinsic personality traits, learned leadership skills, and characteristics of the situation. The function of a leader is to guide people and groups to accomplish common goals. For example, an effective nurse leader is able to inspire others on the health care team to make patient education an important aspect of all care activities.

It is important to note that leaders may not have formal authority granted by the organization but are still able to influence others. The job title such as "nurse manager" will not make a nurse a leader. The nurse's behavior determines his or her ability to be viewed as a leader (Marquis and Huston, 2009).

Management Defined

Management refers to the activities involved in coordinating people, time, and supplies to achieve desired outcomes and involves problem-solving and decision-making processes. Managers maintain control of the day-to-day operations of a defined area of responsibility to achieve established goals and objectives. Managers plan and organize what is to be done, who is to do it, and how it is to be done. A nurse manager will have:

- An appointed management position within the organization with responsibilities to perform administrative tasks, such as planning staffing, performing employee performance reviews, controlling use of supplies and time, and meeting budget and productivity goals
- A formal line of authority and accountability to ensure that safe and effective patient care is delivered in a manner that meets the organization's goals and standards

Leadership Versus Management

Although leadership and management are intertwined and it is difficult to discuss one without the other, these concepts are different. Leadership is the ability to guide or influence others, whereas management is the coordination of resources (time, people, supplies) to achieve outcomes. People are led, whereas activities and things are managed. Leaders are able to motivate and inspire others, whereas managers have assigned responsibility for accomplishing the goals of an organization. A good manager should also be a good leader, but this may not always be the case. A person with good management skills may not have leadership ability. Similarly a person with leadership abilities may not have good management skills. Leadership and management skills are complementary; both can be learned and developed through experience and improving skills in one area will enhance abilities in the other.

Power and Authority

Leadership and management require power and authority to motivate people to act in a certain way. Authority is the legitimate right to direct others and is given to a person by the organization through an authorized position, such as nurse manager. For example, a nurse manager has the authority to direct staff nurses to work a specific schedule. Whereas authority is the legitimate right to direct others granted by the organization, power is the ability to motivate people to get things done with or without the legitimate right granted by the organization. The primary sources of power identified by Hersey, Blanchard, and Natemeyer (1979) are described as follows:

- *Reward power* comes from the ability to reward others for complying and may include such rewards as money, desired assignments, or acknowledgment of accomplishments.
- *Coercive power*, the opposite of reward power, is based on fear of punishment for failure to comply. Sources of coercive power include withheld pay increases, undesired assignments, verbal and written warnings, and termination.
- *Legitimate power* is based on an official position in the organization. Through legitimate power, the manager has the right to influence staff members, and staff members have an obligation to accept that influence.
- *Referent power* comes from the followers' identification with the leader. The admired and respected nurse manager is able to influence other nurses because of their desire to be like their nurse manager.

♦ *Expert power* is based on knowledge, skills, and information. For example, nurses who have expertise in areas such as physical assessment or technical skills, or who keep up with current information on important topics will gain respect and compliance from others.
♦ *Information power* is based on a person's possession of information that is needed by others.
♦ *Connection power* is based on a person's relationship or affiliation with other people who are perceived as being powerful.

An individual may also have informal power resulting from personal relationships, being in the right place at the right time, or unique personal characteristics, such as attractiveness, education, experience, drive, or decisiveness. By understanding the authority of an assigned position and the sources of formal and informal power, the nurse manager will be better able to influence others to accomplish goals.

Formal and Informal Leadership

Both formal and informal leadership can exist in every organization. Formal leadership is practiced by the nurse who is appointed to an approved position (e.g., nurse manager, supervisor, charge nurse, coordinator) and given the authority to act by the organization. Informal leadership is exercised by the person who has no official or appointed authority to act, but is able to persuade and influence others. The informal leader, who may or may not be a professional nurse, may have considerable power in the work group and can influence the group's attitude and significantly affect the efficiency and effectiveness of workflow, goal setting, and problem solving.

The nurse manager must learn to recognize and effectively work with informal leaders. Informal leadership may be positive if the informal leader's purpose is congruent with that of the nursing unit and organizational goals. For example, the informal leader of a patient care group may be highly supportive of a new nursing care delivery model being implemented on the unit, and as a result, the other team members will be more willing to accept the change. However, an informal leader who is not supportive of the nursing unit's goals can create an uncomfortable work environment for the nurse manager and the entire team. Following are some strategies the nurse manager can use to work with informal leaders:

♦ Identify the informal leaders in the work team and develop an understanding of their source of power (see sources of power in the previous section).
♦ Involve the informal leaders and other staff members in decision-making and change-implementation processes.
♦ Clearly communicate the goals and work expectations to all staff members.
♦ Do not ignore an informal leader's attempt to undermine teamwork and change processes. Coaching and counseling the person and setting clear expectations may be required.

LEADERSHIP THEORY

Understanding the development and progression of leadership theory is a necessary building block for developing leadership and management skills. Researchers began to study leadership in the early 1900s in an attempt to describe and understand the nature of leadership. The following sections provide a brief description of key leadership theories. Readers are encouraged to learn more about these theories, especially as they advance in their nursing career.

Leadership Trait Theory

Early leadership theory centered on describing the qualities or traits of leaders and has been commonly referred to as trait theory (Stogdill, 1974). Leadership trait theory was based on the assumption that leaders were born with certain leadership characteristics. Traits found to be associated with leadership include intelligence, alertness, dependability, energy, drive, enthusiasm, ambition, decisiveness, self-confidence, cooperativeness, and technical mastery (Stogdill, 1974). Although trait theories have been important in identifying qualities that distinguish today's leaders, these theories have neglected the interaction between other elements of the leadership situation. Trait theories also have failed to recognize the possibility that leadership traits can be learned and developed through experience. However, by keeping in mind these traits associated with effective leadership, the new nurse can identify areas in which he or she should improve and develop.

Interactional Leadership Theories

Researchers progressed from developing trait theory to studying the interaction between the leader and other variables of the leadership situation. Contemporary theories of leadership, such as situational and behavioral theories, have attempted to integrate the dynamics of the interaction among the leader, the worker, and elements of the leadership situation, arguing that effective leadership depends on several variables, including (1) organizational culture, (2) values of the leader and values of the followers, (3) influence of the leader or manager, (4) complexities of the situation, (5) work to be accomplished, and (6) environment (Marquis and Huston, 2009).

Transformational Leadership

In a contemporary concept of leadership, Burns (1978) identified and defined transformational leadership. Burns contends that there are two types of leaders: (1) the transactional leader, who is concerned with the day-to-day operations of the facility and (2) the transformational leader, who is committed to organizational goals, has a vision, and is able to empower others with that vision. The transformational leader is able to guide employees to feel pride in the work of the organization and to inspire them to be actively engaged to achieve the mission and goals of the organization. Transformational leaders spend time teaching and coaching, seek differing perspectives when faced with problems to solve, and seek new ways of improve the work environment. Box 16-1 compares characteristics of Burns' (1978) transformational and transactional leadership styles.

Studies have reported that nurse managers who demonstrate more transformational leadership characteristics achieve higher levels of staff satisfaction and work group effectiveness (Dunham-Taylor, 2000; Failla and Stichler, 2008; Raup, 2008). The implication for nurse managers is that transformational leadership is very effective in increasing staff satisfaction and work effectiveness. The student is encouraged to read more about transformational leadership

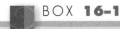

BOX **16-1**

Comparison of Transformational and Transactional Leaders

TRANSFORMATIONAL LEADERS	TRANSACTIONAL LEADERS
• Identify and clearly communicate vision and direction	• Focus on day-to-day operations and are comfortable with the status quo
• Empower the work group to accomplish goals and achieve the vision; impart meaning and challenge to work	• Reward staff for desired work ("I'll do X in exchange for your doing Y")
• Are admired and emulated	• Monitor work performance and correct as needed *or*
• Provide mentoring to individual staff members based on need	• Wait until problems occur and then deal with the problem

and to seek out transformational leaders as mentors. However, it is important to note that even the most effective transformational leader will fail without possessing the day-to-day management skills of transactional leaders (Bass, Avoliio, and Goodheim, 1987).

LEADERSHIP SKILLS

Hersey and Blanchard (1988) identified three major areas required for effective leadership:

1. Technical skills—for nurses this includes clinical expertise and nursing knowledge
2. Human skills—the ability and judgment to work with people in an effective leadership role
3. Conceptual skills—the ability to understand the complexities of the overall organization and to recognize how and where one's own area of management fits into the overall organization

At the staff nurse level of management a considerable amount of technical skill and clinical expertise is needed because the nurse generally is involved in direct supervision of patient care and may be required to help train and mentor nurses and other health care providers. As one advances from lower levels to higher levels in the organization, more conceptual skills are needed. Box 16-2 provides examples of technical, human, and conceptual practices required for nurse leaders.

BOX **16-2**

Effective Leading and Managing: Technical, Human, and Conceptual Practices

TECHNICAL PRACTICES
- Keep your own clinical skills and knowledge current.
- Train staff members adequately—be certain they are competent to perform their assigned responsibilities.
- Act as a willing consultant for clinical problems, contribute to sound nursing judgments, and teach others.

HUMAN PRACTICES
- Maintain honesty and integrity in work and relationships—trust is essential for effective leadership.
- Create a teaching and learning environment—earn a reputation for exceptional training and mentoring.
- Develop and role model a commitment to excellence.
- Create an open, nonthreatening environment—share information, keep staff informed, and encourage them to discuss issues.
- Make an emotional investment—give of yourself in a way that the staff understands your commitment to quality patient care. Care as much as you would like others to care.
- Become a proactive problem solver—knowing how to solve problems is more important than knowing all the answers.
- Get out of the office and into the patient care areas—listen to patients and staff.
- Maintain a confident, positive outlook—identify areas in which you are weak and seek help to learn and grow.

CONCEPTUAL PRACTICES
- Make a commitment to support the mission, vision, and goals of the organization.
- Accept the realities of complex health care systems, which are under pressure to improve patient safety and quality while cutting costs.
- Understand the needs of external customers (patients, families, physicians, referring facilities) and internal customers (staff, administrators, executives, and other departments).

BOX **16-3**

Management Styles

AUTOCRATIC/AUTHORITATIVE	DEMOCRATIC/PARTICIPATIVE	LAISSEZ-FAIRE
• Determines policy and makes all decisions	• Encourages staff participation in decision making	• Does not provide guidance or direction
• Ignores subordinates' ideas or suggestions	• Involves staff in planning and developing new ideas and programs	• Unable or unwilling to make decisions
• Dictates the work with much control	• Believes in the best in people	• Does not provide feedback
• Gives little feedback or recognition for work	• Communicates effectively and provides regular feedback	• Initiates little change
• Makes fast decisions	• Builds responsibility in people	• Communicates by memos or e-mail
• Successful with employees with little education or training	• Works well with competent, highly motivated people	• May work well with professional people

MANAGEMENT THEORY

Behavioral theories emerged to explain aspects of management based on behaviors of managers, leaders, and followers. Three prevalent management behavior styles were identified by Lewin (1951) and White and Lippit (1960): authoritarian, democratic, and laissez-faire. Box 16-3 presents characteristics of these management styles, which vary in the amount of control exhibited by the manager and the amount of involvement that the staff has in decision making. At one extreme the autocratic manager makes all decisions with no staff input and uses the authority of the position to accomplish goals. At the opposite extreme is the laissez-faire manager, who provides little direction or guidance and will forgo decision making. Democratic management is also often referred to as participative management because of its basic premise of encouraging staff members to participate in decision making.

Depending on the situation, the nurse manager may need to use different types of management styles. This concept of situational leadership requires consideration of staff members' needs and experiences, the manager's abilities, and the goals and tasks to be accomplished. For example, in a life-threatening situation, such as treating a patient in cardiac arrest, autocratic management might be appropriate. However, in structuring the weekend call schedule for a home health agency, a participative style of management would be more effective.

Today's health care system requires the use of a democratic or participative management style that involves the staff in patient safety, quality improvement, and problem solving. Health care settings are driven to become increasingly cost-effective while continuing to improve quality, customer satisfaction, and positive patient outcomes. Staff directly involved in the challenges presented by patient care often can suggest the most workable, practical solutions.

Organizational Theory

Just as leadership and management theories have evolved to provide a framework for understanding leadership and management, organizational theory has evolved to provide a framework for understanding complex organizations. A brief review of bureaucracy theory, systems theory, and chaos theory can provide the reader with insight into the value of using organizational theory to understand management processes within today's dynamic, complex health care organizations.

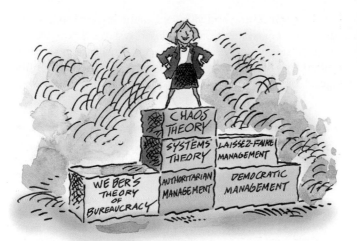

Leadership, management, and organizational theories provide the building blocks for effective nursing management practices.

Weber's Theory of Bureaucracy. Max Weber, known as the father of organizational theory, began his work in the 1920s when he observed the growth of large organizations and predicted that this growth required a formal set of procedures. Weber, in his classic work on defining the characteristics of bureaucracy, argued that the great benefit of bureaucracy was in its ability to apply general rules to specific cases, making the actions of management fair and predictable. The basis of Weber's concepts of bureaucracy revolves around explaining authority within organizations. He postulated that authority—the right to issue commands within an organization—is based on impersonal rules and rights granted by virtue of the management position rather than related to the person who occupies that position. Weber's conceptualization of bureaucracy emphasized rules instead of individuals and competency instead of favoritism as important for effective organizations. Other characteristics of organizations identified by Weber include the following:

- Managers are chosen because they have demonstrated knowledge, skill, and ability to fill the position.
- The division of labor, authority, and responsibility is clearly defined.
- Impersonal rules govern the actions of superiors over subordinates.
- All personnel are chosen for their competence and are subject to strict rules that are applied impersonally and uniformly.
- A system of procedures for dealing with work situations is in place.

Although the structure of bureaucracy described by Weber is still present in most organizations today, his work failed to recognize the complexity of human behavior and the constantly changing environment of today's organizations. As discussed, current leadership and management theories (i.e., participatory management, transformational leadership) recognize the importance of supportive, respectful relationships between managers and employees, with employees being involved in decision making and problem solving.

Systems Theory. The systems theory views the organization as a set of interdependent parts that together form a whole (Thompson, 1967). The interdependent nature of the parts of the organization suggests that anything that affects the functioning of one aspect of the organization will affect the other parts of the organization. Open systems suggest that the organization is affected not only by internal changes among any of its parts, but also external environmental forces that will have a direct influence on the organization and vice versa—the internal forces will affect the external environment. In contrast to open systems theory, closed systems theory views the system as being totally independent of outside influences, which is an unrealistic view for health care organizations. To be successful, today's health care organizations must be able to continually adapt to internal and external changes. Consider the following example to help explain systems theory.

CASE STUDY

The hospital in which William Scoggins, RN, works has reduced the number of RNs employed by the hospital and now requires that the remaining RNs work overtime "at the request of administration." The quality of patient care, patient safety, and the individual nurses' professional practice and personal health have been negatively affected by this change. William and his fellow RNs seek advice from their state nurses association about their professional responsibility to work mandatory overtime. The state nurses association is responding to the situation, which is occurring more frequently across the state and nation, by proposing legislation to mandate nurse-patient ratios and limits to mandatory overtime. The state government may now require hospital administrators to respond to the need for increased staffing levels.

This example demonstrates open systems theory. As internal forces in one department (hospital administration) mandated changes that affected another area (RNs and patient care), internal forces (RNs) pushed for changes from the external environment (state nurses association and state government). The external environment may now force changes to the organization (hospital administration).

Systems theory has provided nurse managers with a framework to view nursing services as a subsystem of the larger organization and to realize the interrelatedness and interdependence of all the parts of the health care organization. Open systems theory suggests that shared responsibility among all groups is necessary to help patients gain and maintain health and wellness (McGuire, 1999). The nurse will be wise to consider open systems theory and the effect a change in one area will have in another area, internal as well as external to the organization.

Chaos Theory. The chaos theory is a more recently developed organizational theory that attempts to account for the complexity and randomness in organizations. Despite the implications of the word *chaos*, the theory actually suggests that a degree of order can be attained by viewing complicated behaviors and situations as predictable. Nurse managers may wish for balanced and steady work environments, but in reality they are dealing with, what seems at best, a chaotic system. Chaos theory says that variation is a normal part of managing health care systems. Based on chaos theory, a nurse manager knows that staff absences as a result of illness, sick children, and family emergencies are a fact of life, requiring the nurse manager to have backup plans in place in the event that staff members "call in" and are not able to report for their assigned shift. Other examples of variation in health care are cultural diversity, constantly fluctuating patient census, and staffing shortages. Until nurses understand that these variations are a normal, predictable state in the organization and should be planned for, they may continue to experience excessive anxiety with the daily events that occur in health care organizations (McGuire, 1999).

MANAGEMENT FUNCTIONS

Classic theories of management suggest that the primary functions of managers are planning, organizing, and controlling (Stogdill, 1974). Leaders in nursing management have added two more functions to this list and now recognize five major management functions (Figure 16-1)

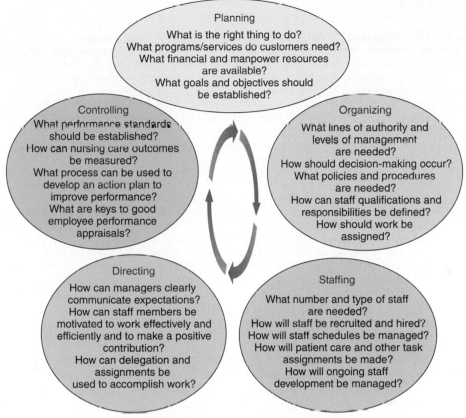

Figure 16-1 *Management functions.*

as necessary for the management of nursing organizations: (1) planning, (2) organizing, (3) staffing, (4) directing, and (5) controlling (Marquis and Huston, 2009).

1. *Planning* includes defining goals and objectives, developing policies and procedures, determining resource allocation, and developing evaluation methods.
2. *Organizing* includes identifying the management structure to accomplish work, determining communication processes, and coordinating people, time, and work.
3. *Staffing* includes those activities required to have qualified people accomplish work, such as recruiting, hiring, training, scheduling, and ongoing staff development.
4. *Directing* encourages employees to accomplish goals and objectives and involves communicating, delegating, motivating, and managing conflict.
5. *Controlling* processes include performing employee performance reviews, analyzing financial activities, and monitoring quality of care.

These management functions are interrelated; different phases of the process occur simultaneously, and the processes should be circular, with the manager always working toward improving the quality of health care, patient safety, and staff and customer satisfaction. Because understanding these five management functions is essential for success as a nurse manager, they will be discussed in further detail.

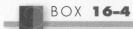

BOX **16-4**

Sample Mission, Values, and Philosophy Statement

The mission of Community Hospital is to provide high-quality, cost-effective health services that patients and families recommend; physicians prefer; employees, volunteers, and board members are proud of; health profession students learn and excel from; and the community values.

The philosophy and values of Community Hospital are:

- Commitment to professional and individual excellence with support for personal and professional growth.
- Continual quality improvement by identifying the key needs of our customers, assessing how well we meet those needs, continually improving our services, and measuring our progress.
- Ethical and fair treatment for *all* through a commitment to forming and maintaining relationships of fairness and trust with our patients, purchasers of our services, and our employees. Our business is conducted according to the highest ethical standards.
- Teamwork consistently demonstrated as we work together to provide ever-improving customer service. People at all levels of the organization will participate in decision making and quality improvement.
- Compassion is our highest priority, we will always provide care and comfort to people in need, and our patients and families will receive respectful and dignified treatment from all of our people at all times.
- Innovation in service delivery is accomplished by investing in the development of new and better ways to deliver services.

Planning

Planning is the first management function and involves several steps: (1) identify goals and objectives to be achieved; (2) identify resources (people, supplies, equipment, etc.) needed; (3) determine action steps; and (4) establish a timeline for the action steps and goal achievement. All management functions are based on planning. *Without effective planning, the management process will fail.* Effective planning requires the nurse manager to understand the following elements:

- Mission statement and philosophy of the organization
- Organizational strategic plan
- Goals and objectives for the entire organization
- Operational plan for the individual unit or facility

Mission and Philosophy. The mission statement, the foundation of planning for any organization, describes the purpose of the organization and the reason it exists. Most health care organizations exist to provide high-quality patient care, but emphasis may be on different concepts, such as research, teaching, preventive care, spiritual care, or community service. The philosophy is the set of values and beliefs that guides the actions of the organization and thus serves as the basis of all planning. New nurses should be aware of the mission and philosophy of the employing organization and understand the relationship between their own personal value system and that of the organization. Box 16-4 provides an example of an organization's mission and philosophy statement.

Strategic Planning. Strategic planning is long-range planning (extending 3 to 5 years into the future) and results from an in-depth analysis of (1) the business, community, the regulatory, and political environment outside the organization; (2) customer and patient needs; (3) technologic changes; and (4) strengths, problems, and weaknesses internal to the organization. The purposes of strategic planning are to:

- Identify strategies to respond to changes in customer needs, technology, health care legislation, the business environment, and the community.

- Dedicate resources to important services and new programs.
- Eliminate duplication, waste, and underused services.
- Establish a timeline for a goal achievement.

The strategic plan is a written document that details organizational goals, allocates resources, assigns responsibilities, and determines timeframes. Responsibility for development of the strategic plan rests with upper-level management, although there is increasing emphasis to include employees at all levels in strategic planning processes. Consider the following example.

CASE STUDY

Gina DellaValle, RN, nurse manager for the Quality Care Home Health Agency, noticed the office had been receiving several calls per week for skilled nursing care for pediatric oncology patients. The agency did not provide services for pediatric patients. Gina reported the situation to the administrator. Gina soon was involved in gathering information about the number of home health agencies that offered pediatric oncology care, the standards of nursing care recommended for pediatric oncology patients, how pediatric oncology patients were receiving home care, how many pediatric patients in the area might need such services, and what reimbursement was available for such services. Within the next few months, the management team for Quality Care Home Health Agency decided that as part of the agency's strategic plan, a program for pediatric oncology services would be developed.

Goals and Objectives. Goals and objectives state the actions necessary to achieve the strategic plan and are central to the entire management process. Goals should be measurable, observable, and realistic. Objectives are more specific and detail how a goal will be accomplished with an established target date.

Goals and objectives serve as the manager's road map; without them it is difficult to know where one is going. Organization-wide goals are established in the strategic planning process, and then unit goals that support the organization-wide goals are developed. Nurse managers should be able to clearly articulate both the organization-wide goals and the goals of the nursing unit. Additionally, goals and objectives must be communicated to everyone who is responsible for their attainment. Consider the following case example.

CASE STUDY

Michele Walker, RN, recently has been appointed as nurse manager in a 150-bed long-term care facility. The mission and philosophy of the organization is to "respect the dignity and worth of the individual and to provide care that will help restore the individual to the best possible state of physical, mental, and emotional health while maintaining his or her sense of spiritual and social well-being." Kenneth Cole, administrator, has asked Michele to develop a set of goals that she views as priorities to accomplish in the next year. After gathering data about resident needs, costs, and staffing levels and meeting with the medical director, direct-care staff, and rehabilitation therapy, social services, dietary, and maintenance staff, Michele develops the following goals: (1) increase by 25% over 12 months the level of satisfaction related to emotional well-being and socialization expressed by residents and family members on the quarterly quality of life satisfaction survey; this will be accomplished by increasing coordination of care activities among nursing, therapy, and social services; (2) reduce resident falls by 50% over 6 months through the implementation of an evidence-based guideline for falls prevention; and (3) increase by 30% in 12 months the number of nursing staff who achieve national certification as a gerontologic nurse through the American Nurses Credentialing Center. To accomplish this goal, the facility will offer certification review courses over the next 6 months. Together Michele and Kenneth review the goals, and agree that they fit with the overall organizational plan and address needs identified in Michele's facility assessment activities.

Operational Planning. The nurse manager is most likely to be responsible for operational planning or the short-range planning that encompasses the day-to-day activities of the organization. For example, short-range planning for a medical-surgical unit in a hospital might include maintaining an overall patient-to-staff ratio of 6:1, with 60% of the staff being RNs. As part of accomplishing organizational goals and objectives, the nurse manager involved in operational planning must be concerned with the following:

◆ Number, type, and location of patients to be cared for
◆ Qualifications and abilities of nursing and other health care staff
◆ Type and amount of supplies and other physical resources available
◆ Allocation of resources (staff, supplies, time) to meet budgetary requirements

The nurse manager also must plan for a variety of other activities, such as staff development, regulatory compliance, and quality improvement and patient safety projects (see Chapter 21).

Organizing

Organizing is the second management function. At the organizational level, organizing is necessary to establish a formal structure that defines the lines of authority, communication, and decision making within an organization. The formal organizational structure helps define roles and responsibilities of each level of management. The organizational chart provides a visual picture of the organization and identifies lines of communication and authority. All nurses should be familiar with the organizational chart of their employing institution. Organizing also involves developing policies and procedures to help outline how work will be done and establishing position qualifications and job descriptions to define who will do the work.

At the unit level, the nurse manager must determine how to best organize the work activities to meet organizational goals in an efficient and effective manner. Organizing involves:

◆ Using resources (people, supplies, time) wisely
◆ Assigning duties and responsibilities appropriately
◆ Coordinating activities with other departments
◆ Effectively communicating with subordinates and superiors to ensure a smooth workflow

Models for staffing and organizing the delivery of patient care are discussed in Chapter 20.

Staffing

Staffing is the third management function. The provision of health care is labor intensive, with a workforce composed of people with a variety of education and skill levels (i.e., professional nurses, physicians, pharmacists, social workers, therapists, dietitians, licensed vocational or practical nurses, technicians, and unlicensed assistive personnel). Hiring and managing staff to accomplish the work of the institution are important functions for all levels of managers.

Marquis and Huston (2009) have described steps in the staffing function as follows:

1. Determine the number and type of staff needed based on goals and budget requirements.
2. Recruit, interview, select, and assign personnel based on job description requirements and performance standards.
3. Get new employees off to a good start by offering excellent orientation, training, and socialization programs.
4. Implement an ongoing staff-development program to ensure employees at all levels have opportunities to develop personally and professionally and to enhance knowledge and skill levels.

5. Implement creative and flexible scheduling based on patient care needs, employee needs, and organizational productivity requirements.

The staffing process most likely will prove to be one of the most time-consuming and challenging functions for the nurse manager; however, it is probably the nurse manager's most important job. Little can be accomplished without the right people properly trained to do the work.

In the midst of a serious nursing shortage, nursing leaders are concerned with recruiting and retaining a talented RN workforce. Results of studies provide managers with information about several areas in which they can increase nurse satisfaction and thus reduce nursing turnover and improve recruitment and retention efforts. Factors positively associated with RNs' work satisfaction include:

- High level of support, encouragement, and open communication provided by the supervisor (Force, 2005; Kovner, Brewer, and Wu, 2006; Wieck, Dols, and Northam, 2009)
- Input into organizational decision making that affects job satisfaction (Perrine, 2009; Wieck et al, 2009)
- Organizational leaders who actively promote a cohesive work environment with respectful relationships between staff and physicians, peers, administrators, and other departments (Perrine, 2009; Wieck et al, 2009)
- High autonomy—the degree to which RNs control their job performance (Kovner et al, 2006; Sengin, 2003)
- Paid-time-off benefit—helps to reduce work-to-family conflict and increase flexibility in work schedules (Kovner et al, 2006)
- Distributive justice—the perceived fairness of the workload (rather than the actual workload) and perceived fairness of the salary (rather than the actual salary) (Kovner et al, 2006; Sengin, 2003)
- Promotional opportunities—the degree to which the organization offers career advancement structures (Kovner et al, 2006; Sengin, 2003)
- High group cohesion—the degree to which employees have friends and feel a sense of team camaraderie in the immediate work setting (Force, 2005; Kovner et al, 2006)

Staff schedules (days and shifts that staff are assigned to work) and patient assignment schedules (patient care assignment for which each staff member is responsible during his or her workday) are also key to employee satisfaction, recruitment, and retention. While meeting staff and patient scheduling needs, the nurse manager must meet organizational staffing and productivity goals. Productivity is the amount of work produced through the use of a specific amount of resources and is measured as output divided by input. For example, the number of nursing hours worked over a 24-hour period divided by the patient census is a standard productivity measurement used by many hospitals. From a practical perspective, the nurse caring for eight medical-surgical patients during one shift has a higher productivity ratio than the nurse caring for only five patients of similar acuity. Other examples of productivity measurements include number of home visits completed or number of procedures performed. Productivity is a method of measuring and tracking the amount of labor costs as compared with the amount of work produced and is a factor in staffing decisions.

Directing

Directing is the fourth management function. After managers have planned what to do, organized how to do it, and staffed positions to do the work, they must direct personnel and activities to accomplish goals. Directing involves issuing assignments and instructions that allow workers to clearly understand what is expected, in addition to guiding and coaching workers to achieve planned goals. Directing requires the nurse manager to:

- Clearly communicate performance expectations.
- Create a motivating climate and team spirit.
- Model expected behaviors.
- Facilitate feedback.

Communicating Performance Expectations. It is the manager's responsibility to monitor how well staff are performing their jobs. The first step is to ensure that staff clearly understand job expectations. Does the staff member know what problems and issues should be reported to the supervisor and how and to whom to report? Does the staff member know how to perform clinical procedures correctly or how and where to seek help when necessary? Does the nurse clearly understand the expectations for documenting clinical care? Does the nurse know how and when to report to physicians and/or involve other members of the interprofessional team? Is the staff member able to meet patient care needs for the number of patients assigned during a typical shift? Does the nurse know how to communicate effectively with patients as well as family members? These questions represent only a sample of issues that the nurse manager will consider when striving to communicate performance expectations.

Communicating performance expectations is an ongoing process that begins in new-employee orientation and continues throughout the term of employment. An important step in communicating expectations is to directly observe employees performing their jobs; through direct observation, the manager can identify strengths and weaknesses and determine areas where performance expectations need to addressed. The next step is to communicate expectations in a respectful two-way process in which the manager seeks first to understand the staff member's perspective, feelings, and knowledge about the issue and then to clarify the expectations in a nonjudgmental, nonthreatening way. The final step is to determine issues that may be preventing the employee from meeting performance expectations and work with that employee to develop a mutually agreed upon plan so that he or she can achieve expectations.

Creating a Motivating Climate. Motivation is the inner drive that compels a person to act in a certain way. The amount and quality of work accomplished by a person are a direct reflection of his or her motivation. A great deal of research has been undertaken to better understand human motivation. Most researchers will agree that motivation is complex and involves a combination of extrinsic, or external, rewards, such as money, benefits, and working conditions, in addition to intrinsic, or internal, needs for recognition, self-esteem, and self-actualization. Box 16-5 summarizes factors that influence nurses' job satisfaction, dissatisfaction, and motivation.

Positive encouragement and support from the nurse manager are essential to create a motivating work climate. An effective method to demonstrate encouragement and support is a technique known as "*management by walking around*" in which the nurse manager literally walks around the unit with the primary purpose of interacting positively with the staff. Just as it implies, management by walking around allows the nurse manager to interact with many different staff on a day-to-day basis, promote quality patient care, and build positive relationships with not only staff but also patients, families, and the interprofessional team (Forman, 2006).

Positive reinforcement in the form of a sincere "thank you, you did a good job" is one of the most powerful yet most often underused motivational resources available to the manager. To be effective, positive reinforcement should (1) be specific with praise given for a particular task

BOX **16-5**

Factors Influencing Nurses' Job Satisfaction and Dissatisfaction

SOURCES OF SATISFATION

- High level of support, encouragement, and open communication provided by the supervisor
- Supportive supervisors who demonstrate respect, encouragement, and caring for each individual
- Distributive justice: fairness of the workload and salary
- Thanks and positive recognition
- Open communication and being informed
- Guidance, mentorship, and opportunities for professional development and advancement
- Challenging work and responsibility to control job performance and be involved in decisions
- Pleasant work environment with high group cohesion, a sense of team camaraderie, and respectful relationships among staff and physicians, peers, administrators, and other departments
- Adequate staffing; help from managers during stressful times
- Ongoing feedback about performance
- Agreeable working hours, flexibility in scheduling, and benefits including paid-time-off and premium pay

SOURCES OF DISSATISFACTION

- Supervisors who are uninvolved and unsupportive
- Poor communication and unclear expectations
- Vague, inconsistent rules and regulations
- No thanks or recognition
- Not being informed about changes
- No commitment by management to professional development
- Lack of involvement in decision making
- Uncooperative physicians; no support for addressing inappropriate or disruptive behaviors
- No help from managers during crisis
- Inadequate feedback about performance
- Excessive workload negatively affecting quality

Sources: Force MV: The relationship between effective nurse managers and nursing retention, *J Nurs Adm* 35(7/8):336-341, 2005; Kovner C et al: Factors associated with work satisfaction of registered nurses, *J Nurs Scholarsh* 38(1):71-79, 2006; McNeese-Smith D: The influence of manager behavior on nurses' job satisfaction, productivity and commitment, *J Nurs Adm* 27(9):47-55, 1997; McNeese-Smith DK, Crook M: Nursing values and a changing nurse workforce: values, age, and job stages. *J Nurs Adm* 33(5):260-270, 2003;
Perrine JL: Strategies to boost RN retention, *Nurs Manage* April:20-22, 2009; Sengin KK: Work-related attributes of RN job satisfaction in acute care hospitals, *J Nurs Adm* 33(6):317-320, 2003; Wieck KL et al: What nurses want: the nurse incentives project, *Nurs Econ* 27(3):169-201, 2009.

done well or goal accomplished; (2) occur as close as possible to the time of the achievement; (3) be spontaneous and unpredictable (praise given routinely tends to lose its value); and (4) be given for a genuine accomplishment (Peters and Waterman, 1982). Management by walking around puts the manager in a position to observe the employee's work performance and offer immediate praise for a job well done.

Role Modeling. Positive role modeling is another effective tool the nurse manager can use to create a positive team spirit and promote high-quality patient care. Positive role modeling simply means that the nurse performs the job in such a way that he or she demonstrates ideal performance as a professional nurse; others hopefully will follow the example. Obviously nurse managers must be the role model for excellence in patient care; similarly, nurse managers must also model caring and respectful relationships with the staff along with an enthusiastic attitude to promote camaraderie and team spirit. If relationships between nurse leaders and their staff are not mutually respectful and caring, it is doubtful that staff will be inclined to establish caring, therapeutic relationships with their patients (Forman, 2006). Likewise, managers who frequently project unhappiness or a disagreeable attitude contribute greatly to low morale and an unmotivated work team (Marquis and Huston, 2009).

Several other skills are essential as nurse managers function in the directing role, including effective communication and conflict management skills (Chapter 18), delegation skills (Chapter 19), and team-building skills (discussed later). The nurse manager is challenged to create a climate that will generate worker satisfaction and motivate workers to accomplish goals.

Controlling

The purpose of controlling, the fifth management function, is to ensure that employees accomplish goals while maintaining a high quality of performance. Controlling requires the nurse manager to:

- Establish performance or outcome standards.
- Determine action plans to improve performance.
- Evaluate employee performance through performance appraisals and feedback.

Establishing Performance Standards. Performance standards describe a model of excellence for work activities and serve as the basis of comparison between actual and desired work performance. For example, performance standards in an ambulatory outpatient clinic might include that (1) every patient is informed about all lab results within 48 hours, whether normal or abnormal, and (2) all diabetic patients must remove their shoes and socks for a complete foot exam each time they come into the clinic. Nurses can draw on several resources for establishing performance standards, including:

- Written organizational policies and procedures
- Standards for the practice of professional nursing developed by the American Nurses Association (ANA) and published in *Nursing: Scope and Standards of Practice* (ANA, 2004)
- Standards for professional nursing specialty practices, such as the *Cardiovascular Nursing: Scope and Standards of Practice* (ANA, 2008a) and *Pediatric Nursing: Scope and Standards of Practice* (ANA, 2008b)
- Evidence-based practice guidelines

The nurse manager should also continually look for ways to improve individual, team, and organizational performance to achieve established standards of care. Chapter 21 provides more discussion about performance standards and presents an excellent process for measuring performance and planning for improvement.

Evaluating Employee Performance. Evaluating employee performance occurs through the formal annual evaluation process and through frequent feedback and coaching provided to employees. A manager should never wait until the annual performance review to discuss problems or deficiencies with a staff member. Consistent day-to-day feedback and coaching about job performance clarifies expectations, improves the quality of work, and allows the manager to correct problems before they become serious. Feedback and coaching can occur in brief, spontaneous interactions or in planned sessions with the employee. Box 16-6 presents useful tips for effective coaching.

Ongoing documentation about an employee's job performance also is an essential management responsibility. Each health care organization has specific policies related to documentation of employee performance and annual performance evaluations. The result of routine performance evaluations should be mutual goal setting designed to meet the employees' training, educational, and work-improvement needs. Box 16-7 presents useful tips for successful employee performance evaluations.

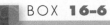

BOX **16-6**

Tips for Effective Coaching

- Discuss situations in a neutral way—avoid judgmental language that will put the other person on the defensive.
- Encourage the other person to provide his or her perspective about the situation (e.g., "What did you think about your exchange with that physician?").
- Encourage the person to reflect on his or her performance through open-ended questions, such as:
  What are your main concerns with this situation?
  What would you like to see happen next?
  What can you learn from this situation?
  What is confusing to you?
  What are some things you could do differently next time?
- Be specific and provide clear examples when possible (e.g., "Next time you are dealing with a difficult family member, you might consider...").
- Share your own experiences if they are relevant and might help.
- Be sincere. Provide coaching and feedback with the clear intent of helping the person improve.
- Be realistic. Focus on factors that the person can control.
- Thank the employee for listening.
- Ask for feedback from your coworkers, subordinates, and peers about your own performance and listen when it is offered.

Sources: Grensing-Pophal L: Give-and-take feedback, *Nurs Manage* 31(2):27-28, 2000; Harvard Business Essentials: *Manager's toolkit: the 13 skills managers need to succeed,* Boston, 2004, Harvard Business School Press.

BOX **16-7**

Tips for Successful Employee Performance Appraisals

- Each employee must understand the standard by which his or her work is being evaluated—at a minimum by receiving a copy of the appraisal form and more effectively by being involved in developing the evaluation criteria.
- Conduct the appraisal during a time when there will be no interruptions for either party; select a comfortable seating arrangement that denotes collegiality, such as side-by-side chairs.
- Avoid surprises—good leaders and managers provide feedback and communicate with staff on a continual basis.
- Focus on the employee's performance and desired outcomes, not on personal characteristics.
- Avoid vague generalities, such as "your performance is fine" or "your attitude needs to improve"—give explicit examples.
- Present a balanced view of the employee's performance—positives and negatives.
- Be selective in reviewing shortcomings or failures—stick to the most important issues.
- Encourage input from the employee.
- Set goals together for continued growth and improvement—identify specific steps as to how goals will be accomplished.
- Be sensitive and caring; demonstrate that you value the employee and his or her contribution to the organization.
- Follow up regularly on progress toward improving performance and meeting goals.

Sources: Harvard Business Essentials: *Manager's toolkit: the 13 skills managers need to succeed,* Boston, 2004, Harvard Business School Press; Marquis BL, Huston CJ: *Leadership roles and management functions in nursing,* ed 6, Philadelphia, 2009, Wolters Kluwer Health/Lippincott Williams & Wilkins.

The management functions of planning, organizing, staffing, directing, and controlling provide the nurse manager with a defined practical set of skills to guide the implementation of management activities. The new nurse manager will be challenged to maintain the different stages of management that occur in the span of just one day. In addition to managing different phases of the process occurring simultaneously, the nurse manager also must function in many different management roles described in the following section.

ROLES OF THE NURSE LEADER AND MANAGER

Nurses assume various roles as they function in leadership and management positions. The first step toward being an effective nurse leader and manager is to clearly understand the job description, roles and responsibilities, and policies and procedures related to the position in which you are employed or assigned. The following discussion presents information about the primary roles that a nurse will assume in any position. By understanding these roles, the nurse can (1) know what is expected to be effective and (2) identify areas that require additional learning and improvement.

Customer Service Provider

Over the past few years, patient satisfaction has moved to the forefront of the nurse's agenda. Nursing shortages, reduced length of stay, more complex patient needs, and national concerns about the quality and safety of patient care have contributed to this growing concern about patient satisfaction and customer service. From how quickly call lights are answered to the extent of family support provided, nurses are challenged to meet a wide spectrum of patient needs. The complex health care environment has created a competitive marketplace in which home health agencies, hospitals, ambulatory clinics, and even hospice agencies compete for patients. To survive and thrive in this competitive environment, the nurse must keep customer service, which includes safety and quality care, first and foremost as the motivator of all plans and activities.

External and Internal Customers. Effective management requires that the health care organization and the nurse develop a comprehensive view of the term customer. Customers can be categorized as external or internal, depending on their relationship to the organization. External customers are not employed by the organization and include patients and families, in addition to physicians and others who serve as referral sources for new patients. For example, home health nurses should view hospital discharge planners as customers and find ways to meet the hospitalized patients' discharge needs. Physicians will not refer patients to a particular hospital or clinic if they are not happy with the nursing services provided by that facility.

Payers (insurance companies, managed care plans) are also being considered as primary external customers. For example, hospitals seek to contract with managed care plans to gain the plan's covered members as customers. Managed care companies seek to contract with hospitals that can demonstrate outstanding service that will please the plan's members. Thus the managed care company becomes the hospital's customer.

Internal customers are employed by the organization and may include patient care staff members, staff members of other departments (e.g., laboratory, dietary), administrators, social workers, dietitians, and therapists. For example, nurse managers should view staff members as "customers" and determine how to meet their needs to facilitate effective and efficient work performance. Other departments—social services, laboratory, maintenance, housekeeping—are essential to manage an effective nursing unit, and the needs of these customers should be considered. If every

BOX **16-8**

Sample Customer Service Commitment for a Health Care Organization

COMMUNITY CLINICS' CUSTOMER SERVICE COMMITMENT
This is our customer service commitment. Translated, it stands for listening, caring, helping, and healing.
- Caring, friendly, professional staff members
- Prompt and personal attention to requests
- Respect for individual preferences
- Timely, convenient services with reasonable wait times
- Confidentiality and privacy respected and upheld
- Serious responses to concerns and complaints
- Ongoing efforts to improve our systems and processes

department in the organization provided great service to both internal and external customers, imagine how much more effective and efficient the entire organization would be.

Customer Service Standards. The customer will define standards for customer service and should have input into the development of standards for customer service. Customers want to feel that their individual preferences are valued and respected. Certainly, all customers have a need to be treated with kindness and respect, to have services provided in a timely and cost-effective manner, and to have effective communication about what is or will be occurring. Further service standards can be defined by listening to and observing customers and analyzing customer surveys, customer complaints, and unsolicited comments or letters. A sample customer service commitment for a health care organization is presented in Box 16-8. Meeting customer needs should be the focus in all planning, organizing, staffing, directing, and controlling activities and in all meetings and communications with superiors and subordinates.

Team Builder

A team is a group of people organized to accomplish the necessary work of an organization. Teams bring together a range of people with different knowledge, skills, and experiences to meet customer needs, accomplish tasks, and solve problems. Team members may include unit secretaries, nursing assistants, social workers, dietitians, therapists, physicians, licensed vocational or practical nurses, and RNs. A team should have clearly defined goals and should be empowered to make decisions within its realm of responsibility. Team building should create synergy. Synergy is the ability of a group of people working together to accomplish significantly more than each person working individually.

Bringing people together to work as a group does not necessarily make them a team. To create synergy, teams must have defined goals and objectives, a commitment to work together, good communication, and a willingness to cooperate. Team members should be encouraged to communicate with one another to identify effective work division and solutions to problems so that synergy is accomplished. The nurse, as team builder, must serve as a role model to encourage and help develop team principles of respect, cooperation, commitment, and a willingness to accomplish shared goals. As a role model for team members, the nurse should:

- Show respect for all members of the team and value their input.
- Clearly define team goals ("What do we want to accomplish?").
- Clearly define the decision-making authority within the realm of the team.

- Encourage the team members to develop a sense of stewardship (or ownership) for the success of the team.
- Exhibit a personal commitment to the team goals.
- Encourage team members to willingly help one another.
- Provide the resources necessary to accomplish goals (i.e., time for team meetings, information, supplies).
- Teach members to exchange constructive feedback for the purpose of meeting team goals.
- Provide relevant and timely feedback to the team.

The leader's behaviors have a significant effect on the behaviors of the team. As Porter-O'Grady stated, "Every moment the leader operates in the leader role, he or she is influencing the roles and actions of other team members" (2003a, p. 105). Thus the nurse as leader must have an astute self-awareness of his or her own emotional patterns and an understanding that negative moods can have a negative influence on relationships with staff members. Learning to recognize and manage one's emotional patterns and negative moods is an important step in team building. The nurse manager who is enthusiastic, caring, and supportive can generate those same feelings among all team members (Porter-O'Grady, 2003a).

Resource Manager

Resources include the personnel, time, and supplies needed to provide patient care and operate the organization. Resources cost money and always will be in limited supply. Unfortunately, no health care organization can afford the luxury of an unlimited number of staff or supplies to accomplish the required work. With health care facilities' focus on cost containment, it is essential that nurses develop an understanding of and expertise in resource management.

Each of the management activities of planning, organizing, staffing, directing, and controlling come into play in the role of resource manager. The nurse needs to learn and develop skills in the following areas:

- Planning for the necessary resources (primarily staff and supplies) to manage the unit
- Organizing the resources to meet identified goals
- Staffing appropriately as determined by patient needs and the budget plan
- Directing to maintain resource allocations within budgetary guidelines
- Controlling by analyzing financial reports and making adjustments where necessary

Budget and financial reports are the primary tools for resource management. Because budget and financial management is a very minimal part of the nursing school curriculum, nurses need to take initiative for on-the-job training about the organization's budget and financial management processes. Nurses are encouraged not to be unsettled by financial and budget reports and conversations. Instead get involved. Do not be afraid to say "I don't understand. Please explain." Review budget and financial reports, ask questions, talk to seasoned nurse managers, talk to the organization's finance department staff, and even consider taking an accounting or finance course at the local college. Understanding financial and budget management is one of the most useful and powerful tools you can have as a nurse manager. Another resource is Chapter 17 of this text, which provides more detailed information about budgets.

Decision Maker and Problem Solver

Problem solving and decision making are essential skills for professional nursing practice. Not only are these skills required in clinical patient care, they also are vital components of effective leadership and management. The nurse leader is continually engaged in decision making while managing the work unit. Problem solving is focused on solving an immediate problem and includes a decision-making step.

Nursing Process as a Guide for Decision Making and Problem Solving. The nursing process, familiar to nurses for addressing patient care needs, can be applied to all management activities requiring decision making and problem solving. The nursing process as a problem-solving process using assessment, analysis and diagnosis, planning, implementation, and evaluation has proven effective to manage the complex decisions required in nursing practice (Howenstein et al, 1996). Table 16-1 summarizes the decision-making and problem-solving activities in each stage of the nursing process.

Assessment. During the assessment stage it is important for the nurse to separate the problem from the symptom by gathering information about the problem or situation. It often is appropriate to involve others—especially those close to the situation—who may be able to provide a different viewpoint or information the manager lacks. For example, the nurse manager concerned about increasingly high absenteeism among the patient care staff may consider implementing a strict policy to punish staff members who call in sick. In this situation the nurse manager may be addressing the symptom instead of the real issue. The following questions should first be asked: What is causing the absenteeism? Are there problems on the unit creating an unhappy work environment? Are several staff members coincidentally having personal problems? Are absentee policies being unfairly administered? The nurse manager must correctly assess and diagnose the problem before developing solutions.

TABLE **16-1**

The Nursing Process Applied to Problem Solving

ASSESSMENT	ANALYSIS AND DIAGNOSIS	PLANNING	IMPLEMENTING	EVALUATION
Gather information about the situation.	Analyze results of information gathering.	Identify as many solutions as possible.	Communicate plans to everyone affected.	Identify evaluation criteria in the planning stage.
Identify the problem; separate the symptoms.	Identify, clarify, and prioritize the actual problem(s).	Elicit participation from people or groups affected.	Be sure plans, goals, and objectives are clearly identified.	Identify who is responsible for evaluation, what will be measured, and when it will take place.
Identify people and groups involved.	Determine whether intervention is appropriate.	Review options and consider safety, efficiency, costs, quality, legal, and ethical aspects.	Maintain open, two-way communication with staff.	Maintain open communication with all involved.
Identify cultural and environmental factors.		Consider positive and negative outcomes of options.	Support and encourage compliance among all staff.	Was the decision successful? What might have made it better?
Encourage input from involved parties.		Remain open minded and flexible when considering options.		

Analysis and Diagnosis. During the analysis stage, decision makers use information gathered in the assessment phase to identify the specific problem to be solved. At this stage managers must also decide whether the situation is important enough to require intervention and whether it is within their authority to intervene. Managers should not attempt to intercede in every situation brought to their attention. It is important to assess why the issue is being called to the manager's attention and what could happen if the manager does not react. Purposeful inaction is an intentional plan on the part of the manager and should not be confused with a "do-nothing approach" taken by a manager who chooses to do nothing when intervention is indicated.

Planning. During the planning stage the goal is to identify as many options as possible and then objectively weigh the options as to possible risks and consequences and positive and negative outcomes, including patient outcomes and staff effectiveness as key considerations. The decision maker should be flexible, creative, and open to suggestions from other staff and peers when reviewing options. Avoid preconceived ideas or rigid thinking such as "there is only one way to do this job" or "that's the way we have always done it." It is also important to remember that decisions made with input from those who will be affected by the decision are more likely to result in positive outcomes. Cost, quality, and legal and ethical aspects of care also should be carefully considered.

Implementation. The implementation stage should include effective communication, delegation, and supervision. It is important for the manager to show positive support for the decision outcome and encourage compliance among all staff. Persons higher in the organizational structure may mandate some decisions, and although not able to control that decision, the nurse manager can influence a positive outcome.

Evaluation. The evaluation stage is necessary to ensure that the implemented plan effectively resolved the problem or the decision situation. Considerable time and energy may be spent on identifying the problem, generating possible options, and selecting and implementing the best solution. However, time for follow-up evaluation must also be allocated. It is important to establish early (during the planning stage) how and what evaluation and monitoring will take place, who will be responsible, and when it will be accomplished.

Staff input should be included in each stage of the decision-making problem-solving process. Additionally, the nurse might seek help from others who are more experienced and knowledgeable in specific areas.

Even the most experienced nurse managers will not be able to effectively solve every problem, nor will any nurse have all the answers. The key to being a good manager is to understand and incorporate the decision-making problem-solving process into all activities; know when and how to access resources; and learn and improve as successes and failures are experienced.

Change Agent

This text frequently has referred to the changing health care environment, and true to that concept, change is an inevitable occurrence in health care organizations. Whether working with individuals, groups, or the entire organization, the professional nurse is certain to be involved in managing change. The nurse as the change agent is responsible for guiding people through the change process. To successfully engage in change, the nurse manager must first be willing to confront the demand for change; staff cannot be expected to embrace change if their nurse leader has not done so. The nurse must also be willing to help others make the change become an integral part of their work (Porter-O'Grady, 2003b).

People often feel threatened by change and may react, especially at first, with resistance and hostility. Change that is carefully planned and implemented slowly with all people continually informed and involved will be more successful in reaching the desired outcome (or change). As Marquis and Huston (2009) have noted, change will often create a wide range of feelings among staff and managers including achievement, loss, pride, and stress. The successful change agent will understand the very real nature of these emotions and manage the change process such that all involved will experience at least some degree of success and pride in the outcome.

In his classic work on change, Lewin (1951) identified several rules that should be followed when change is necessary:

1. Change should be implemented only for good reason.
2. Change should always be planned and implemented gradually.
3. Change should never be unexpected or abrupt.
4. All people who may be affected by the change should be involved in planning for the change.

Change may be indicated for several reasons, including solving an identified problem, implementing a new program, improving work efficiencies, or adjusting to new mandates by regulatory agencies. For example, some states are implementing stricter patient rights regulations that require changes to current patient care practices. Even though a strong reason for change may exist, it almost always will be met with some resistance. Resistance is demonstrated by refusing to cooperate with a course of action or showing active opposition to the change. The effective change agent recognizes that resistance is a natural response to change and does not waste time or energy attempting to eliminate it. Instead the effective change agent identifies and implements effective change strategies that overcome resistance.

Stages of Change. Effective change strategies can be developed through the three classic stages of change identified by Lewin (1951). These stages are:

1. *Unfreezing stage* The change agent promotes problem identification and encourages the awareness of the need for change. People must believe that improvement is possible before they are willing to consider change. The change agent's responsibilities during this stage are to:
   ◆ Gather information about the problem.
   ◆ Accurately assess the problem.
   ◆ Decide if change is necessary.
   ◆ Make others aware of the need for change.
2. *Moving stage*—The change agent clarifies the need to change, explores alternatives, defines goals and objectives, plans the change, and implements the change plan. The change agent's responsibilities during this stage are to:
   ◆ Identify areas of support and resistance.
   ◆ Set goals and objectives.
   ◆ Include everyone affected in the planning.
   ◆ Develop an appropriate change plan with target dates.
   ◆ Implement the change plan.
   ◆ Be available to help, support, and encourage others through the process.
   ◆ Evaluate the change and make modifications if necessary.
3. *Refreezing stage*—The change agent integrates the change into the organization so that it becomes recognized as the status quo. If the refreezing stage is not completed, people may drift into old behaviors. The change agent's responsibilities during this stage are to:
   ◆ Require and enforce compliance with the changed processes.

◆ Support and encourage others until the change is no longer viewed as new but as part of the status quo and well integrated into the daily workflow and communication processes.

In alignment with Lewin's (1951) three stages of change (unfreezing, moving, and refreezing), involvement and education are keys to successful change.

Involvement. The importance of involving all individuals, groups, or departments affected by the change cannot be overstated. Involvement includes clear, two-way communication and a concerted effort to garner information and feedback from all affected parties about the need for change. The effective change agent will take into consideration the needs of external and internal customers and understand that a change in one area almost always will affect another group or department (remember systems theory?). Consider the following case example:

CASE STUDY

As the number of procedures being performed in an outpatient surgery department continued to increase, Kevin Michaels, RN, nurse manager, recognized the need to extend the hours of the department to relieve the tight surgery schedule. When the staff began to complain about working through lunch and staying late some evenings, Kevin encouraged them to accept the need for a new department schedule. Kevin discussed the situation with the administrator and all nursing, technical, and secretarial staff. He carefully assessed the department's scheduling needs, surveyed the surgeons regarding their scheduling preferences, reviewed all options, and finally planned to add a half-day Saturday surgery schedule. Kevin carefully planned the new schedule with the staff and surgeons and was pleased that the plan seemed to be going smoothly. However, Jane Holmes, the housekeeping supervisor who schedules heavy cleaning duties on Saturday mornings when the department is normally closed, was not informed or involved in the schedule change. Much to her dismay, Jane learned through a hallway conversation that she would have to quickly rearrange cleaning schedules and staff schedules to adjust to the new Saturday morning plan.

Peripheral departments (e.g., housekeeping, maintenance, security) are crucial to safe, efficient operations, but they often are forgotten in the planning activities. The change agent should make sure that appropriate individuals and departments are informed and involved to ensure that change is implemented as smoothly as possible.

Education and Training. Education and training also are important components of effective change. People must have appropriate education and training to understand and comply with new policies, procedures, work processes, duties, or responsibilities. Early in the change process the change agent must consider the training needs of all individuals, groups, and departments. Education and training can reduce fear of the unknown and allow the staff to feel prepared and comfortable with taking on new or different responsibilities.

Other Roles

In addition to the roles of customer service provider, team builder, resource manager, and change agent, nurses in leadership and management positions will find themselves functioning in many other roles. Each of the management roles described in this chapter is equally important to performing effectively as a nurse manager.

Clinical Consultant. Staff members look to the nurse leader as a resource for clinical advice. For example, the nurse leader is frequently called on to assess difficult or unusual patient cases and guide the staff nurse to make appropriate nursing judgments. In this role, the nurse manager serves as a role model for excellence in nursing care and provides ongoing staff training and education.

Staff Developer. The nurse manager should be ever mindful of the need for learning and training opportunities to enhance professional and personal growth for all employees he or she supervises. Accessing resources and planning staff development activities that meet the needs of individual staff members, including RNs, LPNs or LVNs, nursing assistants, and clerical staff is a very important role for the nurse manager.

Mentor. As the nurse develops into an effective leader and manager, he or she should accept the responsibility to act as a mentor to new nurses, helping them develop effective leadership and management skills. Mentorship is key to developing our future nursing leaders and managers.

Corporate Supporter. The nurse manager, as a corporate supporter, has a responsibility to embrace the mission, goals, and objectives of the employing organization. In this role as corporate supporter, the nurse manager is a professional representative for the organization and is committed to supporting and accomplishing organizational goals.

CREATING A CARING ENVIRONMENT

Perhaps the most important responsibility for the nurse in any leadership or management role is to create an environment of caring—caring for staff members and for patients and families. Staff members who feel that their manager sincerely cares about them and the work they do are able to pass that feeling of caring on to their patients and other customers. Caring for the staff members can be demonstrated through the following measures (McNeese-Smith, 1997):
- Offering sincere positive recognition for both individuals and teams
- Praising and giving thanks for a job well done
- Spending time with staff members to reinforce positive work behaviors
- Meeting the staff members' personal needs whenever possible, such as accommodating scheduling needs for family events and being flexible in times of illness
- Providing guidance and support for professional and personal growth
- Maintaining a positive, confident attitude and a pleasant work environment

Staff members who feel that their work is valued and that they are respected and cared about as individuals are able to further contribute to a positive, caring environment in which to provide excellent patient care. Creating a caring environment in the highly technical, fast-paced, and extremely stressful environments in which nurses work can be a significant challenge to the nurse manager. However, it is a challenge that is at the heart of nursing if we are to promote the very best in patient care. As Benner has observed, "Failing to attend to caring practices will continue to fuel a technical cure approach to health care rather than attend to illness prevention, care of the chronically ill and health promotion. Sometimes care itself is the most significant outcome, as well as the most significant means to cure, healing and health" (1999, p. 318).

SPECIAL LEADERSHIP AND MANAGEMENT CHALLENGES IN THE TWENTY-FIRST CENTURY

Nurses, as leaders and managers in the U.S. health care delivery system, will face daunting challenges as they move into the second decade of this century. Such challenges include health professional shortages (i.e., nurses, primary care physicians, pharmacists), health care costs that are rising too rapidly to be sustainable, a very large uninsured population, and ongoing concerns about the safety and quality of care. The imperative to reduce costs and improve quality and safety in the nation's health care settings is perhaps the most relevant and important for nurses as they have the opportunity to have a significant effect in these areas on a day-to-day basis. Two national initiatives provide nurse leaders and managers with the framework for making significant changes to address cost, quality, and safety issues: *A Proclamation for Change: Transforming the Hospital Patient Care Environment* (Hendrich, Chow, and Goshert, 2009) and *Keeping Patients Safe: Transforming the Work Environment of Nurses* (IOM and Page, 2003). These initiatives are briefly summarized in the following sections. Nurses are encouraged to read these publications in full and provide leadership in the health care settings in which they work to promote recommended changes.

Transforming the Hospital Care Environment

The *Proclamation for Change* (Hendrich et al, 2009) provides a set of evidence-based recommendations to address inefficiencies that threaten patient safety and to improve retention of the nursing workforce. This proclamation has been endorsed by major health care systems across the nation as well as by professional and consumer organizations. The evidence-based recommendations are based on three major studies to identify the causes of inefficiencies in nursing practice: The time and motion study (Hendrich et al, 2008); transforming care at the bedside (Rutherford, Lee, and Greiner, 2004), and the technology drill down study (Cipriano, 2008). The four basic tenets of the *Proclamation for Change* are (1) patient-centered design to allow patients and families to more easily become engaged in the caregiving process; (2) system-wide, integrated technology to ensure technologic solutions support all clinicians and departments involved in the caregiving process; (3) seamless workplace environments to provide the right medications, supplies and information in the right place at the right time; and (4) vendor partnerships to ensure technology devices that are easy to use and provide patient information across multiple health care settings. Again, nurses are encourage to read more about the *Proclamation for Change* and work within their organizations to promote positive change as recommended in this document.

Patient Safety and the Nurse's Work Environment

Most practicing nurses and students are aware of the Institute of Medicine's (IOM) landmark report *To Err Is Human: Building a Safer Health System* (2000), which reported that up to 98,000 people die each year in our nation's hospitals as a result of medical errors. In follow-up to this landmark report, the IOM's report *Keeping Patients Safe: Transforming the Work Environment of Nurses* (2003), has made a strong connection between the nurse's work environment and medical errors. As the scientific evidence that nurses are essential to patient safety and improved outcomes continues to grow, nurse leaders and managers are challenged to actually implement changes and impart significant improvements in hospitals, nursing homes, home health agencies, ambulatory clinics, and all other settings across the continuum of care.

Although the IOM report has provided guidance and recommendations to improve nurses' work environments, it is up to nurse leaders at all levels, including those in direct patient care, to turn these recommendations into action. Following is a short summary of the IOM's (2003) recommendations for improving nurses' work environments:

Promote Transformational Leadership and Evidence-Based Management. Acquire nurse leaders at all levels in the organization who will:
◆ Participate in executive decision making.
◆ Facilitate mutual trust among management and nursing staff.

- Achieve effective communication among nursing and other clinical leaders.
- Facilitate input from direct-care staff into decision making.
- Actively manage the process of change.
- Have available necessary resources to support and develop staff nurses' knowledge in clinical decision making.

Maximize Workforce Capability. Achieve appropriate staffing levels with nursing staff who have the required clinical knowledge and skills to keep patients safe through the following actions:

- Incorporate patient volume estimates that count all admissions and discharges rather than a patient census at one point of time.
- Involve direct-care staff in identifying appropriate staffing levels, causes of nursing staff turnover, and methods to improve retention.
- Provide for staffing flexibility in each shift's schedule to accommodate variations in patient volume.
- Empower nursing unit staff to set criteria for closing the unit to new admissions as necessitated by workload.
- Ensure that adequate financial and other resources are dedicated to support nursing staff in the acquisition and maintenance of new knowledge and skills.
- Promote interprofessional collaboration through such activities as interprofessional rounds and formal education and training in interprofessional collaboration.

Redesign Work Processes to Prevent Errors. Nurses' work processes and work environments need to be more conducive to detecting and preventing errors. Fatigue has been particularly addressed as a threat to patient safety. Following are some specific recommendations in the area of work redesign:

- Prohibit nursing staff from providing patient care in excess of 12 hours in any given 24-hour period or in excess of 60 hours in a 7-day period.
- Enable nursing staff to collaborate with other health care personnel to identify and redesign high-risk and inefficient work processes to make them safe and efficient.
- Redesign documentation practices with assistance from regulators and oversight organizations (i.e., The Joint Commission, state licensing agencies).
- Address hand hygiene and medication administration among the first work redesign initiatives.

Create and Sustain a Culture of Safety. Patient safety requires a vigilant and strong organizational commitment to prevent errors and to detect, analyze, and rectify errors when they do occur, with organizations placing as high a priority on safety as they do on financial management and revenue generation. To this end the IOM recommends:

- Specify short- and long-term safety objectives.
- Continually review success in meeting these objectives and provide feedback at all levels.
- Conduct an annual confidential survey of nursing and other health care workers to assess the extent to which a culture of safety exists.
- Institute a fair, just, and blameless reporting system for errors and near misses.
- Engage in ongoing employee training in error detection, analysis, and reduction.
- Implement procedures for analyzing errors and providing feedback to direct-care workers.
- Institute rewards and incentives for error reduction.

The IOM report emphasizes that a piecemeal approach to improve patient safety and nurses' work environments will not work—all of the areas described previously must be addressed if we are to create a safe and effective health care system in which nurses feel very good about the care they are able to provide. It is up to nurse leaders at all health care organizations to begin this long yet exciting process of redesigning work environments. The IOM's *Keeping Patients Safe* can be obtained online (www.nap.edu).

SUMMARY

In every area of health care, the professional nurse is expected to provide leadership and management expertise to help manage complex and ever-changing health care organizations. The multifaceted set of theories, functions, roles, and skills presented in this chapter may at first seem overwhelming to the novice nurse. However, by learning and understanding the principles and concepts involved, the graduate nurse can become a successful nurse leader and manager.

Leadership, management, and organizational theories provide a framework on which to build effective nursing management practices. Although there is no one "best" leadership theory, professional nurses should maintain an awareness of their own behavior and how the key elements of the leadership situation influence outcomes.

The management functions of planning, organizing, staffing, directing, and controlling provide the nurse manager with a defined, practical set of skills to guide management activities. Professional nurses can apply these management functions to perform effectively in various management roles, including customer service provider, team builder, resource manager, change agent, clinical consultant, staff developer, mentor, and corporate supporter.

Developing effective leadership and management skills is an ongoing process that continues throughout one's career as a professional nurse. Nurses in management positions should routinely analyze personal strengths and weaknesses in each of these management roles and identify areas in which learning and development are needed. Modeling effective nurse managers and reading relevant professional journal articles and books can increase leadership and management knowledge and skills (Box 16-9 provides nursing leadership and management resources). Management and leadership roles are challenging and exciting and present a wonderful opportunity to grow professionally and personally.

ᏋᐺᎾᒪᐺᏋ Additional resources are available online at: http://evolve.elsevier.com/Cherry/

BOX 16-9

Helpful Websites and Online Resources

NURSING LEADERSHIP AND MANAGEMENT ONLINE RESOURCES
American Organization of Nurse Executives
   www.aone.org
American Nurses Association
   www.nursingworld.org
National Academy Press (copies of the IOM's *Keeping Patients Safe* and *Transforming the Work Environment of Nurses* available)
   www.nap.edu
Transforming Care at the Bedside
   www.ihi.org/IHI/Programs/StrategicInitiatives/TransformingCareAtTheBedside.htm

NURSING MANAGEMENT AND LEADERSHIP JOURNALS
American Journal of Nursing
   www.nursingworld.org/ajn
Journal of Nursing Administration Quarterly
Nursing Management
Journal of Nursing Administration
Nursing & Health Care Perspectives
The Journal of Clinical Systems Management

REFERENCES

American Nurses Association: *Nursing: scope and standards of practice*, Washington, DC, 2004, ANA.

American Nurses Association: *Cardiovascular nursing: scope and standards of practice*, Washington, DC, 2008a, ANA.

American Nurses Association: *Pediatric nursing: scope and standards of practice*, Washington, DC, 2008b, ANA.

Bass BM, Avoliio BJ, Goodheim L: Biography and the assessment of transformational leadership at the world-class level, *J Manage* 13(1):7–19, 1987.

Benner P: Nursing leadership for the new millennium: claiming the wisdom and worth of clinical practice, *Nurs Healthcare Perspect* 20(6):312–319, 1999.

Burns J: *Leadership*, New York, 1978, Harper & Row.

Cipriano P: Technological solutions to workflow inefficiencies on medical/surgical units. Presented at HIMSS annual conference, February 24-28, 2008, Orlando, FL.

Dunham-Taylor J: Nurse executive transformational leadership found in participative organizations, *J Nurs-Adm* 30(5):241–250, 2000.

Failla KR, Stichler JF: Manager and staff perceptions of the manager's leadership style, *J Nurs Adm* 11(38):480–487, 2008.

Force MV: The relationship between effective nurse managers and nursing retention, *J Nurs Adm* 35(7/8):336–341, 2005.

Forman H: From cheerleader to patent processor, *J Nurs Adm* 36(7/8):346–350, 2006.

Grensing-Pophal L: Give-and-take feedback, *Nurs Manage* 31(2):27–28, 2000.

Harvard Business Essentials: *Manager's toolkit: the 13 skills managers need to succeed*, Boston, 2004, Harvard Business School Press.

Hendrich A, Chow MP, Goshert WS: A proclamation for change: transforming the hospital patient care environment, *JONA* 39(6):266–275, 2009.

Hendrich A, et al: A 36-hospital time and motion study: how do medical-surgical nurses spend their time? *Permanente J* 12:25–34, 2008.

Hersey P, Blanchard K: *Management of organizational behavior: utilizing human resources*, ed 4, Englewood Cliffs, NJ, 1988, Prentice-Hall.

Hersey P, Blanchard K, Natemeyer W: Situational leadership, perception and impact of power, *Group Organ Stud* 4:418–428, 1979.

Howenstein MA, et al: Factors associated with critical thinking among nurses, *J Contin Educ Nurs* 27(3):100–103, 1996.

Institute of Medicine: *To err is human: building a safer health system*, Washington, DC, 2000, National Academy Press.

Institute of Medicine, Page A, editors: *Keeping patients safe: transforming the work environment of nurses*, Washington, DC, 2003, National Academy Press.

Kovner C, Brewer C, Wu YW: Factors associated with work satisfaction of registered nurses, *J Nurs Scholarsh* 38(1):71–79, 2006.

Lewin K: *Field theory in social sciences*, New York, 1951, Harper & Row.

Marquis BL, Huston CJ: *Leadership roles and management functions in nursing*, ed 6, Philadelphia, 2009, Wolters Kluwer Health/Lippincott Williams & Wilkins.

McGuire E: Chaos theory: learning a new science, *J Nurs Adm* 29(2):8–9, 1999.

McNeese-Smith D: The influence of manager behavior on nurses' job satisfaction, productivity and commitment, *J Nurs Adm* 27(9):47–55, 1997.

McNeese-Smith DK, Crook M: Nursing values and a changing nurse workforce: values, age, and job stages, *J Nurs Adm*, 33(5):260–270, 2003.

Perrine JL: Strategies to boost RN retention, *Nurs Manage* April:20–22, 2009.

Peters T, Waterman RH: *In search of excellence*, New York, 1982, Harper & Row.

Porter-O'Grady T: A different age for leadership, part 1: new context, new content, *J Nurs Adm* 33(2):105–110, 2003a.

Porter-O'Grady T: A different age for leadership, part 2: new rules, new roles, *J Nurs Adm* 33(3):173–178, 2003b.

Raup G: The impact of ED nurse manager leadership style on staff nurse turnover and patient satisfaction in academic health center hospitals, *J Emerg Nurs* 34(5):403–409, 2008.

Rutherford P, Lee B, Greiner A: *Transforming care at the bedside. IHI innovation series white paper*, Boston, 2004, Institute for Healthcare Improvement.

Sengin KK: Work-related attributes of RN job satisfaction in acute care hospitals, *J Nurs Adm* 33(6):317–320, 2003.

Stogdill RM: *Handbook of leadership: a survey of theory and research*, New York, 1974, The Free Press.

Thompson JD: *Organizations in action*, New York, 1967, McGraw-Hill.

White RK, Lippit R: *Autocracy and democracy: an experimental inquiry*, New York, 1960, Harper & Row.

Wieck KL, Dols J, Northam S: What nurses want: the nurse incentives project, *Nurs Econ* 27(3):169–201, 2009.

Budgeting Basics for Nurses

Barbara Cherry, DNSc, MBA, RN, NEA-BC

*e*volve Additional resources are available online at: http://evolve.elsevier.com/Cherry/

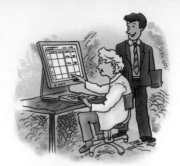

The budget serves as the financial guideline that enables the clinical team to provide quality patient care.

VIGNETTE

Todd Schultz, the nurse manager for the cardiac telemetry unit, returned to his office from a very uncomfortable meeting with the chief financial officer (CFO), the chief nursing officer (CNO), and his immediate boss, Kristy Harris, Director of Critical Care. Todd was very worried. By tomorrow morning he had to complete a detailed variance report for several items in his departmental budget that were out of line with budget expectations. Todd also had to develop a plan for correcting the unfavorable variances in the current month of July. As a new manager Todd was not involved in developing his budget because Kristy told him that she would take care of everything. At the time, Todd appreciated Kristy's willingness to complete the budget without his help, but now he regrets not being more involved. Throughout the meeting, the CFO and CNO reminded Todd that his signature was on the budget for labor and expenses, essentially agreeing to meet the goals. Unfortunately Todd believes his telemetry unit is unable to meet the aggressive budget goals developed by Kristy. Now faced with this challenge, Todd wonders how he should deal with this complex issue. One thing is for sure, Todd is going to be completely involved in developing his departmental budget from now on and will make every effort to learn more about budgets to prevent this situation from happening next year.

■ QUESTIONS TO CONSIDER WHILE READING THIS CHAPTER:

1 Who should be concerned about unit or department budgets?

2 What is the primary purpose of developing a unit or departmental budget?

3 When does the budget development process begin and end, or does it end?

4 How can nurses and nurse managers improve clinical care with better budgeting skills?

We thank Patrick A. Palmieri, MBA, MSN, ACNP, RN, CPHRM, FACHE, and Stephen W. Forney, MBA, CPA, FHFMA, FACHE for their contributions to this chapter in the 4th edition.

KEY TERMS

Budget Financial plan for the allocation of the organization's limited resources and a control for ensuring that results comply with the plan.

Budget assumptions Statements that reflect issues affecting the future performance of the organization; used as the framework for developing the budget, budget assumptions address questions, such as the following: Are supply prices likely to increase or decrease? What salary range will ensure that the organization is able to recruit and retain quality employees? What are the competitors offering in terms of new services? Is the patient census likely to increase or decrease over the next year?

Capital expenditures Amount spent on items that will have long-term (greater than 1 year) value to an organization. Typically includes property and equipment.

Expense An event or item that requires the outlay of money for purchase or the incurrence of a liability for future payment; major expenses for health care organizations include salaries, medical supplies and equipment, and facility maintenance.

Fiscal year A 12-month period used for calculating annual (yearly) financial reports in business; the fiscal year does not have to constitute the calendar year (January to December) but may be any 12-month period (i.e., August through July) established and maintained consistently by the business.

Full-time equivalent (FTE) The number of hours worked or paid that is equal to that expected of a full-time employee working a 40-hour workweek; annual work hours for 1 FTE equal 2080 hours and monthly equal 173.33 hours. One FTE position may be occupied by one employee working full time or shared by two or more employees working part time.

Incremental budgeting An approach to budget development that extrapolates from the prior period's budget and adjusts for future growth or decline in revenues or expenses to determine the budget for the next period.

Revenue Money that a health care organization receives in exchange for providing health care or other related services through normal business activities; synonymous with income.

Salaries, wages, and benefits (SWB) Budget category that typically includes direct payment for hours worked, bonuses, accrued vacation, health benefits, employer portion of payroll taxes, and workers' compensation.

Supplies Materials used in performing tasks within the organization. Typically includes clinical disposables, pharmaceuticals, and office supplies.

Variance The difference between the planned budget and the actual results.

Variance analysis The process of analyzing the differences in the planned budget results and the actual results; involves quantitative and qualitative analysis.

Zero-based budgeting An approach to budget development that begins as though the budget were being prepared for the first time.

LEARNING OUTCOMES

After studying this chapter, the reader will be able to:

1 Understand the basic terminology of budgeting in the health care industry.

2 Contribute to the budget development process for a nursing or clinical department.

3 Contribute to the capital budget development process for a nursing or clinical department.

4 Explain aspects of monitoring financial performance against an operational budget.

5 Understand the overall role of nursing in a health care organization's budget process.

CHAPTER OVERVIEW

The budget serves as the financial guideline that enables a health care organization to achieve its goal of providing high-quality patient care services. Just as nurses learn about clinical guidelines for the care of patients with various diseases, it is also essential that nurses have a working knowledge of the guidelines that ensure the organization is able to operate in a stable financial environment through effective budget management. As nurses advance into supervisory and management positions, they will have financial responsibility for a business unit of a health care organization and must be competent in the financial aspects of operating that unit. Additionally, the focus on cost and quality initiatives in today's health care settings requires that even staff nurses have a basic understanding of budgeting. This chapter introduces the basic concepts of budgeting in health care organizations, but for a deeper understanding of budgeting, nurses are encouraged to continue to build their knowledge by using a health care finance text and/or other resources suggested at the end of the chapter.

WHAT IS BUDGETING?

As a nursing student you are probably more aware of budget concepts than you realize. When you decided to become a registered nurse (RN), you had a goal to graduate from nursing school within a specified time period. You had to make a budget plan by predicting your expenses for that period, such as tuition, books, and living expenses. You also predicted your revenue from areas such as student loans, part-time jobs, savings, or parental or spousal support. After predicting your expenses and your revenues, you most likely planned your budget for how much you could spend on a weekly or monthly basis during this time and eventually achieve your goal of graduating from nursing school. Similarly, health care organizations develop budgets for a specified period by determining what goals they want to achieve, predicting expenses and revenues, then planning the annual budget and monitoring it on a monthly basis. For example, a hospital may plan its annual budget to maintain staffing and supplies to operate its current number of beds, provide a raise for all staff, and open a new outpatient surgical center.

Basically the health care organization's budget is a document that details how financial resources will be allocated to ensure that the organization is able to conduct its daily business and achieve strategic goals. The budget itemizes the organization's predicted expenses and expected revenues for a given period of time. More important, budgets require ongoing attention to ensure that the organization's financial needs are met. Just as nursing students most likely have to make decisions to adjust their budgets during nursing school to meet unexpected changes in revenues or expenses, the health care organization invariably experiences the same challenges during the year. Thus the budget becomes a dynamic action plan that guides the allocation of resources and expenditures and influences the nurse manager's decision making on a day-to-day, week-to-week, or month-to-month basis.

Budgets perform four basic functions to make certain the organization can achieve its strategic goals and permit continued operations from an economic point of view. The four budgeting functions are: (1) planning, (2) coordinating and communicating, (3) monitoring progress, and (4) evaluating performance. The following sections describe each of these important budgeting functions.

Planning

Planning is the most important function of the budgeting process (Foley, 2005). During the planning phase managers first decide on the goals to achieve for a specified period and identify resources (staff, supplies, equipment, etc.) needed to achieve those goals. Next they predict revenues and expenses based on those goals and budget assumptions to use in planning the budget. Budget assumptions allow the managers to answer various questions that will have an effect on the budget, such as:

- What should nursing salaries be in the coming year to reward and retain nurses and to remain competitive with other health care organizations in the area?

♦ How will new services being offered by other health care organizations in the area affect our organization?

Budgets are most often developed for a 1-year period based on predicted amounts of services. For example, hospitals will predict patient census for the coming year and then allocate funds for nursing salaries based on this predicted census.

Consider the following example: The hospital management team has decided to establish a chest pain center as part of the emergency department (ED). In planning the annual budget for the ED and its new chest pain center, the managers have developed the following assumptions:

♦ The chest pain center will see 12 patients every 24 hours. Of the 12 patients, 75% of the daily census (8 patients) are patients directed from the current ED census and 25% (4 patients) are patients new to this hospital.

♦ Four beds will be dedicated to the chest pain center and will require remodeling of an underused section of the current ED.

♦ The chest pain center will be staffed with RNs dedicated to the center.

The management team has planned to include the following expenses in the annual budget for the new chest pain center: salaries for nurses and support staff, supplies, monitoring equipment, equipment maintenance, funds for marketing the new program, and funds to remodel an area in the current ED for the program. Managers also need to think about the other areas that will be affected by the new chest pain center, such as the cardiac catheterization suite, echocardiogram, laboratory, electrocardiogram (ECG), and materials management, which all deserve budgetary consideration as a result of the wide-reaching effect of this seemingly small service expansion.

Historically, nursing has had limited input into fiscal (or financial) planning and development of the organization's budget. Administrators with no nursing background and little understanding of nursing values, beliefs, and care requirements traditionally made decisions about resource allocations related to nursing. Today participating in the budget process to determine resource allocation is a fundamental responsibility of the nurse manager. Involving staff nurses in the budget planning is also highly recommended. Managers and staff who participate in budget planning are more likely to be cost-conscious and appreciate how their unit should function to meet the overall financial goals.

Coordinating and Communicating

Although not commonly associated with budgets, coordination and communication are very important functions of budgeting. The budget process, by necessity, requires that many different groups within an organization come together to discuss the resources necessary to accomplish the goals of a business unit. Therefore, think of the budget process as the best opportunity to discuss concerns about resource allocation with the organization's leaders who are capable of resolving issues.

Consider the new chest pain center described earlier. To plan how the center will establish itself as a center of excellence for emergency care of patients with chest pain, nurses and physicians with experience in caring for chest pain patients must offer input about equipment and supply needs, room layout and design, staffing models, electronic medical record needs, and support staff; the financial officer needs to offer input about reimbursement rates and other financial considerations related to caring for this population; the hospital marketing staff needs to offer input about how the program can be advertised to inform the community about the new service; and other hospital administrators and department managers need to offer input as to how this new center will affect other areas of business both inside and outside the hospital.

Just as coordination and communication among these many groups and departments are essential to develop and manage the budget for the new chest pain center, such coordination and communication are also essential for developing and managing the budgets for all units within the hospital.

Monitoring Progress

Monitoring progress is one of the most vital functions of the budget—and the function that the nurse manager will be most involved with on a daily basis. It is through the comparison of actual performance against expected, or budgeted, performance that an organization measures the effectiveness of its budget. The ongoing monitoring of the budget allows timely corrective action or, if the budget plan is right on target, no adjustments are required.

Consider our chest pain center again. The budget was developed on an anticipated volume of 12 patients every 24 hours, and staffing was implemented to serve this volume of patients. At the end of its first month of operation, the nurse manager reviews the budget information and sees that the actual patient volume is averaging only 8 patients per 24 hours, and the associated revenue for the center is approximately 70% of the planned revenue. The nurse manager has several issues to consider: Does staffing need to be reduced to better reflect the number of patients being treated by the center? Are the patients being seen of higher acuity and thus require a higher intensity of nursing care? Is the low volume a reflection of the new program that is not yet widely appreciated in the community, and as its reputation grows, will the volume also grow? If no immediate changes are made, how will the reduced revenue affect the financial status of the center? Fortunately the nurse manager can consult others involved in developing the budget to address these important issues and make decisions to ensure the success of the center.

The difference between the planned budget and the actual results is called a *variance*. A variance is favorable when the results are better than expected or unfavorable when the results are worse than expected. The lower than planned revenue in the chest pain center is an example of an unfavorable variance. *Variance analysis*, the process by which deviations from budgeted amounts are examined, is discussed in more detail later.

Evaluating Performance

Budget results can also be used as part of the manager's performance evaluation, including the staff bonus structure for some hospitals. Evaluating the manager's performance based on budget results is becoming more widely used because of the growing trend toward accountability and compliance in the business world. By looking at the budget results for a given period, an evaluator can determine the manager's overall success in achieving goals. Nurse managers are frequently evaluated based on their effectiveness in managing nursing overtime costs and supply use, both of which are reflected in the nursing unit's budget. Performance evaluations based on budget results can motivate managers to effectively control budgets and will serve as a basis for salary decisions and career advancement for the manager (Harvard Business Essentials, 2004). Even though the manager is the captain of the unit and is ultimately accountable for the unit's budgetary performance, a lack of staff ownership and involvement in the unit's operation usually leads to problems for the manager.

TYPES OF BUDGETS

The three types of budgets for which a nurse manager typically has responsibility are operational, labor, and capital budgets (Box 17-1).

BOX **17-1**

Three Types of Budgets

Operating budget	Allocates funds for daily expenses, such as salaries, utilities, repairs, maintenance, and patient care supplies
Labor budget	A subset of the operating budget; allocates funds for salaries, overtime, benefits, and staff development and training
Capital budget	Allocates funds for construction projects and/or long-life medical equipment, such as cardiac monitors, defibrillators, and computer hardware

Operational Budget

The operational, or operating, budget represents revenues and expenses for an operational unit, such as a product line, unit, department, or overall organization. The chest pain center previously discussed is considered a product line; an example of a nursing unit is the intensive care unit or medical-surgical unit; an example of a department is dietary or human resources. Whereas the product line, unit, department, and overall organization have designated operational budgets, each operational unit has similar categories of expenses and revenues. The expenses in the operational budget are those necessary to operate on a daily basis, such as salaries, patient care supplies, and overhead expenses such as utilities and administrative costs. The revenues in the operational budget are those paid to the organization from health insurance companies, Medicare, Medicaid, other government programs, and patients' out-of-pocket payments for health care services provided (see Chapter 7 for more information about sources of payments for health care services).

Labor Budget

The labor budget is a subset of the operational budget. Its purpose is to provide detailed documentation of salaries, wages, and benefits with respect to the operational unit. Factors that affect the personnel budget include salary rates, overtime, benefits (e.g., paid time off, health insurance), staff development and training, and employee turnover. The labor budget is virtually always the largest expense item in an operational budget for a health care organization, typically 55% to 65% of the total expenses (Berger, 2005; Shactman et al, 2003). The labor budget is also used to provide managers with a productivity metric, which is the amount of work produced (i.e., hours of nursing care per patient day) by a specific amount of input or resources (i.e., nursing hours worked).

The productivity metric is necessary to give managers a measurement of the number of nursing hours worked in comparison with the amount of patient care provided. Low productivity (high nursing hours worked with low patient census) is not desirable because it means higher staff salaries combined with lower revenues for patient care services. High productivity (high patient census with low nursing hours) means that there are fewer staff to take care of more patients and they may not be able to provide safe and quality patient care. Most health care organizations have a recommended productivity measure that allows for a balance between financial efficiency and quality and safety of patient care. To achieve this balance, nursing must be at the table to ensure the discussion about quality and safety is voiced along with productivity and financial efficiency.

One of the primary difficulties encountered in managing the labor budget is accurately predicting future staffing needs. Because budgets are based on a predicted amount of services (i.e., patient census), variances between actual staffing levels and budget levels occur if the facility experiences an unanticipated increase or decrease in patient services. Another concern related to the budget and labor expense is balancing the patient acuity, or degree of patient illness, with the nurse-to-patient ratio.

An important aspect of labor budgeting is understanding the 12-month historical trend for labor hours and patient days. As a general rule, organizations expect nurse managers to control the number of worked hours versus the actual salary expense. Wage levels, benefit costs, and other related expenses are often controlled at the leadership level. The operational aspect of scheduling staff, measured in worked hours, to meet the needs of patient volume, measured by patients in the unit at midnight, is best controlled and budgeted at the departmental level.

Capital Budget

The capital budget represents funds allocated for construction projects and major equipment purchases (e.g., cardiac monitor, defibrillator, computer hardware). The capital budget is developed separately from the operating budget because capital purchases usually require multiple years to pay out. The main requirements for a purchase or acquisition to be considered as part of the capital budget is that it has a useful life expectancy of more than 1 year and it costs more than a minimum dollar amount established by the organization, usually from $500 to $2000.

The term "capital" simply refers to the funds used to purchase long-term investments, such as major medical equipment, computer systems, or newly constructed buildings. A capital budget item is an expensive purchase that will be used by the organization for many years. Capital budget items are often referred to as capital assets, long-term investments, capital investments, or capital acquisitions. These capital assets are treated differently from the operating budget expense because of their multiyear value. Because capital purchases are often considered investments, they are scrutinized more carefully during the budgeting process.

Planning capital budget requests will test the nurse manager's long-range planning skills. The nurse manager must be able to look down the road from 1 year to several years in advance to identify capital budgeting needs and to bring those needs to the attention of senior management. The unit or department need for a capital purchase must be weighed against the financial implications when considering the organization's entire capital budget. The nurse manager has a critical role in helping to plan the capital budget, justify priorities, and ensure the needs of the facility and patients are met. In addition, nursing staff are vital to a successful capital planning process because their "frontline" equipment needs must be made known to management for purchase consideration. Capital expenditures necessary for ensuring patient safety should be addressed with urgency.

BUDGET METHODS

There are two basic methods for budgeting: the incremental approach and the zero-based approach. Both of these approaches have particular strengths and weaknesses compared with one another, and both are completely sound approaches in most situations.

Incremental Budgeting

The incremental approach is the most commonly used budgeting method primarily because it is relatively simple to apply to most circumstances. The incremental approach is simply a forward trend of current or recent performance with adjustments for future growth or decline in revenues or expenses. For example, the nursing unit's budget would be based on the actual costs from the previous budget period with a small increase for planned salary raises and an increase in the cost of supplies. It is also possible that the incremental budget might include a decrease in all expenses.

Strengths of Incremental Budgeting. The incremental approach has unique strengths and weaknesses. Its primary strength is its simplicity. It is relatively easy to take current revenues or expenses and assume a small inflationary or growth factor. This is essentially how many organizations prepare their budgets irrespective of the apparent complexity of those organizations.

Another strength is its compatibility with most corporate organizational practices. In most cases budgetary amounts are developed at the corporate level of health care organizations and then pushed down to the facility level. It is much easier to allocate the overall budget change on an incremental basis across all departments or units than it is to build departmental budgets to fit a corporate derived number.

Finally the incremental approach is extremely efficient and effective when applied to a well-run department that is supporting organizational goals. Such a department would not expect to see dramatic changes from one budget period to another. Changes would only occur from relatively predictable external sources (e.g., inflation or growth).

Weaknesses of Incremental Budgeting. The weaknesses of the incremental approach stem from the simplicity that is its primary strength. Its primary weakness is that it does not take into account significant changes that may need to be made within the department. It simply perpetuates the current operating assumptions whether they are correct or incorrect. This situation is problematic when departments are not well run or require significant change to support organizational goals.

Finally the incremental approach does not address past mistakes that have been incorporated into the budgeting process. It is not uncommon for certain statistics, relationships, or amounts to be budgeted in error. The incremental approach simply builds on those mistakes and does not correct them.

Zero-Based Budgeting

Zero-based budgeting is used far less frequently than incremental budgeting. This method builds a budget from the assumption of no volume and no resources allocated; in other words, it is developed as though the budget were being prepared for the first time. Each budget cycle begins with a critical review of budget assumptions and proposed revenues and expenditures. Then core resources necessary for one unit of service are identified, and from there resource allocation is determined on a variable basis tied to volume.

Again, consider the chest pain center example. If the nurse manager is developing a zero-based budget, he or she would start each new budget planning cycle by determining the revenue and expenses for caring for one chest pain patient and then predict the average volume for the center and from there determine total revenues and expenses for the budget period. In developing the budget, the nurse manager understands that whereas one nurse is necessary to care for one patient, that nurse may also be able to care for two or three other patients at the same time. Thus the cost of nursing salaries is variable based on the volume of patients being treated in the center.

This process works somewhat differently with nonvariable departments, such as nursing administration and human resources, which are non-revenue generating departments (i.e., departments that do not provide a billable healthcare service). In nonvariable departments, expenses do not vary based on patient volume. Such departments do not base their budgets on a variable volume of patient visits, but rather on a set core of expenses to run the department. Their expenses are allocated to revenue generating departments.

Strengths of Zero-Based Budgeting. The zero-based approach has strengths and weaknesses that are essentially the mirror of the incremental approach. There are two significant strengths associated with this approach. The first strength is that this approach does not build on prior or incorrect assumptions. It requires building each budget from scratch. This places the focus on the current or future environment for which the budget is being created and lessens the likelihood that outdated information will be incorporated.

The second strength is that the complexity of the process yields a number of beneficial results. The process tends to encourage clinical and financial personnel to work closely together in developing a budget because neither group will have all of the information necessary to complete the task. Therefore, the process engenders buy-in and acceptance from both groups and increases the chances that the budget will be adhered to. Additionally, this interaction tends to encourage creative thinking because each side challenges the other in the process. Finally the level of analysis necessary to complete a zero-based budget tends to develop more accurate information about the unit being examined than does the incremental approach.

Weaknesses of Zero-Based Budgeting. The weaknesses of the zero-based approach are what one would expect from such an involved process. This approach is extremely time consuming and resource intensive. Developing an annual budget for a typical health care organization would likely take a minimum of 2 to 3 months of interaction between the finance department and the operational departments or units.

Furthermore, the approach requires that a common frame of reference be shared by all participants to be truly effective. In other words, finance personnel need to understand clinical terminology and processes, and clinical personnel need to understand financial principles.

Finally the zero-based approach may be too complex for a given circumstance. A well-run organization that is not undergoing significant change may find this approach to be far too resource intensive relative to the marginal improvement it would yield.

DEVELOPING A BUDGET

Developing a budget is actually a continual process. Organizations are constantly making projections for future budgets, implementing current budgets, and analyzing month-to-month variances in relation to the budget. The current budget usually covers a 12-month period, also known as the organization's fiscal year. The development of the budget for the new fiscal year occurs a few months ahead of the start of the new fiscal year so that the budget can be developed and approved at all levels before it becomes effective. For example, if the hospital's fiscal year is from September 1st to August 31st, then budget development for the new fiscal year will begin sometime in early summer—or perhaps even earlier depending on the size and complexity of the organization. Large health systems usually begin the budget process much earlier than smaller systems or single facilities as a result of the number of approval layers.

Health care organizations usually have a defined procedure in place for budget development. This defined procedure tells managers if the budget development will use the incremental method, zero-based method, or some other method defined by the organization. Organizations will also define if they use a "top-down," "participatory," or "iterative" approach to budgeting. In the top-down approach, upper management sets budget goals and imposes those goals on the rest of the organization. In the participatory approach, the people responsible for achieving the budget goals are included in goal setting. The iterative approach is a combination of the top-down and the participatory approach with upper management defining strategic goals and then unit leaders developing their operating budgets to incorporate their individual goals in conjunction with the organization's strategic goals (Harvard Business Essentials, 2002).

One key to understanding budgets is to know the *unit of service* on which costs and revenues are based. "Patient-days" is the common unit of service for inpatient facilities; patient visits or visits by categories (short, intermediate, long) are the units of service for ambulatory clinics and home health agencies. Budgets are then developed based on the units of service predicted for a given period. For example, the nurse manager in a hospital intensive care unit will base his or her budget on the average number of days that patients will be on the unit over the course of 12 months. The director of the home health agency will base his or her budget on the number of home visits that will be made during a 12-month period. The unit of service may vary depending on the organization, setting, and financial policies; thus it is essential that the nurse understands the unit of service in the area in which he or she is employed.

Following are the basic steps for developing a budget:

1. Review the organization's strategic plan to identify goals and objectives for the organization, department, or defined operational units. The budget is developed to accomplish these goals and objectives.
2. Set budget assumptions on which to base budgeting decisions. Budget assumptions address issues that affect the future performance of the organization and address questions, such as: Are supply prices likely to increase or decrease and by what percent? What salary range will ensure that the organization is able to recruit and retain quality employees? What will the cost of the health insurance plan be in the coming year? What are the competitors offering in terms of new services? Is the patient census likely to increase or decrease over the next year? Budget assumptions should be developed by a team of managers from different departments and areas of expertise to be certain consideration is given to all issues that will affect the budget.
3. Gather information about past results and use the information in combination with budget assumptions to set reasonable expectations about future performance.
4. Predict the units of service that will be provided during the budget period.
5. Project expected revenues based on the units of service.
6. Project expenses based on the units of service. Determine expenses for the labor budget first based on the predicted units of service and the number of FTEs needed to provide the predicted service volume. Each full-time employee is considered one FTE or 2080 hours per year (40 hours per week). In some organizations, nurses are scheduled for three 12-hour shifts each week, 36 hours per week or 1872 hours per year, and are considered 0.9 FTE. After determining units of service and related FTEs, other expenses are fairly straightforward to project.

Developing the budget is generally a process that involves many discussions among many different managers, from finance to nursing. It is important that nursing have a strong and knowledgeable voice in the budget process so that nursing and patient care needs are appropriately addressed. Box 17-2 lists hints to improve your budgeting skills.

VARIANCE ANALYSIS

The primary use of a budget is to evaluate the progress of the department or unit. Variance analysis is the process by which deviations from budgeted amounts are examined by comparing actual performance results against expected, or budgeted, performance. Through this process

BOX **17-2**

Hints to Improve Your Budgeting Skills

- Understand your organization's budgeting process. What guidelines do you need to follow? What is the timing of the budget process? What key managers can serve as a resource to help you understand the budget process?
- Learn your department's unit of service and exactly how it is defined.
- Build a relationship with a finance person in the organization and collaborate routinely on improvement projects; invite finance staff to your unit meetings and ask to participate in theirs; communicate regularly.
- Review financial reports with the finance person to make sure you are correctly interpreting the reports.
- Understand each line in your budget. If you do not know what something means or where a number comes from, find out.
- Have ongoing discussions with your management team throughout the budget process. The more you participate in the planning process, the better you will understand the budget and your responsibilities related to it.
- Learn your organization's capital budgeting process and what qualifies a purchase as a capital expenditure.
- Do not look for excuses when performing below budget. Instead look for new opportunities to exceed budget.
- Attempt to develop a reasonable budget that improves on previous performance. This will engender respect with financial personnel.

variances are evaluated on a quantitative and qualitative basis. Quantitative analysis focuses on numerical variances to the budget. In other words, are you over or under budget for labor, supply usage, or revenue generated? See Table 17-1 for a sample budget and variance report.

Qualitative analysis of budget variances focuses on reconciling the underlying assumptions on which the budget was based with current conditions. In many cases the operating environment for a department or unit changes in ways that the budget assumptions are rendered invalid. For example, a unit may be budgeted for labor at 10-hour/patient-day based on a given patient acuity level. Then the hospital gets a new internist that attracts large numbers of patients with significantly higher acuity levels, and these patients are admitted to this unit. The labor used rises to 12-hour/patient-day based on the new acuity level. This sort of qualitative change can make budgets difficult, if not impossible, to adhere to without modification. Nurse leaders in the clinical department or unit are best positioned to determine why variances have occurred because variances are almost always related to a clinical issue, such as the one just described.

Variance information typically is presented by means of certain standard reports. Labor budget variances are usually presented on a pay-period basis and provide information on performance against the budgeted standard. Overall budget variances will be presented on a monthly, quarterly, or annual basis and typically provide information to compare current performance against budget and current performance against the previous year's performance as seen in Table 17-1.

COST CONCEPTS RELATED TO BUDGETING

When considering the budget, it is necessary to have a basic understanding of how much health care services cost and how to predict changes in costs. Consider this question: How much does it cost to provide nursing care to one patient for one 12-hour shift? Unfortunately, the answer

TABLE **17-1**

Sample Budget and Variance Report

HOMETOWN GENERAL HOSPITAL: DEPARTMENT PERFORMANCE ANALYSIS—MED-SURG FOR PERIOD ENDING 09/30/20XX

	PRIOR YEAR ACTUAL 9/XX	CURRENT MTD (MONTH)			CURRENT YTD (YEAR-TO-DATE)			PRIOR YEAR	
		ACTUAL 9/XX	BUDGET 9/XX	MTD VAR (VARIANCE) 9/XX	ACTUAL 9/XX	BUDGET 9/XX	YTD VAR. 9/XX	PRIOR YR 9/XX	PRIOR YR VARIANCE
Gross revenue									
Inpatient revenue	1,276,525	1,300,122	1,322,904	-22,782	11,087,012	12,575,946	-1,488,934	12,733,822	-1,646,810
Outpatient revenue	0	0	0	0	0	0	0	0	0
Other revenue	0	0	0	0	0	0	0	0	0
Total gross revenue:	1,276,525	1,300,122	1,322,904	-22,782	11,087,012	12,575,946	-1,488,934	12,733,822	-1,646,810
Operating expenses									
Total productive labor	241,270	293,541	257,954	35,587	2,375,340	2,419,097	-43,757	2,376,009	-669
Total nonproductive labor	29,012	40,031	37,352	2679	359,759	359,453	306	328,128	31,631
Employee benefits and taxes	40,372	38,483	41,133	-2650	366,203	401,616	-35,413	398,766	-32,563
Total SWB (salaries, wages, and benefits)	310,653	372,055	336,439	35,616	3,101,302	3,180,166	-78,864	3,102,903	-1601
Supplies	25,687	20,506	22,628	-2123	193,223	213,853	-20,630	219,267	-26,044
Medical and clinical fees	0	0	0	0	0	0	0	0	0
Contracted dept and other fees	298	0	41	-41	506	371	135	929	-424
Repairs and maintenance	0	0	20	-20	0	184	-184	242	-242
Utilities and telephone	0	0	0	0	0	0	0	0	0
Rent, lease, equipment rental	0	0	0	0	1485	0	1485	0	1485

Continued

TABLE 17-1

Sample Budget and Variance Report—cont'd

HOMETOWN GENERAL HOSPITAL: DEPARTMENT PERFORMANCE ANALYSIS—MED-SURG FOR PERIOD ENDING 09/30/20XX

	PRIOR YEAR ACTUAL 9/XX	CURRENT MTD (MONTH)			CURRENT YTD (YEAR-TO-DATE)			PRIOR YEAR	
		ACTUAL 9/XX	BUDGET 9/XX	MTD VAR (VARIANCE) 9/XX	ACTUAL 9/XX	BUDGET 9/XX	YTD VAR. 9/XX	PRIOR YR 9/XX	PRIOR YR VARIANCE
Other controllable expenses	883	1232	953	279	8617	8741	-124	14,041	-5424
Other noncontrollable expenses	0	0	0	0	0	0	0	0	0
Total operating expenses	337,520	393,792	360,081	33,711	3,305,132	3,403,315	-98,183	3,337,382	-32,249
Gross margin	939,005	906,330	962,823	-56,493	7,781,880	9,172,631	-1,390,751	9,396,440	-1,614,561
Gross margin percentage	73.56	69.71	72.78	-3.07	70.19	72.94	-2.75	73.79	-3.6
Department patient-days	841	853	871	-18	7283	8280	-997	8384	-1101
Average daily census	28	28	29	-1	27	30	-4	31	-4
Observation days	1.67	3.5	5.5	-2	41.54	49.38	-7.83	48.17	-6.63
Total department patient-days	842.67	856.5	876.5	-20	7324.54	8329.38	-1,004.83	8,432.17	-1,107.62

The budget report shows dollar performance comparing actual revenues and expenses to budgeted revenues and expenses for the same month of the prior year, current month, current YTD and the annual totals and variances for the prior year. YTD is the totals for the prior months plus the current month in the fiscal year. The department has spent $33,711 (shaded in yellow) more than budgeted for expenses for the current month, but for the current YTD, the department has spent less than budgeted for expenses by $98,183 (shaded in green).

is not simple because many factors affect how much something costs. An important step to understand costs is to review the primary types of costs that accountants consider when determining the cost of services in a health care setting:

- ◆ *Service unit or unit-of-service:* The basic measure of the product or service being produced. The unit-of-service varies by the health care setting and type of service being provided. Examples include patient-days (hospital), home care visits (home health agency), patient visits (outpatient clinic), and operating room time (outpatient surgical center).
- ◆ *Direct costs:* Costs that can be traced directly to the production of the unit-of-service. Examples include nursing care and supplies to provide direct patient care. The important concept to remember about direct costs is that they vary with the volume of services. As the patient census increases, the need for additional nursing care and supplies also increases.
- ◆ *Indirect costs:* Costs that are incurred as a result of the organization's operating expenses but are not directly related to providing the unit-of-service. Examples include salaries for administrative personnel and expenses for security, housekeeping, and building maintenance. Indirect costs are sometimes referred to as overhead.
- ◆ *Full cost:* The total of all costs associated with a unit-of-service and includes direct and indirect costs.
- ◆ *Fixed costs:* Costs that do not change as the unit-of-service volume changes. For example, administrative salaries do not change regardless of the patient census on the nursing units. The important point to remember about fixed cost is that they remain steady regardless of the change in units-of-service (i.e., patient-days). As the units-of-service increase, the greater the number to share fixed costs. Conversely, as the units-of-service decrease, the fewer number to share fixed costs. An organization's finance leaders are always interested in increasing volume to provide additional revenue to help cover fixed costs.
- ◆ *Variable costs:* Costs that vary directly with changes in the volume of units-of-service. For example, in an ambulatory clinic, the cost of immunizations varies directly with the number of patients who receive immunizations.

This list provides only a basic introduction into cost terminology; it does not provide a comprehensive range of cost accounting terminology and concepts. However, it does demonstrate the complexity of assessing and managing costs.

IMPROVING THE COST AND QUALITY OF CLINICAL CARE

Nurses face challenging situations given the nursing shortage, the rise of the national patient safety agenda, the focus on evidence-based practice, and the increasing acuity of patients in all settings from hospitals to home health agencies to nursing homes. At the same time, organizational leaders are faced with challenging economic times, declining reimbursements, and increasing costs in all areas. Changes to improve quality and reduce costs must be made! How can nurses collaborate with organizational leaders and financial managers to make a difference? Nurses are at the front lines of health care and are key to enhancing the *value* of health care, with value being the combination of quality + cost + service (Esposito-Herr, 2009). Nurses can truly affect the quality and cost of care in significant ways:

- ◆ As discharge advocates, nurses can ensure appropriate discharge instructions and proper follow-up to reduce costly readmissions to the hospital and significantly reduce costs (Jack et al, 2009; Nickitas, 2009).
- ◆ As advocates for evidence-based practice, nurses can engage in robust evidence-based practice programs that will lead to increased quality and lower costs by identifying

less-expensive care alternatives and balancing the effectiveness of treatments with the associated costs (Wurmser, 2009).

◆ As advocates for efficient operations, nurses must be proactive in evaluating staffing patterns and care delivery models along with delegating non-nursing tasks to ancillary personnel to ensure high-quality care and reduce unnecessary costs (Hader, 2009).

◆ As advocates for appropriate supply usage, nurses can become involved in identifying the most cost-effective medical-surgical supplies that can replace more expensive products (Hader, 2009).

◆ As advocates for quality patient care, nurses can contribute to reduced complications and reduced length of stay and thus reduce the overall cost of care while also increasing the quality of care (Hader, 2009).

◆ As advocates for patient safety, nurses can have a significant effect on the hospital's bottom line by preventing hospital-acquired conditions such as injuries from falls and hospital-acquired infections. Commonly referred to as never events, hospitals are no longer paid by Medicare for the cost of treating 28 medical errors that are largely preventable and have serious consequences for patients (a full list of never events is available online at: www.cms.hhs.gov/apps/media/press/factsheet.asp?Counter=3043).

As nurses step up to the challenge of enhancing the *value* of health care—improved quality and lower costs—they must be able to measure and document their contributions. Only by understanding the basics of budgeting and costs can nurses demonstrate their contributions toward reduced readmissions, reduced complications, reduced never events, reduced length of stay, improvements in supply use costs, and overall lower costs per patient combined with increased quality.

SUMMARY

The financial well-being of health care organizations—and the value of health care—rests largely in the hands of the clinical team, with the budget serving as the financial guideline that enables the clinical team to provide quality patient care and achieve strategic goals. This chapter has reviewed the four major functions of the organization's budget: planning, communicating and coordinating, monitoring progress, and evaluating performance. Elements of the three basic types of budgets—operational, labor, and capital—have been described along with the two primary approaches to budgeting—incremental and zero based. The nurse's role in affecting the organization's financial performance by being an advocate for proper patient discharges and follow-up, evidence-based practice, efficient operations, appropriate supply use, and preventing complications and hospital-acquired conditions is reviewed.

The reader is cautioned that this chapter merely provides a general overview of budgeting basics to serve as a framework on which nurses can continue to build their knowledge of health care finance and budgeting. As nurses advance into supervisory and management positions, it is essential that they further develop their skills and knowledge in budgeting through personal study, working with mentors, attending classes, reading books and journals, and joining professional organizations that promote health care finance and budget knowledge. This chapter serves as a good first step in learning about budgets and lists several resources (Box 17-3) that the learner can use to continue developing budgeting and financial management skills.

⊖volve Additional resources are available online at: http://evolve.elsevier.com/Cherry/

BOX **17-3**

Helpful Websites and Online Resources

WEBSITES

Healthcare Financial Management Association
  www.hfma.org
American College of Healthcare Executives
  www.ache.org
American Organization of Nurse Executives
  www.aone.org
Health Affairs: The Policy Journal of the Health Sphere
  www.healthaffairs.org
Modern Healthcare
  www.modernhealthcare.com
American Hospital Association
  www.aha.org

BOOKS

Cleverly WO, Cameron AE: *Essentials of health care finance,* ed 5, Boston, 2003, Jones and Bartlett.
Davis N, ed: *Essentials of health care finance,* Chicago, 2006, American Health Information, Management Association.
Finkler SA, Kovner CT, Jones CB: *Financial management for nurse managers and executives,* ed 3, Philadelphia, 2007, Saunders.

Gapenski LC: *Understanding health care financial management,* ed 5, Chicago, 2006, Health Administration Press.
Hankins RW, Baker JJ: *Management accounting for health care organizations: tools and techniques for decision support,* Boston, 2004, Jones and Bartlett.
Harvard Business Essentials: *Finance for managers,* Boston, 2002, Harvard Business School Press.

JOURNALS AND NEWSLETTERS

HFM Magazine
  A publication of the Healthcare Financial Management Association.
  The Business of Caring: Business Essentials for Nurse Leaders
  A joint publication of the Healthcare Financial Management Association and the American Organization of Nurse Executives.
  Available free at: www.hfma.org/publications/business_caring_newsletter.

REFERENCES

Berger S: Analyzing your hospital's labor productivity, *Healthcare Finance Manage,* April, 2005.
Esposito-Herr MB, Persinger KD, Hunt SS: Partnering for better performance: the nursing-finance alliance, *Am Nurse Today* 4(4):29–31, 2009.
Foley R: Learn to speak finance, *Nurs Manage* Aug:28–34, 2005.
Hader R: Tightening the belt in 2009, *Nurs Manage,* Jan:6, 2009.
Harvard Business Essentials: *Finance for managers,* Boston, 2002, Harvard Business School Press.

Harvard Business Essentials: *Manager's toolkit: the 13 skills managers need to succeed,* Boston, 2004, Harvard Business School Press.
Jack BW, et al: A reengineered hospital discharge program to decrease re-hospitalization: a randomized trial, *Ann Intern Med* 150(3):178–187, 2009.
Nickitas DM: Nursing on the right side: why nurses must step to the right (of our left brains), *Nurs Econ* 27(3), 141, 168, 2009.
Shactman D, et al: The outlook for hospital spending, *Health Aff* 22(6):12–26, 2003.
Wurmser T: The financial case for EBP, *Nurs Manage* (Feb):12–14, 2009.

18

Effective Communication and Conflict Resolution

Anna Marie Sallee, PhD, RN, CCRN

e)volve   Additional resources are available online at: http://evolve.elsevier.com/Cherry/

"The greatest problem of communication is the illusion that it has been accomplished."

—GEORGE BERNARD SHAW

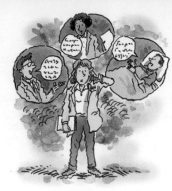

How is your message being received?

■ VIGNETTE

Stacy Shannon, registered nurse (RN), the charge nurse on 4-East, receives a phone call from the secretary in the emergency department (ED) to inform Stacy that a patient is ready for transfer. Stacy was expecting this patient, but had not anticipated the transfer would occur so soon and had not yet informed the nurse who would be assigned to the patient. The ED secretary explains that there are many patients waiting to be seen in the ED and it is becoming increasingly chaotic. Stacy replies that she will locate the nurse who will be assigned to the patient and facilitate the transfer as soon as possible. As Stacy goes down the hallway to locate this particular nurse, she learns that the nurse has left the unit on a short break and is expected back within 10 minutes.

Stacy calls the ED secretary to arrange for the transfer to occur in 20 minutes. To her surprise she finds out that the patient has left the department and is being brought to 4-East immediately. Within a few moments the patient and ED nurse arrive. The ED nurse states that he wants to give report on this patient quickly because he needs to return to the ED right away. Stacy assists him in transferring the patient to a bed and making the patient as comfortable as possible.

As Stacy completes this process, the nurse who was on break returns to the unit, learns that she has a new patient she did not expect, and immediately has to receive report from the ED. Stacy notes through both body language and tone of voice that the interaction between the two nurses is less than cordial.

Within 10 minutes Stacy receives a phone call from the ED charge nurse wanting to discuss this incident. Negative comments are made about the 4-East nurse who left the unit "unannounced" and that "there is a concern for patient safety." How can Stacy best facilitate a positive outcome in this situation?

■ **QUESTIONS TO CONSIDER WHILE READING THIS CHAPTER:**

1 What communication strategies should Stacy use to respond to the accusations being made by the ED charge nurse to help resolve the conflict?

2 What strategies can Stacy use to build a trusting relationship between herself and the ED charge nurse?

3 What positive communication techniques could have prevented this situation from occurring?

4 What nonverbal cues might Stacy have observed between the two nurses during the report exchange?

5 Should Stacy have intervened when she observed the interaction between the two nurses? If so, how?

6 What strategies can Stacy implement to increase the communication skills of her staff?

KEY TERMS

Active communication A participatory form of communication that promotes change.

Active listening The process of hearing what others are saying with a sense of seriousness and discrimination.

Aggressive communication A manner of communicating that limits the focus on or understanding of the opinions, values, or beliefs of others.

Assertive communication A form of communication that enables a person to act in his or her own best interest without denying or infringing on the rights of others.

Blocking Obstructing communication through noncommittal answers, generalization, or other techniques that hamper continued interaction.

Communication A process of relaying information between or among people by the use of words, letters, symbols, or body language.

Conflict An experience in which there is simultaneous arousal of two or more incompatible motives.

Decode A process whereby the receiver takes the message and interprets its meaning.

Empathy An attempt to experience another person's point of view without losing one's own identity.

Encode A process of translating an idea already conceived into a message suitable for transmission.

Equality An attitude that relays acceptance and approval of another person.

Feedback Response from the receiver, which can be verbal or nonverbal.

Filtration Unconscious exclusion of extraneous stimuli.

Information Data that are meaningful and alter the receiver's understanding.

Interpretation Receiver's understanding of the meaning of the communication.

Negative communication techniques Behaviors that block or impair effective communication.

Nonassertive communication Communicating in a timid and reserved manner resulting in limited concern for one's own rights regardless of the situation.

Nonverbal communication Unspoken cues (intentional or unintentional) from the communicant, such as body positioning, facial expression, or lack of attention.

Openness An attitude of willingness to self-disclose, react honestly to the messages of others, and own one's feelings and thoughts.

Passive communication A form of communication in which the individual fails to say what is meant

Perception The manner in which one sees reality.

Positive communication techniques Behaviors that enhance effective communication.

Receiver The destination for or receptor of a message.

Sender Anyone who wishes to convey an idea or concept to others, to seek information, or to express a thought or emotion.

Supportiveness The concern that is fostered by being descriptive rather than evaluative and provisional rather than certain.

LEARNING OUTCOMES

After studying this chapter, the reader will be able to:

1 Outline factors that can influence the communication process.

2 Communicate effectively with diverse intergenerational and interprofessional team members.

3 Apply positive communication techniques in diverse situations.

4 Recognize negative communication techniques.

5 Evaluate conflicting verbal and nonverbal communication cues.

6 Examine constructive methods of communicating in conflict situations.

7 Respond to inappropriate use of logical fallacies in communication.

CHAPTER OVERVIEW

Effective communication is a foundational component of professional nursing practice. The development of effective communication skills can only enhance each nurse's professional image while building strong relationships with patients and colleagues. Understanding communication processes and principles is required for nurses to interact professionally with patients, families and significant others, nursing peers, managers, student nurses, physicians, other members of the interprofessional team, and the public. Nurses communicate through a variety of media including the spoken and written word, demonstration, role modeling, and on occasion, public appearances. The exchange of ideas and feelings is hardly limited to verbal communication. There are many types of nonverbal communication that are often as meaningful as, and in many instances more meaningful than, audible expression. Because communication is such a complex process, there are infinite opportunities for sending or receiving incorrect messages. All too frequently communication is faulty, resulting in misperceptions and misunderstandings.

This chapter reviews the communication process and components, communication styles, and principles of effective communication in professional nursing, including special communication issues related to documentation, cultural diversity, gender and generational differences, and interprofessional teams. A major focus of this chapter is describing effective, positive communication techniques that can prevent or reduce conflict. This chapter also provides techniques that can be used to effectively manage conflict situations when they do occur.

OUR PROFESSION SPEAKS

"Nurses must be as proficient in communication skills as they are in clinical skills."

—**Standard 1, Standards for Establishing and Sustaining Healthy Work Environments, American Association of Critical-Care Nurses (2005, p. 14).**

"Goal 2: Improve Effective Communication. Effective communication, which is timely, accurate, complete, unambiguous, and understood by the recipient, reduces errors, and results in improved patient safety."

—**2009 Patient Safety Goals, The Joint Commission (2009, p. 4)**

THE COMMUNICATION PROCESS

Communication is a process requiring certain components. There must be a sender, a receiver, and a message. Effective communication is a dynamic process: with a response (feedback), the sender becomes the receiver, the receiver becomes the sender, and the message changes (Figure 18-1). The method of delivery influences the effectiveness of communication. In addition, communication is affected by many subcomponents, both environmental and in the mind of the communicators (Figure 18-2). When communication with another person occurs, verbally or nonverbally, a typical pattern develops that includes the actual message being sent, the receiver's belief or interpretation of that message, and the reaction to the message.

Think about the communication activities that occur in the health care setting. There is often much to communicate in a limited period of time and sometimes during very high-stress situations. In addition to the actual message, personal goals or hidden agendas can influence the way a message is delivered or received. Because of this, it is very important to understand the many elements that influence the communication process.

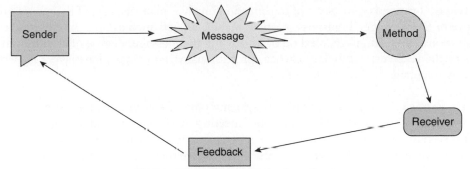

Figure 18-1 *The communication process.*

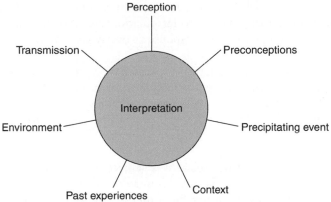

Figure 18-2 *Factors influencing interpretation of messages.*

Interpretation

Interpretation of information can be influenced by such factors as context, environment, precipitating event, preconceived ideas, personal perceptions, style of transmission, and past experiences. Because of the interaction of these factors, the sender's message may mean to the receiver something that was entirely unplanned or unexpected by the sender (see Figure 18-2).

Context and Environment. Context refers to the entire situation relevant to the communication, such as the environment, the background, and the particular circumstances that led to the discussion. Environment can denote physical surroundings and happenings and the emotional conditions involved in the communication.

Precipitating Event. Precipitating event refers specifically to the event or situation that prompted the communication. A precipitating event is a specific single event, whereas context describes the whole ambiance of the situation with the inclusion of multiple circumstances that have led to the precipitating event.

Preconceived Ideas. Preconceived ideas are conceptions, opinions, or thoughts that the receiver has developed before the encounter. Such ideas can dramatically affect the receiver's acceptance and understanding of the message.

Style of Transmission. Style of transmission involves many aspects of the manner of conveyance of the message. Transmission styles include aspects such as open or closed statements or questions, body language, method of organizing the message, degree of attention to the topic or to the receiver, vocabulary chosen (professional jargon versus language a layperson could easily understand), and intonation.

Past Experiences. Each person comes to any type of communication, whether it is friendly conversation, informational lecture, staff meeting, performance evaluation, or any other possible scenario, with baggage in terms of past experiences. Because past experiences are a variety of positive, neutral and negative events, the influence that the experiences can and will have on communication may be positive, neutral, or negative. **The importance of recognizing that any reaction from the receiver may be biased by previous experiences cannot be overstated.** An astute sender will begin to investigate such a possibility if the receiver reacts in an unexpected or inappropriate manner to information that was not expected to produce such a response, which may range from nonresponse to overly vehement response.

Personal Perceptions. Personal perceptions can have a profound effect on the quality of communication. Perception is awareness through the excitation of all the senses. Perception can be described as all that the person knows about a situation or circumstance based on what each of the senses—taste, smell, sight, sound, touch, and intuition—discover and interpret.

Filtration

The most concise delivery of information is subject to some amount of filtration. Think of the process as similar to washing vegetables in a colander. A large amount of water is poured over the produce. Some of the water flows quickly through the colander holes, some water drips through more slowly, and some water hangs on the contents or settles in the solid portions of the colander and never filters through. If people were not able to filter out a portion of the stimuli that bombard them daily, the clutter would be unmanageable! At the same time, however, it is possible to filter out some part of intended communication that is essential to facilitate understanding.

Feedback

Feedback, simply put, is the response from the receiver. However, as with all communication, feedback is a dynamic process. As the receiver interprets and responds to the original message, the sender begins the same process of feedback to the receiver. Because of this circular property, the process frequently is referred to as the "feedback loop" (van Servellen, 1997). As with the original message, feedback is not confined to verbal responses alone. Both communicants constantly assess nonverbal communication as well. Feedback is formed based on all the components of interpretation and filtration.

VERBAL VERSUS NONVERBAL COMMUNICATION
Verbal Communication

Verbal communication is the most common form of interpersonal communication and involves talking and listening. An important clue to verbal communication is the tone or inflection with which the words are spoken and the general attitude used when speaking. Suzette Haden Elgin refers to the "tune the words are set to" (1993, p. 186). The key to the true meaning of a statement may be contained in the emphasis placed on a specific word.

Consider how differently the following phrase could be perceived based on the inflection or the emphasis on the wording:

◆ You are going to **bed**.
◆ **You** are going to bed.
◆ You **are going** to bed.

With an emphasis on bed, the first phrase most likely will be perceived as an inquiry. The second phrase might imply that you are going to bed, but no one else is. The last phrase, an imperative (or command), gives the impression of increased emotion, such as anger or frustration.

Another element central to verbal interaction is the concept of attitude. Being aware of and learning to understand the concept of attitude is key to effective communication. Attitude involves a predisposition or tendency to respond in one way or another. Often the attitude that accompanies a verbal interaction, which can be positive or negative, is much more meaningful than the actual words spoken. Although we may hear "attitude" in a person's tone of voice, it is most often communicated loud and clear through nonverbal communication.

Nonverbal Communication

Nonverbal communication involves many factors that either confirm or deny the spoken word. Facial expression, the presence or absence of eye contact, posture, and body movement all project a direct message. Indirect nonverbal messages might include dressing style, lifestyle, or material possessions. Never presume that external trappings and physical presentation do not influence the quality of communication. Preconceived ideas and expectations interpret input from all such sources, often on an almost subconscious level.

Consider the following scenario: Rhonda, a young wife and mother, was admitted through the emergency department with significant abdominal pain. As the nurse inquires about her symptoms, Rhonda repeatedly glances at her husband, Tommy, before she answers. Although she denies any pain at this time, you observe that she guards her stomach, has a clenched jaw line, and does not make eye contact with you. As you assess and question Rhonda, Tommy often interrupts with comments such as, "She's just fine. It was only a stomachache, and it's gone this morning, isn't it, dear?" Which message seems more likely to be true—the verbal or the nonverbal? How will you address the nonverbal cues? As you read the remainder of this chapter, consider strategies that you can use to enhance communication between this husband and wife.

The inability to make eye contact may be construed to mean that the speaker is shy, scared, or not telling the truth. The judgment of which condition is correct is based on all the factors that feed into the receiver's interpretation—perception, preconceptions, precipitating event, context, past experiences, environment, and transmission. Faced with the many opportunities for incorrect interpretation, is it any wonder that misunderstandings occur?

An important concept to remember is that when the verbal message and the nonverbal message do not agree, the receiver is more likely to believe the nonverbal message. Jan Hargrave (2009) tells us that our bodies give "hidden messages" all the time. We can't get away from what our bodies say; they do not lie! In fact, Hargrave (2009) states that when we are talking to someone, 55% of our message is nonverbal, 38% is voice inflection, and only 7% is the actual words we say.

An understanding of the importance prescribed to body language and other nonverbal clues to the intent of the message explains the advantage of face-to-face communication whenever possible. Although a telephone conversation supplies verbal messages, intonation, and feedback, other signals are missing such as facial expression, body position, and environmental clues. The perils inherent in written and electronic communication are discussed later.

POSITIVE COMMUNICATION TECHNIQUES

Effective, positive communication is characterized by (1) openness—a willingness to self-disclose, react honestly to incoming stimuli, acknowledge, and assume responsibility for one's own thoughts and actions; (2) empathy—experiencing another person's point of view without judgment or losing one's own identity; (3) supportiveness—maintaining a nonthreatening, non-judgmental attitude; (4) positiveness—affirmative regard for self, others, and the interaction; and (5) equality—acknowledging that each individual is valuable and should be heard (Gibb, 1961). Following are techniques that the nurse can use to put positive communication into practice.

Developing Trust

Trust between the nurse and the patient is essential to good communication and often must be cultivated. Factors that enhance the development of trust include openness on the part of the nurse, honesty, integrity, and dependability. These can be achieved by:

- Communicating clearly in language that a layperson can understand
- Keeping promises
- Protecting confidentiality
- Avoiding negative communication techniques such as blocking and false reassurance, which are discussed later
- Being available to the patient

The need for trust is not limited to the nurse-patient relationship, but rather pervades all associations. Care is more effective when the nursing team and the interprofessional team share the essential element of trust.

Using "I" Messages

The use of "I" messages is a fundamental component in acceptable communication. Consider the following exchange:

> *Laura:* "You make me so mad, Donald."
> *Donald:* "I don't mean to make you mad."
> *Laura:* "Well, you do. You never think about how I feel. You know I hate it when you leave a patient's room as cluttered as 103."
> *Donald:* "You don't have the vaguest idea what went on here last night! That's what I hate about you—always so quick to judge. You are so critical. You must think that you are perfect!"

When a comment starts with "you," most commonly the receiver's defenses will promptly go on alert. The use of "you" in such a context sounds—and most probably is meant to be—accusatory. Notice how the emotions quickly escalate to anger. Also notice that although the receiver initially tries to sound conciliatory, he soon begins to respond in a similar accusatory form. Instead of using accusatory and defensive language, the sender should frame the comment in terms of how it makes her or him feel. Consider this alternative: Laura says, "Donald, I feel so upset when I find a cluttered room like 103 at the beginning of my shift. I feel as if I am behind when I start."

The difference is obvious. When "I" messages are used, they become less likely to sound accusatory. By using such an opening, the sender allows the receiver to respond to the true message rather than start to mount a defense. It allows for more effective communication because the receiver is more likely to offer an explanation such as the following: Donald says, "I'm really sorry about room 103, Laura. I guess the wheel that doesn't squeak doesn't get oiled, as they say. Our shift started last night with a patient coding right after he arrived from the ED. There was no family here. It took forever to find them and then to support them through the shock. About the time things settled down, the patient in room 110 coded. It was quite a night."

In this instance, the "I" message enhances communication by giving Donald the opportunity to address the real concern. In addition, if Laura is truly astute, she has a wonderful opportunity to support her colleague by voicing appreciation for the working circumstances of his shift. Most people respond gratefully to recognition and commiseration. The exchange could build collegiality between the two coworkers and perhaps between the two shifts.

Establishing Eye Contact

As mentioned, avoiding eye contact can be interpreted in a number of different ways. A person who does not make eye contact may be thought to be shy, scared, insecure, preoccupied, unprepared, dishonest—the list could go on and on. None of these qualities is likely to be appreciated in a primary caregiver. By making direct eye contact, the nurse gives undivided attention to the patient, and the patient is likely to feel valued and understood by the nurse. Eye contact in essence says, "I am wholly available to you. What you are saying is important to me."

Eye contact is equally important in communication with coworkers and other members of the interprofessional team. This quality is lost in telephone conversations or written communications.

Keep in mind, however, that the use of direct eye contact is a Western value. In some cultures avoidance of eye contact is considered more appropriate social behavior. By careful observation, the nurse quickly will recognize whether direct eye contact is interpreted as inappropriate or disrespectful. Nurses must make every effort to be sensitive to the cultural values of the client and their coworkers to enhance effective communication.

Keeping Promises

Little else can destroy the fragile trust developing in any interpersonal relationship as quickly as making and then breaking promises. Inherent in the concept of promise keeping are the qualities of honesty and integrity. Once a commitment is made, every effort must be expended to fulfill the expectation. Sometimes the request is impossible to satisfy. If this happens, the nurse must explain the situation or circumstances. The fact that the patient understands the nurse has made a sincere effort to meet his or her needs or desires often is more important than whether the goal is accomplished. If the nurse responds, "I'll check on that," and then finds the request impossible to fulfill, but never returns with an explanation, the lack of dependability perceived by the patient (or colleague) will surely drive a wedge into the relationship.

Expressing Empathy

Empathy is the ability to mentally place oneself in another person's situation to better understand the person and to share the emotions or feelings of the person. Empathy is not feeling sorry for another; it is understanding the experiences of the other person, and it is integral to the therapeutic relationship. The nurse is able to perceive and address the needs of the patient without emotional involvement to the point of becoming inappropriately immersed in the situation.

Using Open Communication

Certain styles of phrasing questions and statements lend themselves to obtaining more information. For example, suppose Chris asks Mr. Barrow, "Do you know where you are?" and Mr. Barrow responds, "Yes." Can Chris assume that Mr. Barrow knows he is in the hospital? Not necessarily. Chris may be surprised to hear a completely unexpected response if he rephrases the inquiry:

Chris: "Mr. Barrow, tell me where you are."
Mr. Barrow: "Why, I'm in the honeymoon berth of the *Titanic,* of course. Have you seen my lovely bride?"

Using open-ended questions or statements that require more information than "yes" or "no" can help gather enough facts to build a more complete picture of the circumstances. Questions or statements that are phrased to require only one- or two-word responses may miss the mark entirely.

Clarifying Information

Both communicants have a responsibility to clarify anything not understood. The sender should ask for feedback to be certain the receiver is correctly interpreting what is being said. The receiver should stop the sender anytime the message becomes unclear and should provide feedback regularly so that misinterpretation can be identified quickly. Such phrases as "What I hear you saying is…" or "I understand you to mean…" help communicate to the sender what is being perceived. Other techniques of clarification include using easily understood language, giving examples, drawing a picture, making a list, and finding ways to stimulate all the senses to enhance the ability to understand.

Being Aware of Body Language

Body positioning and movement send loud messages to others. The nurse can imply openness that facilitates effective communication by awareness of body position and movement. In addition to eye contact, effective communication is enriched through an open stance, such as holding one's arms at the side or out toward the patient, rather than crossed, or leaning toward the patient as if to hear more clearly, rather than away from the patient.

Using Touch

Most people have a fairly well-defined personal space. It is important for the nurse to be sensitive to each patient's personal preference and cultural differences in terms of touch. However, for many people, a gentle touch can scale mountains in terms of demonstrating genuine interest and concern. A pat on the back, a hand held, a touch on the shoulder—these are all behaviors that indicate availability and accessibility on the part of the nurse.

NEGATIVE COMMUNICATION TECHNIQUES

Several negative communication techniques have been alluded to in the previous discussion. Closed communication styles, such as asking "yes or no" questions or making inquiries or statements that require other single-word answers, potentially limit the response of the person and may prevent the discovery of pertinent facts. Closed body language can also hinder effective communication. Crossed arms, hands on the hips, avoidance of eye contact, turning away from the person, and moving away from the person impose a sense of distance in the relationship.

Three other techniques detrimental to good communication are blocking, false assurances, and conflicting messages.

Blocking

Blocking occurs when the nurse responds with noncommittal or generalized answers. For example:

> "Nurse, I've never had surgery before. I'm afraid I might not ever wake up." Mr. Clayton is twisting the bed sheet as he speaks.
> "Oh, Mr. Clayton, many people feel that way. It'll be okay." Makayla Butler, RN, smiles brightly, pats his hand, picks up the dirty linen bag, and bounces out of the room.

Does Mr. Clayton feel reassured? Not likely. Will he be inclined to broach the subject with Makayla again? Probably not. Makayla has incorporated some important aspects of positive communication into her response—cheerfulness and touch—but she has not truly communicated. She has effectively blocked Mr. Clayton's attempt to get the reassurance he wanted from her. He may be too intimidated to ask anyone else, assuming that his fear is invalid.

By generalizing in this way, Makayla has trivialized Mr. Clayton's concerns. He is not "many people." He needs to be validated as an individual experiencing a legitimate feeling. Makayla can validate his fear and put it into perspective at the same time with a different approach.

> *Makayla:* "What makes you think you might not wake up, Mr. Clayton?"
> *Mr. Clayton:* "Well, my wife's cousin's husband had surgery about 25 years ago, and he never woke up."
> *Makayla:* "What kind of surgery did he have?"
> *Mr. Clayton:* "Uh, it was some kind of heart surgery, and he had another heart attack on the table and died right there."
> *Makayla:* "It sounds like his condition was critical going into surgery."
> *Mr. Clayton:* "Yes, ma'am. He'd been sick for a long time."
> *Makayla:* "It's not uncommon to feel afraid of having anesthesia, especially if you have never had surgery before. There are rare cases in which complications do occur during surgery. That's why we put the disclosures on the consent form, so that you will know just what the risks are. Thankfully, though, most surgeries are without such drastic problems. Although your gallbladder certainly has made you uncomfortable, you are otherwise in good health. The tests that were done before surgery, like the chest radiograph and the laboratory work, show that you are healthy and should do well with the anesthesia. That drastically decreases the chance for complications in your case. I would be glad to answer any other questions you have or to ask the anesthetist to come and talk with you some more."

Makayla has validated Mr. Clayton's feeling as legitimate, provided an explanation with reasonable reassurances, and offered to explore the issue with him further or to have someone else talk with him.

False Assurances

False assurances are similar to blocking and have about the same effect. When someone is trying to get real answers or express serious concerns, answers such as "don't worry" or "it'll be okay" send several unintended messages. Such answers can be interpreted by the patient as placating or showing a lack of concern or a lack of knowledge. The patient might even conclude that the nurse is being neglectful through trivialization of an issue that is important to him or her. At the very least, the nurse has neither recognized the need the patient has expressed nor provided validation.

Conflicting Messages

Conflicting messages also have been alluded to in the previous discussion. If a person professes pleasure at seeing someone but draws back when that person extends a hand of greeting, the nonverbal message speaks more loudly than the words spoken. If a nurse enters a room and goes through the routine greeting by rote (even with a smiling face and a bouncing step), a patient can quickly perceive this and consider the nurse less approachable.

The nurse's statement that the patient's condition is important to the nurse followed by failing to answer the call bell in a timely manner or by forgetting to bring items promised to the patient sends a double message. Such behavior can leave the patient confused, frustrated, or angry. Carrying through with a commitment, no matter how unimportant it may seem, is a premier method of saying to the person, "You are important to me."

LOGICAL FALLACIES

Logical fallacies are related to an individual's culture, gender, background, and personal experiences and are barriers to meaningful communication. Individuals often cannot separate moods, thoughts, and perceptions because they become interconnected in one continuous evaluation process, involving feeling, thinking, and responding. In times of increased stress, as is common in health care settings, it is more likely that people will employ faulty thinking that affects the communication process. Recognition of distortions and faulty logic promotes effective communication and reduces confusion or even prevents conflict. Following are examples of frequently encountered logical fallacies.

Ad Hominem Abusive

Ad hominem abusive is an argument that attacks the person instead of the issue. The speaker hopes to discredit the other person by calling attention to some irrelevant fact about that person. Perhaps a nurse has just had a disagreement with a physician about lab results that were not properly reported. The nurse makes the following comment to colleagues: "She thinks she's so smart just because she's a doctor." What does that have to do with the disagreement? Nothing. It is an unwarranted attack on the doctor. Does it accomplish the purpose? Very likely, the group will be influenced by the disparaging comment. They may also become angry at the physician, who had legitimate cause to be upset about not receiving lab results. Ultimately, the issue of unreported lab values is lost in the personal attack against the physician.

Appeal to Common Practice

Appeal to common practice occurs when the argument is made that something is okay because most people do it. This logic is likely to be faulty in two ways: (1) Do "most" people really do it? (2) Does common practice really make an action okay? It's easy to imagine a situation in which using an explanation that you did something because you'd seen someone else do it that way, rather than checking the organization's policy and procedure manual, could lead to significant professional and legal problems.

Appeal to Emotion

Appeal to emotion is an attempt to manipulate other people's emotions in order to avoid the real issue. For example, consider Deb, RN, who has repeatedly failed to document patient care properly. She has been called into the nurse manager's office to discuss the incident and receives a written warning. She comes out tearful. It is obvious to her colleagues that she has been reprimanded. She begins to discuss the problem and makes the following statements: "I am the first person in my family to even go to college. I'm a single parent, and I've worked so hard to get where I am. Our manager doesn't care anything about that. She just wants to pass out written warnings to cover herself. She doesn't care about us as individuals." After a bit of this type of talk, the entire staff is probably becoming angry with the nurse manager—who may feel bad that she had to give the written warning because she does indeed care about her staff. However, Deb has successfully deflected the attention away from the real issue, failure to document properly, which was legitimately addressed.

Appeal to Tradition

Appeal to tradition is the argument that doing things a certain way is best because they've always been done that way. This argument is often expressed as "that's just how it's done here." Another version would be, "Oh, we tried that once and it didn't work so we went back to the old way." Change always brings some uncertainty, but choosing to continue a practice just because "that's the way we've always done it" is not very sound reasoning. Health care is a dynamic arena. The old ways of doing things seldom work out to be the best in this time of rapid change.

Confusing Cause and Effect

Confusing cause and effect occurs when one assumes that one event must cause another just because we often see the two events occur together. Jasmine and Chyane are nurses in labor and delivery. One night shift, two mothers delivered babies with significant birthmarks. It happened to be a night with a full moon. Jasmine states, "Wow! Babies born on a night during the full moon are more likely to have birthmarks." She makes an assumption that because the moon was full and two babies were born with birthmarks, some cause-and-effect relationship must exist.

Hasty Generalization

Hasty generalization involves coming to a conclusion based on a very small number of examples. A hasty generalization occurs when an assumption is made that a small group represents the whole population. Jordan and Paige are discussing the high number of pediatric patients on their unit who have respiratory syncytial virus (RSV). Paige notices that most of the babies with the disorder were born during the summer months. She remarks to Jordan, "Babies born in the summer months are much more likely to develop RSV." Making an assumption about all babies born everywhere based on a small number of babies in a single hospital is a hasty generalization.

Red Herring

Red herring is the introduction of an irrelevant topic in order to divert attention from the real issue. Two nurses, Brian and Nikoah, are having an argument regarding Brian's failure to complete his assigned tasks. Brian states, "It's not my work that you're really mad about. It's that I'm a guy. You just don't like male nurses." Nikoah then begins to defend herself, denying any prejudice against male nurses. The focus of the argument has been turned from the real issue, Brian's failure to complete his assigned tasks, to a situation in which Nikoah is on the defensive about her opinion of male nurses.

Slippery Slope

Slippery slope is the belief that one event will inevitably follow another without any real support for that belief. In fact, this type of logic often leads from a fairly harmless situation to an assumption akin to the notion that the sky is falling. Kathy and Janet are talking in the nurses' lounge over lunch. Kathy is upset over the recent announcement that the unit is going to convert to computerized bedside charting. Kathy makes the following statement: "It was bad enough having to chart all we do. Now, we have to learn to use computers and make all kinds of entries. We'll probably have just as much paperwork. We'll end up spending even less time with the patients. The next thing you know, nurses will be sitting at a computer terminal and someone else will be taking care of patients. Then, they'll decide they don't really need nurses at all!" Kathy's logic takes her from a simple unit change to the end of nursing as we know it! All too frequently we hear this kind of "escalating disaster" logic when change is introduced.

Straw Man

Straw man occurs when a person's position on a topic is misrepresented. April, a nurse manager, encourages everyone to be cost-conscious during a staff meeting. In a later discussion with other nurses, Sydney makes the following statement, "April is so worried about saving money that she wants us to avoid using supplies that are necessary for patient care." Sydney then begins to make a case against April and her leadership by implying April is not interested in quality patient care. Sydney creates a straw man by promoting the idea that April's plea for cost-conscious nursing care is really an attempt to support cost cutting at the expense of the patient. Sydney's tactics leave April in a bad light when compromising care was never her intent.

Understanding cognitive distortions and logical fallacies should help the nurse recognize the difference between legitimate and faulty reasoning. A clear understanding and use of sound logic will help health care providers resolve problems and stay focused on the true issues.

LISTENING

> "Nature has given men one tongue and two ears, in token that we should listen twice as much as we speak."
>
> —**Epictetus**

Listening certainly is as important an element in clear and effective communication as any other component. Many distracters contribute to poor listening habits. Framing an answer while the other person is still talking interferes with receiving the entire message. Environmental disturbances can provide major disruption. A crying baby, a call light buzzing, or multiple concurrent conversations in a busy nurses' station are a few of the interruptions that jumble the simplest of instructions. Preexisting concerns or worries can block absorption of conversation because of the preoccupation. Attempts to continue work in progress lead to inattention. Ineffective engagement or peculiar mannerisms on the part of the speaker can be distracting. A person who does not make eye contact, shuffles through papers while talking, or overuses hand movements actually can deter communication. Listening involves three purposeful steps: *Hearing* is listening enough to know what was said. *Understanding* is processing the information you heard. *Judging* is making a decision about what you heard. Does it make sense? Do you believe it? Can you respond appropriately to it (Pearson Education, 2005)?

A number of techniques can be used by the receiver to facilitate the ability to listen:

◆ Give undivided attention to the sender by moving to a more quiet area to avoid distractions and stopping the speaker to clarify any points not understood.

◆ Provide feedback in terms of perceived meaning of the message rephrased in the receiver's own words.

◆ Give attention to positioning to face the sender and make eye contact.

◆ Note nonverbal messages, such as body language and respond to them.

◆ Finish listening before you begin to speak.

If you have accomplished each of these steps, you have engaged in active listening. Active listening dramatically improves the likelihood of receiving the correct message. Equally important, active listening implies a respect for the speaker and communicates a regard for what the speaker has to offer. The nonverbal message that active listening delivers is, "I value you, and what you have to say is important to me."

WRITTEN COMMUNICATION

The professional nurse must interface with many forms of written communication on a daily basis. Nursing documentation includes a variety of reports, such as the nurse's notes in patient charts, memos, e-mails, Kardexes, incident reports, discharge teaching forms, and written shift reports, to name a few. Many of the forms that nurses use for documentation are part of the legal record and require careful consideration. Unclear instructions or reports either written or read by the nurse can lead to misunderstandings, errors, and the potential for litigation. Most profoundly, misinformation can lead to patient harm or injury. Therefore, special attention must be paid to communicating effectively in writing.

Accuracy

Absolute accuracy is paramount in recording legal documentation. For a nurse this most specifically applies to the nursing notes or any other entry in the patient's chart. Every effort should be made to report concisely, descriptively, and truthfully. To write "Patient walked today" is not adequate. A more concise and descriptive entry reads, "Patient walked to the nurses' station and back three times this shift, a total distance of 96 yards." Many hospitals have distance measures marked in the hallway for this purpose.

Consider the following example. Cody Johnson, RN, entered a patient's room and found her agitated and speaking loudly into the phone as she twisted her hair with her free hand. She was crying and periodically pounded the bedside table with her fist. Later the patient told Cody that she had been talking with her mother. Would it be appropriate for Cody to chart, "Patient became very angry with her mother while talking on the phone"? No. The nurse must be diligent not to include personal judgments or quantify the patient's emotional state in such terms.

More objectively, Cody could chart, "Patient found crying while talking on the phone in a loud tone to her mother. Patient was twisting her hair and hitting bedside table with her fist." The information is descriptive and states exactly what Cody observed factually without any judgmental conclusions. If, however, the patient had said, "My mother makes me so mad," Cody could have charted the statement as a direct quote (enclosed in quotation marks).

Attention to Detail

In addition to absolute accuracy, written documents should be descriptive. As mentioned, information should be quantified whenever possible. How many feet did the patient walk? How many times was the patient out of bed? How many mL of fluid did the patient drink? Precisely what did the patient say?

Words can be used to depict a verbal picture of a wound, rash, bruise, or any type of injury or situation. Illustrative terms can create a mental image for the person reading the notes, memo, or other communication. Descriptive categories can include measurement, color, position, location, drainage, or condition when speaking of a physical condition; or time, setting, people present, issues or goals discussed; or direct quotes when speaking of a meeting, conference, evaluation, or other interchange. Consider the differences between the following written communications:

- ◆ "1000: Dressing change completed. Site healthy."
- ◆ "1000: Dressing change completed. Edges of 4-inch surgical wound approximated, no drainage noted. Skin pink without any redness or edema."

The second entry allows the reader to "see" the wound mentally and follow the progress of healing even when unable to be present at the time of the dressing change. A good rule when describing any kind of break in skin integrity—whether from a stabbing, a surgical wound, an intravenous line, and so on—is to describe color, drainage, and presence or absence of edema.

Consider the e-mail written in Box 18-1. What does this message really tell the nurse manager? Not much—only that there is some kind of perceived problem between Lucas and the students. The nurse manager does not know based on the information provided if the problem is "real," if it is based on Jessica's bias or a student bias, if the problem has occurred more than once, if an interpersonal communication problem or misunderstanding exists, or if obvious mistreatment of a student or students has occurred.

Now consider the e-mail written in Box 18-2. Carefully constructing a factual e-mail of this length is more time consuming initially, but it will save a lot of frustration in the long run. The nurse manager now has a clear picture of what has occurred and knows that an ongoing problem exists. Most appropriately Jessica will speak to Bonnie about the problem, even if only briefly, when she is on the unit. However, a written account of the incident must be submitted and should be composed promptly while the facts are freshly remembered. Additionally, written communication often is the first source of contact because the nurse manager is not likely to be immediately available on all shifts.

The skill of writing concisely yet descriptively must be developed. Over time, nurses build a repertoire of phrases and illustrative terminology that are useful and effective. Often when a nurse is stumped as to how to express a situation, she or he will ask a colleague, "How would you write…?" Accessing the experience and expertise of nursing peers is productive problem solving and demonstrates respect for the colleague.

Thoroughness

The e-mail example in the previous section also illustrates the need for thoroughness. In addition to being descriptive in terms of the incident, Jessica's e-mail in Box 18-2 reported her interview with other nursing students. By doing so, Jessica is thorough in describing and

BOX **18-1**

Incomplete E-Mail Message

E-MAIL MESSAGE DATED 08/18/2010
To: Bonnie Thompson, RN, BSN, Nurse Manager
From: Jessica Lindsay, RN, BSN, Charge Nurse
Subject: Lucas Alfred, RN
   I have had lots of complaints about Lucas Alfred's treatment of students. I do not think he should be assigned as a preceptor anymore and do not plan to do so from now on.

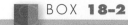

BOX **18-2**

Descriptive, Thorough E-Mail Message

E-MAIL MESSAGE DATED 08/18/2010
To: Bonnie Thompson, RN, BSN, Nurse Manager
From: Jessica Lindsay, RN, BSN, Charge Nurse
Subject: Student precepting
   Today (Monday, August 18) at 0710 I observed what appeared to be an animated conversation between Lucas Alfred, RN, and John Roberts, a student nurse from North Hills University. As I moved toward them, I heard Lucas say loudly, "Well, you better stay with me because I am not going to come looking for you all day. I know how lazy students are." I asked Lucas, "Is there a problem?" He replied, "Oh, no problem. I just hate having students, that's all. They're more trouble than they're worth." I asked Lucas, "Would you prefer that I reassign the student?" He shrugged his shoulders and walked away. I suggested to the student that I assign him to another nurse for the day. He responded, "I'd really appreciate that. Mr. Alfred has let me know since I arrived that he didn't want to work with me."
   Because this group of students has been on the unit 2 days a week for the past 3 weeks, I spoke to other students who had worked with Lucas and asked them how things had gone. The other three students who have worked with him reported similar experiences.
   I would like to arrange a time to meet with you and Lucas to address this problem.

reporting the extent of the problem she has discovered. Providing such completeness of information helps to prevent communication breakdown. Anticipating and answering relevant questions before they are asked exemplifies thoroughness and clarifies communication.

Conciseness

Written communication must be concise. The message must state the necessary information as clearly and as briefly as possible. Consider the e-mail written in Box 18-3. Whew! Extraneous details tend to confuse more than clarify. An inherent dilemma often develops as the nurse attempts to determine how to be descriptive and concise at the same time. One must determine what facts are pertinent to enable the reader to understand the true message. When in doubt and when appropriate, the writer can ask another party to read the message and provide feedback as to what the reader believes the message means. However, the right to confidentiality and privacy of the people involved must be observed. This basic principle applies to patients, families, students, members of the health care team—to everyone. Consequently the nurse must be as judicious in handling written material in a confidential matter as with any other form of communication.

Electronic Communication

More and more communication is computer based using e-mail, text messages, chat rooms, attachments, and other electronic modes. The computer-based written record can be somewhat more transient than other written documents. For example, e-mails are often read and then deleted. However, remember that communication via the computer can be saved and is often retrievable even after deletion. As with any form of written communication, computer-based interaction loses nonverbal cues. Therefore, it is important for the sender to elicit feedback and/or for the receiver to ask for clarification if the meaning of the communication is not clear. Box 18-4 offers guidelines for using e-mail as an effective, time-saving communication tool.

BOX **18-3**

Unclear, Rambling E-mail Message

E-MAIL MESSAGE DATED 08/18/2010
To: Bonnie Thompson, RN, BSN, Nurse Manager
From: Jessica Lindsay, RN, BSN, Charge Nurse
Subject: Student precepting

Today at about 0730 (it may have been earlier because I don't remember whether the breakfast trays had been served or not), I observed what appeared to be an animated conversation between Lucas Alfred, RN, and John Roberts, a student nurse from North Hills University. I thought they might be arguing, but I couldn't tell for sure, so I decided to go over and see what the conversation was about. It really seemed like Lucas was angry because he was talking loudly and not smiling and neither was the student smiling and I heard Lucas say, "Well, you better stay with me because I am not going to come looking for you all day. I know how lazy students are." Well, I could just imagine how that made the student feel, so I asked, "Is there a problem?" even though it was pretty obvious that something was wrong. Lucas said, "Oh, no problem. I just hate having students, that's all. They're more trouble than they're worth." I asked Lucas, "Would you prefer that I reassign the student?" He shrugged his shoulders and walked away. Well I don't know for sure about the student, but I really thought that was rude. I suggested to the student that I assign him to another nurse for the day. He responded, "I'd really appreciate that. He has let me know since I arrived that he didn't want to work with me." Well I know how that would make me feel—to be a student and be treated that way.

The same group of students has been on the unit 2 days a week for the past 3 weeks (maybe a month, I'm not sure, and some of them may have been here on makeup days too), so I talked to other students who had worked with Lucas and asked them how things had been going. They said he'd acted the same way to them. We need to talk to him.

COMMUNICATION STYLES

Communication is influenced by a myriad of individual characteristics learned over a lifetime. However, communication specialists generally recognize four basic communication styles: (1) assertive, (2) aggressive, (3) passive, and (4) passive-aggressive (Rose, 2007).

Assertive Communication

The healthiest form of communication is the assertive style. Assertive individuals choose and make decisions for themselves with sensitivity toward the needs and rights of others. Assertive communicators are honest and direct while valuing and respecting other individuals' views and seeking a win-win solution without the use of manipulation or game-playing. Assertiveness includes active listening and reflective feedback so that other individuals recognize that their opinions are valued as the assertive communicator seeks to find an acceptable solution without compromising his or her own needs.

Assertive communication requires self-confidence and the ability to set limits rather than succumbing to pressure to avoid disappointing or hurting others at the expense of one's own needs and expectations. While it is the most effective style of communication, healthy assertiveness is difficult for many people to develop. Therefore, assertive communication is the style most people use least (Angelfire, 2009).

Aggressive Communication

Aggressive communicators make decisions for themselves and others with the intent of always coming out the winner. Aggressive individuals want their needs met exclusively and immediately, using guilt, hurt, anger and a repertoire of other manipulation tools. Aggressiveness

BOX **18-4**

Tips on Using E-mail Effectively

- The subject line should be meaningful, clear and get the receiver's attention. For example: "draft delegation policy attached."
- Remember, e-mail is meant to be quick; an important point or question may be lost in a long message.
- When sending an e-mail with specific questions to be answered, write the questions on one line so they clearly stand out to the reader; questions risk getting lost if placed among long lines of text.
- Use the "reply to all" option only when necessary.
- Do not overuse the high-priority option.
- If a timely response is important, pick up the phone and call the person or leave a voice message (for example: "Jane, this is Tom, I just sent you an important e-mail. I hope you can read it and respond by early afternoon. Thank you.").
- When replying to a message, include enough of the original message to provide a context.
- Do not write in capitals. This may be interpreted as shouting.
- Use common courtesies, such as "please" and "thank you."
- Use the e-mail auto reply function if you are unable to respond to messages for 24 to 48 hours.

- Use proper grammar, spelling, and punctuation; most e-mail programs can be set up to spell check before sending the message. However, do not depend exclusively on spell check or grammar check. Homonyms, such as "sew" and "so" or "their," "there," and "they're," can be troublesome. Nothing takes the place of a good proofreading of your work.
- Attach files only when necessary—do not overwhelm the receiver with many files that may not be needed.
- When first establishing relationships with coworkers, colleagues, or friends, verify if e-mail is a good way to communicate. Many people may not use or check e-mail regularly.
- Do not copy or forward a message or attachment without permission.
- Do not use e-mail to discuss confidential information.
- Do not send personal or sensitive information by e-mail; remember there is no such thing as a "secure" mail system; e-mail can be forwarded without your knowledge, and delicate or embarrassing messages may fall into the wrong hands.
- Always provide your name and contact information at the bottom of each message.
- Review the message and be certain it is appropriate before clicking "send."

may include honesty but in a hurtful, manipulative way. Aggressive individuals commonly feel superior to others and behave in very controlling ways. Persons with whom they communicate often feel humiliated, defensive, resentful and hurt. Aggressive behavior often leads to and certainly escalates conflict.

Passive Communication

Passive communicators are the polar opposite of aggressive communicators. They allow others to make decisions for them in the hope of avoiding confrontation or difficult situations. Passive communicators are typically inhibited, indirect, and self-denying because they feel that is the safer route. If they win in a situation, it is purely by chance, typically because they happen to share the opinion of the more aggressive person in the exchange. Passive individuals are dishonest because they would rather succumb than state their true feelings or needs.

Passive-Aggressive Communication

Passive-aggressive communicators combine the worst of both styles. These individuals avoid direct confrontation while manipulating others in order to achieve their personal goals. They appear to be honest but "come in the back door" by undermining other individuals through gossip, pouting, playing the victim, and other manipulative behaviors that create or escalate conflict. They win in situations by making other individuals look bad.

SPECIAL INFLUENCES ON COMMUNICATION

Development of truly effective communication necessitates understanding various circumstances that influence communication. In addition to the concepts discussed up to this point, characteristics exist that might impede efficacious exchange of information. Issues such as gender differences, generational differences, cultural diversity, and dissimilarities in the professional approach of the various health care disciplines contribute to disparate understandings and interpretations.

Communication and Gender Differences

A significant clarification must be made regarding communication between men and women. Gender differences resulting from socialization, although based on research and many years of observations and writings, are generalizations and should be viewed from that perspective. Attributes described do not necessarily apply to all persons or all of the time. Nevertheless, a plethora of observations indicates that men and women solve problems, make decisions, and communicate from different perspectives based on socialization that begins shortly after birth (Cummings, 1995; Elgin, 1993; Heim, 1995). Typically, boys are taught to be tough and competitive; girls are taught to be nice and avoid conflict. Pat Heim (1995) suggests, "Playing team sports boys learn to compete, be aggressive, play to win, strategize, take risks, mask emotions, and focus on the goal line." Regarding girls' play, Heim comments, "Relationships are central in girls' culture and therefore they learn to negotiate differences, seek win-win solutions, and focus on what is fair for all instead of winning."

Clearly, learning to approach life on such different terms—with different rules—can lead to frustration, sometimes a sense of total defeat in the communication arena. For the most part, women work toward compromise even when it means relinquishing some of the original goal. Preserving relationships is usually of paramount importance to women. The role of peacemaker and nurturer has been a traditional expectation of women throughout the ages.

Generally men work toward winning. Traditional role expectations of men have included provider and protector. Men learn early in life how to focus on goals and move aggressively toward accomplishment. Team sports teach men that relationships are not destroyed in the "battle" (Heim, 1995). Consequently, men have been socialized to behave assertively when such performance is needed in pursuit of the goal and then move on without loss of friendships. Women have been socialized that assertive behavior will endanger relationships and that conflict should be avoided to preserve friendships.

Men typically use communication as a tool to deliver information, whereas women value the process of communication itself as an important part of the relationship. Therefore in an effort to improve communication, men might try spending more time in discussion, and women might try to phrase comments more succinctly. Consider the following conversation:

> *Nurse:* "Dr. Vernon, this is Holly Michaels, RN. I'm calling to talk to you about Mrs. Guevara. She says she's having more pain and feels a little dizzy. I've given her pain medicine as soon as I can each time. She says she's a little nauseated. Her husband's in the room, and he says she feels worse too. She did not sleep much last night and has not been able to nap today."
> *Physician:* "I have patients to see. Just give me the facts."
> *Nurse:* "Okay, she has received her medication every 4 to 5 hours this shift. I do not know if she needs a higher dose or just needs the medication more frequently, or maybe we should try a different medicine."

Physician: "What are her vitals? Does she have any drug allergies?"
Nurse: "Just a second, and I'll get the chart."
Physician: "Confound it, when you get your act together, call me back."
Dr. Vernon slams down the phone.

Consider the many communication styles and concepts illustrated by the previous conversation. Preparedness, conciseness, contributing environmental conditions (patients waiting), and even courtesy are issues that could be more competently addressed. The fact that the conversation is by telephone compounds the problem with lack of eye contact and lost potential for additional information through other body language. Telephone conversations are a fact of life in health care. Careful planning and preparation of what will be said facilitate effective information exchange. In the professional setting especially, men are more prone to favor brief, concise information exchange. In the professional setting, women still tend to prefer verbal problem solving as the situation is discussed. Knowledge of the gender differences in communication style could have altered the nurse's telephone call in the following manner:

"Dr. Vernon, this is Holly Michaels, RN, from Fairmont General calling about Mrs. Guevara in room 496. She has been receiving her pain medication exactly every 4 hours and continues to complain of incisional pain. She is complaining of slight dizziness and nausea, although she has had no emesis. Her blood pressure is 135/86; pulse 112; and respirations 24, which are higher than they have been running. Her temperature is 98.8° F. She has no drug allergies. How would you like to change her orders?"

Holly has prepared the information the physician will need and communicates it in an orderly fashion.

Communication and Generational Differences

An awareness of generational differences can help facilitate communication and prevent conflict (Lancaster and Stillman, 2002; Williams and Nussbaum, 2001). Traditionalists, for whom the Great Depression and World War II were critical events, place a high premium on formality and the top-down chain of command. These individuals are more likely to write a memo to relay their thoughts or opinions and can become offended by a direct, immediate approach. Respect from others is preferred including the use of formal titles as opposed to first names and scheduling a meeting rather than dropping in unannounced. Putting things in historical perspective is important because traditionalists are comfortable making decisions based on what worked favorably in the past.

"Baby-boomers" experienced the reshaping of corporate culture. As a group, boomers are considered to be highly competitive people who are willing to sacrifice their own interests and needs to achieve success. Boomers strive for recognition and desire a personable style of communication that builds rapport. Like traditionalists, they desire a top-down organizational approach that places value on earning respect.

On the other hand, "generation-Xers" are associated with a high divorce rate among their parents, working mothers, and the latchkey phenomenon. Their parents sacrificed for the corporation and their career and then were laid off during the 1980s recession. gen-Xers are characterized as skeptics who value a balance in their work and personal life. Most of these individuals would choose to be rewarded with extra time off as opposed to a promotion. They value efficiency and may agree to working extra hours if the reason is deemed beneficial. Expectations are immediate and instantaneous, and the chosen communication pattern includes brevity and directness.

"Millennials" are the newest members of the workforce. They are highly collaborative, optimistic, and strive for a balance between work and home life. It is important that they have a voice in organizational decision making and prefer communication that is framed in a positive manner.

As health professionals from different generations struggle to work collaboratively under stressful conditions, being aware of their various differences can certainly help improve communication and the work environment.

Communication and Cultural Diversity

Although Chapter 10 is devoted to cultural and social issues, it is important to highlight cultural issues specific to communication. Sensitivity to cultural differences is an integral part of a nurse's responsibility. Many cultural beliefs are tightly interwoven with strong religious convictions. Societies throughout the world depend as strongly or even more strongly on a variety of alternative healing sources as on medical science. Some people rarely have an opportunity to interface with medical science as it is known in developed countries.

The obvious difficulty is a potential language barrier. Even if the person speaks English as a second language, the preponderance of slang terms and colloquialisms can confound a literal translation. Additionally the stress associated with illness and possibly hospitalization only adds to the potential for misunderstanding and frustration. Fortunately, most communities have interpreters willing to translate in the health care setting. The variety of language interpreters (including sign language for the deaf) available even in smaller communities is surprising.

Many forms of communication do not carry the same meanings in various cultures. In some instances, direct eye contact is to be avoided if possible. Touch, also considered a positive communication technique in Western culture, may be perceived as a serious invasion of privacy. Some gestures considered innocuous in one culture may represent vulgarity in another. Some cultures strictly adhere to paternalism; unless the male head of the family agrees to a procedure or treatment, the family member will refuse under any circumstance. Although many people share a sense of modesty, some cultures experience a greater feeling of violation at having to expose certain body parts than do others. The consumption of certain foods, the use of blood or blood products—the possibilities of culturally diverse practices are endless. The prudent nurse must become knowledgeable of the specific cultural practices in the region of her or his employment.

Interprofessional Team Communication

The interprofessional team is composed of a variety of disciplines approaching health care from the unique perspective of the theories and therapies of their individual professions. Consider the variety represented by nurses, physicians, dietitians, respiratory therapists, pharmacists, occupational therapists, physical therapists, psychologists, and social workers. Then add to the mosaic the sublevel of specialists: cardiologists, endocrinologists, oncologists, orthopedists, clinical nurse specialists, recreational therapists, nurse anesthetists, nurse practitioners, and nurse scientists. RNs with varied educational backgrounds (diploma, associate degree, bachelor or master of science in nursing) and licensed vocational nurses are often found in the same unit with similar assignments. Now add managers, administrators, unlicensed assistive personnel, clerical staff, accountants, and housekeeping, to name a few. Also consider cultural and generational differences among health care professionals and workers. Is it any wonder that communication disasters occur?

All of the positive communication techniques have to be used to clearly understand another's perception. Listening is an essential tool for determination of the intended message as seen from the unique perspective of the other discipline. Frequent clarification and a sense of "safety" are paramount as people explore the meanings that each person attributes to the situation and the discipline-specific suggested solutions. Realization that the fundamental goal of all health care professionals and of ancillary staff is to provide quality patient care should facilitate positive communication.

Confidentiality and Privacy

No discussion of communication is complete without reference to issues of confidentiality and privacy. Breach of confidentiality and the patient's right to privacy through careless gossip has ethical and legal ramifications. Thoughtless conversation in the elevator, the cafeteria, the parking lot, or any other public place has created heartache for the patient and the health care provider alike.

Other sites where communication about confidential or personal patient issues needs to be controlled include the nurses' station, any desks or tables along the halls, and the utility rooms. Such locations are not often viewed as "public" places, but many people pass by these areas and overhear information. Exchange of patient information should occur only between persons with the need and right to know and should take place in private areas.

DIFFICULT CONVERSATIONS

Difficult conversations involve tough issues and, often, high emotions. These discussions can be crucial to the well-being of the patients, their families and significant others, and health care providers. Nurses quite often find themselves in situations that require profound sensitivity and the ability to manage their own emotions while addressing a range of circumstances from delicate to volatile. The proverb "to be forewarned is to be forearmed" is particularly applicable.

Part of being forewarned involves self-examination. How does the nurse feel about death and dying? Has he or she worked through personal issues associated with such a loss? If not, being an empathic listener and meeting the patient's need for information will be very difficult. What has the nurse's personal experience been with conflict management? If conflict cannot be handled successfully in his or her personal life, conflict in the workplace could be disabling. Nurses must therefore do some personal work on values clarification and preparation through self-evaluation and self-actualization before they can communicate truly effectively in the health care environment. This can be accomplished informally through discussions with significant others and colleagues, and formally in coursework.

When faced with a difficult encounter, people often do one of three things: avoid it, face it but handle it poorly, or face it and handle it well (Patterson et al, 2002). For nurses these encounters frequently happen in a high-stress environment with less than optimal timing. All of the positive and negative communication techniques discussed in this chapter come into sharper focus during these challenging conversations.

Responding to Death and Dying

Some things are difficult to talk about with another person. The dying patient may want to talk about how he or she feels, ask questions, or perform a life review. A nurse who is uncomfortable with such topics may consciously or unconsciously block communication through generalizations, closed answers, false assurances, advice giving and a host of other negative responses. Negative communication can be particularly destructive to the patient or family members at such a vulnerable time. Additionally, nurses may be afraid of causing psychologic harm because they are not well prepared to have such a discussion. Until the nurse is able to provide the open communication the patient needs, he or she must promptly defer to other personnel who are more comfortable in the situation.

When engaged in a conversation about a poor prognosis or impending death with the patient or significant others, the nurse must be able to maintain the discussion with the use of every positive communication technique in his or her communication arsenal. The nurse particularly needs to use active listening. Patients and families may hesitate to ask questions because they are afraid of acknowledging their lack of knowledge or because they don't want to be interpreted as a "difficult" patient (Kuebler, Heidrich, and Esper, 2007). The nurse should encourage questions and avoid the tendency to interrupt. Most people have trouble with prolonged silences and have an innate need to fill quiet moments. However, it is important to allow the patient or significant others time to process information and formulate their next question or comment. The emotional stress of the situation is quite likely to interfere with the patient and significant others' ability to understand and even to remember all the information they receive initially. The nurse should provide the opportunity for multiple discussions and planned redundancy and expect to repeat and reinforce information over time.

Talking openly with patients who are working through life's final journey can be profoundly successful using honesty, respect, openness, sensitivity, appropriate reflection, and active listening. The nurse may well be the single most important health care provider in terms of bridging the gap for the patient and reducing a sense of isolation as well as supporting his or her grief. Patients and their families usually have previous experiences with death and dying that they now have to apply to a new and very personal situation. These experiences affect their expectations and ability to process their circumstances. Remember that the patient or significant others don't necessarily want an answer or solution; they just need to talk through their situation with someone who is knowledgeable and sensitive.

Understanding and Managing Conflict

A major goal of communication is to establish understanding and cooperation with others. However, much of our social environment is characterized by interactions that involve conflict, misunderstanding, and a failure to communicate. When more than one person is involved in an interaction, a potential exists for disagreement and misunderstanding. When the interaction becomes stressful, taking on a competitive, hostile, or oppositional nature, it can be classified as conflict (Mayer, 2000).

Conflict is a disagreement through which individuals perceive a threat to the needs, interest, or concerns of themselves or others. As soon as small children are able to express their opinion, they are taught to be good and get along with others. Learning to manage one's own needs and desires without infringing on the rights of others is a fundamental goal of socialization. In the process, the notion of conflict is usually associated with negative behaviors and events.

However, conflicts stemming from differences in goals or desires are not good or bad. The two fundamental bases for conflict are information (one person has information that another does not have, or two individuals have different sets of information) and perception (people see things differently based on their unique belief systems). Despite the discomfort, disparate points of view can result in constructive behavior and positive outcomes.

Conflict, like stress, can have beneficial and detrimental consequences to an individual. Some of the benefits include (Mayer, 2000) (1) recognizing talents and innovative abilities; (2) identifying an outlet for expression of aggressive urges; (3) introducing innovation and change;

(4) diagnosing problems or areas of concern; and (5) establishing unity. Harmful consequences of prolonged conflict can include a negative effect on emotional and physical well-being, an emphasis on personal welfare over that of the group, a diversion of time and energy from important goals, financial and emotional costs, and personal fatigue.

Most of us experience abundant opportunities for conflict, which may be related to the fact that we bring to our relationships an accumulation of attitudes, beliefs, opinions, and habits. Thus conflict is normal and is not necessarily something to avoid. Although uncomfortable, conflict signals the presence of diverse points of view, which can spark creativity, nourish growth, and strengthen relationships. Maintaining an environment supportive of professional, clear, and sensitive communication enables individuals to fight more productively, with less hurt, and with a greater chance of resolving differences and disagreements.

People avoid dealing with conflict similarly to their general communication style. Some styles of conflict resolution are healthy, some are not:

- **Avoidance:** A passive response that tends to cause greater problems as issues remain unresolved over time.
- **Accommodation:** Another passive response in which the individual gives in to others rather than acknowledging his or her own needs and expectations. This approach often escalates conflict over time as well.
- **Competition:** Either an aggressive or a passive-aggressive response depending on the type and style of manipulation used by the individual. Again, this will likely lead to further or prolonged conflict.
- **Compromise:** An assertive response in which individuals participate in mutual give and take.
- **Collaboration:** Another assertive response in which individuals work together to accomplish goals successfully.

Self-awareness of one's usual conflict resolution style goes far in helping understand how one's own behavior contributes to disagreements. Having analyzed one's style of conflict management, the individual can identify behavior tools to improve his or her response to difficult situations.

Remember, don't make it—or take it—personal. Use "I" rather than "you" messages to avoid defensive responses. Keep the focus on the issue, not personalities. Do not create an environment in which other individuals respond defensively in order to protect themselves. Do not respond to conflictive situations as a personal attack—even if it feels like one. Focus and refocus on the issue or behavior rather than the individual.

It is imperative to recognize the importance of perception in conflict management. Regardless of one's intent, the most critical aspect of successful resolution is how an individual is perceived by others involved in the conflict event. Once again, every positive communication technique must come into play. Of these, active listening is critical. If other individuals perceive that they are being heard—rather than silenced—they will feel valued and respected regardless of the eventual outcome. Some excellent active listening techniques and examples are provided in Table 18-1.

The principle that underscores successful conflict resolution is that all people involved must view their conflict as a problem to be solved mutually so that each has a sense of winning or discovering options that are acceptable to all. Although this is an easy principle to understand, it can be challenging to put into practice. If both people can remain open, honest, and respectful of the each other's position, feelings of resentment may be minimized. Box 18-5 presents some basic strategies that can augment a professional response to conflict. The principles listed are

TABLE **18-1**

Active Listening Techniques

TECHNIQUE	WHY DONE	HOW DONE	EXAMPLE
Paraphrase the content of the message	Shows that you are listening, checking meaning, and interpreting the content	Restate basic ideas and facts in your own words	"What I hear you saying is that you weren't consulted" or "So you weren't consulted about this?"
Reflect the emotion of the message	Shows understanding of how the person feels; reflects what is observed rather than what is heard; helps the other person evaluate his or her own feelings after hearing them expressed by someone else	Listen to voice tone and watch for nonverbal cues that indicate feelings; listen to what the person tells you he or she is feeling; restate how you perceive the feeling	"So you are angry about what happened?"
Open questioning	To get more information and avoid any assumptions abut what the other person is thinking; encourages the other person to talk	Ask questions that begin with what, how, when, and where; use questions that begin with "why" cautiously	"What happened after you spoke with her?"
Acknowledging	To convey that you appreciate the other person's perspective; acknowledges his or her worth and actions	Acknowledge the value of the person's issues and feelings; shows appreciation for his or her efforts and actions	"That must be very frustrating."
Summarizing	To review progress; pull together important ideas and information; establish a foundation for further discussion	Restate the central ideas and feelings you heard	"So what is most important to you is…"
Framing	To communicate your message in a way that the other person will be more open to hearing; to increase the opportunity of meeting his or her goals	Present your message in a hopeful, nonjudgmental, and open-ended way; point to common ground and away from differences	"I think it would be best to speak to your supervisor directly about these issues because she is more directly involved with implementation than I am. What do you think about this idea?"

Used with permission from The Neutral Zone, Vancouver, BC, Canada. http://www.theneutralzone.ca/index.html, 2008.

remarkably effective and will help the nurse present herself or himself as a confident and competent professional who will not react to inappropriate behavior in like form, but also will not withdraw from the issues. As always the focus should be kept on the delivery of quality patient care. Box 18-6 lists additional resources for conflict management and resolution.

In conclusion, situations arise when no positive communication skill appears to work. No one is obliged to endure personal attack, humiliation, uncontrolled anger, or other hurtful behaviors. A person who operates on that level expects an opponent to respond in like manner, thereby creating an environment in which escalation is "justified." One simply does not have to

BOX **18-5**

Professional Response to Verbal Conflict

1. Maintain an open and empathic tone of voice.
2. Maintain eye contact (keeping cultural differences in mind). This may be difficult, but it conveys to the other party that you are confident and competent.
3. Maintain an open body stance with your hands at your side or open toward the person (but not invading the other person's space). Do not cross your arms, tap your toe, wag your finger, or perform any body language that is commonly associated with anger.
4. Do not physically back away unless you perceive you actually are in physical danger. By standing your ground, your carriage will convey the message of assurance.
5. Be aware of your own values, beliefs, and cultural perspectives.
6. When a conversation is obviously escalating, move to a more private location.
7. Listen actively and carefully without criticizing or being defensive.
8. Focus on the problem or issue, not the person(s) involved.
9. Use "I" messages that state your thoughts, feelings, and beliefs in an open and clear manner.
10. Use nonjudgmental, noninflammatory language, such as "It seems to me...."
11. Establish ground rules to maintain a safe environment for dialogue, such as "only one person speaks at a time; the other listens."
12. Offer explanations, but do not make excuses.
13. Be redundant, summarize, and convey the same idea in more than one way.
14. Try to understand the intended meaning of what other people are saying.
15. Identify ideas that clarify your own issues, concerns, and are helpful to identify solutions.
16. Avoid unhelpful responses to conflict, such as arguing, sarcasm, moralizing, disbelief, contradiction, criticism, ridicule, and threats.
17. Use metaphors and analogies as gentle ways to create and maintain rapport.
18. Maintain a positive context by stating what you want and avoid stating what you do not want.
19. Repeat, or play back, what you believe you are hearing.
20. If you say you will take care of something, report something, or change something, do it. Then seek out the person to whom you made the commitment and report your action and the result. Little else will go as far as demonstrating that you are dependable and want to work toward a solution.
21. In more difficult situations, consider using a neutral facilitator who understands his or her role.

BOX **18-6**

Helpful Websites and Online Resources

Basics of Conflict Management
   http://managementhelp.org/intrpsnl/basics.htm
Conflict Resolution Skills
   www.helpguide.org/mental/eq8_conflict_resolution.htm
List of Conflict Resolution Organizations
   www.pbs.org/ralphbunche/education/teach_conflict.html
Resolving Conflict Rationally and Effectively
   www.mindtools.com/pages/article/newLDR_81.htm
Success Tips
   www.mlmsuccesstips.com/4types.html

MORE INFORMATION ABOUT LOGICAL FALLACIES
www.nizkor.org/features/fallacies.

TEST YOUR COMMUNICATION STYLE:
http://trainingpd.suite101.com/article.cfm/communication_styles

"take the bait." Ask the aggressor to moderate voice level, language, and nonverbal behaviors. Present a sense of confidence through open styles such as unwavering eye contact, open body position, moderated voice tone, and not shrinking back. Responding to such a person with increasing voice level, similar language, and personal attack simply feeds the inappropriate behavior. If no positive communication techniques work, advise the aggressor in a professional manner that the conversation can be continued in the presence of a third party or when the emotionally charged atmosphere can be dispelled. More often than not, such a professional response engenders increased respect from the aggressor as well as others in the immediate environment.

SUMMARY

In today's health care environment, where high stress levels are all too common and patient safety, quality care, and financial constraints are everyday concerns, nurses play a vital role in promoting a productive work environment in which trust and rapport among the health care team members are common and all are working toward the same goal—delivery of safe, timely, efficient, effective, and patient-centered health care. Professional, clear, and sensitive communication provides the foundation for creating such supportive, effective health care environments. The first step toward developing a professional communication style is understanding the many complex and varied factors that influence the communication process, such as gender, cultural, generational, and interprofessional differences, each of which present many challenges for the nurse who must strive to understand and to be understood. The second step is adopting positive communication techniques that include developing trust, using "I" messages, establishing eye contact, keeping promises, feeling empathy, using an open communication style, clarifying information, and being aware of body language. The third step is for each nurse to reflect on his or her use of negative communication techniques, such as blocking, false assurances, conflicting messages, logical fallacies, and cognitive distortions, that may interfere with effective relationships with patients and coworkers. Recognizing—then avoiding—the use of these negative communication techniques is essential if a nurse is to move toward a more professional communication style. The next step in developing a professional communication style is learning to address and resolve conflict in a positive way. Role-playing with trusted colleagues using the conflict resolution techniques discussed in this chapter can help the nurse become more adept at managing conflict. Finally the nurse's professional communication style can be further developed and enhanced through ongoing study, using the various Internet resources suggested in this chapter. Demonstrating a professional, clear, and sensitive communication style is essential to the professional nursing skill set. As the foundation for effective, supportive work environments and excellent patient care, professional communication must be one goal every nurse strives to achieve.

evolve   Additional resources are available online at: http://evolve.elsevier.com/Cherry/

REFERENCES

American Association of Critical-Care Nurses: *Standards for establishing and sustaining healthy work environments.* 2005. Available at: www.aacn.org/WD/HWE/Docs/HWEStandards.pdf.

Angelfire: *Styles of communication.* 2009. Available at: www.angelfire.com/az2/webenglish/commstyles.html.

Cummings SH: Attila the Hun versus Attila the hen: gender socialization of the American nurse, *Nurs Adm Q* 19(2):19–29, 1995.

Elgin SH: *Genderspeak: men, women, and the gentle art of verbal self-defense,* New York, 1993, John Wiley & Sons.

Gibb J: Defensive communication, *J Comm* 11:141–148, 1961.

Hargrave J: *Nonverbal communication.* 2009. Available at: www.janhargrave.com/index.html.

Heim P: Getting beyond "she said, he said", *Nurs Adm Q* 19(2):6–18, 1995.

The Joint Commission: *Accreditation program: hospital national patient safety goals.* 2009. Available at: www.jointcommission.org/NR/rdonlyres/31666E86-E7F4-423E-9BE8-F05BD1CB0AA8/0/HAP_NPSG.pdf.

Kuebler KK, Heidrich DE, Esper P: *Palliative end-of-life care: clinical practical guidelines,* St Louis, 2007, Saunders.

Lancaster LL, Stillman D: *When generations collide,* Boston, 2002, Harvard Business.

Mayer B: *The dynamics of conflict resolution,* San Francisco, 2000, Jossey-Bass.

Patterson K, et al: *Crucial conversations: tools for talking when stakes are high,* New York, 2002, McGraw-Hill.

Pearson Education: *Infoplease: homework center-listening skills.* 2005. Available at: www.infoplease.com/homework/listeningskills1.html.

Rose J: *Communication styles.* 2007. Available at: http://trainingpd.suite101.com/article.cfm/communication_styles.

van Servellen G: *Communication skills for the healthcare professional: concepts and techniques,* Gaithersburg, MD, 1997, Aspen.

Williams A, Nussbaum JF: *Intergenerational communication across the lifespan,* Mahwah, NJ, 2001, Lawrence Erlbaum.

Effective Delegation and Supervision

Barbara Cherry, DNSc, MBA, RN, NEA-BC
Margaret Elizabeth Strong, MSN, RN, CNA, NEA-BC

@volve Additional resources are available online at: http://evolve.elsevier.com/Cherry/

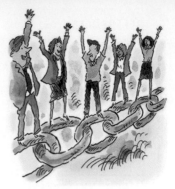

Delegation—linking together for better patient care.

VIGNETTE

Glenda Miller, BSN, RN, is the charge nurse on a medical-surgical floor of a hospital. She has just received report from the 7 PM to 7 AM shift and is about to make assignments for the 7 AM to 7 PM shift. The philosophy of the unit is that the registered nurse (RN) coordinates all patient care. Today on this 12-bed unit there are eight patients and 4 empty beds. The nursing staff consists of Ms. Miller, one RN, one licensed practical nurse, one nursing assistant, and one unit secretary. The following interprofessional team members are available for specific patient care needs: respiratory therapist, physical therapist, occupational therapist, speech therapist, medical social worker, nutritional support nurse, and chaplain. The patients are medically complex with extensive nursing care needs including psychosocial and emotional support. The patients are described to Ms. Miller as follows:

502: Mr. A. is ventilator dependent with an infection that requires IV antibiotics every 12 hours. He needs to be out of bed in a chair twice a day. He has a stage I sacral decubitus ulcer and a PEG tube with bolus feedings. He is very hard of hearing, tries to speak, and becomes very frustrated and uncooperative.

503: Mrs. B., age 77, is on day 2 of 40 days of antibiotics for osteomyelitis. She is dehydrated with a central line in her right subclavian and on TPN. She needs to be out of bed and ambulated in the room. She receives a respiratory treatment every 4 hours and needs assistance with AM care. Her daughter is at her bedside and very upset that her mother may need to go to a nursing home.

504: Mr. C., age 52, is to be discharged to a rehabilitation hospital today. Discharge records need to be prepared for the transfer. The family is at his bedside and extremely anxious.

507: Mr. D., age 64, has TPN infusing into a left subclavian catheter and is on multiple antibiotics. He has vancomycin-resistant Enterococcus in his urine and a stasis ulcer on his left leg that requires Pulsavac every day.

508: Mr. E., age 72, is a ventilator-dependent patient who will start weaning this AM. He is on continuous tube feedings and IV antibiotics and needs to be assessed for a PICC line. He is to begin ambulation in the hall twice a day per physician's orders. He also needs to have a pharyngeal speech evaluation scheduled.

509: Mrs. F., age 66, is 3 days after a CVA and unable to move her right extremities. She has an IV infusing via her left arm. Her blood pressure is 170/100. She needs total care with personal hygiene and feeding. The physician just ordered range of motion exercises every day. Her husband is at her bedside crying continually and asking, "What am I going to do now?"

510: Mr. G., age 52, has been off the ventilator for the past 24 hours and is doing very well. He continues on respiratory treatments every 4 hours. His TPN is being decreased, and his PEG feedings are increasing. He has glucose monitoring ordered every 4 hours, an indwelling urinary catheter to gravity drainage, and IV antibiotics every 12 hours. He needs to be out of bed, ambulating in the hall with assistance. If he stays off the ventilator, he will be discharged in 5 days. The family needs to find a nursing home for him; however, the family has not visited Mr. G. since his admission 18 days ago.

511: Mr. H., age 49, is a new admission that will be coming from ICU sometime during the shift.

In addition to the tasks mentioned, routine activities of taking vital signs, giving scheduled medications, updating care plans, and answering call lights must be assigned. When reviewing the tasks to be accomplished, Ms. Miller must consider several issues to make safe and effective assignment and delegation decisions.

■ QUESTIONS TO CONSIDER WHILE READING THIS CHAPTER:

1 Which of the above tasks must the RN perform as required by your state's nurse practice act?

2 Which of the above tasks can be delegated to the nursing assistant?

3 How can the training, skills, and competencies of the licensed practical nurse (LPN) or licensed vocational nurse (LVN) and nursing assistant be determined?

4 How can other members of the interprofessional health care team contribute most effectively to meet patients' needs?

KEY TERMS

Accountability In the context of delegation, accountability means bearing responsibility for both the action and inaction of the nurse and those to whom he or she delegates tasks (National Council of State Boards of Nursing [NCSBN], 2005).

Assignment The distribution of work that each staff member is responsible for during a given work period; when making assignments, the RN supervisor directs a staff member to do something that he or she is authorized to do and is within the staff member's scope of practice and/or job description (American Nurses Association [ANA] and NCSBN, 2006).

Competency The ability to clearly demonstrate the knowledge, skills, values, attitudes, abilities, and professional judgment required to practice safely and ethically in a designated role and setting (Nurses Board of South Australia, 2004).

Delegation Transferring to a competent staff member the authority and responsibility to perform a selected nursing task that the staff member would not normally be allowed to perform; the RN retains accountability for the delegated task (ANA and NCSBN, 2006).

Nursing assistive personnel (NAP) An unlicensed individual who is trained to function in an assistive role to the RN by performing patient care activities as delegated by the nurse (ANA, 2005).

Supervision The active process of directing, guiding, and influencing the outcome of an individual's performance of an activity or task (ANA, 2005).

LEARNING OUTCOMES

After studying this chapter, the reader will be able to:

1 Evaluate the effect of changes in the current health care system on nurse staffing patterns and responsibilities.

2 Outline six topic areas that the professional nurse should consider when making delegation decisions.

3 List nine essential requirements for safe and effective delegation.

4 Incorporate principles of delegation and supervision in professional nursing practice to ensure safe and legal patient care.

CHAPTER OVERVIEW

The delivery of patient care is the fundamental goal of every health care organization. To accomplish this goal cost-effectively, teams of diverse professionals and assistants are used to deliver care. Because the RN is most often responsible for coordinating care provided by the various team members, he or she must clearly understand and be able to effectively use the management processes of delegation and supervision to ensure high-quality safe patient care. This chapter highlights issues that influence staffing patterns and delegation and supervision processes. The chapter also discusses the RN's role and responsibility in delegating to and supervising staff members including nursing assistive personnel (NAP) and LPNs or LVNs and provides useful guidelines for establishing a safe and effective delegation and supervision practice.

DELEGATION AND SUPERVISION IN THE HEALTH CARE SYSTEM

Several factors influence staffing patterns and the provision of patient care in today's health care systems. First, reduced reimbursement from Medicare, Medicaid, and private insurance companies has led to cost-cutting measures. Second, the growing uninsured population is forcing health care organizations to provide care in the most cost-efficient manner possible. Third, the strong focus on safety and quality is requiring health care systems to make rapid changes for continual improvement. Fourth, advances in medical technology are causing a sharp increase in the cost of providing care. Finally, the nursing shortage combined with an increase in patient acuity and complex treatments contribute to health care environments struggling to address multiple complex priorities with dwindling resources. Using NAP, such as nursing assistants and patient care technicians, is one strategy to increase cost-effectiveness of providing patient care.

As the use of NAP increases, the RN is forced to delegate more tasks to a person who does not have clearly defined parameters for education, training, job responsibilities, and role limitations. Therefore, it is up to the RN to know the laws and regulations that govern nursing practice. It is also important that the RN work closely with nonclinical administrators and managers to make sure they understand the assessment and decision-making activities that must be performed by the RN according to state law.

There is a growing concern that the roles and responsibilities of care providers, including RNs, LPNs or LVNs, and NAP, are significantly overlapping. In some practice settings, LPNs or LVNs are functioning as managers and supervisors and are performing more complex and invasive procedures. In some states, NAP are trained to perform complex procedures, such as venipunctures and catheter insertions. This trend has prompted many nurses, nursing organizations, and state boards of nursing to reexamine the scope of nursing practice and the nurses' delegation and supervision responsibilities.

More recently the issue of health care errors and the RN's essential role in keeping patients safe has been brought to the nation's attention through the Institute of Medicine's (IOM) report *Keeping Patients Safe: Transforming the Work Environment of Nurses*. This report effectively highlights how nurses improve patient outcomes through the ongoing monitoring of patients' health status, coordinating care, educating patients and families, providing essential therapeutic care, and intercepting health care errors before they can adversely affect patients (IOM, 2004). RNs must learn to delegate nursing tasks safely and effectively so that they will be available to deliver these most important aspects of professional nursing care.

In support of the role of NAP in delivering patient care, the Joint Statement on Delegation (ANA and NCSBN, 2006) states, "There is a need and a place for competent, appropriately supervised, unlicensed assistive personnel in the delivery of affordable, quality health care" (p. 2). As the nursing shortage worsens and health care facilities continue to seek more cost-effective ways to provide care, RNs will remain in short supply. Thus it is imperative that nurses learn new ways of managing care and delegating tasks.

Because the use of NAP and LPNs or LVNs is a reality in today's health care system, RNs are becoming increasingly responsible for delegation and supervision. Therefore, it is imperative that RNs have confidence in their delegation skills and understand the legal responsibility that they assume when delegating to and supervising licensed personnel and NAP. RNs should know what aspects of nursing and health care can be delegated and what level of supervision is required to ensure that the patient receives safe, competent, and effective care.

WHAT IS DELEGATION?

Delegation is a legal and management concept that involves assessment, planning, intervention, and evaluation. Delegation as defined by the American Nurses Association (ANA, 2005) is "the transfer of responsibility for the performance of an activity from one individual to another while retaining accountability for the outcome" (p. 4). Although RNs can transfer the responsibility and authority for the performance of an activity, they remain accountable for the overall nursing care. The essential aspects of delegation are the nursing process, task identification and transfer, communication, supervision, and accountability for outcomes. When delegating tasks, the nurse should understand the delegatee's competencies, communicate succinctly, offer clear guidelines in advance, monitor progress, and remain accountable for the final outcomes of care.

Delegation is a two-way process in which the RN requests that a qualified staff member perform a specific task. When a task is delegated, the delegator shares with the delegatee the ultimate responsibility and authority for the accomplishment and outcome of the task. However, the RN delegator remains accountable for the patient outcomes. When delegating, the RN delegator is accountable for:

- The act of delegation
- Supervising the performance of the delegated task
- Assessment and follow-up evaluation
- Any intervention or corrective actions that may be required to ensure safe and effective care

The delegatee is accountable for:

- His or her own actions
- Accepting delegation within the parameters of his or her training and education
- Communicating the appropriate information to the delegator
- Completing the task

Delegation is a management strategy that when used appropriately can ensure the accomplishment of safe and effective health care.

WHAT SHOULD AND SHOULD NOT BE DELEGATED?

Unfortunately there is no easy answer as to what can and cannot be delegated. The answer varies, depending on the (1) nursing practice acts and other applicable state laws, (2) patient needs, (3) job descriptions and competencies of staff members, (4) policies and procedures of the health care organization, (5) clinical situation, and (6) professional standards of nursing practice. To establish a safe, effective delegation practice, the RN must seek guidance and integrate information regarding each of these areas as discussed in the following paragraphs (Figure 19-1).

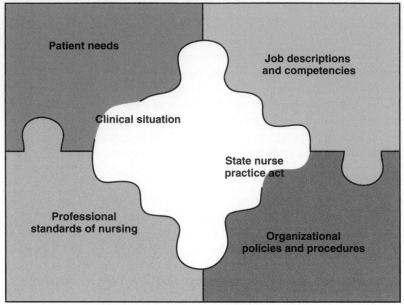

Figure 19-1 *Solving the delegation puzzle.*

State Nurse Practice Acts

Each state's nurse practice act provides the legal authority for nursing practice, including delegation. However, each state's nurse practice act expresses delegation criteria differently, and the criteria often are not clearly spelled out in the act, or they may be presented in various parts of the act. It is absolutely essential that every RN be familiar with his or her state nurse practice act and know the delegation criteria contained within the act. Johnson (1996) has identified 10 essential elements related to delegation criteria in nurse practice acts, as follows:

1. Definition of delegation
2. Items that cannot be delegated
3. Items that cannot be routinely delegated
4. Guidelines for the RN about what can be delegated
5. Description of professional nursing practice
6. Description of LPN or LVN and unlicensed nursing assistant roles
7. Degree of supervision required
8. Guidelines for decreasing the risks associated with delegation
9. Warnings about inappropriate delegation
10. Restricted use of the word nurse to licensed nurses only

Although not every state's nurse practice act contains all 10 elements, the RN can use this list to assist in understanding delegation criteria in his or her own nurse practice act and apply the information to enhance delegation activities. Box 19-1 presents policies common to many nurse practice acts.

If the nurse practice act does not provide clear direction regarding delegation, the state board of nursing may be able to offer guidance. The board of nursing may have developed definitions, rulings, advisory opinions, or interpretations of the law to provide guidance regarding delegation activities. Many state boards of nursing may also have practical tools available, such

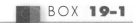

BOX **19-1**

Policies Common to Many State Nurse Practice Acts

- Only nursing tasks can be delegated, not nursing practice.
- The RN must perform the patient assessment to determine what can be delegated.
- The LPN or LVN and NAP do not practice professional nursing.
- The RN can delegate only what is within the scope of nursing practice.
- The LPN or LVN works under the direction and supervision of the RN.
- The RN delegates based on the knowledge and skill of the person selected to perform the tasks.
- The RN determines the competency of the person to whom he or she delegates.
- The RN cannot delegate an activity that requires the RN's professional skill and knowledge.
- The RN is accountable and responsible for the delegated task.
- The RN must evaluate patient outcomes resulting from the delegated activity.
- Health care facilities can develop specific delegation protocols, provided they meet the state board delegation guidelines.
- Delegation requires critical thinking by the RN.

From Johnson SH: Teaching nursing delegation: analyzing nurse practice acts, *J Contin Educ Nurs* 27(2):52-58, 1996.

as delegation decision trees or delegation checklists. Figure 19-2 is a delegation decision tree recommended by the NCSBN and provides an excellent framework for the four steps in the delegation process—assessment and planning, communication, surveillance and supervision, and evaluation and feedback.

Most states also have a practice act to govern practice by LPNs or LVNs. Because the practice of LPNs or LVNs varies significantly from state to state, RNs should know the LPN or LVN practice act in the state in which they practice and understand the LPN or LVN's legal scope of practice. State law generally does not define practice by NAP, although such practice should be governed by the health care organization's standards.

Patient Needs

When deciding to delegate, the RN must remember that tasks can be delegated, but nursing practice cannot. The functions of assessment, evaluation, and nursing judgment cannot be delegated. Generally the more stable the patient, the more likely delegation is to be safe. However, it also is important to remember that many tasks that can be delegated may also carry with them a nursing responsibility. Taking vital signs on a physiologically stable patient after a CVA could be delegated to NAP, but the task presents an opportunity for the RN to assess the patient's cognitive functioning. In the vignette presented at the opening of this chapter, Ms. Miller should not delegate any care for the newly admitted patient until the nursing assessment is complete and the plan of care is developed.

Job Descriptions and Competencies

The RN who is delegating has the responsibility of knowing the background, skill level, training received, and job requirements of each person to whom tasks are delegated. The job description provides important information about what a staff member is allowed to do and delineates the specific tasks, duties, and responsibilities required of the person as a condition of employment. Job descriptions generally comply with state laws and the health care organization's standards of care. However, in all cases, legal requirements related to delegation supersede any organizational requirement or policy.

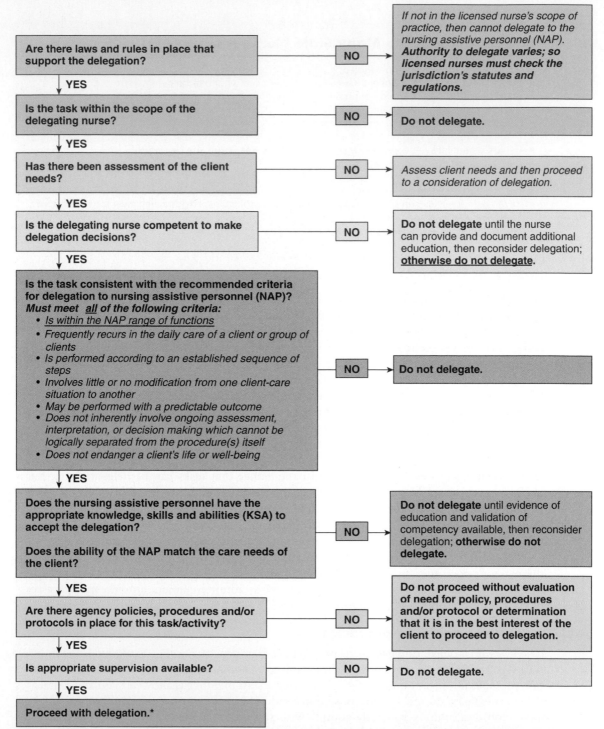

Figure 19-2 *Decision tree for delegating to nursing assistive personnel. (From the Joint Statement on Delegation, Appendix B, National Council of State Boards of Nursing. Used with permission from the American Nurses Association [ANA] and the National Council of State Boards of Nursing [NCSBN], 2006.)*

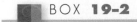

BOX **19-2**

Annual Competencies to be Demonstrated by RNs and LVNs in a Family Practice Ambulatory Care Clinic

- Safety rules and regulations
- HIPAA policies and procedures
- Patient safety goals
- Infection control
- Telephone triage
- Glucose testing

- Patient education and health literacy
- Medication management
- Reporting abuse and neglect
- Documentation in the medical record
- Handling emergencies in the outpatient setting

HIPAA, Health Insurance Portability and Accountability Act.

The RN should be aware of what type of education and training the person received to function as described in the job description and when possible, be involved in training programs. The RN should also know what kind of orientation is provided to new employees. In the opening vignette, the LPN's job description most likely would include duties, such as "perform dressing changes" and "administer oral medications," but Ms. Miller also should know the LPN's knowledge and skill level for the population of patients on the unit.

In addition to requiring job descriptions for care providers, health care organizations also require employees to demonstrate that they are competent to perform certain technical procedures and to apply specific knowledge to safely care for patients. Written documentation of those skills and knowledge for which the employee has demonstrated competency is maintained in the employee's personnel file. Most health care organizations require employees to undergo annual competency training for aspects of care unique to the population of patients generally being cared for in the nursing unit. Box 19-2 provides an example of annual competencies to be demonstrated by nurses in a family practice ambulatory care clinic. Various regulatory and accrediting agencies, such as The Joint Commission (TJC) require written documentation of staff competencies. It is important for the RN to be aware of the documented competencies for all staff members whom he or she supervises.

Organizational Policies and Procedures

When delegating, the RN should comply with the specific skill requirements designated in the organization's written policies and procedures, which usually describe the supervision required for a specific task and how problems or incidents should be reported and documented. Again it is important for the nurse to remember that the legal requirements related to delegation supercede any organizational requirement or policy. The RN should also know the organization's general standards of care, such as infection control, and ensure that the delegatee has the necessary knowledge and skills to comply with the standards. In the opening vignette, Ms. Miller should be aware of the hospital's policy regarding the orientation process. All clinical staff members should have received training about the unit's infection control, emergency, and safety procedures.

Clinical Situation

Each delegation opportunity presents the RN with a variety of considerations, including the delegatee's current workload and the complexity of the task in relationship to the patient. Does the staff member realistically have time to accomplish the task? Is the staff member familiar with characteristics of the patient population (i.e., pediatrics or geriatrics) and with the task to be performed? Is the RN able to provide the appropriate level of supervision? Other considerations include the availability of resources, such as supplies and equipment.

Professional Standards of Nursing Practice

Professional standards of nursing practice, as established by professional nursing organizations, exist to guide the RN in providing patient care. According to the ANA (2004), "Standards are authoritative statements by which the nursing profession describes the responsibilities for which its practitioners are accountable. Standards reflect the values and priorities of the profession and are based on research and knowledge from nursing and various other sciences and disciplines. Standards provide direction for professional nursing practice and a framework for the evaluation and improvement of practice" (p. 12). To practice safe delegation, the RN should be familiar with the standards of practice outlined in ANA's *Nursing: Scope and Standards of Practice* (2004) and with the standards for any specialty area in which the RN practices. (Refer to Appendix A on the Evolve website for a list of most of the specialty nursing organizations in the United States.)

As an accepted standard of care, the RN should use professional judgment to determine activities that are appropriate to delegate based on the concept of providing safe and effective patient care and protecting the public. In delegation the RN considers the following:

- Assessment of the patient condition
- Capabilities of the nursing and assistive staff
- Complexity of the task to be delegated
- Amount of clinical oversight (supervision) the RN will be able to provide
- Staff workload

The RN *cannot* delegate activities that include the core of the nursing process and require specialized knowledge, judgment, and/or skill (ANA, 2005) including:

- Initial nursing assessment and any subsequent assessment that requires professional nursing knowledge, judgment, and skill
- Determination of nursing diagnoses, establishment of nursing care goals, development of the nursing plan of care, and evaluation of the patient's progress with the nursing plan of care
- Any nursing intervention that requires professional knowledge, judgment, and skill

Box 19-3 presents a list of questions to assist the nurse in making delegation decisions.

DEVELOPING SAFE DELEGATION PRACTICES

For the RN to make safe, effective delegation decisions and develop a sound delegation practice, he or she must have a strong foundation of knowledge related to the legal criteria and standards of practice governing delegation decisions. In addition to having a good understanding of what should and should not be delegated based on the previous discussion, the RN also must know the patient, the staff members to whom he or she is delegating, and the tasks to be performed. The RN must provide for effective outcomes by clearly communicating expectations, supporting and appropriately supervising the delegatee, evaluating the outcomes, and reassessing the patient after the delegated task is completed. Following is a brief discussion about these essential requirements for safe and effective delegation.

Know the Patient

A nursing assessment must be completed before delegation—know the level of care required by the patient, considering the clinical, physiologic, emotional, cognitive, and spiritual status. Is the patient's condition considered stable? Generally the more stable the patient, the more

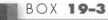

BOX **19-3**

Questions to Guide Delegation Decision Making

A. State nurse practice act
  1. Is the task within the RN's scope of practice?
  2. Does the nurse practice act address delegation of the task?
  3. Does the task to be delegated require the exercising of nursing judgment?
  4. Is the RN delegator willing to accept accountability for the performance of the delegated task?
B. Job description and competencies
  1. Does the RN delegator understand the nature of the task and have the knowledge, skills, and competency required to perform the task?
  2. Does the delegatee have the appropriate education, training, skills, and experience to perform the task?
  3. Is there documented or demonstrated evidence that the delegatee is competent to perform the task?
  4. Does the delegatee perform the task on a routine basis?
  5. Is the delegatee familiar with the patient population?
C. Organizational policies and procedures
  1. What skill level and level of supervision are required for the task as stated in the procedure manual?
  2. What is the policy or procedure for documenting tasks and reporting results, observations, problems, or unusual incidents?
  3. Does the delegatee have the necessary knowledge and skills to comply with general standards of care, such as infection control?
D. Clinical situation and task
  1. Is adequate supervision by the delegator available?
  2. Are adequate resources available, including supplies and equipment, to the delegatee?
  3. What is the delegatee's current workload? Does the person realistically have time to perform the task?
  4. How complex is the task? Does it frequently recur in the daily care of patients? Does it follow a standard and unchanging procedure?
E. Patient needs
  1. Has the nursing assessment and plan of care been completed by the RN?
  2. What is the patient's clinical, physiologic, emotional, cognitive, and spiritual status?
  3. Is the patient's condition considered stable?
  4. What is the potential for change in the patient's condition as a result of the delegated task?
  5. Can the patient's safety be maintained with delegated care?
F. Professional standards of nursing practice
  1. What specific standards of nursing practice apply to the specific situation?
  2. Does the delegated task include health counseling, teaching, or other activities that require specialized nursing knowledge, skill, or judgment?

likely delegation is to be safe. What is the potential for change in the patient's condition as a result of the delegated task? If there is moderate to high risk that the task will result in a change in the patient's condition, delegation should not be considered. Can the patient's safety be maintained with delegated care? The answer to this question must be a firm "yes" for delegation to be considered.

Know the Staff Member

Before the task is delegated, the delegatee must have the skills and knowledge necessary to perform the task, as evidenced by the person's job description, training program, and documented competencies. Experience and past job performance should also be considerations. Is the staff member knowledgeable and trained to perform the task? Does the staff member perform the task routinely? Select the right person for the right task. It is very helpful for the RN to be involved in development of job descriptions, training programs, and competency documentation for staff members.

Know the Task(s) to Be Delegated

The RN delegator must be competent and skilled in performing any task he or she is considering delegating, and the task must be in the RN's scope of practice. Routine, standardized tasks that are performed according to a standard and unchanging procedure and have predictable outcomes are the safest to delegate. These routine tasks are most likely to have been documented in the staff member's competencies and may require fewer directions and less supervision. Complex tasks or activities that pose a high risk for patient complications or unpredictable outcomes should be examined closely before delegation is considered.

Explain the Task and Expected Outcomes

The RN should explain the delegated task, what must be done, and the expected outcomes. If necessary outline the task in writing. Failure to effectively communicate what is expected may result in unsatisfactory performance, errors, and possible harm to the patient. Directions should be provided clearly and concisely. Demonstration and return demonstration by the delegatee or other in-service education may be required. The delegated task is acceptable only when the staff member understands the task and is adequately prepared to carry it out.

Expect Responsible Action from the Delegatee

When the staff member accepts and understands the task, he or she should then be allowed to perform the task. The staff member becomes responsible for his or her own actions and is obligated to complete the task as mutually agreed. The RN should provide appropriate supervision, but should not intervene in task performance unless assistance is requested or an unsafe situation is recognized. Interfering with the delegatee's task will negate his or her responsibility and obligation. The RN should expect responsible actions, give authority, and retain accountability.

Assess and Supervise Job Performance

Supervising job performance provides a mechanism for feedback and control. Job performance is assessed by making frequent rounds, observing, and communicating (ask about progress and determine whether there are any questions or concerns). Determine the appropriate level of supervision. The RN should be available to the delegatee if there are any questions or unexpected problems. Supervise in a positive and supportive manner to reassure the staff member that his or her work is important and appreciated. Intervene immediately if the task is not being performed in a safe and appropriate manner. Poor performance must be documented and reported to the nurse manager. Never ignore poor performance. When a mistake is made, use it as a learning opportunity for all staff involved.

Evaluate and Follow Up

Once the task is complete, evaluate the staff member's performance and reassess the patient to ensure that the expected outcomes were achieved. Follow up with any interventions that may be required based on the patient's care outcomes or the delegatee's job performance. Review

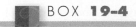

BOX **19-4**

From Deciding to Delegate to Actual Delegation: Steps to Remember

A. Communicate effectively
  1. The delegatee accepts the delegation and accountability for carrying out the task correctly.
  2. The RN delegator provides clear directions to the delegatee, including what specific task is to be performed, for whom the task is to be done, when the task is to be done, how the task is to be performed, what data are to be collected, and any patient-specific instructions.
  3. The RN delegator clearly communicates expected outcomes and timelines for reporting results.
B. Provide appropriate supervision
  1. Monitor performance to ensure compliance with established standards of practice and organizational policies and procedures.
  2. Obtain and provide feedback.
  3. Intervene if necessary.
  4. Ensure proper documentation.
C. Evaluate and reassess
  1. Reassess the patient.
  2. Evaluate the performance of the task and the delegatee's experience.
  3. Reassess and adjust the overall plan of care as needed.

and document the skills that were learned. Appropriate evaluation and follow-up will ensure a positive outcome for both patient and staff member. Box 19-4 presents some important steps to remember after the decision to delegate has been made.

Understand High-Risk Delegation

The RN often expresses concern about legal liability—"putting my license on the line"—when delegating to unlicensed staff members. How does the RN know whether he or she might be at risk when delegating? The RN may be at risk if the (ANA, 1996):

◆ Delegated task can be performed only by the RN according to law, organizational policies and procedures, or professional standards of nursing practice.

◆ Delegated task could involve risk or harm to a patient.

◆ RN knowingly delegates a task to a person who has not had the appropriate training or orientation.

◆ RN fails to adequately supervise the delegated activity and does not evaluate the delegated action by reassessing the patient.

One method to avoid high-risk delegation and simplify the delegation process is referred to as the five rights of delegation (ANA and NCSBN, 2006):

1. *The right task:* Delegated tasks must conform to the established guidelines.
2. *The right circumstances:* Delegate tasks that do not require independent nursing judgment.
3. *The right person:* Delegate to someone who is qualified and competent.
4. *The right direction and communication:* Give clear explanation about the task and expected outcomes and indicate when the delegatee should report back to the RN.
5. *The right supervision and evaluation:* Invite feedback to assess how the process is working and how to improve the process. Also evaluate the patient's outcomes and results of the tasks.

RNs can prevent being placed into unsafe, risky delegation situations by adhering to the safe delegation practices recommended in this chapter. See the following case study demonstrating excellence in delegation practice in a home health setting.

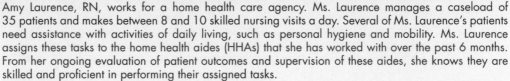

CASE STUDY: Excellence in Delegation Practice

Amy Laurence, RN, works for a home health care agency. Ms. Laurence manages a caseload of 35 patients and makes between 8 and 10 skilled nursing visits a day. Several of Ms. Laurence's patients need assistance with activities of daily living, such as personal hygiene and mobility. Ms. Laurence assigns these tasks to the home health aides (HHAs) that she has worked with over the past 6 months. From her ongoing evaluation of patient outcomes and supervision of these aides, she knows they are skilled and proficient in performing their assigned tasks.

Five of Ms. Laurence's patients are newly diagnosed with diabetes and need extensive assistance with monitoring blood glucose levels and administering insulin. The home health agency where Ms. Laurence works has recently adopted a diabetic delegation policy. This policy allows HHAs that have been specifically trained and certified to perform glucose testing and give insulin from prefilled, labeled syringes. Ms. Laurence actively participates in the training classes to certify HHAs in diabetic care.

In caring for her patients with diabetes, Ms. Laurence does extensive diabetic teaching with each of her patients and sees them weekly to assess their learning, monitor their physiologic status, evaluate and adjust their individualized plans of care, and provide ongoing education and support as needed. During the weekly visits Ms. Laurence fills and labels the exact number of insulin syringes with the correct doses of insulin to last the week. Ms. Laurence is then able to delegate the daily insulin administration and glucose monitoring to the HHAs certified in diabetic care. During the initial delegation process, Ms. Laurence makes supervisory visits to each patient's home to ensure that the HHA is performing the tasks correctly and has been carrying them out according to the patient's plan of care. To provide appropriate supervision of these delegated tasks, Ms. Laurence plans her weekly skilled nursing visits to coincide with the HHA's daily visit. During these visits, Ms. Laurence observes each HHA perform the glucose testing and insulin administration and reinforces any specific training needed. Following these supervisory visits, Ms. Laurence is confident that the HHAs are competent to perform the delegated tasks.

In this case Ms. Laurence is following all of the criteria essential for safe delegation in her state. She is adhering to the agency's policy, which also is in line with the state board of nursing rules for delegation in a home setting. She has actively participated in the training programs for the HHAs and provided clear direction during the initial delegation process. Ms. Laurence provides ongoing patient assessment, care evaluation, and supervision of the HHAs. In performing appropriate delegation, Ms. Laurence is able to focus her energy on skilled nursing services, such as providing patient education, assessing and monitoring patients' physiologic condition, and coordinating the care for the interprofessional home health team.

SUPERVISION

Supervision is defined by the ANA (2005) as "the active process of directing, guiding and influencing the outcome of an individual's performance of a task" (p. 4). Supervision may be categorized as on-site, in which the nurse is physically present or immediately available while the activity is being performed or off-site, in which the nurse has the ability to provide direction through various means of written, verbal, and electronic communication (ANA, 2005). On-site supervision generally occurs in the acute care or ambulatory care settings where the RN is immediately available. Off-site supervision may occur in home health practice, community settings, and long-term care facilities.

Hansten and Jackson (2004) have identified levels of supervision based on the task delegated and the education, experience, competency, and working relationship of the people involved:

◆ **Unsupervised:** One RN is working with another RN in a collegial relationship, and neither RN is in the position of supervising the other. Each RN is responsible and accountable for his or her own practice. However, the RN in a supervisory or management position (e.g., team leader, charge nurse, nurse manager), as defined by the health care organization, will be in a position to supervise other RNs.

◆ **Initial direction and/or periodic inspection:** The RN supervises a licensed or unlicensed caregiver, knows the person's training and competencies, and has developed a working relationship with the staff member. For example, the RN has been working with the nursing assistant for 6 months and is comfortable in giving initial directions for a delegated task and following up with the assistant once during the shift.

◆ **Continuous supervision:** The RN has determined that the delegatee will need frequent to continual support and assistance. This level of supervision is required when the working relationship is new, the task is complex, or the delegatee is inexperienced or has not demonstrated an acceptable level of competence.

It is absolutely essential that the RN understands and provides the appropriate level of supervision whenever tasks are delegated. Box 19-5 provides a list of online resources for more information about delegation and supervision.

ASSIGNING VERSUS DELEGATING

Assigning tasks is not the same as delegating tasks. Assignment, as defined by ANA, is "the distribution of work that each staff member is responsible for during a given work period" (2005, p. 4). An assignment designates those activities that a staff member is responsible for performing as a condition of employment and is consistent with the staff member's job position and description, legal scope of practice, and training and educational background. The staff member assumes responsibility and is accountable for completing the assignment.

Assignment Considerations

Assigning groups of patients to various care providers, including NAP and LPNs or LVNs, is not appropriate. For example, NAP cannot be assigned to a patient or group of patients, but rather should be assigned to an RN. Typical assignments for NAP include passing trays, assisting patients with activities of daily living, transporting patients, stocking supplies, and completing delegated tasks for the RN. The LPN or LVN may be assigned specific patients for whom to perform care, but the RN remains responsible for all nursing practice activities, including patient assessment, care planning, and patient teaching.

BOX **19-5**

Helpful Websites

American Nurses Association
 www.nursingworld.org
National Council of State Boards of Nursing
 www.ncsbn.org
Position Paper *Working with Others: A Position Paper. www.ncsbn.org/Working_with_*
 Others.pdf
Individual states' board of nurse examiners
 Many states provide online access to their nurse practice act.

The RN is also responsible for assignments made to personnel in the clinical setting. Several factors should be considered when making assignments.

◆ **Patient's physiologic status and complexity of care:** Are vital signs unstable? Is the patient's condition changing rapidly? Does the patient have multisystem involvement? Does the patient need extensive health education? Does the patient need extensive emotional support? What technology is involved in the care (e.g., cardiac monitor, intravenous pump, patient-controlled analgesia pump)? Patients with more unstable physiologic status or complex care requirements need a higher level of skilled care.

◆ **Infection control:** To what extent are isolation procedures required? Which patients could be adversely affected as a result of cross-contamination? For example, a new patient is admitted with a history of night sweats and chronic cough. The results of a sputum culture are pending. Another patient on the unit was admitted with complications resulting from chemotherapy. The same caregiver should not be assigned to a potentially infectious patient and an immunosuppressed patient.

◆ **Degree of supervision:** What level of supervision, direct or indirect, is required based on staff members' education, experience, skill level, and competence? Is the appropriate supervision available? The on-call RN who works an occasional weekend may require more supervision than the LPN who has worked in the unit full time and has demonstrated competence in caring for the patient population on the unit.

Note that the most experienced skilled staff members should not be exclusively assigned to the most complex, difficult cases. Assignments should be used as a staff development tool. Assigning a less experienced nurse to a more complex patient, but at the same time increasing the level of supervision, increases that nurse's skill level, competence, and confidence while maintaining safe, effective patient care.

Working with Interprofessional Health Care Team Members

Other health professionals who are members of the interprofessional health care team, including respiratory therapists, physical therapists, occupational therapists, speech therapists, nutritionists, medical social workers, and chaplains, are very valuable in helping meet patient care needs. In the vignette, Ms. Miller will need to coordinate the efforts of each of the interprofessional team members available to her unit to accomplish the many and varied tasks needed by the patients for whom she is responsible and accountable.

The RN must be knowledgeable about the scope of practice and training background of the interprofessional team members to ensure the very best patient care. The RN also needs to understand how the work is delegated or assigned to the team members and where they fit in the unit's organizational structure. In some organizations some or all of the interprofessional team members report to the RN, and it is the RN who is responsible for assigning and delegating patient care tasks to the team members. In other organizations the interprofessional team members report to supervisors in their individual disciplines and work collaboratively with the RN to provide patient care based on their individual legal scope of practice, knowledge, and experience.

The RN is generally responsible for coordinating the efforts of the interprofessional team. In the opening vignette, the interprofessional team members do not report directly to Ms. Miller, but to a supervisor in their respective disciplines. However, each team member is available and willing to work collaboratively with Ms. Miller to meet the needs of the patients on the unit. For example, the respiratory therapist monitors all patients on ventilators and assists in the weaning process. The medical social worker provides valuable assistance to identify family support and assists with nursing home placement for Mr. G. The speech therapist can work on communication techniques with Mr. A, the ventilator-dependent patient who becomes very frustrated when he tries to speak.

BUILDING DELEGATION AND SUPERVISION SKILLS

Effective delegation is an underlying quality for the success of working with others efficiently and being able to provide safe, cost-effective care to patients. Delegating can be very difficult, especially for the novice nurse. Some of the struggles the nurse has are the fear of being disliked, losing control, taking risks, making mistakes, lack of confidence, and lack of knowledge of the delegation process itself. Because delegation and supervision involve interactions between two people, the RN needs to develop strong interpersonal skills and a supportive work environment to guarantee an effective delegation situation. Following are management skills RNs need to develop to become proficient at delegation and supervision.

Communicate Effectively

Clear communication is the key to successful delegation. The first step toward effective communication is for the RN to know exactly what needs to be done and what outcomes are expected. What is the specific task to be done? For whom is the task to be done? When is the task to be done? How is the task to be performed? What is the expected outcome? What feedback is expected? Why does the task need to be done in a certain way?

Maintaining self-control and confidence is an important communication skill. New RNs often have expressed concern about delegating to more seasoned LPNs or LVNs or NAP. "I have been working here for 12 years, and I do not need you telling me what to do" might be a typical response directed to the new RN. The RN's correct response is to maintain composure and confidence and remain positive. "I appreciate your experience and knowledge, and I need you to ... [describe the task clearly]."

It also is important to listen carefully to the delegatee's response. Did the delegatee appear to listen and understand the directions? Did he or she appear to be hesitant to accept the task? Angry? Uninterested? Frustrated? If a delegation action elicits a negative response from the delegatee, ask for feedback using open-ended, nonthreatening statements, such as, "You seem unsure about performing this task." Always provide an opportunity for the delegatee to ask questions. The positive communication techniques discussed in Chapter 18 provide additional guidelines for the reader to enhance delegation skills.

Create an Environment of Trust and Cooperation

Staff members will report problems more quickly if they know that the reaction from the supervisor will be nonthreatening and nonjudgmental. When mistakes occur, the person should not be blamed or criticized, but rather the supervisor should look for root causes and system issues, such as inadequate training or an overly heavy workload. Encouraging staff members to report and discuss problems is an excellent method of improving patient care and maintaining a helpful, supportive attitude. Just as the RN establishes trust and rapport with patients, he or she should strive for the same type of supportive relationships with staff members.

Provide Feedback and Follow-Up Evaluation

The delegation process is not complete until the RN reassesses the patient and adjusts the plan of care as indicated. The RN also should provide honest feedback to the delegatee about his or her performance. An easy, although often overlooked, delegation skill is to praise good performance. Often more difficult for the RN, and sometimes ignored, is the duty to address poor job performance.

The RN should tell the staff member about mistakes in a supportive manner—in private—with a focus on "learning from mistakes." However, if the staff member performs in an inappropriate, unsafe, or incompetent manner, the RN must intervene immediately and stop the unsafe activity, document the facts of the performance, and report to the nurse manager or supervisor. In addition, the RN should request additional training or other appropriate action for the staff member to ensure that patient safety is protected. The RN has a professional responsibility to intervene appropriately when poor performance is observed.

SUMMARY

Effective delegation and supervision are essential skills for the professional nurse in any practice role or setting, especially with the increased use of NAP to provide health care services. Although there is no definitive list of what can and cannot be delegated, the RN is guided to safe, effective delegation and supervision through an assessment of (1) the clinical situation; (2) patient needs; (3) the job descriptions and competencies of the assistive and vocational or practical nursing personnel; (4) the health care organization's policies and procedures; (5) nurse practice acts and other regulations and applicable state laws; and (6) professional standards of nursing practice. This chapter presents information to assist the RN with delegation decisions and also discusses effective delegation and supervision skills, including communicating effectively, creating an environment of trust and cooperation, and providing feedback and follow-up evaluation. These activities and skills provide the tools the RN needs to provide safe and legal delegation in practice.

 evolve   Additional resources are available online at: http://evolve.elsevier.com/Cherry/

REFERENCES

American Nurses Association: *Nursing: scope and standards of practice*, Washington, DC, 2004, ANA.

American Nurses Association: *Principles for delegation*, Silver Spring, Md, 2005, ANA.

American Nurses Association and National Council of State Boards of Nursing: *Joint statement on delegation*. 2006. Available at: www.ncsbn.org/Joint_statement.pdf.

American Nurses Association: *Registered professional nurses and unlicensed assistive personnel*, ed 2, Washington, DC, 1996, ANA.

Hansten RI, Jackson M: *Clinical delegation skills: a handbook for professional practice*, ed 3, Sudbury, MA, 2004, Jones and Bartlett Publishers.

Institute of Medicine (IOM): *Keeping patients safe: transforming the work environment of nurses*, Washington, DC, 2004, National Academies Press.

Johnson SH: Teaching nursing delegation: analyzing nurse practice acts, *J Contin Educ Nurs* 27(2):52–58, 1996.

Nurses Board of South Australia: *Standards: delegation by a registered nurse or midwife to an unregulated healthcare worker*, 2004, Unpublished manuscript.

National Council of State Boards of Nursing (NCSBN): *Working with others: a position paper*. 2005. Available at: www.ncsbn.org/Working_with_Others.pdf.

Staffing and Nursing Care Delivery Models

Barbara Cherry, DNSc, MBA, RN, NEA-BC

 evolve Additional resources are available online at: http://evolve.elsevier.com/Cherry/

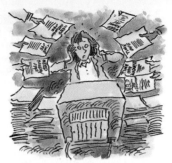

Staffing and assigning work are two of the nurse manager's most important and challenging roles.

VIGNETTE

As a student nurse, John Knox noticed during rotations through the different clinical areas that the registered nurses (RNs) had various types of responsibilities and duties. On the medical-surgical units, RNs supervised a group of licensed practical nurses (LPNs) and nursing assistants who provided direct patient care, and the RNs performed patient assessments, care planning, and education. In the critical care unit, RNs provided all the care required by the patient with little help from any other caregivers. In the obstetric unit, two RNs worked as a team to provide care to laboring mothers. In the outpatient health clinic, each RN was assigned to perform specific tasks; one nurse was assigned to do all diabetic teaching, and another was assigned to triage all telephone calls from patients. Some of the clinical areas used a mostly RN staff, whereas other clinical units had a variety of staff, from RNs to nursing assistants. John had many questions about why care delivery was very different in the different clinical sites.

■ QUESTIONS TO CONSIDER WHILE READING THIS CHAPTER:

1 Why is the RN's work assignment different in different units—obstetrics, critical care, medical-surgical, and the outpatient clinic?

2 Who decides how many nurses and other personnel are needed to staff a clinical site?

3 How do nurse managers on nursing units decide how assignments will be made?

4 Who has responsibility and authority for making patient care assignments?

KEY TERMS

Clinical pathway Clinical management plans that specify the optimal timing and sequencing of major patient care activities and interventions by the interprofessional team for a particular diagnosis, procedure, or health condition and are designed to standardize care delivery (Coffey et al, 2005); clinical pathways may also be called critical paths, practice protocols, or care maps; clinical pathways support the implementation of clinical practice guidelines.

Clinical practice guidelines Recommendations for appropriate treatment and care for specific clinical circumstances; guidelines are developed though a systematic process to integrate the best evidence for treating specific medical conditions and assist health care providers to make decisions about appropriate treatment (Institute of Medicine [IOM], 1990).

KEY TERMS—cont'd

Multiskilled worker Unlicensed caregiver trained to perform multiple tasks, such as phlebotomy, vital signs, housekeeping, and assisting patients with hygiene and ambulation.

Nursing assistive personnel (NAP) Unlicensed individuals who are trained to function in an assistive role to the RN by performing patient care activities as delegated by the nurse (American Nurses Association [ANA], 2005).

Nursing care delivery model Also called care delivery system or patient care delivery model; details the way work assignments, responsibility, and authority are structured to accomplish patient care; depicts which health care worker is going to perform what tasks, who is responsible, and who has the authority to make decisions.

Patient acuity Indication of the amount and complexity of care required for any particular patient; high acuity indicates a need for more intense, complex nursing care as compared with lower acuity, which indicates a need for moderate, less complex nursing care.

Patient classification system Method used to group or categorize patients according to specific criteria and care requirements and thus help quantify the amount and level of nursing care needed.

Staff mix Combination of categories of workers employed to provide patient care (e.g., RNs, LPNs, or licensed vocational nurses [LVNs], nursing assistants, multiskilled workers, or nursing assistive personnel [NAP]).

Staffing Ensuring that an adequate number and mix of health care team members (e.g., RNs, LPNs or LVNs, NAP, clerical support) are available to provide safe, quality patient care; usually a primary responsibility of the nurse manager.

LEARNING OUTCOMES

After studying this chapter, the reader will be able to:

1 Outline key issues surrounding staffing for a health care organization.

2 Evaluate lines of responsibility and accountability associated with various types of nursing care delivery models.

3 Analyze the advantages and disadvantages of nursing care delivery models in relation to patient care in various settings.

4 Integrate essential components of the critical pathway model into patient care planning.

5 Differentiate among several nursing care delivery models by evaluating their defining characteristics.

6 Explain the purpose and components of nursing case management.

7 Summarize criteria to be considered in developing future models of nursing care delivery.

CHAPTER OVERVIEW

Of all the nurse manager's varied and complex roles, staffing and assigning work is probably the most challenging and certainly the most important to the delivery of safe, quality patient care. Staffing ensures that an appropriate number and level of staff members are available to provide care; assigning is the method used to divide work tasks among the various staff members. This chapter presents a brief introduction to staffing and its surrounding issues, such as acuity levels and staff satisfaction. A description follows of various nursing care delivery models, which details how work assignments are structured. Also discussed are telehealth and case management as nursing care delivery models, in addition to the use of clinical pathways and clinical practice guidelines. The chapter attempts to answer the following questions related to staffing and nursing care delivery models:

- ◆ *How does staffing affect patient care, staff satisfaction, and the organization's financial status?*
- ◆ *What staff mix (e.g., combination of RNs, LVNs or LPNs, NAP, multiskilled workers, technicians) is required to provide quality patient care?*
- ◆ *Who is responsible for making work assignments?*
- ◆ *What factors should be considered when making patient care and other work assignments?*
- ◆ *Is the work assigned by task or by patient?*
- ◆ *How is communication about patient issues managed?*
- ◆ *What factors are considered when choosing a nursing care delivery model?*
- ◆ *What is case management, and how is it used to provide patient care?*

STAFFING

Staffing can be defined as the activities required to ensure that an adequate number and mix of health care team members (e.g., RNs, LVNs or LPNs, NAP, clerical support) are available to meet patient needs and provide safe, quality care. Important research is validating the contribution and value of RNs to improving patient outcomes, reducing complications and length of hospital stay, and preventing premature mortality (Aiken et al, 2002, 2003; Dall et al, 2009; Kane et al, 2007; Needleman et al, 2002). The Institute of Medicine's report titled *Keeping Patients Safe: Transforming the Work Environment of Nurses* (2004) is an extensive analysis of nurses' work environments and staffing issues; this report strongly affirms nurses' essential roles in achieving quality patient care and safety. In order for nurses to have the greatest opportunity to achieve safe, quality care, staffing systems must address patient acuity levels, provide nurses time to exercise professional judgment, and acknowledge that patient needs can change from moment to moment (ANA, 2009a). While appreciating the overall value of the RN in providing patient care, several specific considerations regarding staffing are reviewed related to (1) patient needs, (2) staff satisfaction, and (3) organizational needs.

Staffing and Patient Needs

The primary considerations for staffing a specific nursing unit are the number of patients; the level of intensity of care required by those patients (commonly referred to as patient acuity); contextual issues, such as architecture, geography of the environment, and available technology; and the level of preparation and experience of the staff members providing the care (ANA, 2009b). Knowing only the number of patients that require care is an ineffective way to plan staffing because of the wide range of care requirements needed by individual patients. To account for the diverse care needs and quantify the intensity of care required by a group of patients, nurse managers responsible for staffing use various patient classification systems.

Patient Classification Systems. Patient classification systems group or categorize patients according to specific criteria and care needs and thus help quantify the amount and level of care needed. This may be referred to as the acuity level. The higher the acuity level, the more intense the patient's nursing care needs. For example, patients may be grouped in such categories as "uncomplicated postpartum" or "ventilator dependent." As the reader can easily visualize, these two groups of patients require very different levels and amounts of care and therefore are categorized at different acuity levels. Imagine the many different kinds of patients treated by a health care facility and you can begin to picture the complexity of patient classification systems.

Because of this complexity and the differences in patient populations across different health care facilities, patient classification systems vary from organization to organization. However, the ANA (2009b) has recommended that the following physical and psychosocial factors be considered when determining the intensity of care required for any group of patients:

- Age and functional ability
- Communication skills
- Cultural and linguistic diversities
- Severity and urgency of the admitting condition
- Scheduled procedures
- Ability to meet health care requisites
- Availability of social supports
- Other specific needs identified by the patient and by the RN

Understanding the intensity of care required by individual patients and groups of patients based on these factors is the first step in developing effective patient classification systems and planning for appropriate staffing levels. The second step is knowing the level of preparation, skill, and experience of the staff members who are available to provide patient care.

Level of Staff Preparation and Experience. It is of critical importance that the staff members available to provide patient care have the educational preparation, skill, and experience necessary to meet patient care needs. Another consideration in staffing is the clinical competencies that are required to care for the population being served. The nurse who is responsible for making staffing decisions must be aware of each individual staff member's educational level, competencies, experience, skill, and training. Ideally, clinical support from experienced RNs should be available to support and advance the skills of those RNs and other staff members with less experience. Unfortunately, this is not always possible in times of nursing shortages. If the nurse manager does not believe that adequate numbers of appropriately skilled and experienced staff members are available to provide safe patient care, the nurse should immediately address those concerns with his or her supervisor.

Staffing and Staff Satisfaction

Nurses who are satisfied with their work generally provide higher-quality more cost-effective care. Staffing systems should address the quality of work life for the nursing staff as equally important as the quality of patient outcomes (ANA, 2009a). Attention to staff schedules is a major responsibility for the nurse manager, especially in light of the 24-hour/day, 365-day/year staffing needs in many health care facilities. Creative staffing options are available to meet the varied needs of staff members, including:

- 10-hour shifts/4 days per week
- 12-hour shifts/3 days per week
- Premium pay or part-time staff for weekend work
- Job sharing, flextime, and/or staff self-scheduling

Each of these options has various advantages and disadvantages. For example, long shifts over consecutive days may result in clinical errors when nurses become fatigued (IOM, 2004). Self-scheduling is a popular staffing technique in which the responsibility for staffing the unit is delegated to the employees on the unit who work collectively to design the schedule based on preestablished staffing criteria and some guidance from the manager. No one scheduling system has proven to be best overall for staff satisfaction. However, staffing methods that gain staff input and enhance staff autonomy seem to be a major key to staff satisfaction (Wieck, Dols, and Northam, 2009).

Staffing and Organizational Needs

The three basic organizational needs that are significantly affected by staffing are: (1) financial resources, (2) licensing regulations and The Joint Commission (TJC) standards, and (3) customer satisfaction.

Financial Resources. Productivity, the ratio of the amount of outputs produced (i.e., home visits) to the specific amount of input (nursing hours worked), is the measure of staffing efficiency. Because staff salaries are by far the largest expense for any health care organization, productivity—or the efficient use of staff—has a direct effect on the organization's bottom line. Fortunately, even though RNs represent the highest-paid staff in a facility, research has yet again demonstrated the value of RNs in improving patient outcomes and increasing hospital profitability (Dall et al, 2009; McCue, Mark, and Harless, 2003). However, it is important to remember that most health care organizations continue to function under tight financial constraints, making efficient management of staff essential to ensure the organization's financial solvency. The nurse manager is accountable for appropriately managing staffing to stay within budgetary guidelines for the following:

- ◆ Numbers of staff working at any given time to provide care to a given number of patients
- ◆ Staff mix, the combination of types of workers present to provide patient care (e.g., RNs, LVNs or LPNs, nursing assistants, multiskilled workers, or NAP)

Licensing Regulations and Accreditation. Health care facility licensing agencies, such as a state health department, and accreditation agencies, such as TJC, address minimum staffing levels. However, TJC and state licensing agencies do not impose mandatory staffing ratios (with the exception of California, which enacted legislation mandating specific nurse-patient ratios). Licensing regulations for long-term care facilities stipulate minimum RN coverage for the unit, but do not mandate specific nurse-to-patient ratios. However, these agencies do look for evidence that patients receive adequate care, which can only occur with adequate staffing. They also require documentation of staff training and competency to care for the organization's specific patient population.

Customer Satisfaction. Perhaps most critical to an organization's success in a competitive health care environment is customer (patient) satisfaction. The key to customer satisfaction is the patient's personal interaction with the organization's employees. According to Kenagy and associates (1999), "Interactions with patients and their families have remarkably strong effects on clinical outcomes, functional status and even physiologic measures of health" (p. 663). Appropriate staffing within budget constraints with well-trained, competent, professional staff members who are committed to providing safe, high-quality care is the nurse manager's number-one challenge.

This section has provided the reader with a brief introduction to staffing issues, such as scheduling options, patient classification systems, productivity and staff mix, and the RN's contribution to improved patient outcomes. These issues related to staffing in a health care organization are much more complex than may appear from this introduction. The reader, especially the person interested in entering nursing management, is encouraged to learn more about staffing and these related issues. Box 20-1 lists online learning resources related to staffing.

NURSING CARE DELIVERY MODELS

Nursing care delivery models, also called care delivery systems or patient care delivery models, detail the way task assignments, responsibility, and authority are structured to accomplish patient care. The nursing care delivery model describes which health care worker is going to perform

BOX **20-1**

Helpful Staffing Websites

ANA's Safe Staffing
  www.safestaffingsaveslives.org
Institute of Medicine Report: *Keeping Patients Safe: Transforming the Work Environment of Nurses*
  www.nap.edu/books/0309090679/html
National Database of Nursing Quality Indicators
  www.nursingquality.org/Default.aspx

what tasks, who is responsible, and who has the authority to make decisions. The basic premise of nursing care delivery models is that the number and type of caregivers are closely matched to patient care needs to provide safe, quality care in the most cost-effective manner possible.

The four classic nursing care delivery models used during the past five decades are: (1) total patient care, (2) functional nursing, (3) team nursing, and (4) primary nursing. During the 1990s, in an effort to continually improve both the quality and cost-effectiveness of patient care, variations of these four classic models were adopted, including modular nursing and the partnership model (or coprimary nursing). Other variations on nursing care models include patient-centered care, telehealth nursing, and case management. As the health care system continues to evolve in the twenty-first century with a focus on rapid patient turnover in acute care settings, extensive use of outpatient and community-based settings, and evidence of the RN's valuable role in patient safety and improved outcomes, the need for new models of nursing care delivery is emerging. Thus considerations for future care delivery models also are presented.

Total Patient Care

The oldest method of organizing patient care is total patient care, sometimes referred to as case nursing. In total patient care, nurses are responsible for planning, organizing, and performing all care, including personal hygiene, medications, treatments, emotional support, and education required for their assigned group of patients during the assigned shift. A diagram of the total patient care model is shown in Figure 20-1.

Advantages of the total patient care model are:

♦ The patient receives holistic, unfragmented care by only one nurse per shift.
♦ At shift change, the RN who has provided care and the RN assuming care can easily communicate about the patient's condition and collaborate about the plan of care to ensure continuity because so few caregivers are involved.

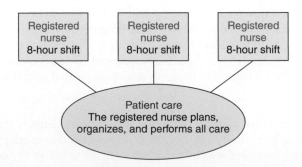

Figure 20-1 *The total patient care (case method) delivery model.*

♦ The nurse maintains a high degree of practice autonomy.

♦ Lines of responsibility and accountability are clear.

Disadvantages of the total patient care model are:

♦ The number of RNs required to provide total patient care may simply not be available because of the nursing shortage or financial constraints.

♦ The RN performs many tasks that could be performed by a caregiver with less training at a lower cost.

Today the total patient care method is commonly used in the hospital's critical care areas, such as intensive care units and postanesthesia care units, where continuous assessment and a high degree of clinical expertise are required at all times. This method is less widely used in other patient care settings as health care organizations move to more efficient, interprofessional team approaches to patient care, allowing RNs to concentrate on aspects of care essential to good patient outcomes, such as providing patient teaching and evaluating the patient's response to the plan of care. However, variations of the total patient care method exist. When reviewing other methods of nursing care delivery, you may see similarities to the total patient care model.

Functional Nursing

In the functional nursing method of patient care delivery, staff members are assigned to complete certain tasks for a group of patients rather than care for specific patients. For example, the RN performs all assessments and care planning, and administers all intravenous medications; the LVN or LPN gives all oral medications; and the assistant performs hygiene tasks and takes vital signs. A charge nurse makes the assignments and coordinates the care. A diagram of the functional nursing care model is shown in Figure 20-2.

Advantages of the functional nursing model are:

♦ Patient care is provided in an economic and efficient manner because less-skilled, lower-cost workers are used in areas where task completion is the focus.

♦ A minimum number of RNs is required to supervise and to perform strictly nursing duties.

♦ Tasks are completed quickly, and there is little confusion about job responsibilities.

Disadvantages of the functional nursing model are:

♦ Care may be fragmented, and the possibility of overlooking priority patient needs exists because several different workers focus only on performing specific patient care tasks.

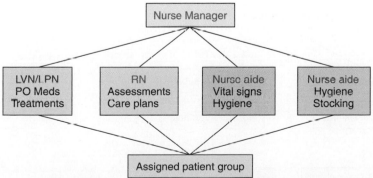

Figure 20-2 *The functional nursing care delivery model.*

- ◆ The patient may feel confused because of the many different individuals providing different aspects of care.
- ◆ Caregivers may feel unchallenged and unmotivated when performing repetitive functions.

Although the functional nursing model is considered efficient and economical, the patient is treated by many caregivers who are not able to give personalized care because they are focused on performing a task, not on meeting patient needs. This model may not fit well in the new health care system, which focuses on customer service. However, functional nursing care delivery is still appropriate in some care settings and may be used in the operating room.

Team Nursing

In team nursing, the RN functions as a team leader and coordinates a small group (no more than four or five) of ancillary personnel to provide care to a small group of patients. As coordinator of the team, the RN must know the condition and needs of all the patients assigned to the team and plan for individualized care for each patient. The team leader also is responsible for encouraging a cooperative environment and maintaining clear communication among all team members. The team leader's duties include planning care, assigning duties, directing and assisting team members, giving direct patient care, teaching, and coordinating patient activities. A diagram of the team nursing model is shown in Figure 20-3.

Advantages of the team nursing model are (Marquis and Huston, 2009):

- ◆ High-quality comprehensive care can be provided with a relatively high proportion of ancillary staff.
- ◆ Each member of the team is able to participate in decision making and problem solving.
- ◆ Each team member is able to contribute his or her own special expertise or skills in caring for patients.

Disadvantages of the team nursing model are:

- ◆ Continuity of care may suffer if the daily team assignments vary and the patient is confronted with many different caregivers.
- ◆ The team leader may not have the leadership skills required to effectively direct the team and create a "team spirit."
- ◆ Insufficient time for care planning and communication may lead to unclear goals. Therefore, responsibilities and care may become fragmented.

Team nursing is an effective, efficient method of patient care delivery and has been used in most inpatient and outpatient health care settings. However, for team nursing to succeed,

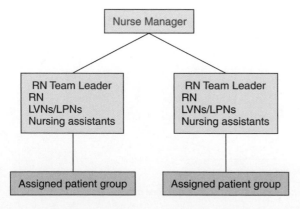

Figure 20-3 Team nursing model.

the team leader must have strong clinical skills, good communication skills, delegation ability, decision-making ability, and the ability to create a cooperative working environment. In an attempt to overcome some of its disadvantages, the team nursing design has been modified many times since its original inception, and variations of the model are evident in other methods of nursing care delivery, such as modular nursing.

Modular nursing is a modification of team nursing and focuses on a smaller team assigned to a geographic location in the nursing unit. The nursing unit is divided into modules or districts, and the same team of caregivers is assigned consistently to the same geographic location. The concept of modular nursing calls for a smaller group of staff providing care for a smaller group of patients. The goal is to increase the involvement of the RN in planning and coordinating care. To maximize efficiency, each designated module should contain all the supplies needed by the staff to perform patient care.

Primary Nursing

In primary nursing, the RN, or "primary" nurse, assumes 24-hour responsibility for planning, directing, and evaluating the patient's care from admission through discharge. This model differs significantly from the total patient care model in that the "primary nurse" assumes 24-hour responsibility for directing the patient's plan of care. While on duty the primary nurse may provide total patient care or delegate some patient care tasks to LPNs or LVNs or NAP. When the primary nurse is off duty, care is provided by an associate nurse who follows the care plan established by the primary nurse. The primary nurse, who has 24-hour responsibility, is notified if any problems or complications develop and directs alterations in the plan of care. A fundamental responsibility for the nurse in the primary nursing model is to maintain clear communication among all members of the health care team, including the patient, family, physician, associate nurses, and any other members of the health care team. A diagram of the primary nursing model is shown in Figure 20-4.

Advantages of the primary nursing model are (Marquis and Huston, 2009):
 ◆ Direct patient care provided by a few nurses allows for a one-to-one relationship to be established between nurse and patient.
 ◆ Nurses are able to practice with a high degree of autonomy and feel challenged and rewarded.
Disadvantages of the primary nursing model are (Marquis and Huston, 2009):
 ◆ Implementation may be difficult because the primary nurse is required to practice with a high degree of responsibility and autonomy.
 ◆ An inadequately prepared primary nurse may not be able to make the necessary clinical decisions or communicate effectively with the health care team.

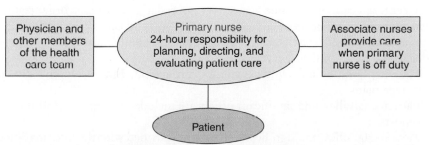

Figure 20-4 *Primary nursing model.*

◆ The RN may not be willing to accept the 24-hour responsibility required in primary nursing.
◆ The number of nurses required for this method of care may be difficult to recruit and train.

The primary care nursing model lends itself well to home health nursing, hospice nursing, and long-term care settings in which the patient requires nursing care for an extended period. Primary nursing may be more difficult to provide in acute care settings, where stays are short, and the nurse may see the patient for only 1 or 2 days. Because the concept of primary nursing is sound, some organizations have modified this nursing care model and implemented partnership models that use a wider staff mix.

Partnership Model

The partnership model, sometimes referred to as coprimary nursing, is a modification of primary nursing. This model was designed to make more efficient use of the RN, who delegates nonprofessional tasks to the partner, thus providing more time for the RN to address professional demands, such as assessment and patient education (Lookinland, Tiedman, and Crosson, 2005). In the partnership model, the RN is partnered with an LVN, LPN, or NAP, and the pair work together consistently to care for an assigned group of patients.

Advantages of the partnership model are:
◆ The model is more cost-effective than the true primary care nursing system because fewer RNs are needed.
◆ The RN can encourage the training and growth of his or her partner.
◆ The RN can perform the nursing duties and the partner can perform the nonnursing tasks.
Disadvantages of the partnership model are:
◆ The RN may have difficulty delegating to the partner.
◆ Consistent partnerships are difficult to maintain based on varied staff schedules.

Patient-Centered Care

Patient-centered care has been a core nursing value since the beginning of professional nursing; however, it is receiving renewed attention as a result of the IOM's focus on safety and quality in health care (Mitchell, 2008). The IOM (2001) defines patient-centered care as "providing care that is respectful of and responsive to individual patient preferences, needs, and values and ensuring that patient values guide all clinical decisions" (p. 40). Delivering patient-centered care means that nurses, physicians, and other health professionals partner with patients and families to ensure that health care decisions respect patients' wants, needs, and preferences and patients have the education and support they need to make decisions and participate in their own care (IOM, 2001).

As the reader can see, patient-centered care is more a philosophy of care rather than a typical nursing care delivery model as discussed in the previous sections. However, because patient-centered care has become a core focus in today's health care organizations, it needs to be incorporated as an essential component of any nursing care delivery model. Following are some practical methods for ensuring that patients and families are actively engaged as partners and decision makers in their health care:
◆ Patients, families and significant others are included in developing care plans and discharge plans.
◆ Patients, families, and significant others are included in change of shift or other hand-off reports.
◆ Patients, families, and significant others are provided with the information and education they need to make informed decisions.

♦ "Family advisory councils" are established to engage patients and families in decision making (Ponte et al, 2003)

The nurse, as coordinator of the interprofessional team, is responsible for making the patient and family an integral part of the team, keeping the patient involved in decision making, and promoting an environment respectful of patient's wants, needs, and preferences.

TELEHEALTH NURSING

Telehealth, or telephone nursing, has emerged as an important method of providing nursing care to clients in ambulatory settings. The American Academy of Ambulatory Care Nursing (AAACN) defines the practice of telehealth nursing as "using the nursing process to provide nursing care and access to health care for individual patients or patient populations over the telephone" (2009, p. 1).

Nurses began to formally use the telephone to interact with patients in the early 1970s. As the efforts of health care organizations to balance quality care with cost control have increased, the use of telehealth and telephone nursing services has increased as well. These services may be referred to as telephone triage, telephone nursing, or telehealth, a term that encompasses all tele-communication methods, including e-mail, Internet, facsimile, and telephone nursing practice.

Nurses' roles in telehealth nursing include triage, interventions, consultation, surveillance, and follow-up. Challenges for telehealth nursing include multistate licensure that opens doors for nurses to provide care for clients across state lines, regulation of telehealth for nursing and medicine, legal issues, and Medicare reimbursement.

The AAACN has defined the following criteria for telehealth nursing practice (AAACN, 2009):

♦ Using protocols, algorithms, or guidelines to systematically assess and address patient needs
♦ Prioritizing the urgency of patient needs
♦ Developing a collaborative plan of care with the patient and his or her support systems, which may include wellness promotion, prevention education, care counseling, disease state management, and care coordination
♦ Evaluating outcomes of practice and care

Telephone nursing may be an integral part of an outpatient clinic practice or the function of a centralized call center. Centralized telephone services are typically used by managed care groups and operate to provide nursing advice after clinic hours. This centralized service uses nursing time efficiently and facilitates appropriate management of the services; however, processes must be carefully evaluated to ensure nurses are able to practice as intended to meet patient needs (Valanis et al, 2003). Telephone nursing in medical offices may be enhanced by the availability of interaction with the medical professional.

To guide interventions with callers, telephone nurses may use standardized protocols or protocols developed for their particular setting. Optimal outcomes are fostered when nurses are involved in decisions about telehealth practices and protocols, have communication with other telephone nurses, and can educate health care providers about their role and function (Valanis et al, 2003). More information about telehealth nursing is available online from the AAACN (www.aaacn.org).

CASE MANAGEMENT
Evolution of Case Management

Case management is a model of care delivery in which an RN case manager coordinates the patient's care throughout the course of an illness. The concept of case management was first introduced in the 1970s by insurance companies as a method to monitor and control expensive health insurance claims, usually created by a catastrophic accident or illness. Today virtually every major health insurance company has a case management program to direct and manage the use of health care services for their clients. Case management by payer organizations (e.g., health insurance companies, health maintenance organizations [HMOs]) is known as external case management.

By the mid-1980s, hospitals had recognized the need for a case management model to manage the treatment plans and lengths of stay of hospitalized patients. When the Medicare prospective payment program was implemented in 1983, hospitals were reimbursed a set payment based on the patient's diagnosis, or diagnosis-related groups (DRG), regardless of how long the patient was hospitalized or what treatment was provided. To keep costs lower than the diagnosis-related payment, the hospitals had to efficiently manage the treatment provided to a patient and reduce the patient's length of stay. Thus internal case management, or case management "within the walls" of the health care facility, was created to maintain quality care while streamlining costs.

Definition of Case Management

Nursing case management is defined as a "dynamic and systematic collaborative approach to provide and coordinate health care services to a defined population. Nurse case managers actively participate with their clients to identify and facilitate options and services, providing and coordinating comprehensive care to meet patient-client health needs, with the goal of decreasing fragmentation and duplication of care, and enhancing quality cost-effective clinical outcomes. Nurse case managers continually evaluate each individual's health plan and specific challenges and then seek to overcome obstacles that affect outcomes" (American Nurses Credentialing Center [ANCC], 2009, p. 1). The framework for nursing case management includes five components: assessment, planning, implementation, evaluation, and interaction.

Other disciplines, most notably social work, have been involved in developing case management programs and have identified themselves as case managers. It is common to see the term "case manager" used for many types of caregivers in many different health care settings. However, when clinical knowledge and experience are required, the RN is most effective in the case management role. Variations of case management models now are found in almost all health care organizations, including home health agencies, rehabilitation and long-term care facilities, hospitals, and ambulatory care organizations.

Components of Case Management

The nurse case manager manages a caseload of patients from preadmission (or onset of illness) to discharge (or resolution of illness). Although case managers generally do not perform direct care duties, they assume a planning and evaluative role and collaborate with the interprofessional health care team to ensure that goals are met, quality is maintained, and progress toward discharge is made. The goal of case management, whether internal or external, is to focus attention on the quality, outcomes, and cost of care throughout the patient's episode of illness and to assist the patient to move through the continuum of care.

For example, the nurse case manager coordinates arrangements to move the patient from acute care to rehabilitation to home health to independent living, as determined by patient needs.

Case Management Related to Other Nursing Care Delivery Models

Nursing case management in a health care facility supplements nursing care and does not take the place of the nursing care delivery model in place to provide direct patient care. For example, if a hospital's medical-surgical unit uses a team nursing approach to patient care, a

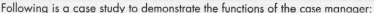

CASE STUDY

Following is a case study to demonstrate the functions of the case manager:

Mr. Smith, 58 years old, was diagnosed with lung cancer 1 year ago. He has been in Medical Center Hospital with multiple complications for more than 3 weeks. Debra Welch, RN, the internal case manager assigned to Mr. Smith's case, is working with the patient, family, physician, other members of the health care team, and the insurance company to determine a timely cost-effective discharge plan. Debra has performed a comprehensive health assessment and understands the patient's condition and the available support systems. The physician, patient, family, and health care team agree that Mr. Smith's prognosis is grave, and the treatment plan should be for palliative care only. Pain management is most important at this stage of the disease. Mr. Smith has a strong desire to go home, and his wife and adult daughter are willing to share the responsibility for home care. Debra also has identified the family's need for emotional support to deal effectively with the terminal illness.

After contacting Mr. Smith's insurance company, Debra learns that the company does not provide home health or hospice benefits, but that the patient could be transferred to a subacute facility for continued care. Knowing Mr. Smith's strong desire to go home and the support systems in place, Debra identifies all the costs for home care (hospital bed, bedside commode, oxygen, wheelchair, and hospice support with pain management) and reports the comparative costs of home care versus subacute care to the insurance company. By demonstrating that home care is slightly less expensive than inpatient, subacute care, Debra is able to negotiate successfully a payment for home care from Mr. Smith's insurance company.

As case manager, Debra's next responsibilities are to coordinate Mr. Smith's discharge and to arrange for home services needed, including hospice care and medical equipment. The home plan of care is developed by the health care team and approved by the physician. Debra communicates the plan of care to the home care providers to ensure unfragmented care. As a result of case management, Mr. Smith and his family are able to go home with continued support and a smooth transition of care.

---

system of case management also might be in place to assist with coordinating the patient's total care through discharge. Case management is not needed for every patient in a health care facility and generally is reserved for the chronically ill, seriously ill or injured, and long-term, high-cost cases.

CLINICAL PATHWAYS

Clinical pathways, also called critical paths, practice protocols, patient care protocols, or care maps, are clinical management plans that specify major patient care activities and interprofessional interventions and desired outcomes within a specified time period for a particular diagnosis or health condition. The advantage of the clinical pathway is that it provides a means of standardizing care for patients with similar diagnoses. Clinical pathways differ from clinical practice guidelines in that clinical pathways define key processes and patient goals in the day-to-day management of care, whereas clinical practice guidelines guide broader decision making and focus on the decisions to perform a procedure or service. Clinical pathways are usually developed within the health care facility and are based on broader clinical practice guidelines. Because clinical pathways dictate the type and amount of care given, they have financial implications for the health care facility.

In essence the clinical pathway can be viewed as a road map the patient and health care team should follow to guide the patient's care management and recovery. As the patient progresses along the path, specified goals should be accomplished. If a patient's progress deviates or leaves the planned path, a variance has occurred. A positive variance means that the patient has progressed ahead of schedule, and a negative variance means that the identified goals are not accomplished as planned. The RN generally identifies that a variance has occurred and mobilizes the interprofessional team members to create an action plan to address the problem or issue.

Clinical pathways were developed in response to the need to identify quality, cost-effective care plans to reduce the patient's length of stay in the hospital. The Joint Commission (TJC) now stipulates that health care facilities use clinical pathways to meet accreditation standards (TJC, 2007).

Clinical Pathway Terminology

Understanding the following terminology related to clinical pathways is necessary to be able to effectively use this clinical management tool:

◆ Patient outcomes are the end result of intervention by the health care team.
◆ Interprofessional intervention is the collaborative effort by all disciplines (e.g., nursing, physician, dietitian, physical therapy, occupational therapy, pharmacy), along with the patient and the family, to help the patient reach the desired health outcomes.
◆ Variance is any event that may alter the patient's progress through the clinical pathway.
◆ Triggers alert the caregiver that an unexpected event has occurred and identify potential and actual variations in the patient's response to the planned intervention (Birdsall and Sperry, 1997).

Components of Clinical Pathways

Components of a clinical pathway include physical assessment guidelines, laboratory and diagnostic tests, medications and procedures, safety and self-care activities, nutrition requirements, patient and family education, discharge planning, and milestones the patient should achieve through the progression of care. Many clinical pathways also address triggers, which are events that identify potential or actual variations in the patient's response to the planned interventions. The most commonly used clinical paths in acute care settings are for treatment of community-acquired pneumonia, total hip or knee replacement, and stroke or transient ischemic attack (Darer, Pronovost, and Bass, 2002).

Developing Clinical Pathways

Clinical pathways most often are developed for the health care facility's most common or costly diagnoses. For example, a general hospital may develop pathways for the treatment of congestive heart failure from admission in the emergency department, to care in the coronary care unit, to care on the general floor, to discharge home. It is important that the clinical pathway be individualized to meet unique patient needs. Clinical pathways should also be based on accepted standards of practice as recommended by specialty nursing organizations.

A team supported by management, with representatives from various disciplines, including nursing, medicine, therapy, pharmacy, and dietary, develops clinical pathways for the organization. As a starting point, samples of clinical pathways can be found in the literature. In addition, professional medical and nursing associations and the Agency for Healthcare Research and Quality (AHRQ) (www.guidelines.gov) are excellent sources for currently recommended clinical practice guidelines, which provide the foundational information for developing the clinical pathway. The success of clinical pathway development and implementation depends on input and support from all disciplines, including physicians, involved in using the pathway and caring for the patient.

CHOOSING A NURSING CARE DELIVERY MODEL

The nursing care delivery models presented in this chapter can be integrated into a variety of health care settings, including acute care, long-term care, ambulatory care, home care, and hospice. The organizational structure, patient needs, and staff availability influence which delivery system will be used.

Acute care settings may use different types of care delivery models for various patient care units. Emergency departments often use functional approaches to care because emphasis is on efficient assessment and immediate treatment. Team nursing frequently is used in medical-surgical units, whereas total patient care is common in critical care units. One study found that more than 50% of staff from 26 hospitals reported using two or three nursing care delivery models, sometimes over the course of one shift (Kramer and Schmalenberg, 2005). As identified in this chapter's opening vignette, acute care hospitals demand that RNs understand and be able to function in the diverse patterns of care that are in place throughout the organization.

In long-term care settings, such as nursing homes, skilled nursing facilities, and rehabilitation settings, patients remain in the care settings for extended periods. Therefore, the care delivery models may be structured differently than in the acute setting. Because of its economy and efficiency, functional nursing may be used for daily care tasks, whereas a form of primary care nursing is used for assessment, care planning, and evaluation.

The variety of ambulatory care settings continues to grow as health care moves out of the more expensive inpatient settings to the less costly outpatient settings. Outpatient surgery centers, minor emergency clinics, outpatient cancer centers, outpatient dialysis units, outpatient birthing centers, health clinics, and physicians' offices are examples of ambulatory care settings. The nursing care delivery model used in ambulatory settings varies widely, depending on the type of patients being treated and their particular needs. For example, in outpatient dialysis units, a combination of functional and primary care nursing usually works well. Patient care technicians are assigned to perform specific patient care functions, such as dialysis machine setup and treatment initiation, whereas the RN is assigned primary nurse responsibilities for a group of patients to ensure effective assessment, care planning, and care coordination with the interprofessional team. Telephone nursing is becoming increasingly important as a method of care delivery in ambulatory settings.

Home health agencies often use a variation of the primary care model. Although in home care the RN does not provide 24-hour care, he or she is responsible for the patient's needs for a 24-hour period and will coordinate intermittent care provided by others, including the home health aide and therapists involved in the patient's care. In the home health setting, the RN may also function in the role of case manager for his or her assigned patients.

In every care setting a nurse manager must carefully evaluate the nursing care delivery model to ensure safe, efficient, and effective patient care. When evaluating nursing care delivery models, the following questions should be asked:

- ◆ Is patient safety ensured while achieving optimal patient outcomes in a timely, cost-effective manner?
- ◆ Are patients and families happy with the care they are receiving?
- ◆ Are nurses, physicians, and other health team members satisfied with the safety and quality of care they are able to provide?
- ◆ Does the system allow for implementation of the nursing process in a timely and efficient manner?
- ◆ Does the system facilitate communication among all members of the health care team?

FUTURE NURSING CARE DELIVERY MODELS

Without a doubt, the ways in which nursing care is delivered over the next 20 years will change dramatically as a result of the following factors:

- Rapid technologic advances in medical care with less invasive procedures for disease treatments
- Fast-paced patient turnover in acute care settings; the rapid discharge and admission cycle is now referred to as "churning" and is estimated to range from 25% to 70% on a typical medical-surgical unit (Spader, 2008)
- Evidence of the RN's value in promoting patient safety and quality of care
- Ongoing shortages of nurses and other health professionals
- Strong focus on safety and outcomes of care
- Consumers' demands for instant access to care and information
- Need to engage people to focus on the underlying determinants of their individual health that are affected by lifestyle and personal choice

Because acute care settings now admit only the most seriously ill or injured individuals with a focus on stabilization and transition, the traditional models of nursing care may no longer apply. In the past, nurses provided care based on comprehensive knowledge of the patients' needs, which were learned by caring for the patients over an extended period. Now nurses may have an entirely new group of patient to care for every shift or even more than once during a shift. Nurses of the future must learn to conduct focused assessments and set priorities to be resolved before the patient is quickly transitioned to another level of care (Deutschendorf, 2003).

Nurses in outpatient and community-based settings are challenged with similar problems in attempting to address (1) patients' demands for instant access to care and information, and (2) patients' needs for support and education to address lifestyle and personal choices that may affect their health. These challenges in acute-care and outpatient settings are further complicated by the nursing shortage, which is only expected to worsen over the next decade.

Relationship-based care must also be considered as part of the care delivery model in high-tech fast-paced environments where nurses struggle to provide care that is consistent with nursing values of compassion, caring and healing. Manthey (2003) translated relationship-based care to mean that "regardless of how high-tech, short-term, or financially driven the health system becomes, no one can tell nurses they cannot practice within a conceptual framework of 'intentional presence in a therapeutic relationship with the patient,' where the outcome is competent care that is oriented toward empowering patients to accept responsibility for living their lives with maximum health" (p. 370). Nurse leaders will be challenged to identify new models of care delivery that are cost-effective and will improve the quality and safety of care provided, and facilitate the practice of relationship-based nursing.

SUMMARY

Managers of health care organizations are concerned that patient care is delivered in the most efficient and cost-effective method possible and that staffing is appropriate to ensure safe, high-quality care and contributes to staff satisfaction. For this reason, nursing care delivery models have undergone tremendous change throughout the past decade and will continue to evolve as organizations look for ways to improve patient safety and outcomes in complex health care systems that are challenged by nursing shortages, reduced reimbursement, rapidly advancing technology, rapid patient turnover, and consumer demand for instant access and information.

SUMMARY—cont'd

Regardless of changes that are certain to occur, the RN will retain responsibility to evaluate nursing care delivery models to ensure that patient care is delivered safely and efficiently, that caregivers are competent and legally qualified to perform the duties they have been assigned, and that safe quality care and staff satisfaction are maintained.

 Additional resources are available online at: http://evolve.elsevier.com/Cherry/

REFERENCES

Aiken L, et al: Hospital nurse staffing and patient mortality, nurse burnout, and job dissatisfaction, *JAMA* 288(16):1987–1993, 2002.

Aiken L, et al: Educational levels of hospital nurses and surgical patient mortality, *JAMA* 290(12):1617–1623, 2003.

American Academy of Ambulatory Care Nursing: *Telehealth nursing practice SIG*. 2009. Available at: www.aaacn.org.

American Nurses Association: *Principles for delegation*, Silver Spring, MD, 2005, Author.

American Nurses Association: *Safe staffing saves lives*. 2009a. Available at: www.safestaffingsaveslives.org.

American Nurses Association: *Principles for nurse staffing*. 2009b. Available at: www.nursingworld.org/MainMenuCategories/ThePracticeofProfessionalNursing/NursingStandards/ANAPrinciples/Principles-on-Nurse-Staffing/Nurse-Staffing.aspx.

American Nurses Credentialing Center: *Nursing case management certification*. 2009. Available at: www.nursecredentialing.org/Eligibility/CaseMgmtNurseEligibility.aspx.

Birdsall C, Sperry SP: *Clinical paths in medical-surgical practice*, St Louis, 1997, Mosby.

Coffey RJ, et al: An introduction to critical paths, *Qual Manag Health Care* 14:46–55, 2005.

Dall TM, et al: The economic value of professional nursing, *Med Care* 47(1):97–104, 2009.

Darer J, Pronovost P, Bass EB: Use and evaluation of critical pathways in hospitals, *Effect Clin Pract* 5(3):114–119, 2002.

Deutschendorf AL: From past paradigms to future frontiers: unique care delivery models to facilitate nursing work and quality outcomes, *J Nurs Adm* 33(1):52–59, 2003.

Institute of Medicine, Field MJ, Lohr KN, editors: *Clinical practice guidelines: directions for a new program*, Washington, DC, 1990, National Academies Press.

Institute of Medicine: *Crossing the quality chasm: a new health system for the 21st century*, Washington, DC, 2001, National Academies Press.

Institute of Medicine, Page A, editors: *Keeping patients safe: transforming the work environments of nurses*, Washington, DC, 2004, National Academies Press.

Kane RL, et al: The association of registered nurse staffing levels and patient outcomes: systematic review and meta-analysis, *Med Care* 45(12):1195–1204, 2007.

Kenagy JW, Berwick DM, Shore MF: Service quality in health care, *JAMA* 281(7):661–665, 1999.

Kramer M, Schmalenberg C: Revisiting the essentials of magnetism tool: there is more to adequate staffing than numbers, *J Nurs Adm* 35(4):188–198, 2005.

Lookinland S, Tiedman ME, Crosson AE: Nontraditional models of care delivery: have they solved the problems? *J Nurs Adm* 35(2):74–80, 2005.

Manthey M: Primary nursing, *J Nurs Adm* 33(7/8): 369–370, 2003.

Marquis BL, Huston CJ: *Leadership roles and management functions in nursing*, ed 6, Philadelphia, 2009, Wolters Kluwer Health/Lippincott Williams & Wilkins.

McCue M, Mark B, Harless D: Nurse staffing, financial performance, and quality of care, *J Health Care Finance* 29(4):54–76, 2003.

Mitchell PH: Patient-centered care—a new focus on a time-honored concept, *Nurs Outlook* 56(5):197–198, 2008.

Needleman J, et al: Nurse-staffing levels and the quality of care in hospitals, *N Engl J Med* 346(22):1715–1722, 2002.

Ponte PR, et al: Making patient-centered care come alive: achieving full integration of the patient's perspective, *J Nurs Adm* 33(2):82–90, 2003.

Spader C: Rapid turnover: admission RNs make fast-paced admits/discharges less stressful for everyone, *NurseWeek* Aug 11:32–33, 2008.

The Joint Commission (TJC): *Comprehensive accreditation manual for ambulatory care*, Oakbrook Terrace, IL, 2007, Author.

Valanis B, et al: Making it work: organization and processes of telephone nursing advice services, *J Nurs Adm* 33(4):216–223, 2003.

Wieck KL, Dols J, Northam S: What nurses want: the nurse incentives project, *Nurs Econ* 27(3):169–201, 2009.

Quality Improvement and Patient Safety

Kathleen M. Werner, MS, BSN, RN

evolve Additional resources are available online at: http://evolve.elsevier.com/Cherry/

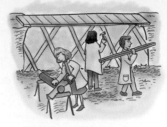

Nurses are building bridges to patient safety and quality care.

VIGNETTE

It was a typical day on 4 East, a busy med-surg unit in General Hospital. Patients were being admitted, discharged, and transported to surgery at a brisk pace. For Maureen Harper, RN, the day was like most others, until one of her patients was to be discharged. All of the necessary paperwork was completed, the patient's belongings were packed, and all discharge instructions were completed. But Maureen's patient could not be discharged until the pharmacy delivered the newly prescribed medication that was to be taken at home. This was not the first time a patient had to wait for a prescription, and for Maureen it was becoming a repeated pattern in the normal course of discharge preparations. The patient eventually received the medication after an hour's wait and was sent home, but Maureen began to ponder the effect of this repeating set of circumstances.

Maureen calculated the additional cost that resulted from this patient's delayed discharge. This 1-hour delay meant an extra hour of hospital care, an extra hour of nursing care, and because this occurred during lunchtime, it also meant that an extra meal needed to be served to the patient while he waited. Although each of these individual costs was small, Maureen began to think of the implications of these costs as they multiplied across dozens of patients throughout the many different nursing units at General Hospital. More important, Maureen was beginning to see the effect this delay had on patients' perceptions of the hospital. Family members often arrived early in the morning to take patients home, only to find they had to wait. Likewise, patients were not pleased when told they would need to wait. An entire positive hospital stay could be tainted with the experience of having to wait for discharge medication. Would that perception stay with them as they spoke to other friends and family about their hospitalization? Maureen began to feel more pressed to do something about the situation.

The next week Maureen approached her nurse manager and expressed concern about delayed discharges. Maureen's manager thanked her for the feedback and expressed similar interest in resolving this problem. Pharmacy staff members already had been in preliminary conversations with Maureen's manager about the discharge medication process and were willing to work collaboratively with the nursing staff to find a solution to this problem. Maureen eagerly volunteered to participate in a work group that was charged with understanding the common causes of delays in filling discharge medication prescriptions and implementing key changes to eliminate delays.

The team met regularly for several weeks and gained a clear understanding of what was contributing to medication delays. This was accomplished through creation of a detailed picture of what typically happened in filling discharge medication prescriptions and working on constructive ways to prevent breakdowns in this process. The project involved data collection to validate the sources of the breakdowns; what surfaced were surprises for staff members in each of the major departments involved, who always thought that someone else was to blame for the problems. In reality the interaction of multiple departments led to delays. Over time, with constant monitoring of the turnaround time between the writing of the discharge medication order and delivery of drugs back to the units, progress toward reducing the delays was demonstrated. Maureen now knows that the proper steps are in place to guarantee an efficient way for medication orders to be tracked and filled. When her patients are ready for discharge, so are their medications, and Maureen feels like she is a vested part of this success.

■ QUESTIONS TO CONSIDER WHILE READING THIS CHAPTER:

1 What key principles of quality improvement are demonstrated in the vignette?

2 What quality improvement tools did Maureen and the team most likely use to identify the causes for delays in filling discharge medications?

3 What resources are available to help Maureen and others in her organization learn more about improving the quality of health care?

KEY TERMS

Cause-and-effect diagram A tool that is used for identifying and organizing possible causes of a problem in a structured format. It is sometimes called a "fish-bone" diagram because it looks like the skeleton of a fish.

Clinical indicators Measurable items that reflect the quality of care provided and demonstrate the degree to which desired clinical outcomes are accomplished; clinical indicators help identify the goals of quality improvement.

Core measures Standardized sets of valid, reliable, and evidence-based quality measures used by The Joint Commission (TJC) to integrate performance measures into the accreditation process.

Customer Individual or group who relies on an organization to provide a product or service to meet some need or expectation. It is these customer needs and expectations that determine quality.

Failure mode and effects analysis (FMEA) A systematic process for identifying potential design and process failures before they occur, with the intent to eliminate them or minimize the risk associated with them.

Flowchart Picture of the sequence of steps in a process. Different steps or actions are represented by boxes or other symbols. A top-down flowchart shows the sequence of steps in a job or process. It can have different levels of detail. A deployment flowchart shows the detailed steps in a process and the people or departments that are involved in each step.

IOM National Academy of Sciences Institute of Medicine; a nonprofit organization with a mission of advancing and disseminating scientific knowledge to improve human health. The institute provides objective, timely, authoritative information and advice concerning health and science policy to government, the corporate sector, the professions, and the public.

ISMP Institute for Safe Medication Practices; a nonprofit organization that is well known as an education resource for the prevention of medication errors.

Lean methodology An integrated system of principles, practices, tools, and techniques focused on reducing waste, synchronizing workflows, and managing variability in production flows. Originally developed by Toyota and other Japanese companies and now adopted by the health care sector.

NCQA National Committee for Quality Assurance; an accreditation body that has become the primary group that accredits health maintenance organizations.

KEY TERMS—cont'd

Never events Serious adverse events during an inpatient stay that should never occur or are reasonably preventable through adherence to evidence-based guidelines. The Centers for Medicare & Medicaid Services, through revisions in coverage and payment policies, provide hospitals with financial incentives to reduce the occurrence of never events.

Pareto chart A graphic tool that helps break down a big problem into its parts and then identifies which parts are the most important.

Process Series of linked steps necessary to accomplish work. A process turns inputs, such as information or raw materials, into outputs, such as products, services, and reports. Clinical processes are a series of linked steps necessary for the provision of patient care. It is through the improvement of processes that an organization improves its work and sustains itself.

Process variation The differences in how the steps in a work process might be accomplished and/or the variables that may affect each step in the process. Variation results from the lack of perfect uniformity in the performance of any process. Understanding variation in a process is necessary to determine the direction that improvement efforts must take.

Quality management (QM) Philosophic framework for managing organizations that recognizes quality is determined by customer needs and expectations. Attention is paid to how the work is done, with an emphasis on involving the people who best understand the detail of the work processes with which they are involved. Health care QM is specifically related to the quality of health care services provided.

Root cause analysis Defined by TJC (2008) as a process for identifying the basic or causal factors that underlie variation in performance, including the occurrence or possible occurrence of a sentinel event. A root cause analysis focuses primarily on systems and processes, not individual performance.

Run chart A graph of data in time order that help identify any changes that occur over time; also called a time plot. A run chart that has a centerline and statistical control limits added is known as a control chart. Control limits help detect specific types of change in a process.

Sentinel event Defined by TJC (2008) as an unexpected occurrence involving patient death or serious physical or psychologic injury or the risk thereof. Serious injury specifically includes loss of limb or function. The phrase "or the risk thereof" includes any process variation for which a recurrence would carry a significant chance of a serious adverse outcome. Such events are called sentinel because they signal the need for immediate investigation and response.

Six Sigma A concept for company-wide quality improvement first introduced by the Motorola Corporation in 1987, characterized by its customer-driven approach, emphasis on decision making based on careful analysis of quantitative data, and a priority on cost reduction.

Standardization Approach to process improvement that involves developing and adhering to best known methods and repeating key tasks in the same way, time and time again, until a better way is found, thereby creating exceptional service with maximal efficiency.

TJC (The Joint Commission) A national agency that conducts surveys of inpatient and ambulatory facilities and certifies their compliance with established quality standards.

LEARNING OUTCOMES

After studying this chapter, the reader will be able to:

1 Apply principles of QM to the role of the professional nurse.

2 Analyze the basis for the increasing emphasis on health care quality and medical errors.

3 Analyze the role of health care regulatory agencies and how they have embodied the principles of QM.

4 Critique key evolutionary facts that led to the development of QM in health care.

5 Discuss the role process improvement can play in ensuring patient safety and improving quality in the health care system.

6 Describe the tools and skills necessary for successful QM activities.

7 Discuss the professional nurse's role in reducing medical errors and improving health care quality.

CHAPTER OVERVIEW

Although Maureen Harper's story depicted in the vignette seems credible and would be a logical way for any organization to begin addressing customer concerns, far too often that has not been the case. Hospitals and health care organizations have been slow to recognize the necessity of a true customer perspective and to emphasize quality in a proactive manner. Porter and Teisberg (2006), making the case for why competition alone has not resulted in quality care, wrote:

> *"How could the U.S. health care system, which is largely a private system and characterized by arguably more competition than any other health care system in the world, be performing so poorly? Why are U.S. costs among the highest in the world even though many citizens do not have health coverage? How could costs, already so high, still be rising so rapidly? Why is quality so uneven? Why is there growing evidence of alarming quality problems in the system?" (Preface).*

The intention of this chapter is to make the reader aware of the pressing nature of the nation's quality health care crisis and to address the following questions:

- ◆ *What is quality in health care?*
- ◆ *Who determines the degree to which quality is evident in our health care system?*
- ◆ *How should the health care system be redesigned to improve quality?*
- ◆ *What do the potential answers to the first three questions mean in relationship to professional nursing accountability?*

The responses to these questions, particularly in relation to nursing's commitment to become involved with QM and to participate in its implementation, provide the elements of hope in determining and implementing sustainable, positive improvements in the design and delivery of health care.

THE URGENT CASE FOR QUALITY IMPROVEMENT IN THE U.S. HEALTH CARE SYSTEM

In an alarming 2000 report by the National Academy of Science's Institute of Medicine (IOM) titled *To Err Is Human: Building a Safer Health System*, authors extrapolated and summarized data from two major studies and concluded that up to 98,000 patients are killed each year from medical errors, confirming that poor quality of care is a major problem in the United States (IOM, 2000). Contributing factors cited in the report included the following:

- ◆ Overuse of expensive invasive technology
- ◆ Underuse of inexpensive care services
- ◆ Error-prone implementation of care that could harm patients and waste money

Following this report, the IOM released *Crossing the Quality Chasm: A New Health System for the 21st Century* (2001) to define a vision for improving the quality of our nation's health care. This report states:

> "The U.S. health care delivery system does not provide consistent, high quality medical care to all people. Americans should be able to count on receiving care that meets their needs and is based on the best scientific knowledge—yet this frequently is not the case. Health care harms too frequently and routinely fails to deliver its potential benefits. Indeed between the health care that we now have and the health care that we could have lies not just a gap, but a chasm" (p. 1).

The quality chasm report details a number of factors that have contributed to this chasm, including the unprecedented advancement of science and technology, growing complexity of health care, changing public health care needs, and a poorly organized and uncoordinated health care delivery system. Following are selected indicators from recent IOM reports that indicate just how wide the quality chasm is between what we know is good care and what is current practice:

◆ Between 44,000 and 98,000 Americans die from medical errors annually (IOM, 2000).
◆ Medication-related errors for hospitalized patients cost roughly $2 billion annually (IOM, 2000).
◆ 45 million Americans remain uninsured and experience gaps in health care, which results in needless illness, suffering, and even death (IOM, 2009).
◆ The lag between the discovery of more effective forms of treatment and their incorporation into routine patient care averages 17 years (IOM, 2003).
◆ Forty percent of patients are not receiving care that is recommended; on average, patient safety measures declined by nearly 1% annually in each of the last 6 years (Agency for Healthcare Research and Quality [AHRQ], 2008).
◆ The 2008 National Healthcare Quality report notes that U.S. health care quality is suboptimal and continues to improve at a slow pace, reporting of hospital quality is leading improvement but patient safety is lagging, and health care quality measurement is evolving but much work remains (AHRQ, 2008).

The quality chasm report details six guiding aims for improvement that should be adopted by every individual and group involved in the provision of health care, including health care professionals, public and private health care organizations, purchasers of health care, regulatory agencies and organizations, and state and federal policymakers. These six guiding aims are collectively referred to by the acronym STEEEP. Individually, these aims are for health care to be (IOM, 2001):

◆ **S**afe: Preventing injuries to patients from the care that is intended to help them
◆ **T**imely: Reducing waits and sometimes harmful delays for both those who receive and those who give care
◆ **E**ffective: Providing services based on scientific knowledge to all who could benefit and refraining from providing services to those not likely to benefit
◆ **E**fficient: Preventing waste, including waste of equipment, supplies, ideas, and energy
◆ **E**quitable: Providing care that does not vary in quality because of personal characteristics, such as gender, ethnicity, geographic location, and socioeconomic status
◆ **P**atient centered: Providing care that is respectful of and responsive to individual patient preferences, needs, and values and ensuring that patient values guide all clinical decisions

To help establish a framework for accomplishing the significant redesign of the health care system, the authors of the quality chasm report formulated a set of 10 simple rules to guide improvement initiatives. Professional nurses must serve as role models for all health care professionals, caregivers, and administrators in practicing these 10 rules:

1. *Care is based on continuous healing relationships.* Patients should receive care whenever they need it and in many forms, including face-to-face visits, over the Internet, by telephone, and by other means as needed.
2. *Care is customized according to patient needs and values.* The system should be designed to meet the most common needs, but should also be responsive to individual choices and preferences.
3. *The patient is the source of control.* Patients should be given the necessary information and opportunity to exercise the degree of control they choose over health care decisions that affect them.

4. *Knowledge is shared and information flows freely.* Patients should have unfettered access to their own medical information and to clinical knowledge with clinicians communicating effectively and sharing information.

5. *Decision making is evidence based.* Patients should receive care based on the best available scientific knowledge, and care should not vary illogically from clinician to clinician or place to place.

6. *Safety is a system property.* Patients should be safe; reducing risk and ensuring safety require greater attention to systems that help prevent and mitigate errors.

7. *Transparency is necessary.* The system should make available to patients and families information that allows them to make informed decisions, including information describing the system's performance on safety, evidence-based practice, and patient satisfaction.

8. *Needs are anticipated.* The system should anticipate patient needs rather than simply react to events.

9. *Waste is continually decreased.* The system should not waste resources (i.e., supplies, health professionals' time and energy) or patient time.

10. *Cooperation among clinicians is a priority.* Actively engage in collaboration and communication to ensure an appropriate exchange of information and coordination of care.

The remainder of this chapter provides the reader with a set of principles and skills necessary to implement improvements and move toward a system of health care that is safe, timely, effective, efficient, equitable, and patient centered.

PRINCIPLES OF QUALITY MANAGEMENT

Many buzzwords describe activities associated with QM. The most prevalent are total quality management (TQM), continuous quality improvement (CQI), continuous process improvement, statistical process control, and performance improvement (PI). The terms themselves are not as important as the principles they embody: assessment and improvement of work processes while focusing on what customers want and need. In the example of Maureen and her patient waiting for discharge medication, the work process would be that of filling discharge prescription medication orders. The customer in this situation would be Maureen's patient, who wants to receive the medication quickly so that he can go home as soon as possible. Essentially the cornerstones of QM are:

◆ **Quality:** Recognition and understanding by all who serve a customer that it is the customer who defines quality. In health care, primary customers are patients, and they are the ones who determine what quality is, not those who are in the position of providing the care and service. Historically, caregivers frequently have assumed the role of determining what is best for the patient. With QM, patients become involved in helping to determine what is best for them.

◆ **Scientific approach:** Organizational support for all employees to develop quality knowledge and skills and to begin thinking of their work as a series of processes that can be more deeply understood and improved through data measurements. As employees within an organization work to improve their work processes, they begin to understand the interrelationship and effect of process work across departments, such that ultimately the final product or service offered to the customer can be vastly improved. This chapter's vignette demonstrated this concept through Maureen's participation on a work team in which pharmacy and nursing staff studied their contribution to the discharge medication process and found ways to better meet the patients' expectations of timeliness.

◆ **"All one team":** Belief in the people who are working to serve the customer. By recognizing the insight and knowledge held by those who are closest to the work and allowing them to be involved with the study and improvement of their own work, the potential for dramatic improvements can be realized.

Maureen's example is one that demonstrates these three principles of QM:

1. Maureen began to consider the patient as the one who would define the quality of his hospital stay. She recognized that the perceived quality of the entire hospital stay could suffer if the timeliness of delivering discharge medications could not be improved.

2. Maureen was supported organizationally by her manager, who provided the opportunity for Maureen to collaborate with other key department employees to better understand the current series of processes that were in place for medication delivery. This group's work led to a clearer understanding of the interrelationship of the processes across multiple departments, which together affected the overall timeliness of medication delivery and enabled the group to make the necessary improvements to achieve the desired result.

3. Managers in Maureen's hospital had faith in the people who were working on the medication delivery team. These people were recognized as those who had the best understanding of how the medication delivery "work" was happening and where the system was breaking down.

Quality

To provide a better appreciation of the importance of these three QM cornerstones, customers' perspective of quality must be considered, including the personal interactions they experience with an organization's personnel in addition to the products or services they receive. The products or services provided to the customer are not made up of just the physical items or a one-time experience that the customer encounters, but rather of all the services that go with it. Organizations actually provide a "bundle" of products and services to customers to satisfy some need. If the service and product or outcomes together are perceived as a good value, a loyal customer following will be established. Or as in the case presented in the vignette, Maureen's patient might view the entire hospital stay negatively because of the delay in receiving the medications before discharge.

Scientific Approach

The scientific approach, the second cornerstone of QM, emphasizes that to make significant improvements in an organization's processes, decisions must be based on sound, valid data, and the people managing the processes must have a clear understanding of the nature of variation in processes. Remember that a process is a series of linked steps necessary to accomplish work. For example, the steps necessary to complete a new medication order from the time the order is received until the medication is administered to a patient is a process. Understanding variation—the differences in how the steps in the process might be accomplished and/or the variables that may affect each step in the process—is necessary to identify the direction that improvement efforts must take.

Two types of variation in processes can occur: common cause variation and special cause variation. Processes that demonstrate common cause variation are stable, predictable, and statistically in control. Processes that demonstrate both common cause and special cause variation are unstable, unpredictable, and not in statistical control. The actions that should be taken to implement improvements under each type of variation are significantly different.

The best way to understand common cause and special cause variation is to use Maureen's example again. Maureen's team members collected data over time regarding the length of time it took from the writing of the discharge medication order to delivery of the drugs back to the clinical unit. Overall the time interval showed variability because of numerous factors associated with this process, one example being the total volume of orders written on any given day. The team recognized the total volume of orders written as common cause variation and realized that to minimize the degree of this variation, the overall process would need to be studied to determine the best ways to change the medication delivery system, regardless of the total order volume.

The team was aware of a significant time delay in medication delivery during the week of the computer system conversion. This variation was special cause, one of extreme impact, but related to a clearly identified single source. If the team had modified the overall medication delivery process based solely on the special cause factor, the computer conversion, the underlying problem most likely would not have been improved for the long term.

All One Team

Effective team functioning is the third QM cornerstone, which embodies the principles of believing in people; treating everyone in the workplace with dignity, trust, and respect; and working toward win-win situations for all customers, employees, shareholders, suppliers, and perhaps even the broader community as a whole. For people to work this way, they must believe it is in their best interest to cooperate; they need to be more concerned with how the system as a whole operates rather than optimizing their own contributing area. In other words, all team members must rely more on cooperation and less on competition.

THE ROLE OF REGULATORY AGENCIES IN QUALITY MANAGEMENT

Quality management in the United States did not begin to grow until well after World War II, following Dr. W. Edwards Deming's work with the Japanese in their postwar reconstruction efforts (Neave, 1990). The Western business world was slow to embrace Deming's philosophy, but, by the time of his death, it was evident that quality efforts in U.S. industry were more than a passing fad. As QM moved from manufacturing to service industries, penetration into the health care environment began.

From Quality Assurance to Quality Management

Initially hospitals were some of the first health-related organizations to seriously explore the potential value in adopting a total quality mindset in the 1980s and wrestled with more traditional models of quality assurance versus those of quality improvement. Health care leaders began to recognize that quality improvement was not necessarily a replacement for existing quality assurance activities, but rather an approach that broadened perspectives on quality, and therefore they introduced tools that helped facilitate the improvement process previously lacking in quality assurance (Box 21-1).

Another way to think about this shift from quality assurance to QM is that health care quality was historically gauged through "inspection" methods, frequently relying on retrospective reviews of patient incidences or adverse outcomes. For example, an adverse patient response to a medication would have been reviewed through quality assurance auditing with a review of the circumstances surrounding this one particular adverse event. This historical approach focused on specific incidents rather than on widely sweeping improvements that could address the more common causes of declining quality care and lead to preventing problems and improving care.

BOX **21-1**

Quality Assurance Versus Quality Improvement

QUALITY ASSURANCE	QUALITY IMPROVEMENT
Inspection oriented (detection)	Planning oriented (prevention)
Reactive	Proactive
Correction of special causes	Correction of common causes
Responsibility of few people	Responsibility of all involved with the work
Narrow focus	Cross-functional
Leadership may not be vested	Leadership actively leading
Problem solving by authority	Problem solving by employees at all levels

From Koch MW, Fairly TM: *Integrated quality management: the key to improving nursing care quality,* St Louis, 1993, Mosby.

Regulatory Agencies

Equally important in driving this movement from quality assurance to QM was the incorporation of quality principles into health care regulatory standards and requirements in the early 1990s (Bliersbach, 1992). Almost all regulatory and voluntary accrediting agencies now require QM in some form. The Centers for Medicare & Medicaid Services (CMS), which administers the U.S. Medicare program, has "conditions of participation" for its quality foundation, and many state licensing authorities also have required QM standards.

Voluntary accrediting organizations, such as the Commission on Accreditation of Rehabilitation Facilities and the Accreditation Council of Developmental Disabilities, promote QM requirements primarily for community-based providers serving various populations. The National Committee for Quality Assurance (NCQA) is becoming the primary voluntary accreditation body for managed care organizations, including outpatient clinic and medical practice group settings. This committee's emphasis revolves around performance measures of patient outcomes and results of practice patterns. The NCQA has grown significantly during the 1990s and now surveys at least half of the U.S. health maintenance organizations (HMOs).

The Joint Commission (TJC). TJC was one of the first regulatory agencies to embrace quality improvement principles in hospital-based settings. TJC standards address the organization's level of performance in key functional areas, including patient rights, patient treatment, and infection control. TJC accreditation system not only focuses on an organization's ability to provide safe high-quality care but now also requires evidence of actual performance and continued improvement.

Core Measures. TJC introduced their ORYX initiative in 1997, which was the initial integration of outcomes and other performance measurement data as part of the accreditation process. The ORYX measurements were intended to support organizations in their quality improvement efforts as well as supplement their accreditation process. In 2002, accredited hospitals began collecting data on standardized "core" performance measures and by 2004, TJC and the CMS worked to align their current and future measures common to both organizations. These standardized measures are referred to as National Hospital Quality Measures and the performance data is publicly reported on TJC website at Quality Check (www.qualitycheck.org). The 2009 reporting requirements allow hospitals to collect and submit data on a minimum of four

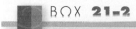

BOX **21-2**

The 2009 Joint Commission ORYX Performance Measurement Sets

Acute myocardial infarction
Heart failure
Pneumonia
Pregnancy and related conditions
Surgical care improvement project (SCIP)
Children's asthma care
Hospital outpatient department
Hospital-based inpatient psychiatric services

Specifications Manual for National Hospital Inpatient Quality Measures: www.jointcommission.org/PerformanceMeasurement/PerformanceMeasurement/Current+NHQM+ Manual.htm.

core measure sets or a combination of applicable core measure sets and non-core measures as described through TJC (Box 21-2).

It is especially important for nurses to be knowledgeable about core measures because they are in the unique position of supporting the overall management of patient care throughout the length of stay in the facility, working collaboratively with other health care professionals to initiate changes, and monitoring ongoing effectiveness of the care provided. For more information on core measures, nurses are encouraged to visit the Performance Measurement section of the TJC website (www.jointcommission.org).

CLINICAL INDICATORS AND PROCESS IMPROVEMENT TOOLS AND SKILLS

The basic foundation of the monitoring and evaluation process required by QM principles is in the use of clinical indicators, measurable items that reflect the quality of care. Clinical indicators are aspects of clinical care that can be measured to show the degree to which care is or is not carried out as it should be. Indicators focus on clinical actions or outcomes of clinical care; indicators should not focus on procedures that support clinical care. For example, replacing the intravenous (IV) solutions on the IV supply cart as they are used is a procedure that supports clinical care. Administering the correct IV solution at the correct rate as prescribed is appropriate clinical care. Both items are measurable, but only the latter is truly a clinical indicator. Indicators are not meant to define quality, but rather to point the way to assessment of areas in which quality issues may be present.

How do process improvement skills and tools fit with clinical indicators? Clinical indicators help to identify the goals of quality improvement, whereas process improvement skills and tools support the quantitative understanding of key work processes. Knowledge of specific improvement strategies and related technical skills such as the Lean Methodology, Six Sigma and Failure Mode and Effects Analysis (Frankel et al, 2009) provides the context and understanding for where and when to apply specific tools. It is not within the scope of this chapter to address these specific improvement strategies but it is important to note that all improvement models generally have the following in common:

- ◆ Analyzing and clearly understanding the process
- ◆ Selecting key aspects of the process to improve
- ◆ Establishing "trial" targets to guide improvement measures
- ◆ Collecting and plotting data
- ◆ Interpreting results
- ◆ Implementing improvement actions and evaluating effectiveness

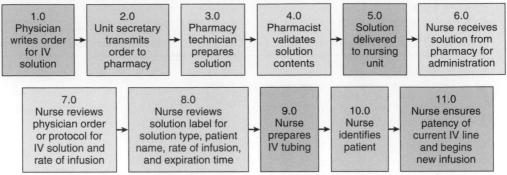

Figure 21-1 *Top-down flowchart of the process for administering intravenous solutions.*

Various tools, such as flowcharts, Pareto charts, cause-and-effect diagrams, and run charts, may be used to accomplish each of these six steps (Joiner Associates, 1995). It will become increasingly necessary for professional nurses to understand improvement models and to develop the ability to apply these tools. A review of the most frequently used tools follows.

Flowcharts

The analysis of a work process usually is initiated through construction of some sort of flowchart or flow diagram. These are indispensable tools in mapping out what actually occurs during the process versus what is intended. There are several different types of flowcharts, each of which is valuable in its own way. A top-down flowchart simply lists the main steps and substeps of a process in a linear fashion (Figure 21-1). A deployment flowchart maps out the steps of a process under headings designating people or departments who actually carry out each step. This type is especially helpful when dealing with processes that cross multiple caregivers or areas and when there is a need for common understanding of what the process is doing as a whole (Figure 21-2). As illustrated in Figures 21-1 and 21-2, top-down and deployment flowcharts can be used to view the process of administering the correct IV solution at the correct rate.

Pareto Charts

In selecting key aspects on which to focus within the process, a Pareto chart may be an appropriate tool. By collecting data on presumed or known problems in a given process, areas of focus or concentration can be achieved. This tool itself is a type of bar graph, with the height of bars reflecting the frequency with which events occur or the effect events have on a process problem. The bars are arranged in descending order so that the most commonly occurring problems are readily visible. Figure 21-3 is based on the Pareto principle, which proposes that 80% of process or system problems are generated from only 20% of the possible causal factors. Therefore, by focusing on the significant few causes, a much broader effect can be achieved in improvement efforts.

Cause-and-Effect Diagrams

Cause-and-effect diagrams are other worthy tools that can help determine the potential sources of a problem. These diagrams essentially are lists of potential causes, arranged by categories to show their potential effect on a problem. The categories usually are broad, with subsequent levels of detail pursued under each as the "might cause" question is asked of each subsequent

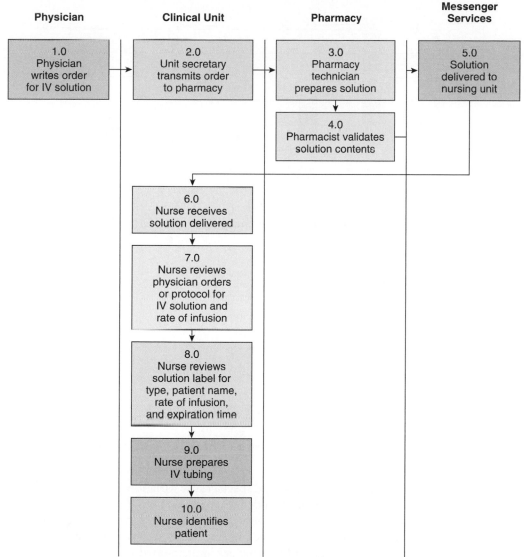

Figure 21-2 *Deployment flowchart of the process for administering intravenous solutions.*

level of detail. This diagram sometimes is referred to as a "fish-bone" diagram because it resembles a fish skeleton when complete. Cause-and-effect diagrams (Figure 21-4) are useful when the major problem areas have been localized using the Pareto chart.

Run Charts

Measuring data over time to evaluate patterns in process variation typically is suited for tools, such as run charts and control charts. Run charts, also known as "time plots," are graphs of data points as they occur over time. Valuable information can be obtained regarding process variation by studying the trends in the run chart. A control chart is a slightly more sophisticated tool

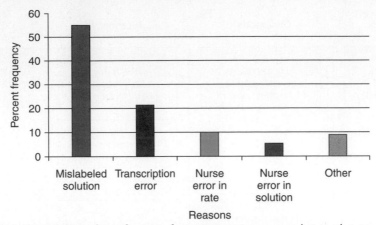

Figure 21-3 *Pareto chart of reasons for incorrect intravenous solution administration.*

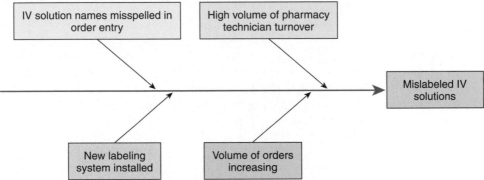

Figure 21-4 *Cause-and-effect diagram of mislabeled intravenous solutions.*

in helping distinguish between common and special cause variation. A control chart is basically a run chart with statistical control limits added (Figure 21-5).

Through use of these tools, results can be analyzed with interpretations subsequently guiding appropriate improvement actions. Once improvements are initiated, ongoing monitoring follows to evaluate the effectiveness of the changes implemented.

UNDERSTANDING, IMPROVING, AND STANDARDIZING CARE PROCESSES

Standardized processes, otherwise referred to as best known methods or best known practices, when effectively managed, have shown themselves to be the foundation for improvements in all areas of business today, but especially in the clinical care setting. There is a typical resistance to standardizing practices, especially when they involve providing patient care and services, but the realistic effect of care without standardization must be considered in the following context as described by Joiner (1994):

- ◆ Most employees receive little training on how to do their jobs. Instead the majority are left to learn by watching a more experienced employee.
- ◆ Most employees have developed their own unique versions of any general procedures they witnessed or were taught. They think, "My way is the best way."

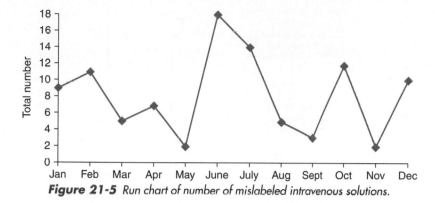

Figure 21-5 *Run chart of number of mislabeled intravenous solutions.*

◆ Changes to procedures happen haphazardly; individuals constantly change details to counteract problems that arise or in hopes of discovering a better method. Tampering is rampant.

Each of the quality management cornerstones could easily be applied to caregiver situations. At first glance it would be assumed that all care practices are based on scientific evidence and research, and although many are, others exist simply because that was how the practitioner originally was educated. Those practices that are research based, even though they represent best known methods, may still not be widely practiced and therefore result in lack of standardization.

During the past few years a number of methods have been used in health care settings for the purpose of supporting standardization of care processes. Clinical guidelines, critical pathways, and case management are standardization methods that are more prevalent and familiar. Although these terms sometimes are used interchangeably, the following is offered as a context in which to understand their potential differences.

Clinical Pathways or Critical Pathways

A clinical pathway or critical pathway typically defines the optimal sequencing and timing of interventions by physicians, nurses, and other interprofessional team members for a particular diagnosis or procedure. These pathways typically are developed through collaborative efforts of the interprofessional team that includes physicians, nurses, pharmacists, and others to improve the quality and value of the patient care provided. Among the most obvious benefits of using clinical pathways are (1) reduction in variation of the care provided, (2) facilitation and achievement of expected clinical outcomes, (3) reduction in care delays and ultimately lengths of stay in the inpatient setting, and (4) improvements in cost-effectiveness of the care delivered while maintaining or increasing patient and family satisfaction. See Chapter 20 for more discussion about clinical pathways.

Clinical Protocols or Algorithms

Clinical protocols or algorithms are different from clinical guidelines because they represent more of a decision path that a practitioner might take during a particular episode or need. For example, common algorithms exist for treatment of hypertension, provision of both basic and advanced life support, and general diagnostic screening (Figure 21-6).

Case Management

Case management embraces somewhat different elements of professional caregiving. Traditionally, case management has been provided by professional registered nurses (RNs) and physicians, although there are appropriate settings in which psychologists or social workers may

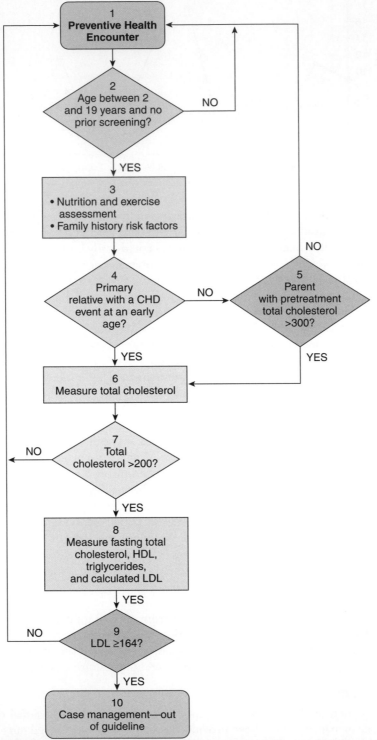

Figure 21-6 *Clinical algorithm—health care guideline: lipid screening in children and adolescents. (From Institute for Clinical Systems Integration [ICSI]: 1996 Health care guidelines, vol 1, Bloomington, MN, 1996, ICSI, p. 141.)*

assume the role. The original intent of case management was to match the most appropriate services to the patient's care needs in the most efficient, effective manner. This could result in reduced costs and lengths of stay, particularly in inpatient settings. Case management is discussed in more detail in Chapter 20.

BREAKTHROUGH THINKING AND PRACTICE INNOVATIONS

Just as standardization is critical to the foundation of health care improvement, so is the notion of breakthrough thinking and swift application of best known methods within the industry. The premise behind breakthrough thinking and its resulting action is threefold: (1) substantial knowledge exists about how to achieve better performance than currently prevails; (2) strong examples already exist of organizations that have applied that knowledge and broken through to substantial results; and (3) the stakes are high and relevant to the most crucial strategic needs of health care (Berwick, 1997).

The Institute for Healthcare Improvement (IHI), a voluntary organization formed to assist leaders in all health care settings actively involved in improving quality, has established and teaches a results methodology that begins with what they term "change concepts." A list of change concepts has been developed by a planning group of national experts in several topic areas, such as reducing cesarean deliveries, reducing patient delays and waiting times, and reducing adverse drug events and medical errors. Organizations use these change concepts to develop specific changes that they test, refine, and implement. For example, hospital systems have tested, refined, and implemented changes that have effectively reduced cesarean section rates while maintaining maternal and infant outcomes.

The model that IHI proposes for improvement essentially is composed of two parts. Part one asks three fundamental questions:

1. What are we trying to accomplish?
2. How will we know that a change is an improvement?
3. What changes can we make that will result in improvement?

Part two uses a sequence of steps, starting with developing an action plan based on the three questions, taking actions to test the action plan, making refinements as needed, and implementing the resulting changes in real work settings. This is known as a "plan-do-check-act" cycle, or PDCA (Figure 21-7). Organizations are supported in determining measurements that provide guidance for further action. The IHI has also established best-practice collaboratives with participating organizations as a way to support implementation of some of the significant IOM safety recommendations (Mechanic, Rogut, and Colby, 2005).

PATIENT SAFETY

Nowhere is the need for quality improvement more evident than in the area of health care errors and patient safety. As discussed previously in this chapter, the IOM report *To Err Is Human: Building a Safer Health System* (2000) placed the issue of medical mistakes on the pages of many national newspapers, on the agendas of health care governing boards, and at the forefront of federal government legislation. In response to the imperative to improve patient safety, leaders of regulatory agencies (i.e., CMS) and accrediting agencies (i.e., TJC) have initiated various programs to promote safer healthcare systems.

Sentinel Event Standard. As one response to the increasing emphasis on patient safety, TJC established its sentinel event standard in 2000. This standard, which continues today, requires organizations to carry out designated steps to fully understand the factors and systems

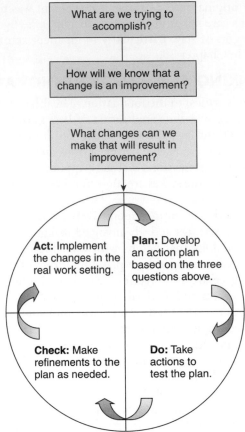

Figure 21-7 *Institute for Healthcare Improvement (IHI) quality improvement model.*

associated with adverse patient events, given that certain defining characteristics have been confirmed. The steps revolve around a "root cause analysis," which is a direct application of the quality improvement principles and methods defined earlier. The intention behind the root cause analysis is to understand the systems at fault within the organization so that improvements can be determined and implemented to prevent any future occurrences. TJC allows organizations a degree of latitude in determining the policy for disclosure of these events to the commission. The commission does validate that organizations have policies and systems in place to address sentinel events.

National Patient Safety Goals. In February 2002, the Sentinel Event Alert Advisory Group was formed to advise TJC in the development of its national safety goals. These goals were to be based on ongoing analyses of reported sentinel events and assessment of the responding recommendations for correcting the identified root causes of these events. An annual review of these goals has resulted in some modification of existing goals and the creation of new ones as evidenced in the published list for 2009 (Box 21-3). Subsequently the purpose of TJC's national patient safety goals has been modified to state that the purpose is to promote specific improvements in patient safety with the goals highlighting problematic areas

BOX **21-3**

The 2010 National Patient Safety Goals for Hospitals

Improve the accuracy of patient identification.
- Use of two patient identifiers
- Eliminating transfusion errors

Improve the effectiveness of communication among caregivers.
- Timely reporting of critical tests and critical results

Improve the safety of using medications.
- Labeling medications
- Reducing harm from anticoagulation therapy

Reduce the risk of health care–associated infections.
- Meeting hand hygiene guidelines
- Preventing multidrug-resistant organism infections
- Preventing central line–associated blood stream infections
- Preventing surgical site infections

Accurately and completely reconcile medications across the continuum of care. **Note:** All requirements for this goal are not in effect at this time.
- Comparing current and newly ordered medications
- Communicating medications to the next provider
- Providing a reconciled medication list to the patient
- Settings in which Medications Are Minimally Used (NPSG.08.04.01)

Reduce the risk of patient harm resulting from falls.

Prevent health care–associated pressure ulcers.

The organization identifies safety risks inherent in its patient population.
- Identifying individuals at risk for suicide

Universal protocol for preventing wrong site, wrong procedure, and wrong person surgery
- Conducting a pre-procedure verification process
- Marking the procedure site
- Performing a time-out

The Joint Commission. *2010 National Patient Safety Goals — Hospitals.* Available at http:www.jointcommission.org/PatientSafety/NationalPatientSafetyGoals/.

and evidence-based solutions to the problems with system-wide solutions wherever possible (TJC, 2008).

Never Events. In 2006 the CMS announced that they would investigate ways that Medicare could help decrease or eliminate the occurrence of never events—serious and costly errors in health care delivery that should never happen. Examples of such events included wrong site surgery or mismatched blood transfusions, which could cause serious injury or death to the patient and result in increased costs to Medicare. The CMS worked with the National Quality Forum (NQF) to determine which events would be included in this category. The initial list included significant and focused events that occurred as a result of surgery, faulty and/or misuse of products or devices, failure to protect patients, care management mishaps, or problems related to environmental or criminal happenings. In 2008, the CMS began selecting hospital-acquired conditions that were determined to be reasonably preventable and would no longer pay the additional cost of hospitalization of such conditions if an extended stay was necessary. As of 2008, the CMS listed eight preventable conditions for which it would not make additional payments. On July 31, 2009, CMS issued a final rule which did not change the list of hospital-acquired conditions but stated plans for evaluating the impact of the existing policy on hospital practices and patient care. For more information on never events, visit the CMS website at: www.cms.hhs.gov/apps/media/press/factsheet.asp?Coun ter=3043.

The Professional Nurse and Patient Safety

Many experts argue that the answers for improved patient safety cannot lie within regulatory agencies alone. The answers reside in care providers pulling together to review critical circumstances and learning from key events. Basic improvement principles can help direct possible solutions within an organization by pinpointing warning flags through analyzing data, applying tools and methods to address the concerns, and continually evaluating the resulting patient outcomes.

For nurses the challenge starts with making patient safety improvement and reducing errors not just an organizational priority, but a personal one as well. This means buying into a state of mind that recognizes the complexity and high-risk nature of modern health care and subscribing to implementing standardized best practices and eliminating never events. Two significant nursing functions that clearly have an effect on patient safety, quality of care, and resulting outcomes are:
1. Monitoring for early recognition of adverse events, complications and errors
2. Initiating deployment of appropriate care providers for timely intervention and response and rescue of patients in these situations

A critical factor in supporting a nurse's ability to carry out these two functions is the available level of nurse staffing. Although defining the actual level of staffing is a matter of debate and scrutiny, there is widespread recognition that a strong linkage exists between patient outcomes and nurse staffing resulting from various published studies (Aiken et al, 2008; Mechanic et al, 2005). Chapter 12 presents a thorough discussion about strategies nurses can use to promote quality care and a safe work environment.

Nursing Quality Indicators. The governing body of the American Nurses Association (ANA) established the National Database of Nursing Quality Indicators (NDNQI) in 1998 as part of the ANA's safety and quality initiative. This national database program collects designated indicators (Box 21-4) strongly affecting patient clinical outcomes for two major purposes: (1) to provide comparative data to health care organizations to help support quality improvement activities, and (2) to develop national data to better understand the link between nurse staffing and patient outcomes. As of 2009, 1200 hospitals had joined the database with quarterly reports now being provided to these organizations for analysis of their own care processes and support systems as related to nurse staffing (ANA, 2009).

Interprofessional Team Work. Equally critical in its effect on patient safety is the work environment that supports the interdependence and effective communication of nurses with other health care professionals. Most nurses and other clinical staff assume they already work in teams; however, teamwork concepts are infrequently taught in most basic educational programs and are very limited within a typical medical school curriculum (Mann, Marcus, and Sachs, 2006). Patient care is dependent on effective communication to support the coordination of activities that promote efficiency and safety. The AHRQ and the U.S. Department of Defense have joined forces to create a national training and support network called the TeamSTEPPS (Team Strategies and Tools to Enhance Performance and Patient Safety)

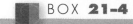

BOX **21-4**

The National Database of Nursing Quality Indicators (NDNQI)

Patient falls and patient falls with injury

Pressure ulcers (community acquired, hospital acquired, unit acquired)

Skill mix (registered nurses [RNs], licensed practical nurses [LPNs] or licensed vocational nurses [LVNs], unlicensed assistive personnel)

Nursing hours per patient-day

RN surveys (job satisfaction, practice environment scale)

RN education and certification

Pediatric pain assessment cycle and intravenous infiltration rate

Psychiatric patient assault rate

Restraints prevalence

Nurse turnover

Nosocomial infections (ventilator-assisted pneumonia, central line–associated blood stream infection, catheter-associated urinary tract infections)

American Nurses Association: Available at: www.nursingquality.org.

project. TeamSTEPPS is an evidence-based teamwork system aimed at optimizing patient outcomes by improving communication and teamwork skills among health care professionals. Four major strategies used in the TeamSTEPPS project to produce higher-quality safer patient care are:

1. "Producing highly effective medical teams that optimize the use of information, people, and resources to achieve the best clinical outcomes for patients
2. Increasing team awareness and clarifying team roles and responsibilities
3. Resolving conflicts and improving information sharing
4. Eliminating barriers to quality and safety" (AHRQ, 2009, par. 2)

ROLE OF PROFESSIONAL NURSES IN QUALITY IMPROVEMENT

There are lessons for all nurses from one of the original patient safety and quality improvement mentors, Florence Nightingale. Nightingale used data to support her efforts to reduce the incidence and spread of infections in the patient wards she was accountable for during the Crimean War. What resulted from her work was a broader shift in the culture of health care at that time. Culture is defined as a system of shared beliefs, values, customs, behaviors, and material objects that members of a society use to cope with their world and with each other that is passed on from generation to generation through learning. Culture may be viewed as almost any form of behavior that is learned rather than instinctive or inherited (Bates and Fratkin, 1999).

What can result from the current emphasis on quality and patient safety is a shift in the health care culture. "Building health care systems that do no harm" will increasingly be the shared value and goal of all those involved in patient care delivery. Nurses are in the perfect position to lead this cultural change. Quality improvement should not be considered a separate function within the role of care provider, but rather an ongoing part of the professional role for all health care professionals. Box 21-5 presents a list of online resources to help the professional nurse seek more information about how to improve the quality of care for all patients.

BOX **21-5**

Helpful Websites and Online Resources

The Institute for Healthcare Improvement (IHI)
 www.ihi.org
The Agency for Healthcare Research and Quality(AHRQ)
 www.ahrq.gov
National Association for Healthcare Quality (NAHQ)
 www.nahq.org
The Joint Commission (TJC)
 www.jointcommission.org
The Institute for Safe Medication Practices (ISMP)
 www.ismp.org
American Society for Quality (ASQ)
 www.asq.org
National Patient Safety Foundation (NPSF)
 www.npsf.org
Picker Institute
 www.pickerinstitute.org
Partnership for Patient Safety (p4ps)
 www.p4ps.org
Hughes RG: *Patient safety and quality: an evidence-based handbook for nurses.* 2008. AHRQ
Publication No. 08-0043. Available free at:
 www.ahrq.gov/qual/nurseshdbk/docs/FrontMatter_NursesHandbook.pdf

SUMMARY

For today's graduating nurses the challenge is to find whatever means are available to refine the knowledge and skills fundamentally necessary to enter a partnership with all other interprofessional team members in the ongoing improvement of health care. Just as essential to professional nursing practice as knowing, for instance, the symptoms of diabetic ketoacidosis or how to give an injection, are understanding the basic principles of quality management, process improvement, and variation; using clinical indicators, process improvement tools, and standardized care processes; and addressing patient safety in every aspect of care. Every nurse should enter practice accepting accountability for the quality of care provided by the health care organization and taking a leadership role to implement improvements to achieve health care that is safe, timely, effective, efficient, equitable, and patient centered.

⊖volve Additional resources are available online at: http://evolve.elsevier.com/Cherry/

REFERENCES

Agency for Healthcare Research and Quality (AHRQ): *National healthcare disparities report*, 2008. Available at www.ahrq.org.

Agency for Healthcare Research and Quality (AHRQ): *TeamSTEPPS: National implementation*, 2009. Available at http://teamstepps.ahrq.gov/about-2cl_3.htm.

Aiken LH, et al: Effects of hospital care environment on patient mortality and nurse outcomes, *JONA* 38(5): 220–226, 2008.

American Nurses Association: *The National Center for Nursing Quality*, 2009. Available at www.nursingworld. org/MainMenuCategories/ThePracticeofProfessional Nursing/PatientSafetyQuality.aspx.

Bates D, Fratkin E: *Cultural anthropology*, ed 2, Toronto, Canada, 1999, Prentice-Hall.

Berwick D: The breakthrough series, *Qual Connect* 6(2):11, 1997.

Bliersbach CM: *Guide to QM*, Skokie, IL, 1992, National Association for Healthcare Quality.

Frankel AS, et al: *The essential guide for patient safety officers*, Oakbrook Terrace, IL, 2009, Joint Commission Resources, Inc.

Institute of Medicine, Kohn L, Corrigan J, Donaldson M, editors. *To err is human: building a safer health system*, Washington, DC, 2000, National Academies Press.

Institute of Medicine: *Report brief: crossing the quality chasm: a new health system for the 21st century*, 2001. Available at www.nap.edu/html/quality_chasm/reportbrief.pdf.

Institute of Medicine, Greiner AC, Knebel E, editors: *Health professions education: a bridge to quality*, Washington, DC, 2003, National Academies Press.

Institute of Medicine: *American's uninsured crisis: consequences for health and health care*, Washington, DC, 2009, National Academies Press.

Institute for Safe Medication Practices: *Medication self-assessment for automated dispensing cabinets*, 2009. Available at www.ismp.org/selfassessments/ADC/Survey.pdf.

Joiner Associates: *Plain and simple: introduction to the tools*, Madison, WI, 1995, Joiner Associates.

Joiner BL: *Fourth generation management*, New York, 1994, McGraw-Hill.

Mann S, Marcus R, Sachs B: Lessons from the cockpit: how team training can reduce errors on L&D, *Contemp Ob/GyN* (1):1–7, 2006.

Mechanic D, Rogut LB, Colby DC: *Policy challenges in modern health care*, Piscataway, NJ, 2005, Rutgers University Press.

Neave HR: *The Deming dimension*, Knoxville, TN, 1990, SPC Press.

Porter M, Teisberg E: *Redefining healthcare: creating value-based competition on results*, Boston, 2006, Harvard Business School Press.

The Joint Commission (TJC): *Accreditation program: hospital chapter: national patient safety goals*, Oakbrook Terrace, IL, 2008, TJC. Available at www.jointcommission.org/PatientSafety/NationalPatientSafetyGoals/09_hap_npsgs.htm.

Quality and Safety Education in Nursing (QSEN)

Gwen Sherwood, PhD, RN, FAAN

Rodney (Rod) W. Hicks, PhD, RN, FNP-BC, FAANP, FAAN

evolve Additional resources are available online at: http://evolve.elsevier.com/Cherry/

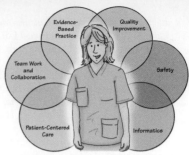

Transforming practice through quality and safety competencies.

VIGNETTE

Glenda Rogers is a senior student nurse and is doing a clinical rotation at a leading academic medical center on a busy medical unit. The unit uses electronic medication administration records, automated dispensing cabinets, and "smart pumps" to regulate many intravenous fluids. The unit staff is composed of 70% registered nurses (RNs) and 30% other licensed individuals.

On this particular day Glenda checked her patient's morning medications with the assigned RN preceptor and helped withdraw the medications from the automated dispensing cabinet. The RN preceptor verified the medications and was reasonably comfortable with Glenda's performance and attention to detail because she was able to give a verbal summary of why each medication was appropriate for the patient and confirmed the name and the dose. Given that Glenda's nursing instructor was also available, the RN preceptor left to provide care to her other assigned patients. Glenda went to the patient's room and observed that the hospital's intravenous team members were in the final steps of initiating a new intravenous catheter in the patient's left forearm. As soon as the intravenous nurse provided report on the procedure, Glenda began to administer the morning medications. Her instructor entered the room and noticed instantly that she was administering 5 mL of guaifenesin through the intravenous line instead of the patient's feeding tube.

The instructor stopped the intravenous infusion, attempted to aspirate contents, and immediately notified the RN preceptor and nurse manager. The nurse manager quickly contacted the drug information center in the hospital's pharmacy for advice on management options. The attending physician was also contacted. Within minutes it was determined that no additional treatment could be given to the patient and the patient's condition was considered stable.

Within the hour the physician, drug information specialist, nurse manager, nursing instructor, RN preceptor, risk manager, chief nursing officer, and Glenda met to review the incident. According to hospital policy an incident report was required given the practice variance. The risk manager led the completion of the incident report by exploring questions about the general conditions on the unit at the time of the incident and the personnel involved in the care of the patient. The risk manager also inquired about the medication error and the supplies associated with the error. The preliminary conclusion was that the guaifenesin was contained in a syringe with a Luer-lock connection and was connected to the intravenous tubing instead of the feeding tube adapter. It was determined that if the medication had been contained in an oral dosing syringe, it would not have been possible to administer the medication intravenously. The team also agreed that it was of utmost importance to inform the patient and family members about the incident as soon as possible.

■ QUESTIONS TO CONSIDER WHILE READING THIS CHAPTER:

1 What could Glenda, the nursing instructor, or the RN preceptor have done to prevent this error?

2 What ways can nurses examine system failures to increase awareness and surveillance to prevent potential errors?

3 How can nurses transform their practice by incorporating the six quality and safety competencies as defined by the Institute of Medicine: patient-centered care, teamwork and collaboration, evidence-based practice, continuous quality improvement, safety, and informatics?

4 How can nurses integrate continuous quality improvement as an ongoing part of their professional role?

KEY TERMS

Adverse event Any injury caused by medical care (Agency for Healthcare Research and Quality [AHRQ], 2009a).

Benchmark An attribute or achievement that serves as a standard for providers or institutions to emulate (AHRQ, 2009a).

Checklist Algorithmic listing of actions to be performed for a given clinical procedure designed to ensure that no matter how often performed by a given clinician, no step will be forgotten (AHRQ, 2009a).

Competency The ability to clearly demonstrate the knowledge, skills, attitudes, and professional judgment required to practice safely and ethically in a designated role and setting (Nurses Board of South Australia, 2004).

Electronic health record (EHR) The medical record in digital format that serves as the primary source of information for health care, meeting all clinical, legal, and administrative requirements for medical records; the EHR is capable of being shared electronically among health care providers and patients.

Error reporting system A formal system, either voluntary or mandatory, that collects data pertaining to adverse events for purposes of learning, accountability, or effecting change.

Human factors The study of human abilities and characteristics as they affect the design and smooth operation of equipment, systems, and jobs (AHRQ, 2009a).

Incident reporting The identification and reporting of occurrences that could have led, or did lead, to an undesirable outcome (AHRQ, 2009a).

Just culture An organizational culture that promotes patient safety by acknowledging that competent health care professionals may make mistakes but should not be held accountable for system failings over which they have no control. However, the just culture does not tolerate reckless behavior or a conscious disregard of risk to patients; thus it is not considered a "no blame" culture (AHRQ, 2009a).

Quality and Safety Education in Nursing (QSEN) A national program that addresses the challenge of preparing future nurses with the knowledge, skills, and attitudes (KSA) necessary to continually improve the quality and safety of the health care systems in which they work.

SBAR (Situation-Background-Assessment-Recommendation) A communication technique that provides a framework for communication among members of the health care team about a patient's condition.

Sentinel event Defined by The Joint Commission (2008) as an unexpected occurrence involving patient death or serious physical or psychologic injury or the risk thereof. Serious injury specifically includes loss of limb or function. The phrase "or the risk thereof" includes any situation for which a recurrence would carry a significant chance of a serious adverse outcome. Such events are called sentinel because they signal the need for immediate investigation and response.

Standard of care The knowledge and skill the average prudent clinician would possess and exercise in the same or similar circumstances based on evidence (AHRQ, 2009a).

After studying this chapter, the reader will be able to:

1 Describe driving forces for quality and safety competency in nursing.

2 Define the six core quality competencies integrated into nursing curricula to prepare nurses for working in systems focused on quality.

3 Base nursing care delivery on the knowledge, skills, and attitudes defining the six core competencies.

4 Evaluate nurses' roles in improving health care quality.

CHAPTER OVERVIEW

A mandate for sweeping changes in the U.S. health care system emerged from a series of revealing reports known as the Quality Chasm Series *issued by the Institute of Medicine (IOM) detailing issues in quality and safety. To accomplish its recommendations for a redesigned health system to improve quality outcomes, the IOM declared education as the bridge to quality through major redesign of health professions education focusing on six core competencies:*

◆ *Patient-centered care*

◆ *Teamwork and collaboration*

◆ *Evidence-based practice*

◆ *Quality improvement*

◆ *Safety*

◆ *Informatics*

These six competencies should form the practice base for all health professionals. This chapter examines how nurses' work is being redesigned in response to the IOM challenges with discussion of the knowledge, skills, and attitudes required in new roles and responsibilities.

Nurses have traditionally focused their care on the patient, adhered to safety concerns, and managed increasingly complex interventions. In redefined nurses' work and professional identity, nurses are implementing continuous quality improvement initiatives, participating in analysis of adverse events, and leading interprofessional teams. What are the knowledge, skills, and attitudes required to fulfill these new opportunities for leadership? This chapter examines each competency to describe new interpretations of the traditional terms of patient-centered care, teamwork and collaboration, evidence-based practice, continuous quality improvement, safety, and informatics

QUALITY AND SAFETY: THE NEW STANDARD FOR NURSING EDUCATION

The United States is considered to have the world's most technologically advanced health care system delivered by a dedicated and highly skilled workforce, state-of-the-art technology, and advanced pharmacologic agents. It is also recognized as the most expensive system in the world (Anderson et al, 2005; Gabel and Fitzner, 2003). Still, failures in the system occur with some regularity. Health care lags behind other high-performance industries such as aviation and nuclear power in focusing on quality and safety as an industry standard (Kohn, Corrigan, and Donaldson, 2000).

Through the *Quality Chasm* reports the IOM has sustained the emphasis on the imperative to transform the U.S. health care system in order to address inconsistent outcomes and prevent errors (Bates et al, 1997; Committee on Quality of Health Care in America, 2001; Kohn et al, 2000). Poor quality outcomes and medical errors erode public confidence, increase health care costs, and increase morbidity and mortality. Simply put, health care errors strike at the heart of the health care system—the responsibility to do good and avoid harm (Mayo and Duncan, 2004).

Recommendations for health professions' education outlined in the 2003 *Health Professions Education: A Bridge to Quality* (Greiner and Knebel, 2003) identify competencies or abilities that all health care professionals should achieve to transform health care systems, reduce errors, and improve quality outcomes. Educators are mindfully altering educational experiences to help students form a professional identity in preparation to deliver *patient-centered care* as members of an *interprofessional team*, emphasizing *evidence-based practice*, *quality improvement*, and *informatics* (Cronenwett et al, 2007; Greiner and Knebel, 2003). The competencies are not discrete concepts but overlap; it is difficult to work on any one without an overlay of the knowledge, skills, and attitudes that define another.

Underlying concepts for redesigned systems recognize that health care organizations, like other high-reliability industries, are complex, internally dynamic, and interactive. They are charged with performing exacting tasks under considerable time pressures and sometimes, extreme conditions, yet work with a focus on where the next adverse event will occur as a major prevention strategy. Such organizations recognize that changing the system requires understanding the circumstances at every step of an event by studying what happened. What is learned is applied to prevent future occurrences. Shifting from an individual blame approach to a system approach allows the integration of all the competencies that include the patient and family as partners in creating a safer system. As systems redesign around quality and safety, nurses have opportunities for helping shape health care and improve outcomes.

History of QSEN

Emerging opportunities for nurses to have key roles in transforming the health care system require new learning experiences and incorporating the six competencies from the IOM's recommendations. Through support from the Robert Wood Johnson Foundation, the national Quality and Safety Education for Nurses (QSEN) project was created to develop and facilitate the execution of changes in nursing education (Cronenwett et al, 2007), offer new opportunities for faculty development, and to learn from a 15-school pilot collaborative (Cronenwett, Sherwood, and Gelmon, 2009).

Leading scholars in each of the six competencies as well as pedagogical experts were selected as QSEN faculty to lead the change. Recognizing that policy changes would be needed to achieve curricula innovation, a QSEN advisory board included leaders from regulatory agencies who define educational standards, physicians to cross-walk with changes in medical education, and innovators with experience in leading other major educational changes (Cronenwett et al, 2007). The groups used an iterative process beginning with a literature review, draft of definitions including the knowledge, skills and attitudes of the IOM competencies relevant to all entry level registered nurses (RNs), and discussion of pedagogies for achieving behavioral changes. Although the IOM identified five competencies, the QSEN faculty determined that quality and safety should be separate competencies because of the science supporting each of these areas.

The six competencies, at first look, appear to be familiar topics to faculty and students, as indicated in a 2007 survey of schools to determine if they are teaching this content (Smith,

Cronenwett, and Sherwood, 2007), yet focus groups indicated the need for faculty development and translation into curricular essentials. The six competencies were incorporated into nursing education standards and the licensure examination (American Association of Colleges of Nursing, 2008; Smith et al, 2007). A robust website, www.QSEN.org, posts information on the competencies, an annotated bibliography for each competency, and peer-reviewed teaching strategies.

The Robert Wood Johnson Foundation supported the Pilot School Collaborative to model how faculty could include the six competencies in prelicensure programs. Fifteen schools, representing BSN, ADN, and diploma programs, were selected to receive grants to support the collaborative work. Each school completed curricular mapping and exemplar projects, which are posted on the QSEN website (Cronenwett et al, 2009). Schools completed a student survey of graduating seniors to determine student self-assessment of their mastery of the competencies (Sullivan, Hirst, and Cronenwett, 2009). Findings reinforced the value that recent graduates and faculty place on the competencies, the need to increase knowledge about patient safety practices, and the opportunities for faculty development and redesigned student learning experiences.

APPLYING THE COMPETENCIES IN PRACTICE

Nurses have traditionally focused their care on the patient, adhered to safety concerns, and managed increasingly complex interventions. In redefining nurses' work and professional identity based on the six competencies, nurses are implementing continuous quality improvement initiatives, participating in analysis of adverse events, and leading interprofessional teams. What are the knowledge, skills, and attitudes required to fulfill these new opportunities for leadership? The following sections examine each competency to describe new interpretations of patient-centered care, teamwork and collaboration, evidence-based practice, continuous quality improvement, safety, and informatics.

Patient-Centered Care

The essential feature of patient-centered care is knowing the patient well enough to be able to see health care situations through the patient lens (Cronenwett et al, 2007) with recognition of the patient's values and health beliefs. It involves eliciting and incorporating patient preferences and values in the plan of care. In a patient-centered care model, patients and families participate in nursing and medical decision making and in care coordination with all members of the health care team (Chapman, 2009). Patient-centered care respects the diversity of the human experience so that nurses must examine their own attitudes about working with individuals and groups whose values differ from their own. Examples of critical questions to ask in a patient-centered care approach include (Day and Smith, 2007):

- ◆ What is the most important thing I could do for my patient at this moment?
- ◆ How can the patient and/or family participate in accurately assessing the patient's pain and determining the best pain management plan that recognizes the patient's attitudes and expectations about pain and suffering?
- ◆ How can I assist family members with visiting hours and access to their family member to allay anxiety and include them as partners in care?

Patient-centered care requires nurses to seek out and apply interventions gleaned from broad-based populations, textbooks, and other reputable sources to the individual patients receiving the care. This broad-to-specific application ensures that standards of care are followed while tailoring the care to the immediate needs of the client and/or family (Boehm and

TABLE **22-1**

Patient-Centered Care

Definition: Recognize the patient or designee as the source of control and full partner in providing compassionate and coordinated care based on respect for patient preferences, values, and needs

KNOWLEDGE	SKILLS	ATTITUDES
Integrate understanding of multiple dimensions of patient-centered care	Elicit patient values, preferences, and expressed needs as part of clinical interview	Value seeing health care situations "through patients' eyes"
Describe how diverse cultural, ethnic, and social backgrounds function as sources of patient, family, and community values	Communicate patient values, preferences, and expressed needs to other members of the health care team	Respect and encourage individual expression of patient values, preferences, and expressed needs

Adapted from Cronenwett L et al: Quality and safety education for nurses, *Nurs Outlook* 55(3):122-131, 2007.

Morast, 2009). Table 22-1 presents the QSEN definition and knowledge, skills and attitudes related to patient-centered care.

Teamwork and Collaboration

Traditional views of teamwork have applied to nursing teams and focus on delegation and team functioning. New views of teamwork recognize the interprofessional nature of coordinating the increasing complexities of patient care among nurses, physicians, pharmacists, therapists, dietitians, social workers, and many other health care team members. The unsettling IOM report, *To Err Is Human* (Kohn et al, 2000), revealed that up to 66% of health care errors are related to poor working relationships and communication (Figure 22-1). Teams with shared communication demonstrate better patient outcomes (Shojania et al, 2001) yet few health professions education programs integrate learning with other disciplines.

One widely used team training approach for health care teams is TeamSTEPPS (Team Strategies and Tools to Enhance Performance and Patient Safety), developed by the U.S. Department of Defense TriCARE Management Activity and customized for broad application by the Agency for Healthcare Research and Quality (AHRQ, 2009b). TeamSTEPPS acknowledges that team training and enhanced communication are among the essential components of a comprehensive patient safety system. Based on the TeamSTEPPS framework, effective interprofessional teams include the following components:

- ◆ Dynamic rather than static membership that changes from patient to patient and even daily for the same patient depending on the care goals and needs for that patient.
- ◆ Team members who consistently use situation monitoring to recognize who needs to be out front as leader in a given circumstance, based on professional role, patient priorities, and unique circumstances.
- ◆ Team leaders who articulate clear goals and make it easy for team members to contribute, to speak up, and to ask questions that ensure appropriate care decisions. Leaders model mutual respect for the whole team, including the patient, and value the team contribution over the individual contribution.
- ◆ Team briefings to plan care together, huddles to problem solve, and debriefings after events to examine what happened and how to improve.

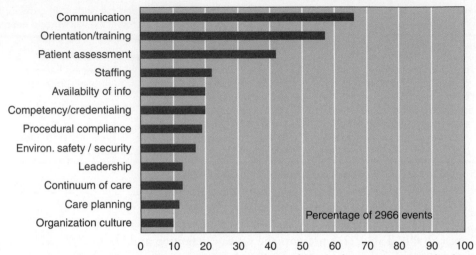

Figure 22-1 *Analysis of sentinel events from 1995 to 2004 indicates failures of communication to be the root cause of the event in about 65% of cases. (The Joint Commission:* Improving America's hospitals: The Joint Commission's annual report on quality and safety, 2007. *Available online at: www.jointcommission.org/Library/annual_report.)*

The TeamSTEPPS curriculum includes a set of standardized communication strategies to help team members share concerns, clarify decisions about care, and ensure accurate and complete information exchange (Box 22-1). Ideally all members of the team recognize and respect these communication strategies so that team members can share a concern by stating, "I need clarity," which essentially means "Stop, we have a potential problem. I see something I think is wrong." It is a way of communicating concerns without alarm in a calm manner.

Team members use situation monitoring to actively scan behaviors and actions to assess elements of the environment and situations as they are happening. Team members monitor safety by monitoring the actions of team members in a system of checks and balances, called "watching each other's backs," and acknowledge the other's help when an error is thus avoided. The shared accountability builds mutual trust across the team. Team members use situational awareness to share mental models of a situation to be sure that everyone is on the same page. Sharing one's perception can avoid confusion and ensure all are working toward agreed-upon patient care goals. With teamwork and collaboration as a core competency for nursing practice, nurses must focus on how to function effectively as members of interprofessional teams. Table 22-2 presents the QSEN definition and knowledge, skills, and attitudes related to teamwork and collaboration.

Evidence-Based Practice

Evidence-based practice has become a core competency for safe, high-quality nursing practice. Nurses must be able to determine the best approach to nursing care interventions by navigating through various levels of constantly changing scientific knowledge, clinical opinions, and time-honored traditions as well as patient and family preferences. As nurses encounter new

BOX **22-1**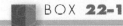

Communication Strategies for Effective Teamwork (TeamSTEPPS) (AHRQ, 2009b)

Structured communication can ensure accurate information exchange and shared decision making and help providers develop shared mental models to know what to expect, synchronize care, and mitigate errors. The nurse's surveillance role often means he or she has information critical to care management.

1. SBAR
   a. Situation: patient information and brief sentence of what is happening now
   b. Background: diagnosis, relevant lab and assessment data, chief complaints
   c. Assessment: analysis of the problem, what is of concern
   d. Recommendation: form as a question of what may be a solution or request for help
2. Call-out: Provider calls out critical information so all team members can hear during urgent situations to help anticipate next steps.
3. Check-back: Repeat back what is heard. For example: "I need 3 mg epinephrine." "Three mg epinephrine, here."
4. Mutual support: Team members cross-monitor and help overloaded team members, redistribute tasks, offer verbal support, encourage others, and share information and safety alerts.
5. Hand-off: Checklists ensure the transfer of information, authority, and responsibility when transferring care along the continuum with an opportunity to ask questions and clarify and confirm information.
6. Critical language: Providers are taught key phrases understood by all team members to mean, "Stop. We may have a problem."
   a. Examples include CUS: "I need some CLARITY. I am UNCERTAIN. I have a SAFETY concern."
   b. Team members assertively voice a concern two times to ensure it was heard using the three C's: "I'm **c**urious; I'm **c**oncerned; I'm still uncomfortable, let's **c**onsult with a third party."

TABLE **22-2**

Teamwork and Collaboration

Definition: Function effectively within nursing and interprofessional teams, fostering open communication, mutual respect, and shared decision making to achieve quality patient care

KNOWLEDGE	SKILLS	ATTITUDES
Describe one's own strengths, limitations, and values in functioning as a team member	Demonstrate awareness of one's own strengths and limitations as a team member	Acknowledge one's own potential to contribute to effective team functioning
Describe examples of the effect of team functioning on safety and quality of care	Follow communication practices that minimize risks associated with hand-offs among providers and across transitions in care	Appreciate the risks associated with hand-offs among providers and across transitions in care

Adapted from Cronenwett L et al: Quality and safety education for nurses, *Nurs Outlook* 55(3):122-131, 2007.

clinical problems in direct patient or population care, they will combine skills from another competency—informatics—to quickly locate information and assess its validity and value for a given situation. Chapter 6 offers guidelines for evidence-based nursing practice including methods to evaluate research studies and determine how results might be applicable to clinical practice. Table 22-3 presents the QSEN definition and knowledge, skills, and attitudes related to evidence-based practice.

TABLE **22-3**

Evidence-Based Practice (EBP)

Definition: Integrate best current evidence with clinical expertise and patient/family preferences and values for delivery of optimal health care

KNOWLEDGE	SKILLS	ATTITUDES
Demonstrate knowledge of basic scientific methods and processes	Participate effectively in appropriate data collection and other research activities	Appreciate strengths and weaknesses of scientific bases for practice
Discriminate between valid and invalid reasons for modifying evidence-based clinical practice based on clinical expertise or patient/family preferences	Consult with clinical experts before deciding to deviate from evidence-based protocols	Acknowledge own limitations in knowledge and clinical expertise before determining when to deviate from evidence-based best practices

Adapted from Cronenwett L et al: Quality and safety education for nurses, *Nurs Outlook* 55(3):122-131, 2007.

TABLE **22-4**

Quality Improvement

Definition: Use data to monitor the outcomes of care processes and use improvement methods to design and test changes to continually improve the quality and safety of health care systems

KNOWLEDGE	SKILLS	ATTITUDES
Describe strategies for learning about the outcomes of care in the setting in which one is engaged in clinical practice	Seek information about outcomes of care for populations served in care setting	Appreciate that continual quality improvement is an essential part of the daily work of all health professionals
Describe approaches for changing processes of care	Design a small test of change in daily work	Appreciate the value of what individuals and teams can do to improve care

Adapted from Cronenwett L et al: Quality and safety education for nurses, *Nurs Outlook* 55(3):122-131, 2007.

Quality Improvement

Consumer demand for quality outcomes in health care has helped drive a quality-focused culture. Health care organizations with a quality culture encourage inquiry, asking questions about what, how, and why health professionals do what they do. Adverse events and near misses are investigated systematically from a system perspective to determine points in the design or protocol when errors can be prevented. Organizations focused on quality use practice standards and protocols based on the latest evidence while considering patient preferences, values, and needs at the moment.

To guide improvement activities, organizations typically adopt a quality improvement (QI) methodology such as Six Sigma or the Institute for Healthcare Improvement (IHI) Model (see Chapter 21). With QI as a core competency for nursing practice, nurses need to clearly understand and be able to use the QI model adopted by their work setting. Chapter 21 provides more detailed information about QI and the use of QI tools and models. Table 22-4 presents the QSEN definition and knowledge, skills and attitudes related to quality improvement.

Safety

In the QSEN project, safety and quality were defined as separate competencies to emphasize patient safety as the new standard of care. This new view of safety is more than monitoring the patient to maintain a safe environment. Health care professionals with a focus on patient safety and error prevention apply the knowledge of human factors, value learning from adverse events through event reporting and analysis, and promote and support a "just culture." Health care organizations focused on safety use constant surveillance to manage the potential for humans (health professionals) to make unintentional mistakes. Organizations with a just culture promote learning from adverse events while recognizing that even competent health care professionals may make mistakes but should not be held accountable for system failings over which they have no control (Mayer and Cronin, 2008).

Factors that contribute to health care errors involve human factors such as circumstances in the workplace, provider characteristics and training, and interactions among providers. For example, adequate staffing is difficult to predict because patients have such variability in needs and patient census fluctuates. Chronic shortages in the nursing workforce often contribute to nurses' overload of responsibilities. To accomplish their work, nurses are subject to frequent interruptions, the need to multitask, and reliance on "work-arounds" because of inadequate system support. Additionally, the high risk nature of nurses' work carries intense physical and emotional tensions. Fixation on completing certain tasks can be a blinder to other developments, thus opportunities to stop an error may be lost. Inconsistent skills in communicating with various members of the health care team (for example, excessive professional courtesy with physicians) can contribute to safety issues.

Another important aspect of safety is how errors are viewed, from the individual approach or from a systems approach (Reason, 2000). Each model yields different philosophies of error management. Reason's error model states that the individual approach to errors blames individuals for forgetfulness, inattention, or moral weakness. A systems approach, on the other hand, examines conditions under which individuals work (as described in the previous paragraph) and sets up defenses to avert errors or mitigate their effects. With patient safety as a core competency for nursing practice, nurses must take responsibility to promote a just culture and systems approach to preventing errors and actively promoting patient safety. Table 22-5 presents the QSEN definition and knowledge, skills, and attitudes related to safety.

TABLE **22-5**

 Safety

Definition: Minimizes risk of harm to patients and providers through system effectiveness and individual performance

KNOWLEDGE	SKILLS	ATTITUDES
Examine human factors and other basic safety design principles as well as commonly used unsafe practices	Demonstrate effective use of technology and standardization practices that support safety and quality	Value the contributions of standardization/reliability to safety
Discuss potential and actual effect of national patient resources, initiatives, and regulations	Use national patient safety resources for professional development and to focus attention on safety in care settings	Value relationship between national safety campaigns and implementation in local practices and practice settings

Adapted from Cronenwett L et al: Quality and safety education for nurses, *Nurs Outlook* 55(3):122-131, 2007.

Informatics

Health care in general has been slow in adapting informatics and information technology (IT) to manage information and to improve communication across systems of care. Cost is a major inhibitor to state-of-the-art IT as organizations struggle with the economics of health care, coupled with the rapid development of technology, making it hard to remain current. Informatics and IT are links to ensure patient safety through improved information access and data management.

Nurses can and should play crucial roles in organizations to help shape the design, purchase and implementation of technology to match clinical needs throughout the organization (McKesson, 2009). In a national survey of nurses employed in an informatics role (n = 432), respondents felt that by contributing to the organization's IT plan, they had a significant effect in areas of patient safety, clinician workflow, and end-user acceptance of the product. Informatics nurses who responded to the survey performed a variety of IT-related job responsibilities including end-user education, workflow analysis, system implementation, and ongoing user support (McKesson, 2009). Competency in informatics means that nurses must have access in their work settings to the expansive areas of clinical knowledge and research to support evidence-based practice, quality improvement strategies, and solving unique clinical problems. Table 22-6 presents the QSEN definition and knowledge, skills, and attitudes related to informatics.

IMPLICATIONS FOR PRACTICE

Health care organizations focusing on quality and safety have defining characteristics that enable nurses to apply the six core competencies (Page, 2004). By encouraging inquiry, making it okay to ask questions, resources are provided to access information needed through various means including informatics. Standards of care are evidence based, quality reporting is benchmarked against industry standards, and critical incidents are investigated within a just culture from a systems perspective. Such organizations value and reward knowledge workers—characterized as those who engage in their work, ask critical questions, and continually seek to improve outcomes of care.

TABLE **22-6**

Informatics

Definition: Use information and technology to communicate, manage knowledge, mitigate error, and support decision-making

KNOWLEDGE	SKILLS	ATTITUDES
Identify essential information that must be available in a common database to support patient care	Navigate the electronic health record	Value technologies that support clinical decision making, error prevention, and care coordination
Describe examples of how technology and information management are related to the quality and safety of patient care	Respond appropriately to clinical decision-making supports and alerts	Value nurses' involvement in design, selection, implementation, and evaluation of information technologies to support patient care

Adapted from Cronenwett L et al: Quality and safety education for nurses, *Nurs Outlook* 55(3):122-131, 2007.

Hospitals nationally recognized for quality report healthier work environments, higher levels of job satisfaction and better retention rates (Ulrich et al, 2007). Focusing on quality can have benefits across the organization and shape the work environment and the workplace culture. Workplace culture is defined by the behavior, beliefs, and values of the group and is built from connecting consequences with behavior, so what is valued is recognized and rewarded. As nurses continually improve their competencies in patient-centered care, teamwork and collaboration, evidence-based practice, quality improvement, safety, and informatics, they can make significant contributions to shaping the quality and safety of the health care systems in which they work. The goal is to alter nursing's professional identity so that when we think of what it means to be a respected nurse, we think not only of caring, knowledge, honesty, and integrity but also of knowledge and commitment to quality and safety as an integral part of the professional role

SUMMARY

This chapter has described the six core competencies identified by the IOM as essential to form the practice base for all health professionals: patient-centered care, teamwork and collaboration, evidence-based practice, quality improvement, safety, and informatics. Each of these competencies is described as intended by the IOM in order to provide nurses with the same framework of understanding as shared by other health professionals. As a group, these competencies contribute to a strong foundation of professional nursing practice and establish nurses as leaders in promoting positive change in today's health care systems. All nurses must embrace the challenge to advance their knowledge, skills, and attitudes related to these six competencies to continually improve the quality and safety of the health care systems in which they work.

 evolve Additional resources are available online at: http://evolve.elsevier.com/Cherry/

REFERENCES

Agency for Healthcare Research and Quality: *AHRQ PSNet patient safety network: glossary*, 2009a. Retrieved November 2009 from: www.psnet.ahrq.gov/glossary.aspx#J.

Agency for Healthcare Research and Quality: *TeamSTEPPS: national implementation*, 2009b. Retrieved November 2009 from: http://teamstepps.ahrq.gov/index.htm.

American Association of Colleges of Nursing: *The essentials of baccalaureate education for professional nursing practice*, Washington, DC, 2008, American Association of Colleges of Nursing.

Anderson GF, et al: Health spending in the United States and the rest of the industrialized world, *Health Aff* 24(4):903-914, 2005.

Bates DW, et al: The costs of adverse drug events in hospitalized patients, *JAMA* 277(4):307-311, 1997.

Boehm H, Morast S: Quiet time: a daily period without distractions benefits both patients and nurses, *Am J Nurs* 109(Suppl 11):29-32, 2009.

Chapman K: Improving communication among nurses, patients, and physicians: a series of changes leads to cultural transformation at a TCAB hospital, *Am J Nurs* 109(Suppl 11):21-25, 2009.

Committee on Quality of Health Care in America: *Crossing the quality chasm: A new health system for the 21st century*, Washington, DC, 2001, National Academies Press.

Cronenwett L, et al: Quality and safety education for nurses, *Nurs Outlook* 55(3):122-131, 2007.

Cronenwett L, Sherwood G, Gelmon S: Improving quality and safety education: the QSEN leaning collaborative, *Nurs Outlook* 57(6):304-312, 2009.

Day L, Smith EL: Integrating quality and safety content into clinical teaching the acute care setting, *Nurs Outlook* 55(3):138-143, 2007.

Gabel J, Fitzner K: New evidence to explain rising healthcare costs, *Am J Manag Care* 9(special issue 1):SP1-SP2, 2003.

Greiner AC, Knebel E, editors: *Health professions education: A bridge to quality*, Washington, DC, 2003, National Academies Press.

Kohn LT, Corrigan JM, Donaldson MS: *To err is human: building a safer health system*, Washington, DC, 2000, National Academies Press.

Mayer C, Cronin D: Organizational accountability in a just culture, *Urol Nurs* 28(6):427–430, 2008.

Mayo AM, Duncan D: Nurse perceptions of medication errors: what we need to know for patient safety, *J Nurs Care Qual* 19(3):209–217, 2004.

McKesson: *HIMSS 2009 Informatics nurse impact survey*: McKesson.

Nurses Board of South Australia (2004). *Standards: delegation by a registered nurse or midwife to an unregulated healthcare worker*. Unpublished manuscript.

Page A, editor: *Keeping patients safe: Transforming the work environment of nurses*, Washington, DC, 2004, National Academies Press.

Reason J: Human error: models and management, *BMJ* 320(7237):768–770, 2000.

Shojania KG, et al: *Making health care safer: A critical analysis of patient safety practices*. Evidence report/technology assessment number 43, Rockville, Md, 2001, Agency for Healthcare Research and Quality.

Smith E, Cronenwett L, Sherwood G: Current assessments of quality and safety education in nursing, *Nurs Outlook* 55(3):132–137, 2007.

Sullivan DT, Hirst D, Cronenwett L: Assessing quality and safety competencies of graduating prelicensure nursing students, *Nurs Outlook* 57(6):323–331, 2009.

The Joint Commission: *Accreditation program: hospital chapter: national patient safety goals*, Oakbrook Terrace, IL, 2008, TJC. Available at: www.jointcommission.org/PatientSafety/NationalPatientSafetyGoals/09_hap_npsgs.htm.

Ulrich B, et al: Critical care nurses' work environments value of excellence in beacon units and magnet organizations, *Crit Care Nurse* 27:68–77, 2007.

Health Policy and Politics: Get Involved!

Barbara Cherry, DNSc, MBA, RN, NEA-BC
Virginia Trotter Betts, MSN, JD, RN, FAAN

evolve Additional resources are available online at: http://evolve.elsevier.com/Cherry/

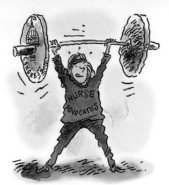

Nurses are powerful advocates for health care.

VIGNETTE

Juan Hernandez is one of only four registered nurses (RNs) now staffing the 7 AM to 7 PM shift in a 12-bed medical intensive care unit after two RNs have been replaced by nursing assistive personnel. Recently a new unit policy was circulated stating, "All RNs will work overtime as necessary and determined by administration." Juan was already concerned about the potential for compromised safe delivery of patient care by the decrease in RN staffing, the increased number of assistive personnel, and the increase in patient load and acuity. Juan feels a professional and moral obligation to ensure that adequate RN coverage is available for patient care and knows that the increased physical and mental strain of working overtime hours will be an additional detriment to quality care and patient safety. Juan understands that by mandating overtime, hospital administrators are failing to address the underlying issue: adequate numbers of RNs are required to provide high-quality, safe patient care. Juan works with other RNs who have these same concerns.

Juan realizes that based on the nurse practice act (NPA) in his state, he has a professional responsibility to "implement measures to promote a safe environment for clients." He further understands that he is individually professionally accountable for his daily practice with each patient. Juan calls his constituent member association to discuss his concerns. Through that call he discovers that other nurses around the state and across the United States are facing some of the same dilemmas. He finds that although he has a professional responsibility to advocate for safe care for patients, issues of working hours are not currently protected under the NPA or through any other policy or regulation in his state. Therefore, Juan makes a commitment to engage in a discussion about political strategies to amend the NPA or promote other viable policy options that will protect himself and other RNs in refusing mandatory overtime assignments without being accused of unprofessional conduct.

■ QUESTIONS TO CONSIDER WHILE READING THIS CHAPTER:

1 What types of local, state, and federal health policies affect Juan's nursing practice?

2 What are the major steps in health policy development that Juan must understand?

3 How can Juan apply the nursing process to develop an effective plan for policy development related to mandatory overtime assignments?

4 What types of grassroots political strategies can Juan use to ensure that policymakers hear his interests and concerns about safe patient care?

KEY TERMS

Constituent A citizen who has the opportunity to vote for candidates in elections for representation at the local, state, and federal level.

Constituent member association (CMA) The state professional organizational member of the American Nurses Association that represents all nurses at the state level (formerly known as the State Nurses Association).

Grassroots lobbying Advocacy by individual constituents—everyday citizens—in support of an organization's official position related to a policy issue.

Health policy A set course of action undertaken by governments or health care organizations that results in a health outcome. Private health policy is made by health care organizations, such as hospitals, whereas public health policy refers to local, state, and federal legislation, regulation, and court rulings that govern health care within a certain arena. Health policy as used in this chapter most often refers to public policies directly related to the health care workforce, service delivery, and/or reimbursement.

Lobbying An act of persuading or otherwise attempting to educate and convince policymakers to comply with a request, support a particular position on an issue, or follow a particular course of action.

Platform The statement of principles and policies of a political party, candidate, or elected official.

Policymaker A local, state, or congressional elected official who can propose legislation, regulations, or programs that can become actualized as public law.

Regulation Rules used to implement legislation and translate concepts into legal action that can be put into practice.

Stakeholders Individuals, groups, or organizations who have a vested interest in and may be affected by policy decisions and actions being taken and who may attempt to influence those decisions and actions.

LEARNING OUTCOMES

After studying this chapter, the reader will be able to:

1 Differentiate between policy and politics.

2 Discuss the roles of the legislative, administrative, and judicial levels of government.

3 Differentiate among federal, state, and local governments and their roles in governing and influencing health care and nursing practice.

4 Identify three policy issues of significant consequence to nurses and nursing.

5 Demonstrate knowledge needed to be a responsible and informed politically active nurse.

6 Use diverse technologic resources to obtain information about current health policy developments and political issues.

CHAPTER OVERVIEW

Perhaps at no other time in the history of the nursing profession has there been such an imperative for strong nursing leadership. The problems currently faced by the U.S. health care system—serious patient safety issues, a severe nursing and health care workforce shortage, strained work environments, a fragmented delivery system, an aging population, the rising number of uninsured, and threats of terrorist attacks and pandemic outbreaks—compromise the health and well-being of patients, families, and communities across the country. Nurses can no longer accept responsibility for the delivery of patient care without also addressing these very serious issues that jeopardize our health care system. Frequently these critical issues can be resolved only through the policy process. Without a doubt, legislation and health policy directly affect how health care is delivered and how the health care system responds to the very real threats it faces. Nurses must get involved now in the policy process and provide strong leadership to ensure the evolution to an efficient, effective health care system that promotes and protects the health and well-being of each person in our society.

This chapter explores the effect of governmental roles, structures, and actions on health care policy and demonstrates how participation in the policy process can shape the U.S. health care system. Local, state, and federal legislative concerns including the involvement of professional nursing organizations in policy and politics are discussed. The nurse's very important role in the policy process and involvement in political advocacy and campaigns is described. This chapter provides the reader with a basic understanding of policy development and political processes, ways to gain political savvy, and methods for getting politically involved.

NURSES' INVOLVEMENT IN HEALTH POLICY AND POLITICAL ACTION

Nurses' involvement in policy and politics has become considerably more important in recent years for the following reasons:

- State and federal governments play an increasingly important role in health care, especially as President Obama's administration embarks on implementation of *The Health Care and Reconciliation Act of 2010*, which was signed into law March 30, 2010.
- Nursing practice is directly affected by policy development which is, in turn, affected by the political action of nurses and others.
- Evidence of serious patient safety issues has received national media attention and has become a major debate among policymakers.
- National attention on the nursing shortage has intensified over the past few years.

Decisions affecting the health care system, patient care, and the nursing profession will be made with or without the input of nurses. According to Mason, Leavitt, and Chaffee, "*Patient care is a highly political endeavor. Politics determine who gets what kind of care from whom and when*" (2007, p. 3). Thus it is absolutely essential that nurses become actively engaged in the policy process and use political action to ensure the development of health policies that are reflective of the nursing perspective.

WHAT IS HEALTH POLICY?

Health policy is a set course of action undertaken by governments or health care organizations to obtain a desired outcome. Private health policy is made by health care organizations, such as hospitals, and includes those policies instituted to govern employee practices and health care services provided by the organization. A hospital policy related to reporting patient care errors is an example of private health policy. Public health policy refers to local, state, and federal legislation, regulations, and funding related to health care service delivery and reimbursement. The mandatory requirement for licensure to practice professional nursing is an example of public health policy. There is a close link between private and public policy in that the policies of health care organizations must conform to and are frequently implemented to comply with a public policy. Although it is vital that the RN be a leader in policy development at the health care organization in which he or she is employed, this chapter focuses on the development of public health policy, which will be referred to simply as "health policy."

Health Policy at the Local, State, and Federal Level

Health policies may be developed and implemented at the local, state, or federal level and are characterized by the fact that they apply to all residents within the jurisdiction of the respective government. Local health policy applies only to those people who are residents of that local community, whereas health policy enacted at the federal level applies to all residents in the United States.

Local Health Policy. At the local level, many cities or counties offer a variety of health care services to meet the needs of their residents. For example, as part of a city's health policy, free or reduced-rate immunizations may be offered to all children in the community. Allocating funds to employ RNs in public schools is another example of local health policy. A more controversial policy is a community's requirement for tobacco-free public areas, such as restaurants and office buildings. Local health policy varies considerably across the United States, with some communities funding an extensive variety of health programs and others offering very limited health services or none at all. However, even the smallest communities are involved to some extent in health policy through partnerships with their state government to provide public health programs, such as safe drinking water, enforcement for seat belt and child restraint laws, and emergency medical systems.

State Health Policy. Health policy at the state level has a powerful influence on the health and safety of each state's residents. In addition to its lead role in governing nursing practice through the state's NPA, each state also has innumerable health policies that may be less visible. These policies include maintaining a safe meat supply through livestock inspections, ensuring safe food storage and preparation in restaurants, and ensuring that health care facilities provide safe, quality care through regulatory compliance. Only when these activities fall short of preventing problems—as in cases of *Escherichia coli* outbreaks—do most states' residents realize the importance of these health policies.

State health policy also involves paying for some individual health care services. The Medicaid program, which pays for health care services for people at (or below) a specific income level and other groups (as defined by a combination of federal or state standards), is funded through a blend of state and federal funds. Most states also have a State Children's Health Insurance Program (SCHIP) that provides health insurance coverage to uninsured children who do not qualify for the Medicaid program. The SCHIP is funded through a partnership between federal and state governments. State and federal governments are also the prime sources of funding for mental health and substance abuse services, long-term care services for older adults and disabled persons, and health care services for prisoners.

Federal Health Policy. Just as state health policies have an enormous effect on people's health and safety, the federal government plays a vitally important leadership role in the health of Americans, including the health policy reforms considered by the 111th Congress. The federal government's role in health care includes significant funding for health and disease research; supplemental funding for education for health professionals, including nurses and physicians; and paying for individual health care services through Medicare, Medicaid, SCHIP, and the Veterans Administration health care system.

Federal health policies have played and continue to play a monumental role in shaping nursing practice. The first federal policy to provide funding for nursing services was the Sheppard-Towner Act of 1921. This act, (which was passed by Congress despite objections from the American Medical Association [AMA]) provided states with matching funds to establish prenatal and child health centers staffed by public health nurses. Their goal was to reduce maternal and infant mortality rates by teaching women about personal hygiene and infant care. Eventually this highly successful program was discontinued when the AMA successfully persuaded Congress that physicians should perform these health activities (Starr, 1982).

Another example of legislation that significantly influenced the context of nursing practice was the Hill-Burton Act, also known as the Hospital Survey and Construction Act, enacted in 1950. This act provided funding that resulted in a boom in the construction of hospitals across the country. As the number of hospitals increased rapidly, so did the need for nurses to staff them. Thus the nurse's role shifted from community and public health settings to the increasing number of acute care settings. Today federal legislation affects nursing practice through expanding reimbursement directly to advanced practice nurses and implementing policies and programs to address the nursing shortage. Table 23-1 provides historic examples of how health policy enacted at the federal level affected nursing practice and health care. Current policy issues affecting nursing practice and health care are addressed later in this chapter.

HOW IS HEALTH POLICY DEVELOPED?

The development of health policy at the state or federal level is a complex, dynamic process that occurs in the following three ways (Mason et al, 2007):

- ◆ Enactment of legislation and the accompanying rules and regulations that carry the weight of law
- ◆ Administrative decisions made by various governmental agencies
- ◆ Judicial decisions that interpret the law

Numerous individuals and groups are involved in developing health policy, including elected officials and their staffs; officials from executive branch governmental agencies; experts in the related area; citizens who may be affected by the policy; stakeholders, such as corporate

TABLE **23-1**

Examples of Health Policies That Have Influenced Professional Nursing Practice

LEGISLATION	INFLUENCE ON PROFESSIONAL NURSING PRACTICE
Nurse practice acts and registration of nurses were established (1910).	Established scope of practice and minimal educational requirements for nurses; implemented by most states.
Sheppard-Towner Act (1921) funded prenatal and child health centers staffed by public health nurses.	First federal policy to provide funding for nursing services.
Hill-Burton Act (1950), also known as the Hospital Survey and Construction Act, provided federal funding for hospital construction.	Caused a boom in hospital construction, which shifted nurses' primary employment setting from public health to hospitals.
Medicare program (1965) provided funding for health care services for older adults and the disabled.	Led to an increased number of hospitalized older adults and increased need for nurses in acute care settings.
Renal Disease Program (1972) provided funding for dialysis treatments and renal transplants for patients with kidney failure.	Led to the development of a new area of nursing practice that is now a recognized specialty—nephrology nursing.
Diagnosis-related groups (DRGs) (1983) changed Medicare reimbursement to hospitals from fee-for-service to a fixed-fee method.	Forced hospitals to reduce patients' lengths of stay, cut costs, and reduce staff, including nurses; led to the development of new nursing roles—nursing case management and utilization review.
Medicare part D (2006) added a prescription drug benefit for Medicare enrollees; the first major change in Medicare since the 1960s.	This much needed benefit for Medicare enrollees will continue to receive attention from policymakers, requiring nurses to stay alert to proposed legislation and advocate for better benefits for the nation's older adults

TABLE **23-2**

The Three Branches of the Federal Government

	EXECUTIVE	LEGISLATIVE	JUDICIAL
Composition	Office of the President and 15 executive departments (State, Treasury, Defense, Agriculture, Energy, Housing and Urban Development, Justice, Commerce, Education, Health and Human Services, Interior, Labor, Transportation, Veterans Affairs, and Department of Homeland Security)	Senate and House of Representatives, known as Congress	U.S. Supreme Court, federal district courts, and U.S. circuit courts of appeals
Role in health policy	Recommends legislation and promotes major policy initiatives	Possesses the sole federal power to enact legislation	Judicial interpretations of the Constitution or various laws may have a policy effect
	Implements laws and manages programs after they have been passed by Congress	Able to originate and promote major policy initiatives	Resolves questions regarding agency regulations that may affect policy
	Writes regulations that interpret statutes (laws) Has the power to veto legislation passed by Congress	Power to override a presidential veto	
Restrictions to power	Unable to enact a law without the approval of Congress (legislative branch)	U.S. Supreme Court may invalidate legislation as unconstitutional	Unable to recommend or promote legislative initiatives

representatives, who may be affected by the policy; and representatives from special interest groups who have a particular interest in the policy. As a special interest group, the American Nurses Association (ANA) represents nurses throughout the United States and carries a strong voice and high visibility in influencing health policy and nursing practice. At the state level, the constituent member associations (CMAs) of the ANA are the policy voice of the profession with governors and the state legislatures.

The development of health policy involves all three branches of government: executive, legislative, and judicial. A basic knowledge of the function of the three branches of government is necessary to understand health policy development. Table 23-2 presents a brief review of the three branches of the federal government and their roles in health policy. Although most state governments parallel the structure and functions of the federal government, there are differences among states. Each nurse is encouraged to learn about the government structure of his or her state. In addition to understanding the branches of government, nurses also need to understand the influence of legislation and regulation on health policy, both of which are discussed in the following sections.

Legislation and Health Policy Development

The development of health policy refers to the steps through which an issue moves from a societal problem to an actual social program that can be implemented and evaluated. The legislative process is fundamental to the movement from a public problem to a public solution: a viable program. Although there are many problems related to health care and nursing practice, problems that will attain policy solutions are those that are brought to the attention of a policymaker who is willing to take definitive action through the legislative process.

Generally, individuals or groups approach policymakers either with a problem to be solved or to suggest a legislative solution to a health problem. However, policymakers may also learn of problems through their personal or constituents' experiences and take action independently. At the federal level only members of Congress can introduce legislation. The congressional member who introduces a specific piece of legislation becomes the prime sponsor of that legislation. Legislation is introduced by a member of Congress only after careful analysis of the problem, which likely includes:

- Public perception of the problem
- Definition of the problem
- Societal consequences of action or inaction and the number of people affected by the problem
- Degree of support and opposition from other members of Congress, special interest groups, business leaders, and the general public

After the problem is thoroughly analyzed and the decision is made to draft a piece of legislation, the staff of the congressman sponsoring the issue translates the idea into legal, technical, and constitutional language, which the congressman then introduces through the appropriate process. Only then does the problem become a bill as a proposed legislative solution.

Steps in the Legislative Process

The official legislative process at the federal level begins when a bill or resolution is introduced by the sponsoring member(s) of Congress and is numbered, referred to committee(s), and printed by the U.S. Government Printing Office. Following are the basic steps a bill follows in the legislative process (ANA, 2009a):

Step 1: Referral to committee. The bill is referred to a standing committee in the house or senate according to carefully defined procedures.

Step 2: Committee action. The bill may be referred to a subcommittee or be considered by the committee as a whole; it is examined carefully and its chances for passage are determined. If the committee does not act on the bill, it is essentially dead.

Step 3: Subcommittee review. Bills may be referred to a subcommittee for study and hearings; hearings provide committee members with the opportunity to obtain written or oral testimony about the bill from the executive branch, experts in the related area, and supporters and opponents of the bill.

Step 4: Markup. After hearings the subcommittee may choose to "mark up" the bill, which means to make changes or amendments before recommending the bill to the full committee. The bill dies if the subcommittee votes not to refer the bill to the full committee.

Step 5: Committee action to report a bill. After the full committee receives the bill from the subcommittee, the committee can conduct further hearings and further study or vote on the subcommittee's recommendations. The full committee then votes on its recommendations to the house or senate, a procedure known as "ordering a bill reported."

Step 6: Publication of a written report. The committee staff members prepare a written report about the bill that includes its intent, effect on existing laws and programs, position of the executive branch, and views of dissenting members of the committee.

Step 7: Scheduling floor action. The bill is scheduled on the calendar in either the House or the Senate. In the House there are several different legislative calendars, and the speaker and majority leader determine whether, when, and in what order bills are to be considered. There is only one legislative calendar in the Senate.

Step 8: Debate. Debate begins when the bill reaches the floor of the House or Senate; various rules govern the conditions and amount of time allowed for debate.

Step 9: Voting. After debate, the bill is passed or defeated by the members voting.

Step 10: Referral to other chamber. After a bill is passed by either the House or Senate, it is referred to the other chamber, where it normally follows the same process through committee and floor action; at this point, the bill may be approved as received or rejected, ignored, or changed.

Step 11: Conference committee action. If only minor changes are made in step 10, the bill will go back to the first chamber for concurrence. However, if the second chamber significantly alters the bill, a conference committee is formed to reconcile the differences between the House and Senate. The legislation will die if the conferees are unable to reach agreement. If members of the conference committee reach agreement, a conference report will be prepared with recommendations for changes to the bill. Both the House and Senate must approve the conference report.

Step 12: Final actions. After the bill is approved by both the House and Senate in identical form, it is sent to the President, who may (a) approve and sign the bill into law; (b) take no action for 10 days while Congress is in session, after which time the bill automatically becomes a law; (c) veto the bill; or (d) take no action after Congress has adjourned, allowing the legislation to die.

Step 13: Overriding a veto. If the President vetoes the bill, Congress may override the veto, which requires a two-thirds roll call vote of the members who are present in sufficient numbers for a quorum.

Although this legislative process appears to be a simple, straightforward method for creating public law, it is actually very complex and convoluted with only a very small fraction of legislation introduced actually making it through the final process to become law. In the 110th U.S. Congress (2007 to 2008), 11,081 bills were introduced; only 442 of those actually became public law (*Congressional Record*, 2009). In other words, only 4% of bills introduced in the 110th Congress actually became public law.

Once a bill becomes a law (a public policy), implementation falls to the jurisdiction of one of the departments under the executive branch of government (see Table 23-2). At the federal level, most health-related policies fall under the jurisdiction of the U.S. Department of Health and Human Services (USDHHS) and its related agencies. The agency that will administer the law develops the regulations to implement the law. Implementation of new legislation can often be very different from what was originally intended when Congress debated and passed the bill. It is extremely important that supporters of any new law take steps to ensure that the law is implemented as intended by the policymakers This leads us to the discussion about regulation and health policy.

HOW ARE HEALTH POLICY AND REGULATIONS CONNECTED?

The regulatory arena is an important but often overlooked area of political action that significantly affects nursing practice. An understanding of regulatory authority and processes provides nurses with the knowledge necessary to become involved and influence the future of nursing. Regulation refers to the written set of rules issued by the executive branch agency that has responsibility for administering the law. Because regulations carry the force of the law, they directly shape the implementation of health policy. Thus it is very important that the regulations reflect the intent of the law as enacted by the legislative body. As stated, supporters of any new law must be vigilant and involved in its implementation through the development of regulations long after the legislation is adopted.

As regulations are being developed by the government agency, public hearings are held to allow individuals to comment on the content of the regulations. At this stage nurses can play an influential role in the final regulations by writing to the regulatory agency or speaking at public hearings. Once the proposed regulations are developed, they must be published and open to public comment for a specified length of time before being adopted. Comment is critical for the development of administrative law. Each comment received must be considered and responded to before final regulations are issued. The time interval between the interim and final rules is critical for assessing the effect of the proposed rules and requires concerted nursing action to react to the proposed rules either positively or negatively. Final published regulations carry the force of the law and will dictate how the law is actually implemented.

At the federal level the proposed (or interim) regulations are published in the *Federal Register*. The *Federal Register* (located online at www.gpoaccess.gov/fr) is the best source of information about proposed new rules and changes to existing rules for federal programs. It is printed each day and contains complete directions about where to send comments, in addition to the deadlines for the public comment period. Most states have a parallel publication (e.g., *Texas Register*) with information about proposed rules and regulations at the state level for state legislation.

A great deal of effort goes into the development of health policy, from the time a public health problem is identified, a legislative solution is conceived, and a health policy is actually implemented. By understanding and becoming involved in these processes, nurses can protect and influence nursing practice and create and direct change throughout the health care system.

HOW ARE HEALTH POLICY AND POLITICS CONNECTED?

Many people view politics as somewhat "shady" activities that occur in federal, state, and local governments to influence the outcomes of candidate elections and/or the passage of legislation. Mason and colleagues have defined politics as "the process of influencing the allocation of scarce resources" (2007, p. 4). Politics can also be defined as the process used to influence decisions and exert control over circumstances and events. As the reader will see, "influence" is the common denominator in any definition of politics. Political influence can come in many forms, including:

- Campaign contributions
- Knowledge
- Relationships
- Information
- Talent
- Perceived control over large groups of votes

Florence Nightingale was the consummate political nurse and understood how to use data (knowledge) to influence the British Parliament to allocate funds to reform British military hospitals and substantially improve the health conditions for the troops through changes in sanitary practices.

Politics is a necessary part of the policy process. Multiple interest groups, such as elected officials, special interest groups, and corporate leaders, are all competing to achieve their potentially different goals. The process becomes even more interesting when the varied agendas of the Democratic, Republican, and Independent parties are added to the mix. Groups and individuals who have a stake in the fate of a piece of legislation (or the election of a candidate) use political strategies to obtain their desired outcome(s). Thus it is through *effective* political action that nurses can positively influence legislative and regulatory decisions and the development of health policies that will affect nursing practice and the health of Americans. Following is a discussion of how nurses can get involved in the political process and use effective political strategies to influence health policy.

Getting Involved Through the Nursing Process

The first step for nurses to get involved in health policy development and politics is to learn to recognize nursing and health care issues that require policy action. During nursing school, students learn the nursing process as the foundation for professional nursing practice. Once nursing students graduate they appreciate the nursing process as the basis for making sound clinical judgments. As nurses commit to being more politically astute, they will find the nursing process as a natural approach to identify broader professional and health care issues:

1. *Assessment:* collection of information
2. *Analysis and diagnosis:* specific, targeted identification of the issue
3. *Planning:* development of a scope for action
4. *Implementation:* action taken to put the plan in place
5. *Evaluation:* evidence that determines the success (or not) of the intervention

Assessment. Collecting information and understanding the information collected are important initial steps in identifying policy issues and how to approach them. As a nurse, one would not care for a patient without first knowing the patient's health problems and other factors that may affect health status. Once the nurse understands the health problems and other possible influencing factors, he or she has enough information to move to the next step in the process: identifying the nursing diagnosis. This same principle applies to health policy and political action. Information and material must be gathered from as many sources as possible before the health care issues amenable to policy intervention can be identified.

An excellent example of health policy assessment is provided by the Institute of Medicine's (IOM) report titled *The Future of Drug Safety: Promoting and Protecting the Health of the Public* (2006a). Because of public concerns over the health risks posed by approved drugs, the U.S. Food and Drug Administration (FDA) requested that the IOM conduct an independent assessment of the current system for evaluating and ensuring drug safety postmarketing (after drugs are available to the public) and make recommendations to improve risk assessment, surveillance, and the safe use of drugs. The assessment and subsequent recommendations are being used by Congress, the pharmaceutical industry, and health care organizations to monitor, evaluate, and improve drug safety.

Analysis and Diagnosis. Once the information is gathered (system symptoms), it must be analyzed to identify the fundamental issue or underlying problem(s) that needs to be addressed. For a patient, the nursing diagnosis is determined after analysis of all objective and subjective data is completed. For an issue that may lend itself to a policy intervention, the collected information is analyzed, and the parameters of the issue are determined.

An excellent example of a health policy diagnosis is related to the nursing shortage. Extensive data about the nursing shortage have been, and continue to be, collected and analyzed, thus providing policymakers and nursing advocates with the information needed to identify the underlying multifaceted problems of the shortage, in addition to its effect on multiple systems to ensure that effective policy interventions are developed.

Planning. After collecting the information and identifying the issue, the nurse is ready to develop a plan. Generally an effective policy plan involves input from many sources and perspectives (positive as well as negative outcomes). The plan includes options and a determination of potential consequences for each option. Just as getting an issue on the agenda for policy action is about competing problems, competing options for policy solutions also occur. Having data and potential positive outcomes helps to ensure movement toward adoption of nursing's preferred solutions or options.

The U.S. health care system's quality and safety issues provide an excellent example of a well-represented and large-scale plan for a policy issue. Based on assessment and diagnosis of patient safety and the quality of care in America's hospitals, national organizations and federal agencies are working together to plan policy interventions to improve the safety and quality of health care. Key among these planning groups are the Agency for Healthcare Research and Quality (AHRQ) and the IOM. The AHRQ and the IOM have worked together to develop the congressionally mandated *National Healthcare Quality Reports*, which monitor the nation's progress toward improved health care safety and quality. These reports can be accessed on the AHRQ website at www.ahrq.gov/qual/measurix.htm.

Implementation. Once a policy option is selected it must be adopted and implemented. Implementing a policy plan requires political action and a set of strategies. In a classic example, a member of the Association of periOperative Registered Nurses learned about a regulatory issue of great importance to perioperative nurses. The issue involved the state administrative code concerning licensure of hospitals and the use of RN circulators in the operating room. As part of a regulation review the state department of health and social services had proposed a change that would have allowed non-RNs to circulate in selected cases. Because of development and implementation of a policy plan by the nurses in that state, the state regulation was addressed and continues to require assignment of an RN to circulating duties, with other personnel allowed only to *assist* with circulating duties (Oxhorn and Rosen, 1992).

This example raises at least two critical issues. First is the special relationship between the nursing profession and society. Nurses have a legal obligation to provide at the minimum a "safe" standard of care to the persons they serve. Allowing use of non-RNs to circulate in even selected operative cases could jeopardize nurses' commitment and obligation to safeguard patients. Second is the connection between standards of practice and standards of education. RN circulators possess advanced skills, knowledge, and judgment that surpass the technical skills of non-RNs (Oxhorn and Rosen, 1992). This case is an excellent example to illustrate a nearly universal concept: what is good for nursing is good for patients and vice versa. Thus nursing advocacy improves health care for all.

Evaluation. After implementing the plan, evaluation of the action must occur. An excellent example of evaluating a public policy can be illustrated by the mandatory staffing rules *(not ratios)* established for Texas hospitals in 2002. The initiative—led by the Texas Nurses Association and enforced through hospital licensing regulations—requires Texas hospitals to adopt, implement, and enforce a written staffing plan. Direct-care nurses must be involved in developing the staffing plan and patient outcomes are used as a guide to assess the adequacy of the staffing plan. After evaluating the effectiveness of the 2002 staffing rules, the Texas Nurses Association again initiated legislation to strengthen the staffing plan and the Texas Safe Hospital Staffing Act was passed into law in June 2009. This new act strengthens the influence of nurses on nurse-to-patient staffing levels, provides for a flexible approach to staffing to match patient needs with characteristics of the nursing staff, and prohibits mandatory overtime (Texas Nurses Association, 2009). The Texas plan illustrates the importance of evaluating staffing legislation and moving forward with new actions as appropriate to ensure the intended outcomes of such legislation—improved patient outcomes and nurse work environments—are realized.

GRASSROOTS POLITICAL STRATEGIES

Grassroots political strategies are actions taken at the local level to influence policymakers. Nurses as political constituents have a right to petition, lobby, or persuade policymakers to ensure that their interests and concerns are heard. Such advocate actions (typically referred to as lobbying) provide those individuals and groups who are stakeholders in a particular issue an opportunity to be heard. The lobbying process also provides policymakers with needed information from health experts on which to base their decisions. Following are various methods through which nurses can be effective grassroots players:

- Registering to vote and voting in *all* elections
- Joining professional nursing organizations
- Working in political candidates' campaigns
- Visiting with policymakers or their staff members
- Attending "meet the candidates" town hall meetings
- Communicating with policymakers by e-mail, fax, and phone

Register to Vote, and Vote in All Elections

Voting is a must for *every* nurse. However, voting is not enough. Informed voting is necessary to enhance nurses' political power to ultimately improve the health of patients and the nursing care that they receive. Becoming informed involves reading legislative newsletters and finding out about policymakers' backgrounds, voting records, and current party and candidate platforms. Discussing your findings on these issues with nurse colleagues and others in the community enhances everyone's understanding of candidates and their positions and facilitates informed voting.

Join a Professional Nursing Organization

Another must for the professional nurse is to join a professional nursing organization. The value of the ANA, its constituent member associations (CMAs), and specialty nursing organizations is that together the nursing profession is much more powerful than any individual RN speaking alone. As professionals in a collective, nurses know more, have more resources, and are able to pool their strengths and direct resources toward winning the health policy "game" and ensuring nurse-friendly public policy.

The ANA is the foremost recognized professional nursing organization for federal health and nursing public policy. ANA speaks for professional nurses, regardless of specialty. All nurses should consider ANA membership as one of their basic professional responsibilities. Nurses who choose to maintain membership in the specialty organization that represents their area of nursing practice have the additional advantage of receiving clinical and health policy information related to that specialty.

Because professional nursing organizations monitor public policy and offer avenues for their members to learn about health policy, they serve as an invaluable resource for reliable information related to policy issues and policymakers. Joining a professional nursing organization that has a political action committee (PAC) can help develop the necessary skills to understand political issues.

A PAC is an arm of a corporation, association, or labor union formed to provide support either to persuade a policymaker to support a certain policy or program or, more often, to ensure the election or reelection of policymakers who support the organization's overall goals/ priorities. Professional nursing organizations may choose to endorse a specific candidate for office. Endorsement simply means that in a particular political race the nursing organization selects a particular candidate to support because of that candidate's platform or record supporting specific issues or goals. Although endorsement does not mean that everyone in the organization must vote for the selected person, it does mean that the organization has carefully screened the candidate, and the nurse can be reasonably sure that the candidate will support the organization's preferred outcomes and interests.

Work in Political Candidates' Campaigns

Most political candidates are not health professionals and do not fully understand health-related issues. By becoming involved in political campaigns, nurses can (and should) educate and inform candidates about health care issues. Other activities that the nurse may undertake on behalf of the candidates include assisting in writing health care position statements, working in campaign offices, attending local debates, displaying the candidates' political buttons and signs, and participating in fundraising events. Nurse supporters may also write letters to and/ or call other nurses in the region to tell them about their support of the candidate and to ask for their vote. Having "nurse-friendly" candidates win and become "nurse-friendly" policymaking officials is critical to achieving nursing's policy agenda.

Visit with Policymakers and Their Staff Members

Personal visits to policymakers and their staff members can be one of the most effective methods of advocacy for or against a health care policy. Nothing is more effective in communicating nursing's position than face-to-face contact between a policymaker and his or her staff and a group of well-informed nurses. Face-to-face meetings provide a great opportunity for nurses to educate policymakers about health care issues. Policymakers are very interested in information that will increase their knowledge about health care and help them develop options for future health care policy. Tips to prepare for a personal visit with policymakers are available in the online *RN Activist Tool Kit* on the American Nurses Association website (www.nursing world.org).

Participate in Meet-the-Candidates Town Hall Meetings

A strategy that nursing associations can use to determine which candidate(s) to endorse is to invite all candidates running for a particular office to a town hall meeting to discuss their platforms directly with nurses. Town hall gatherings with nurses allow the candidates to talk about their platform to a group of interested voters and afford nurses an opportunity to understand the candidate's vision and to voice their experiences, opinions, and concerns about health care issues. Box 23-1 provides the correct titles to use when addressing state elected officials.

BOX **23-1**

Speaking with the Governor, Lieutenant Governor, Legislators, or Staff

Governor: Governor (last name)
Lieutenant Governor: Governor (last name)
Speaker of the House: Mr. Speaker or Madam Speaker
Senator: Senator (last name)
Representative: Representative (last name) or Mr. or Ms. (last name)
Staff: Mr. or Ms. (last name)

Hosting a meet-the-candidates town hall meeting can be an exciting activity for student nurses and faculty. Just as in preparing for a personal visit to a policymaker, nursing students should also prepare carefully to host a town hall meeting:

1. Before the town hall meeting, become familiar with each candidate's background, including his or her voting record on health policy issues, major contributors, personal occupations, family information, and hobbies. This information can provide insight into the candidate's positions on issues.
2. Identify current issues that would be relevant for discussion with the candidates. Collect and review information related to the issues, and then prioritize the issues. Time may not be sufficient to discuss all of the issues of interest.
3. Prepare to give concise examples of how the issue affects the individual, community, health care consumers, and other members of the nursing profession. Be prepared to debate arguments that unfavorably reflect one's position.
4. Plan the agenda for the meeting to allow ample time for discussion.
5. After introductions are made, listen carefully as each candidate presents his or her campaign platform, then be prepared to clearly and concisely discuss the issues with relevant examples.
6. At the conclusion of the meeting, provide the candidate with contact information (names, addresses, telephone numbers, and e-mail addresses) for key members of your group.

Communicate with Policymakers Through E-mail, Fax, and Phone

Contacting policymakers through letters, e-mail, fax, and phone can be effective if properly planned and implemented. The timing of the communication is important; it should be made early before policymakers commit to vote a certain way. It is easier to convince an undecided policymaker than it is to get him or her to switch positions. A second very effective step is to send a follow-up communication immediately before the vote on a particular bill is scheduled. Information about voting schedules can be obtained online in most states.

Because of the anthrax decontamination process now in place, delivery of U.S. mail to Congress and the White House may be delayed by as much as 3 months, making letters an inefficient means of communicating with policymakers. Using e-mail or sending a fax is really the best way to make sure your voice will be heard in time to make a difference. Guidelines for communicating with policymakers include the following (ANA, 2009b):

1. *Be brief.* Short, direct e-mail and faxes are the most effective.
2. *Be specific.* Deal with just one subject or issue in the communication; state your topic clearly in the first paragraph. The subject of an e-mail message should contain the

number of the bill to which you are referring in the message. For example, "In opposition to Senate bill 123" immediately focuses the reader. The message itself should be just a few short lines to relay a clear and strong message related to the issue. Brief examples of how the issue affects the policymaker's constituents are often very effective.

3. *Be personal.* Communication is most effective when it reflects your personal experiences and presents your views in your own words; mass produced letters, e-mails and faxes do not carry as much weight as a communication that you have written yourself.

4. *Provide your name and address.* Policymakers pay most attention to communications that come from their constituents, people who may be voting for or against them. So it is important to let them know you are from their district. Include contact information so that the elected official may respond to your concerns.

5. *Be persistent.* Communicate often, especially if the policymaker is undecided on an issue.

Telephone calls are usually taken by a staff member; ask to speak to the staff person assigned to the bill or issue for which the call is being made. After introducing yourself, give a brief and simple message, such as "please tell Senator or Representative [name] that I support/oppose [bill number]." You may briefly state your reasons for supporting or opposing the bill and ask for the policymaker's position on the bill. Conclude the call by leaving your name, telephone number, and address; if appropriate ask for a written response to your telephone call.

Rosters of state legislators can be found online in most states. The roster contains contact information for each policymaker and usually includes information about his or her committee memberships. Contact information for members of the U.S. House of Representatives is available online at www.house.gov. This site includes committee memberships and links to individual representatives' websites. Similar information for U.S. senators is also available online at www.senate.gov.

THE AMERICAN NURSES ASSOCIATION

The ANA is the professional nursing organization representing the nation's entire RN population—approximately 2.9 million RNs. The ANA is composed of 51 CMAs that represent state and U.S territory nursing associations and includes many organizational affiliates including the American Nurses Credentialing Center, the American Nurses Foundation, the American Academy of Nursing, and specialty organizations such as the American Association of Critical-Care Nurse. A full list of ANA-affiliated organizations and links to their websites can be found on the ANA website at www.nursingworld.org.

The two most recently established ANA organizational affiliates are the United American Nurses (UAN) and the Center for American Nurses (CAN). The UAN is the labor union for nurses representing RNs nationwide and is an affiliate of the AFL-CIO (American Federation of Labor-Congress of Industrial Organizations). Students can learn more about the UAN by visiting their website: www.uannurse.org/who/index.html. The CAN, established in 2003, addresses the needs of individual nurses who are not represented by unions by offering tools, services, and strategies designed to make nurses their own best advocates in their practice environments. Students can learn more about the CAN by visiting: www.centerforamerican nurses.org.

Through political and legislative activities, the ANA has taken firm positions on various issues, including Medicare and Medicaid reform, patients' rights, the importance of safer needle devices, whistle-blower protection for health care workers, adequate reimbursement for health care services, access to health care, and most recently, health care reform. Students are encouraged to spend time browsing the ANA website at www.nursingworld.org to learn more about this most important nursing organization.

Nurses Strategic Action Team

Nurses are impressive in their collective abilities to mobilize and take effective grassroots action in shaping national health care policy through the Nurses Strategic Action Team (N-STAT). N-STAT is an ANA program that unifies nurses' political voices across the country to enact measures to benefit health care for everyone and to defeat measures that would have serious negative effects on the health care system. N-STAT is composed of thousands of nurses around the country who stay informed on issues and contact their legislators about pending issues. Through legislative updates, N-STAT keeps members up-to-date on key bills as they move through the legislative process. Through action alerts, members are informed about when e-mails, phone calls, and faxes will have the most effect. N-STAT makes the political process less intimidating by keeping nurses informed of political issues and providing strategies for making their opinions known. For more information and to sign up as a member of N-STAT, go to: www.rnaction.org.

CURRENT HEALTH POLICY ISSUES

Policy issues come and go as society, health care, and public needs and demands ebb and flow. However, two topics bear watching over the next decade—health care reform and health care safety and quality. The importance of these topics will keep them on the policy agenda for many years to come.

Health Care Reform

As the first decade of the twenty-first century draws to a close, historic health care reform legislation has become a reality with passage of *The Health Care and Education Affordability Reconciliation Act of 2010*. Health care reform is the general term used to refer to health policy initiatives to effect significant changes in how health care is delivered and paid for in the United States. Many Americans and professional health care organizations such as the ANA support bold health care reform to address critical problems facing our health care system: a growing uninsured population, access to care, rapidly rising costs, health professional shortages (i.e., nurses, primary care physicians), and ongoing concerns about the quality and safety of care.

Access to care is perhaps the most significant problem to address through major health care reform. In 2007, 45 million Americans—just over 15% of the population—were without health insurance coverage for a full year (U.S. Census Bureau, 2007). Lack of health insurance is the greatest barrier to accessing health care and has a tremendous negative effect on an individual's health. Studies have consistently found that the uninsured receive less than adequate health care. Consider these findings (Kaiser Family Foundation, 2008):

- More than 50% of the uninsured have no regular source of health care.
- Uninsured individuals are four times more likely to delay or ignore needed care, resulting in conditions being diagnosed at a later stage.
- Uninsured individuals are less likely to receive preventive care and more likely to be hospitalized for avoidable conditions.

The lack of health insurance has serious financial consequences for individuals and families as well. More than 60% of bankruptcies in the United States are related to medical causes or medical debt (Himmelstein et al, 2009). The uninsured populations also generate uncompensated or indigent care costs and bad debt for health care providers requiring providers to increase charges to public and private insurers and making it even more difficult for households and businesses to afford coverage.

On the federal level, historic steps are in process to implement policies that provide affordable and accessible health care coverage for all Americans through the recently passed health care reform bill. Implementation of the 2010 health reform bill will likely challenge the nation's leaders for years to come. As rules and regulations are developed to implement this legislation, nurses and professional nursing organizations need to have a strong and united voice to ensure the legislation will positively affect access to care and cost of care as intended by the policymakers.

The ANA will play a strong role to influence implementation of the new health care reform legislation. The ANA document *Health System Reform Agenda* released in 2008 (available at: www.nursingworld.org) outlines four critical areas of health care reform: access to care, quality of care, cost of care, and workforce shortages. More recently, ANA leaders worked with approximately 18 nursing organizations to develop a set of reform principles and recommendations to serve as a resource for policymakers and their staff. The principles and recommendations address (1) the continuing shortage of RNs; (2) the use of advanced practice nurses to provide comprehensive, cost-effective, and high-quality care; (3) the use of care coordination models to improve quality outcomes and reduce costs; (4) increased emphasis on wellness and health promotion strategies; and (5) implementation of a nationwide health information system (Gonzales, 2009).

It is vitally important that nurses pay particular attention to the new health care reform legislation. The ANA provides the venue for nurses to stay current—and become involved—as health care reform moves forward for our country. Through health care reform initiatives, nurses will be able to advocate for their profession and the safety, quality, and availability of care for all Americans.

Patient Safety and Health Care Quality

The IOM report *To Err Is Human: Building a Safer Health System* (IOM, 2000) placed the issue of medical mistakes and patient safety on the pages of many national newspapers, on the agendas of health care governing boards, and at the forefront of federal government legislation. The report concluded that up to 98,000 patients die each year as a result of medical errors. The IOM's more recent follow-up report, *Keeping Patients Safe: Transforming the Work Environment of Nurses* (Page, 2004) has focused national attention on the very important role nurses play daily in patient safety. Because the IOM is viewed as the nation's foremost authority on health care issues, policymakers pay close attention to their reports and recommendations. Thus it is not surprising that patient safety, health care quality, and nurses' work environments are receiving a great deal of attention and consideration for policy interventions at the state and federal levels.

In 2005 Congress passed the Patient Safety and Quality Improvement Act of 2005 for the purpose of improving patient safety by encouraging voluntary and confidential reporting of events that adversely affect patients. The legislation allows for a confidential reporting structure in which physicians, nurses, hospitals, and other health care professionals and entities can voluntarily report information on errors to patient safety organizations (PSOs). The PSOs then analyze the data to develop patient safety improvement strategies. More information about PSOs can be found on the AHRQ website: www.pso.ahrq.gov/psos/overview.htm.

In the 111th Congress (2009 to 2010), the Nurse and Health Care Worker Protection Act of 2009 (H.R. 2381) has been proposed. This bill would provide for a safe patient handling and injury prevention standard to reduce injuries to patients, direct-care registered nurses, and all other health care workers.

As one can see, proposed legislation has the potential to significantly affect a nurse's daily work environment and patient care. Thus nurses need to stay alert for new and proposed legislation that will affect nursing care, patient safety, and health care quality. Nurses can review and track the progress of proposed bills at the federal level on the Library of Congress's "Thomas" website (www.thomas.loc.gov). Simply enter the bill number, if known, or key words from the bill and use the search button to find information about a particular piece of legislation. It is absolutely essential that nurses stay actively engaged in tracking these important pieces of legislation and advocating for passage of legislation that will improve access to care, patient safety, quality of care, and the work environment of nurses.

BOX **23-2**

Helpful Websites and Online Resources

- AHRQ: Federal agency that sponsors and conducts research on health care outcomes; quality; and cost, use, and access; the information helps patients, clinicians, health system leaders, purchasers, and policymakers make more informed decisions and improve the quality of health care services: *www.ahrq.gov*
- American Nurses Association: Professional nursing organization representing the nation's entire registered nurse population: *www.nursingworld.org*
- Center for American Nurses: ANA-affiliate organization for nurses who are not represented by unions; offers noncollective bargaining workplace advocacy strategies, programs, and services to nurses: *www.centerforamericannurses.org*
- Department of Health and Human Services (HHS): Federal agency responsible for protecting the health of Americans and providing essential human services through more than 300 programs administered by 11 operating divisions: *www.hhs.gov*
- *Federal Register:* Best source of information about proposed rules and regulations for newly enacted legislation and changes to existing rules for federal programs: *www.gpoaccess.gov/fr*
- Institute of Medicine: Part of the National Academy of Sciences with a mission to advance and disseminate scientific knowledge to improve human health; provides objective, timely, authoritative information and advice concerning health and science policy to government, the corporate sector, the professions, and the public: *www.iom.edu*
- Library of Congress's "Thomas" website: Established to make federal legislative information freely available; tracks status of current legislation with historic information available as far back as the 104th Congress (1995): *www.thomas.gov*
- National Healthcare Quality Reports: Monitor the nation's progress toward improved health care safety and quality: *www.ahrq.gov/qual/measurix.htm*
- United American Nurses: Labor union for nurses, representing RNs nationwide; affiliate of both ANA and the AFL-CIO: *www.uannurse.org*
- United States House of Representatives: *www.house.gov*
- United States Senate: *www.senate.gov*

SUMMARY

Nurses must be powerful advocates for health care for all. By understanding the policy and political processes presented in this chapter, nurses can make significant contributions to the development of health policies that promote a healthier society (Box 23-2 lists websites that will help nurses be more knowledgeable and active advocates for health care reform.) A basic professional responsibility is to be involved in professional nursing organizations and to be politically active in supporting meaningful health policies. Just as the first politically active nurse, Florence Nightingale, used health policy to make a difference so can we make a difference in the lives of people we care for, in our own lives, and for the future of our profession.

 Additional resources are available online at: http://evolve.elsevier.com/Cherry/

REFERENCES

American Nurses Association: *Hill basics: the legislative process.* 2009a. Available at: http://nursingworld.org/MainMenuCategories/ANAPoliticalPower/Federal/ToolKit/LegislativeProcess.aspx.

American Nurses Association: *Tips: contacting members of Congress.* 2009b. Available at: www.nursingworld.org/MainMenuCategories/ANAPoliticalPower/Federal/ToolKit/ContactCongress.aspx.

Buerhaus PI: Massachusetts health care reform: lessons for the nation? *Nurs Econ* 27(3):194–196, 2009.

Congressional Record: Bill summary & status for the 110th Congress. 2009. Available at: www.thomas.gov/bss/110search.html.

Gonzales R. Headlines from the hill. health system reform: where is nursing? Where are you? *Am Nurse Today* 4(7):18, 2009.

Himmelstein DU, et al: *Medical bankruptcy in the United States, 2007: Results of a national study.* 2009. Available at: www.washingtonpost.com/wp-srv/politics/documents/american_journal_of_medicine_09.pdf.

Institute of Medicine: *The future of drug safety: promoting and protecting the health of the public.* 2006a. Available at www.nap.edu/catalog.php?record_id=11750.

Institute of Medicine: *To err is human: building a safer health system*, Washington, DC, 2000, National Academies Press.

Kaiser Family Foundation: *Kaiser Commission on Medicaid and the uninsured: the uninsured and the difference health insurance makes.* 2008. Available at: www.kff.org/uninsured/upload/1420-10.pdf.

Mason DJ, Leavitt JK, Chaffee MW: Policy and politics: a framework for action. In Mason DJ, Leavitt JK, Chaffee MW, editors: *Policy and politics in nursing and health care*, ed 5, Philadelphia, 2007, Saunders.

Oxhorn V, Rosen S: Understanding the regulatory arena, *AORN J* 55(2):623–629, 1992.

Page A, editor: *Keeping patients safe: transforming the work environment of nurses*, Washington, DC, 2004, National Academies Press.

Starr P: *The social transformation of American medicine: the rise of a sovereign profession and the making of a vast industry*, BasicBooks, Jackson, TN, 1982, HarperCollins Publishers.

Texas Nurses Association: *Highlights: safe hospital staffing act.* 2009. Available at: www.texasnurses.org/associations/8080/files/SafeHospitalStaffingAct.pdf.

U.S. Census Bureau: *Income, poverty, and health insurance coverage in the United States.* 2008. Available at: www.census.gov/prod/2008pubs/p60-235.pdf.

CHAPTER

24

Making the Transition from Student to Professional Nurse

Tommie L. Norris, DNS, RN

evolve Additional resources are available online at: http://evolve.elsevier.com/Cherry/

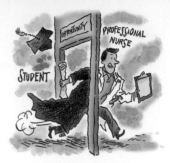

Moving from student to professional can be frightening: plan your strategies.

VIGNETTE

Every nurse has experienced the transition from student to professional nurse. Why can't we learn from our experiences and help our future nurses have a positive first impression of nursing? The cost alone of the revolving door for new nurses should be enough for organizations to reconsider not only how novice nurses are orienting to the facility but also what proactive measures are in place to ensure that experienced nurses stay rather than leave due to violence or burnout.

■ QUESTIONS TO CONSIDER WHILE READING THIS CHAPTER:

1 What could educators incorporate into the curriculum to decrease the "reality shock" of transition from student to professional nurse?

2 What could employers of novice nurses do during the orientation phase to help nurses learn the ropes of their organization, which may differ somewhat from the learning environment?

3 What strategies should novice nurses use to gain self-esteem and prove themselves capable of having the required skills while still needing help with specific tasks and skills that come with experience?

4 Should professional nurses form official task teams to look at the role of mentoring as one means of transitioning novice nurses into the profession?

5 What could orientation for new employees include to help novice nurses be proactive in preventing or reacting to violence at work?

KEY TERMS

Biculturalism The merging of school values with those of the workplace.
Compassion fatigue The gradual decline of compassion over time as a result of caregivers being exposed to events that have traumatized their patients.
Horizontal hostility (also known as lateral hostility) "A consistent (hidden) pattern of behavior designed to control, diminish, or devalue another peer [or group] that creates a risk to health and/or safety" (Hinchberger, 2009). Bullying, negative insinuations, undermining, and exclusion are examples.
Mentoring A mutual interactive method of learning in which a knowledgeable nurse inspires and encourages a novice nurse.

KEY TERMS—cont'd

Novice nurse A nurse who is entering the professional workplace for the first time; usually occurs from the point of graduation until competencies required by the profession are achieved.

Preceptor An experienced professional nurse who serves as a mentor and assists with socialization of the novice nurse.

Reality shock Occurs when a person prepares for a profession, enters the profession, and then finds that he or she is not prepared.

Role model A person who serves as an example of what constitutes a competent professional nurse.

Socialization The nurturing, acceptance, and integration of a person into the profession of nursing; the identification of a person with the profession of nursing.

Transition Moving from one role, setting, or level of competency in nursing to another; change.

Workplace violence Sexual harassment and abusive acts from patients that can be physical, verbal, and emotional and lead to a hostile work environment. It has been suggested that identifying workplace violence is difficult due to its subjectivity by the recipient.

LEARNING OUTCOMES

After studying this chapter, the reader will be able to:

1 Compare and contrast the phases of reality shock.

2 Differentiate between the novice nurse and the expert professional nurse.

3 Design strategies to ease the transition from novice to professional nurse.

4 Differentiate between compassion fatigue and burnout.

5 Make the transition from novice to professional nurse.

CHAPTER OVERVIEW

According to Webster (www.merriam-webster.com), transition is defined as "change" or the "passage from one state, place, stage, or subject to another." As nurses prepare to enter the profession and make the transition from student to registered nurse (RN), they move not only from one role to another, but also from the school or university setting to the workplace. Transition is a complicated process during which many changes may be happening at once. The novice nurse tries to juggle all these changes while continuing a life outside of nursing (e.g., as mother, father, husband, wife, daughter, son, active church leader, or community volunteer.

To help students gain an understanding of the issues involved in the transition from the student role to that of the professional nurse, this chapter discusses the various stages of reality shock. Strategies that may alleviate this shock and ease the transition are also suggested.

REAL-LIFE SCENARIO

The first impression the novice nurse has of his or her chosen profession is valuable and sets the stage for entry into nursing. This first impression occurs during the transition phase from student to professional. Consider the following scenario.

CASE STUDY

Rachel Stevens had wanted to be a nurse for as long as she could remember. As a child she donned a pretend laboratory jacket and set to work providing care to teddy bears and dolls. She softly spoke to her pretend patients, explaining that she was a nurse and would make everything better. After graduation from high school Rachel entered nursing school and visualized her dream coming true. She was

Continued

CASE STUDY—cont'd

a high achiever and received comments from her instructors, such as "shows evidence of applying the nursing process to the clinical environment," "psychomotor skills improving," and "becoming more autonomous." Her patients complimented her nursing abilities and caring attitude. Finally, Rachel graduated from nursing school, passed the national licensure examination, and accepted her first position as an RN. She proudly entered the hospital and felt confident that she would be a caring nurse and assist patients to achieve their highest level of health.

The hospital provided a 2-month orientation period. The first week consisted of classes to explain benefits, safety education, Standard Precaution protocols, and computer classes. Rachel loved her new job. The next step in her employment was orientation to the medical-surgical unit where she would be working. The nurse manager welcomed her to the unit and introduced her to the staff. Because all the seasoned nurses wanted to transfer to the day shift, Rachel was hired to work the evening shift, which had a higher nurse-patient ratio than the day shift. Rachel proudly sat through the shift report, jotting down reminders that were stressed by the previous shift, such as "The patient in room 200 needs a blood glucose test drawn at 6 PM," and "the patient in room 215 is to receive a unit of blood." Rachel's assignment consisted of six patients. The charge nurse encouraged Rachel to ask if she had any questions. The nursing assistants hurried to complete their tasks. Rachel reread her assignment and entered the first room. "Hello, my name is Rachel Stevens, and I'll be your nurse tonight." She assessed her patients and reviewed their medication sheets. No medications were due until 6 PM, so she began researching those medications with which she was not familiar. At 5:30 PM, the charge nurse informed Rachel that the only other nurse on the floor would be going for dinner and that Rachel should respond to her patients during her absence. Rachel was a little nervous about the responsibility, but positively acknowledged the assignment.

Moments later Rachel was paged to respond to a newly admitted patient who was assigned to the nurse on break. As soon as she entered the room, the patient complained of nausea and began vomiting. Rachel assessed and comforted the patient and reviewed the medication record for orders related to antiemetics. The physician had not ordered medication for nausea, so Rachel quickly telephoned his office to report the patient's condition. She received an order to insert a nasogastric tube and place to suction. Rachel was anxious; she had only inserted one such tube with her instructor's assistance. She gathered supplies and reentered the patient's room. She measured for correct placement and was just positioning the patient when she received a page that the blood had arrived for the other patient, and the laboratory assistant could not obtain a blood culture ordered on yet another of Rachel's patients.

After numerous unsuccessful attempts to insert the nasogastric tube, Rachel became more anxious and requested assistance from the charge nurse. The charge nurse replied, "I'm admitting a new patient and can't help you. Don't you know how to insert the nasogastric tube?" Rachel explained that she had made numerous attempts, and the patient was continuing to vomit. Rachel returned to the patient's room and attempted again to insert the tube. The nurse originally assigned to the patient returned to the floor; however, neither the secretary nor the charge nurse informed her of the new admission with orders, so she proceeded to care for her other patients. Finally, Rachel again requested help, and the charge nurse inserted the tube to the relief of Rachel and the patient. Now the medications were late, she had forgotten to check the patient's blood sugar, and she had not completed the charts. "Where are my notes?" Oh, well, she would just have to remember. Finally, at 10 PM, 1 hour before the shift ended, Rachel sat down to chart. She took out scrap paper and began writing her notes, but what time did she start the blood? She became more and more anxious. The clock continued to advance to 11 PM, and Rachel was still charting. "You need to give the shift report to the oncoming shift," said the charge nurse. Rachel complied and 15 minutes later returned to her charting. At 1 AM, Rachel left the unit feeling depressed and incompetent.

REALITY SHOCK

Nursing students are in college for several years and learn that role, many of them becoming expert students (Tingle, 2000). However, when the expert student moves into the novice nurse role, uncertainty takes over, and the support of classmates and the nursing instructors is gone. This time marks the end of one era as a student and the beginning of a new era in a nursing career.

Novice nurses often suffer what Kramer (1974) describes as reality shock, which is the result of inconsistencies between the academic world and the world of work. Reality shock occurs in novice nurses when they become aware of the inconsistency between the actual world of nursing and that of nursing school. As the novice nurse enters the new profession, reality shock begins. The excitement of passing the licensure examination quickly fades in the struggle to move from the student to the staff nurse role. Reality shock leads to stress (Bowles and Candela, 2005), which can threaten the well-being of new nurses resulting in physical illness and mental exhaustion, leading to disillusionment with their career (Hertel, 2009) and ultimately absenteeism and turnover (Jennings, 2008). There are four phases of reality shock: honeymoon, shock or rejection, recovery, and resolution (Kramer, 1974).

Honeymoon Phase

During the honeymoon phase everything is just as the new graduate imagined. The new nurse is in orientation with former school friends or other new graduates who often share similarities. Many novice nurses in this phase are heard making the following comments: "Just think, now I'll get paid for making all those beds" and "I'm so glad I chose nursing; I will be a part of changing the future of health care."

Shock (Rejection) Phase

Then orientation is over, and the novice nurse begins work on his or her assigned unit. This nurse receives daily assignments and begins the tasks. "But wait. I've only observed other nurses hanging blood. Where is my instructor?" Now the shock or rejection phase comes into play. The nurse comes into contact with conflicting viewpoints and different ways of performing skills, but lacks the security of having an expert available to explain uncertain or gray areas. The security of saying, "I am just the student nurse," is no longer valid. During this phase, the novice nurse may be frightened or react by forming a hard, cold shell around him or herself. Vague feelings of discomfort are experienced, and the inexperienced nurse often wonders whether the other nurses care about the patients. After going home from a shift, the new nurse may experience feelings of rejection and a sense of lack of accomplishment. The novice nurse may reject the new environment and have a preoccupation with the past when he or she was in school. A need to contact former instructors, call schoolmates, or visit the nursing school may occur. Others may reject their school values and adopt the values of the organization. In this way, they may experience less conflict (Kramer, 1974); however, there are drawbacks to this approach as well.

During this phase Kramer (1974) suggests that novice nurses must ask themselves two important questions:

1. What must I do to become the kind of nurse I want to be?
2. What must I do so that my nursing contributes to humankind and society?

Dealing with the shock phase can be approached in many different ways. Some common approaches for dealing with it are reviewed in the following sections. After that each nurse must decide which method best allows the previous two questions to be answered.

Natives. Many nurses choose to go "native" (Kramer, 1974, p. 161). That is, they decide they cannot fight the experienced nurses or the administration, thus they adopt the ways of least resistance. These nurses may mimic other nurses on the unit and take shortcuts, such as administering medications without knowing their action and side effects and the associated nursing responsibilities.

Runaways. Others choose to "run away." They find the real world too difficult. These new nurses may choose another occupation or return to graduate school to prepare for a career in nursing education to teach others their "values in nursing."

Rutters. Some adopt the attitude that "I'll just do what I have to do to get by," or "I'm just working until I can buy some new furniture." These nurses are called "rutters." They consider nursing just a job.

Burned Out. These nurses bottle up conflict until they become burned out. Kramer (1974) describes the appearance of these nurses as having the look of being chronically constipated. In this situation, patients may feel compelled to nurse their nurse. Inexperienced nurses may become burned out because they assume too many responsibilities in a short period of time (Domrose, 2000). Some common symptoms of burnout include extreme fatigue, headaches, difficulty sleeping, mood swings, anxiety, poor work quality, depression, and anger (Larsen, 2000). The more intelligent, hard-working nurses are the most prone for burnout, but if you exhibit these symptoms; remember that they can be reduced.

Compassion Fatigue. Not to be confused with burnout or transference, compassion fatigue is the gradual decline of compassion over time as a result of caregivers being exposed to events that have traumatized their patients (Figley, 2001). Even experienced nurses, who commonly have a great deal of empathy, working in environments in which patients have suffered trauma, may develop a reaction in which they have a decrease in compassion. Exposure to traumatic events experienced by their patients may result in compassion fatigue. Nurses who work in emotionally charged environments, such as hospice, emergency departments, and mental health settings, are likely to experience this reaction. The compassion fatigue process is depicted in Figure 24-1.

Loners. These nurses create their own reality. They adopt the attitude of "just do the job and keep quiet." These nurses may prefer night shifts, during which they often are "left alone."

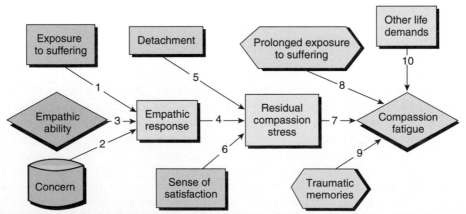

Figure 24-1 *Compassion fatigue process. (Figley CR: Compassion fatigue: an introduction. 2001. Retrieved December 2006 from: www.giftfromwithin.org/html/cmpfatig.html.)*

New Nurse on the Block. These nurses change jobs frequently. They go from the hospital setting to community health to the physician's office. They are always new in their setting and therefore adopt the attitude of "teach me what you want; I'm new here."

Change Agents. These are the nurses who care enough to work within the system to elicit change. They frequently visit the nurse manager or head nurse to suggest change or a better way. They keep the welfare of the patient at the forefront. Unfortunately, Kramer refers to these nurses as "bicultural troublemakers" (1974, pp. 91–93).

Recovery Phase

The return of humor usually is the first sign of the recovery phase. The novice nurse begins to understand the new culture to a certain degree. There is less tension and anxiety, and healing begins. The nurse in this phase may comment, "I'll hang that blood, and I'll bet I can infuse it before 8 hours this time."

Resolution Phase

The resolution phase is the result of the shock phase combined with the novice nurse's ability to adjust to the new environment. If the nurse is able to positively work through the rejection phase, he or she grows more fully as a person and a professional nurse during the resolution phase. Work expectations are more easily met, and the nurse will have developed the ability to elicit change.

Most novice nurses experience each phase of reality shock (honeymoon, shock or rejection, recovery, and resolution); however, the degree of shock is individualized. For example, the new graduates who complete their clinical rotation during school in the same institution as they choose to begin their career may suffer reality shock to a much lesser degree because they already may be familiar with the environment, staff, and overall personality of the nursing unit. However, many students choose another institution for various reasons, such as better hours, better pay, or less travel time to work. Nurses who choose to work in an institution different from the one in which they worked as student nurses may experience a higher degree of shock. This does not imply that all nurses should work in the institution where they received their clinical educational experience. The staff in the institution where novice nurses were educated may continue to see them as only "student nurses," which simply presents another barrier for novice nurses to overcome.

Zerwekh and Claborn (2009) suggest completing a reality shock inventory to make nurses more aware of how they feel about themselves and the situation at present. The higher the score, the better the attitude. It might be helpful to take the test at different times throughout one's career or when trying to decide whether a career change would be advantageous (Box 24-1).

CAUSES OF REALITY SHOCK

Many nurses are familiar with the term "culture shock." Culture shock occurs when people are immersed into a culture different from their own with norms that are unfamiliar and uncomfortable. This is exactly what happens in reality shock. Academia stresses patient-centered nursing, whereas the workforce stresses management of tasks and timelines, which may lead to feelings of failure because of the inability to provide holistic care. Novice nurses who can't complete all their tasks are often classified as unvalued (Farrell, 2001). First, consider how students were taught to think in nursing school. When they prepared a care plan that took all night to complete, how were they to view the patient? Nursing schools teach holistic nursing, or rather "wholistic" nursing, in which students are taught to look at the patient as a whole and even incorporate the family and significant other into the care plan. However, in the real world

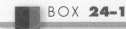

BOX **24-1**

Reality Shock Inventory

Respond to the following statements with the appropriate number.

1—Strongly agree	4—Slightly disagree
2—Agree	5—Disagree
3—Slightly agree	6—Strongly disagree

_____ I think often about what I really want from life.

_____ Nursing school and/or my work has brought stresses for which I was unprepared.

_____ I would like the opportunity to start anew, knowing what I know now.

_____ I drink more than I should.

_____ I often feel that I still belong in the place where I grew up.

_____ Much of the time my mind is not as clear as it used to be.

_____ I am experiencing what would be called a crisis in my personal or work setting.

_____ I cannot see myself as a nurse.

_____ I must remain loyal to commitments, even if they have not proven as rewarding as I had expected.

_____ I wish I were different in many ways.

_____ The way I present myself to the world is not the way I really am.

_____ I often feel agitated or restless.

_____ I have become more aware of my inadequacies and faults.

_____ I often think about students or friends who have dropped out of school or work.

_____ I am still finding new challenges and interest in my work.

_____ My own personal future seems promising.

_____ There is no sense of regret concerning my major life decision of becoming a nurse.

_____ My views on nursing are as positive as they ever were.

_____ I have a strong sense of my own worth.

_____ My sex life is as satisfactory as it has ever been.

SCORING

To compute your score, reverse the number you assigned to statements 1, 3, 9, 10, 11, and 19. For example, if you responded to a statement with a 1, your score for that statement would be a 6. Likewise 2 would become a 5; 3 would become a 4; 4 would become a 3; 5 would become a 2; and 6 would become a 1. Total the numbers. The higher your score, the better your attitude. The range is 20 to 120.

From Zerwekh J, Claborn JC: *Nursing today: transition and trends,* ed 5, Philadelphia, 2006, Saunders.

nurses may function with a partial-person approach. Different members of the health care team divide the patient care into parts.

Partial-Task Versus Whole-Task System

This type of health care, in which different members of the health care team divide the patient care into parts, is termed the partial-task system and only requires partial knowledge (Kramer, 1974). For instance, one nurse may be assigned to administer all medications, whereas another may be assigned to dressing changes. The nursing assistant aids with personal hygiene and grooming; the physical therapist provides range-of-motion exercises, and the respiratory therapist teaches pulmonary hygiene techniques. There are many other nursing care delivery models in which the role of the RN varies considerably. The partial-task system just described is also congruent with the model known as "functional nursing," which places a high emphasis on completion of tasks. It is an efficient method when working with large numbers of patients, but the nurse cannot provide holistic care within such a system (Huber, 2009). With functional nursing and the partial-task system, the nurse is seen as only part of the care picture, but the RN is the central organizer and responsible for follow-through on all care given by other members. This type of system is popular because fewer professional staff members are required, and it is frequently used on the evening and night shifts when staffing is considerably less. This type of partial-task system encourages loyalty to the organization because it forces the nurse to focus on task completion and productivity. The nurse ensures that all tasks are carried out, but is not the sole provider of care. A simple checkmark often assesses quality, with initials being placed by completed tasks (Box 24-2).

Most novice nurses are more comfortable with the whole-task system because it is more consistent with what they were taught in school. The whole-task system requires complete knowledge and encourages loyalty to the profession. The nurse provides total patient care, which incorporates physical, emotional, spiritual, and cultural components. The model of nursing care consistent with the whole-task system is primary nursing, in which the nurse is responsible for all the needs of the patient (Huber, 2009). This model provides increased satisfaction for the patient and the nurse. However, because of the need to use an increasing number of lower-salaried employees and the shortage of RNs, few institutions continue to use this model.

Evaluation Methods

Another inconsistency between the school and work environment is the means of evaluation (Kramer, 1974). The school environment evaluates care from the "correct step" aspect, whereas the evaluation phase in the work environment is based on whether components of care were completed according to established policies and procedures. Were all the steps carried out in a logical, correct, and efficient way? This is exemplified in the following scenario:

CASE STUDY

A graduate nurse was involved in a resuscitation effort. After the incident she exclaimed, "I remembered to keep the time recorded and even had all the needed equipment on hand. I did everything right." But what about the patient? This nurse may have enacted all the steps correctly, but may not have completed the components of care according to policies and procedures.

BOX **24-2**

Whole-Task and Partial-Task Checklist

WHOLE-TASK CHECK LIST (Completed by same nurse)			**PARTIAL-TASK CHECKLIST** (Completed by different members of the health care team)		
Initials		**Task**	**Initials**		**Task**
TN	✓	Nursing history	SJ	✓	Nursing history
TN	✓	Nursing assessment	TN	✓	Nursing assessment
TN	✓	Patient education	BC	✓	Patient education
TN	✓	Medication teaching	CS	✓	Medication teaching
TN	✓	Bed made	CS	✓	Bed made
TN	✓	Intake and output recorded	SJ	✓	Intake and output recorded
TN	✓	Dressing changed	SJ	✓	Dressing changed
TN	✓	IV fluids hung	CS	✓	IV fluids hung
TN	✓	Patient turned	BC	✓	Patient turned

Think back to your first days in the nursing skills course. Can you remember the hours of practice you spent in learning the six rights of medication administration and technique of parenteral medication administration? Remember the stress you felt when the instructor observed you drawing up and administering your first intravenous (IV) push medication? How much error did the instructor allow? Probably not much. This is not to say that you should become lax in your tolerance for error. For example, it is never acceptable to have errors in the six rights of medication administration. You must and will develop your own system and quality check for performing nursing care. Nursing texts often list supplies followed by a flow diagram for procedures in which each step is listed. Let us go back to the resuscitation scenario: even basic and advanced life support courses focus on algorithms that direct, step by step, the care of the patient. Always remember that patient safety comes first.

The transition from student to professional nurse is difficult, and changes in the health care environment have only added to the strain. Socialization of the novice nurse is key to his or her ability to transition or just "survive" at the clinical level (Mooney, 2007). Often new nurses are greeted with open hostility rather than being welcomed (Adler, 2009; DeRung 2004). Nursing administrators may not support the novices' need to learn and may expect them to perform at the same level as experienced nurses. Unfortunately, the novice nurse may become bewildered and discouraged.

FROM NOVICE TO EXPERT

Benner (1984) described the following five stages through which novice nurses proceed to become clinically competent:

- **Stage 1:** The nurse has few experiences with clinical expectations, and skills are learned by rote; this stage usually occurs while completing the nursing educational requirements.
- **Stage 2:** Exemplifies advanced beginners who are able to perform adequately and make some judgment calls based on experience; most novice nurses enter the workforce during this stage.
- **Stage 3:** Includes competent nurses who are able to foresee long-range goals and are mastering skills.
- **Stage 4:** Includes proficient nurses who view whole situations rather than parts and are able to develop a solution.
- **Stage 5:** Includes expert nurses for whom intuition and decision making are instantaneous.

During these five stages of transition from novice to expert, nurses are most likely to experience stress. Stressors common to novice nurses include the following:

- Unrealistic expectations: novice nurses are expected to care for a standard patient workload as soon as orientation is completed (Chesnutt and Everhart, 2007)
- Stressful work environments: patient ratios are unrealistic (Bowles and Candela (2005)
- Powerlessness: novice nurses are not heard when suggesting changes to improve workflow but often are blamed when things go wrong (Mooney, 2007)

SPECIAL NEEDS OF NOVICE NURSES

The following skills have been identified as needing further refinement in novice nurses. Discussion about each of these areas follows.

- Interpersonal skills and communication skills (Ricker, 2008; Tingle, 2000)
- Clinical skills (Gries, 2000; Ricker, 2008)
- Organizational skills (Tingle, 2000)

  ◆ Delegation skills (Huber, 2009; Tingle, 2000)
  ◆ Priority-setting skills (Gries, 2000; Huber, 2009; Ricker, 2008)
  ◆ Assertiveness skills

Interpersonal Skills

Most physicians, administrators, and nurse managers expect the novice nurse to immediately develop interpersonal skills that they take for granted. These feelings probably are rooted in the past when nurses in training spent most of their time on units caring for patients and received little theoretic information or content in the classroom setting. They had time to get to know the members of the health care team and felt comfortable interacting with them. It is difficult for many people, including novice nurses, to be comfortable with interpersonal skills at work when they feel incompetent and inadequate as a member of the interprofessional health care team. They are often uncomfortable making rounds, clarifying orders, and participating in interprofessional team conferences. However, effective communication is critical. For example, the novice nurse receives the following order from the patient's physician: "Give Tylenol as needed for pain." The unit secretary transcribes the order and hands the chart to the new nurse, stating, "You will need to clarify this order: I can't take the new order." Feelings of fear and uncertainty invade the novice nurse as he or she practices what to say to the physician.

> *"Can you clarify the Tylenol order on your patient?" Or possibly, "How much Tylenol did you want your patient to have?" or maybe "Hey stupid, can't you write your orders using the six rights?"*

Well, perhaps the conversation would go as follows:

> *"Dr. Jones, this is the student nurse. I mean the nurse taking care of your patient. I don't understand your order. I mean can you clarify how much Tylenol you want me to take? I mean how much Tylenol do you want the patient to have?"*

The inexperienced nurse hangs up feeling ineffective, and the physician questions the nursing care the patient is being given.

Before asking the physician to clarify the order, it is a good idea to practice what will be said and even write it down so as not to forget. Then when face to face with the person, state the facts simply and allow time to consider the correct answer. A smile during the exchange in conversation might provide the receiver with a little more patience. Gaps in communication may also occur between the experienced staff and the novice nurse because staff are so familiar with the routines that they may leave out information, making the novice unable to complete the task. Novice nurses must listen, ask the appropriate person, and avoid distractions when communicating (Tingle, 2000).

Clinical Skills

Novice nurses often lack trust in experienced nurses to help them problem solve clinical situations (Pine and Tart, 2007). Practice increases the effectiveness, efficiency, and correctness of performing skills. However, until the nurse has experience, there are actions the novice nurse can take. For example, it is wise to be familiar with the procedure manual on the unit. Also during the orientation phase, the novice nurse should ask to observe or assist an experienced nurse with procedures for which there is a lower comfort level or a lesser degree of experience. It is important to remember that no skill is "basic," and step-by-step instructions, such as those found in procedure manuals, are helpful (Gries, 2000). Remember that everyone had to learn these skills. No one was born with a Foley catheter in one hand and the set of directions engraved in memory.

Organizational Skills

The novice nurse may lack organizational skills. This lack of proficiency may be exaggerated by feelings of being "overwhelmed" by the new environment. Typically, student nurses are responsible for a limited number of patients, and although they must answer for their care, they typically are not responsible for as many patients as they will be assigned as new nurses. Someone is usually with students to offer suggestions on how to organize their time. The instructor might question: "Now what do you plan to do, and what supplies will you need to accomplish the task?" New nurses might consider asking these same questions. If unsure the procedure book lists not only the steps to follow but also the supplies that will be needed. List specific time-limited tasks. Avoid scheduling time so tightly that a slight delay causes chaos. Planning and prioritization skills were seen as an area of concern of newly graduated nurses (Lofmark, Smide, and Wikblad, 2006). Chapter 25 offers valuable tips on getting organized, setting priorities, and managing time.

Delegation Skills

Most students have limited exposure to delegation. Uncertainty or feeling uncomfortable with delegation may be a result of the characteristics of the personnel to whom one is delegating. Consider the licensed practical nurse, the nursing assistant, or other nonlicensed staff. Often these personnel are older and more experienced; therefore, the new nurse might feel intimidated when delegating to these individuals. Novice nurses should familiarize themselves with policies concerning which tasks can be performed by which category or level of health care provider. The question "Who can perform this task other than myself?" should be considered. Because of the broad span of responsibility for most nursing jobs, it is impossible for one person to complete all the work alone (Huber, 2009). Delegation relies on trust and leadership skills, both of which may be deficient in the novice nurse. Chapter 19 presents a comprehensive overview of delegation.

There are also times when the novice nurse should decline to accept a delegated responsibility because he or she may not be competent to perform the task even though it is within his or her scope of practice. Remember that patient safety is always the priority. Show your willingness to learn and ask someone to demonstrate the task. Tingle (2000, p. 3) suggests simply stating, "I haven't done this; who can talk me through it?" or "I don't know how to do that, but I am willing to help with it."

Priority-Setting Skills

Priority setting is a skill that all nursing students must demonstrate. The difference between nursing school and the real world is that serious consequences occur if prioritizing is not done effectively in the real world. Flanagan (1997) suggests asking the following questions when prioritizing:

- Will patients be jeopardized if this task is not done?
- Is this task a priority because of time deadlines?
- What other personnel can perform this task?
- Do safety concerns make this task a priority?
- What will be the consequences if this task is postponed?
- What are the legal issues related to the priority of the task?

Many novice nurses need help in organizational skills and saying no is difficult (Gries, 2000). Novice nurses may derive more satisfaction from performing technical skills, such as starting an intravenous (IV) drip, than from cognitive skills, such as developing a plan of care. Once they are comfortable with basic skills, they move on to critical thinking skills. Gries (2000) stresses that with the loss of the graduate nurse role, novice nurses are propelled into practice, where they focus on what they do not know and are seemingly blind to their accomplishments. For further exploration you can visit an online scenario by Gries of how this can happen to a novice nurse at: http://community.nursingspectrum.com/MagazineArticles/article.cfm?AID=800.

Gries (2000) also supports the idea of nurses using an organization sheet to facilitate prioritization and completion. How many people make to-do lists? Many make grocery lists, lists of bills to be paid, or lists of important dates. The same should be done for work—tasks are crossed off as they are completed. At the end of the day, consider what time was spent in unproductive ways, what caused interruptions, and what could have been done to save time. Huber (2009) also suggests determining the urgency of the problem, which allows for prioritization.

Assertiveness Skills

Students are often very gullible when they are told by recruiters, "Come work for us; we offer a 6-month orientation, and you can ask for an extension if you feel uncomfortable. You will not be placed in charge, and only after a full year's experience will you be allowed to independently care for patients requiring advanced technology, such as ventricular assist devices." Students may be misled into feeling that they are "advanced" in their learning and moving ahead of all the others if they agree to shorten their orientation or if, after only 6 months, they take on the responsibility of caring for patients with special equipment.

However, after 6 months, even though novice nurses are becoming more competent and confident, they lack the experience to make instantaneous decisions based on intuition. Unfortunately novice nurses are often employed on the night shift working with nurses with the same or less experience. As newer novice nurses (those who graduated the following semester) are hired, the more experienced novice nurses may even be expected to serve as a preceptor. Faculty should invite recent graduates to speak to classes concerning expectations after employment. Faculty should also inform the students that they will move through many stages during the next year, and they should take full advantage of this learning opportunity.

VIOLENCE AT WORK

When you think of dangerous occupations, law enforcement and military careers may come to mind. However, nursing is four times more dangerous than most other occupations (Gallant-Roman, 2008), second only to law enforcement in violence at work (Duhart, 2001). Workplace violence aimed at nursing is increasing at an alarming rate across the world (Chapman et al, 2009; Hinchberger, 2009) with abusive acts committed by patients increasing (Paniagua, Bond, and Thompson, 2009). Sixty percent of nurses reported being threatened or verbally abused and 90% cited health and safety concerns as influencing their decision to leave nursing (Palmer, 2003). Student nurses are prone to physical assaults as well as those nurses working in the psychiatric and learning disability areas (Wells and Bowers, 2002). Student nurses are also leading recipients of horizontal or nurse-to-nurse violence, which perpetuates the cycle of "lateral violence continuing in nursing because it can" (Sincox and Fitzpatrick, 2008). Four types of workplace violence are identified by Olszewski, Parks, and Chikotas (2007) and a fifth by Baltimore (2006) and Ramos (2006) in Box 24-3.

Baltimore describes the fifth type, horizontal or lateral violence to include such acts as "antagonism, gossiping, criticism, innuendo, scapegoat, undermining, intimidation, passive aggression, withholding information, insubordination, bullying, and verbal and physical

BOX **24-3**

Types of Workplace Violence

Type 1	These violent acts are not committed by employees; rather criminals are the perpetrators of the crime on entering the health care agency/organization.
Type 2	Patients become perpetrators of violent acts.
Type 3	Prior or disgruntled employees commit violence against current employees and/or management.
Type 4	Individuals who have a relationship with a current employee commit a violent act in the health care environment.
Type 5	Violence that occurs between workers; known as horizontal violence.

Baltimore JJ: Nurse collegiality: fact or fiction? *Nurs Manage* 37(5):28-36, 2006; Olszewski K, Parks C, Chikotas NE: Occupational safety and health objectives of *Healthy People 2010:* part II. A systematic approach for occupational health nurses, *AAOHN J* 55(3):115-123, 2007; Ramos MC: Eliminate destructive behaviors through example and evidence, *Nurs Manag* 37(9):34-41, 2006.

aggression (2006, p. 30), and Longo and Sherman add belittling, blocking promotion, and isolation (2007). This type of violence leads to decreased job satisfaction and even turnover. Nurses may exhibit marginality in which the nurse takes on the characteristics of the oppressor (Sofield and Salmond, 2003), directing frustration toward coworkers and subordinates which may unfortunately be the novice nurses (Longo and Sherman, 2007) entering their nursing career. This violence quickly diffuses the novices' enthusiasm for their new profession as they become the object of gossip by more experienced nurses. A new grad describes horizontal violence from nurses, physicians, anesthesia staff, pharmacy, and unit secretaries as the type of environment that pushes novice nurses out of the hospital and profession (DeRung, 2004). Baltimore (2006) suggests incompetence is seldom the culprit, but instead that purposeful omission and lack of guidance from more experienced staff lead to errors made by novice nurses. At a time of a severe nursing shortage, a survey reported by Baltimore (2006) found that 75% of nurses feel novices are indeed the recipients of hostility.

STRATEGIES TO EASE TRANSITION

When interviewing for their first positions, novice nurses should determine philosophies of the agencies and how orientation programs assist new nurses to enter the profession. There are many opinions on the best way to accomplish a smooth transition, and each nurse should evaluate orientation options available.

Novice nurses are even chatting on the Internet about their frustrations with the transition from student to professional nurse. One such novice nurse described herself as in a race, having only 5 minutes for meals, and having to stay overtime (Cybernurse, 2000). She searches the Internet for "words of encouragement for a novice" and to learn how others have dealt with the period of change.

Biculturalism

Biculturalism is the joining of two contradictory value systems, in this context, those of school values with those of the workplace. Biculturalism is designed to enhance a positive self-image and help novice nurses set realistic goals for practice. This strategy, if accepted in the workplace, allows the new nurse to introduce ideas or values brought from nursing school and integrate them into the work environment. Kramer (1974) suggests that the novice nurse apprise both sides of an issue, determine how his or her behavior will have an effect on other members of the interprofessional health care team, and single out accessible objectives.

Role Models and Mentors

Mentoring and role modeling are often considered to be the same, but in fact they are different. Mentoring is an interactive, mutual, and personal experience (Sullivan and Decker, 2009), whereas role modeling is usually not an interactive process (Stone, 2000). Sullivan and Decker (2009) suggest that choosing the correct mentor is one of the most important tasks for the novice nurse.

Mentors are experienced nurses who must be willing to commit to a relationship with novice nurses to help them recognize their weaknesses and strengths. Mentors help novice nurses set and reach realistic goals by reinforcing and recommending appropriate courses of action. Mentors help novice nurses build self-confidence and gain professional satisfaction while helping novice nurses develop as nurses and individuals (Blakeney, 2005). The benefactor of mentoring is termed a protégé. A skilled mentor can be a role model, but also serves as the student advocate (Blakeney, 2005) opening not only the novice's eyes to the profession but also hopefully a few professional doors and career opportunities (Sherman and Murphy, 2009). A patient mentor can also be a positive role model (Lee and Harris, 2007). Vance (2000) lists the characteristics of both the mentor and protégé in Box 24-4. The Florida Nurses Association published a guideline for identifying mentors found in Box 24-5.

Recruitment and retention efforts are often supplemented with mentoring programs, which have become especially important in light of the current nursing shortage (Childers, 2003; Sullivan and Decker, 2009). Some mentoring programs are aimed specifically at pairing male students and male novice nurses with male mentors. Just as females face special challenges when entering a preponderantly male profession, so do men entering the preponderantly female

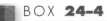

BOX **24-4**

Characteristics of Mentor and Protégé

MENTOR	PROTÉGÉ
Generosity	Takes initiative
Competence	Career commitment
Self-confidence	Self-identity
Openness to mutuality	Openness to mutuality

From Vance C: Discovering the riches in mentor connections, *Reflect Nurs Leadersh* 26(3):24-25, 2000.

BOX **24-5**

Guidelines for Identifying Mentors (Florida Nurses Association)

Knowledgeable in the novice's area of interest.
Honest and trustworthy to allow novice to voice frustrations and maintain confidentiality.
Emotional security demonstrating confidence and steadfastness when communicating with novice nurses.
Maturity to separate self from emotions of the mentee.
Willingness to share helpful hints to ease the transition of the novice or less experienced nurse.

profession of nursing. Networking with other male nurses helps with the socialization and integration of men into the profession.

Preceptorships

Another popular orientation program is the use of preceptors during the final semester of nursing school and on entering the workforce. Preceptor programs have gained popularity as a means to socialize the novice nurse into the profession and to ease the tension of transition from student to nurse. Preceptor programs often are incorporated during the senior nursing student's final practicum, but they also may be used as part of the orientation program in the first work experience. Preceptorship is often viewed as one method of orientation, which usually lasts about 3 weeks (Sullivan and Decker, 2009). Preceptors orient the novice nurse to the specific nursing area, aid in socialization, and teach skills that are deemed necessary. Preceptor programs reduce economic cost by reducing turnover of new graduates and assisting novice nurses in meeting the expectations of their employers and peers.

Self-Mentoring

Ultimately no one is as responsible for the transition into the nursing profession as the novice nurses themselves. Mentors and preceptors can ease the transition, but novice nurses can also help by using self-mentoring when preceptors or mentors are not available. Novice nurses must be willing to learn appropriate references, develop problem-solving skills, and ask questions. Novices should reflect back over times when they were self-reliant and believed in themselves.

Residency Programs

Residency programs are one innovative way to ease the transition from academia to practice and also may be an incentive for graduates when selecting that first job. Residency programs often provide didactic or program activities as well as one-to-one precepted experiences for an extended time, with 12 months being typical. Although residency programs differ, they all focus on retention and increased satisfaction of the new nurse with the added bonus of improved patient outcomes and safety. One such residency program in Colorado provides a 12-month precepted experience first introducing clinical and leadership development, then critical thinking. One novice nurse who participated in a residency program described it as "a starting off point" rather than a "being shoved off" (Ricker, 2008) as she worked one-one with a preceptor.

Preprofessional and Professional Organizations

Students who join preprofessional organizations, such as the National Student Nurses Association (NSNA), gain leadership opportunities and meet not only other students from across the nation and internationally but also leaders in nursing, whom they thought they would only read about. Students participating in the NSNA leadership university network learn how to "work in cooperative relationships with peers, faculty, students in other disciplines, community service organizations, and the public in a service learning environment" (www.nsnaleadershipu. org). These organizations provide another avenue for socialization and a sense of "belonging to an important profession" (Domrose, 2003). The NSNA publishes a magazine with information on job opportunities and legislative issues that affect nursing practice. Participation in preprofessional organizations develops leadership skills that are useful in professional organizations and for potential employers after graduation. The American Nurses Association (ANA) and some state specialty organizations offer reduced rates for new graduates and student nurses and continue with the above-mentioned benefits after graduation. In addition to lobbying efforts, access to up-to-date information on standards of practice, certification, and networking opportunities are also benefits of involvement in the ANA.

Self-Confidence and Self-Esteem

"Even though this is my dream, I can still get discouraged. I can still forget that this is what I want to do" (Klein and Dickenson-Hazard, 2000, p. 21).

A relationship woven with encouragement can inspire self-esteem and self-confidence. It is easy to become discouraged and disillusioned when reality does not quite match our dreams and fantasy. Self-esteem, or belief in oneself, comes as the novice nurse passes through the stages of reality shock and into a career in nursing.

Self-esteem = Self-confidence + Self-respect

Individuals with high self-esteem can critically problem solve, tackle obstacles, take sensible risks, believe in themselves, and take care of themselves (Positive Way, 2000). Nurses with self-esteem are effective and respond to themselves and others in healthy ways (Figure 24-2). They can accomplish more because they feel comfortable with themselves. Take the self-esteem questionnaire in Box 24-6; then go to the Create Positive Relationships website. If your score is low, visit the Positive Way website to learn how to stop the inner critic (http://positive-way. com/stopping%20your%20inner%20critic.htm).

So far we have discussed ways that the employer and novice nurse can use to ease the transition period—implementing biculturalism, preceptorships, mentoring, and self-mentoring. However, each new nurse must begin by evaluating his or her own self-esteem. In addition, the novice nurse must realize his or her uniqueness and rely on instinct and past experiences when maturing and moving to a higher level of responsibility. The new nurse should remember to seek a role model or mentor for guidance through the transition. It is important to remember that it is difficult to be successful if personal and social life are not kept in balance (e.g., in high school it was great to solve all the chemistry equations on an examination, but if "personal chemistry" was neglected, a void was felt that could plague future attempts at maturing).

Violence Prevention

Because new graduates are frequently victims of horizontal violence in their first year of practice, preceptors with zero tolerance for such activities are invaluable. It is also suggested that

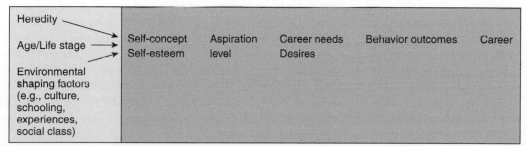

Figure 24-2 *Behavior model. (From Schutz C, Decker PJ, Sullivan EJ: Effective management in nursing: an-experiential/ skill building workbook, Menlo Park, CA, 1992, Addison-Wesley.)*

BOX **24-6**

Self-Esteem Questionnaire

Answer yes or no to the following questions:

_____ Do you have a hard time nurturing yourself?

_____ Have you ever turned down an invitation to a party or function because of the way you felt about yourself?

_____ Do you get your sense of self-worth from the approval of others?

_____ Are you supportive of others who berate you?

_____ When things go wrong in life, do you blame yourself?

_____ Do you react to disappointment by blaming others?

_____ Do you begin each day with a negative attitude?

_____ Do you feel undeserving?

_____ Do you ever feel like an impostor and that soon your deficiencies will be exposed?

_____ Do you have an inner critic who is disparaging or demeaning?

_____ Do you believe that being hard on yourself is the best motivation for change?

_____ Do your good points seem ordinary and your failings all important?

_____ Do you feel unattractive?

_____ Have you ever felt that your accomplishments are due to luck but that your failures are due to incompetence or inadequacy?

_____ Have you ever felt that, if you are not a total success, then you are a failure and that there is no middle ground and no points for effort?

_____ Do you feel unappreciated?

_____ Do you feel lonely?

_____ Do you struggle with feelings of inferiority?

_____ Do other people's opinions count more to you than your own?

_____ Do you criticize yourself often?

_____ Do others criticize you often?

_____ Do you hesitate to do things because of what others might think?

The more yes answers you have, the greater the opportunity exists for improving your self-esteem.

Positive Way, 2000, PO Box 1703, Williamsville, NY 14231 (e-mail: positive-way@positive-way.com).

having nurses on the unit describe their first year may deflect the desire to continue the violence cycle with the new hires (Baltimore, 2006; Longo and Sherman, 2007). Novices who practiced responses to horizontal violence during orientation were better equipped to successfully defend against horizontal violence (Longo and Sherman, 2007). Baltimore (2006) also suggests that nurses should devise a plan to increase socialization of novice nurses with staff; make assignments realistic, role modeling professional behavior, check egos, evaluate attitudes of staff, resist gossiping, and should conflict arise address it directly with the individual. Should incompetence of the novice be apparent, leave this to management to resolve. Perhaps most important is making horizontal violence transparent. DeRung (2004), herself a novice nurse, suggested finding intra and interprofessional coworkers who exhibit healthy working relationships and not dwell on the negative but refuse to accept abusive behaviors. Novice nurses entering the workforce will find the Occupational Safety and Health Administration (OSHA) book *Guidelines for Preventing Workplace Violence for Health Care and Social Service Workers* helpful (www.osha.gov/SLTC/etools/hospital/hazards/workplaceviolence/viol.html) along with the *Framework Guidelines for Addressing Workplace Violence in the Health Sector* (www.osha.gov/SLTC/etools/hospital/hazards/workplaceviolence/viol.html#violenceprevention). In fact, OSHA has called for zero tolerance of workplace violence. "The incidence of lateral violence and bullying in the workplace is on the rise" (Center for American Nurses and AzNA, 2009, p. 6). Due to this increase in workplace violence and conflict, The Joint Commission introduced standards requiring health care organizations to construct a code of conduct that clearly defines "acceptable, disruptive, and inappropriate behavior" (Martin, 2008, p. 22). Novice nurses can access the Conflict Engagement Portfolio for help with managing conflict management (www.centerforamericannurses.org) and should review the ANA position statement for recommended strategies to help eliminate lateral violence (www.centerforamericannurses.org/positions/lateral_violence.pdf). Chapman and colleagues (2009) suggest nurses can predict the risk of workplace violence instigated by patients by using the acronym STAMPEDAR (staring, tone of voice, anxiety, mumbling, pacing, emotions, disease process, assertive/nonassertive behavior, and resources. Adler (2009) suggests having a village of senior nurses who help novice nurses and demonstrate caring can rewrite our legacy from "eating our own" to one of caring and compassion to our fledging nurses. Novice nurses are key to stopping the cycle of horizontal violence by being aware of its existence and refusing to accept it as part of the hazing of new nurses. Novice nurses must report any behavior that undermines them on their job; this may be horizontal violence (Hinchberger, 2009).

KEYS TO SURVIVAL DURING TRANSITION

Tingle (2000) suggests a transition strategy using the analogy NURSES (Box 24-7).

Melissa Groggin (2001) suggests 10 ways to help nurses cope and reduce stress:

1. *Think before answering*—take a few minutes before you answer and decide what is best for you.
2. *Take vacations*—what can seem like a crisis before the break may become manageable with distance.
3. *Get rid of minor things that drain your energy*—bring your lunch and eat in a quiet space rather than spending most of your break waiting in line, only to "swallow your lunch whole" or, even worse, eat on the unit.
4. *Support your coworkers*—be a good listener.
5. *Wear comfortable uniforms and shoes*—you cannot think if your feet hurt and your pants are too tight.
6. *Treat yourself*—do something nice for yourself every week.
7. *Avoid people who irritate or hassle you*—pessimistic people can bring you down.
8. *Keep in touch with yourself*—do not take on everyone else's responsibilities.
9. *Say no*—and don't feel guilty.
10. *Remember that nursing is a noble profession.*

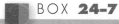 BOX **24-7**

NURSES

Never fail to ask for help.
If you do not ask, you may never receive help. The best way to get help is to ask.

Use available facility resources.
Use other experienced staff, policy, and procedure manuals and staff development personnel.

Reenergize with professional associations.
This helps to keep the novice nurse from losing sight of the profession in favor of the job.

Stay in contact with friends.
Join the alumni association at your nursing school and find out what your peers are doing.

Evaluate your growth realistically.
Develop short-term goals (e.g., open all charts by 9 AM), then long-term goals (e.g., gain certification in your field).

Stay focused on your goals.
Remember: climbing the hill of professionalism is hard, but the pure "pride" becomes your armor.

Tingle CA: *Workplace advocacy as a transition tool.* 2000. Available at: www.lsna.org/newpage12.htm.

John (2006) suggests finding a place to work that "just feels right" (p. 18) and to take time off before starting that important first job to rejuvenate after the countless hours of study. She also encourages the "first time nursing job seekers" to know as much as possible about their future employer by reviewing the job description and population for whom they will be caring. Really get to know your preceptor, the organizational chart, and the policies behind the procedures. Finally, use resources wisely, plan on lifelong learning, and participate in professional organizations to develop networks. Developing a portfolio of positive experiences not only will help you remain positive but also may serve as a source for promotion later in your career.

MEETING SPECIAL NEEDS OF THE NOVICE NURSE

It is important to review some common problems perceived by novice nurses and to offer suggestions to ease the transition period.

Organizational Skills

Lack of organization is common when the novice nurse's assignment becomes much heavier than that of a student nurse. The use of a report sheet can enable the novice nurse to note important information received during the shift report and from other members of the interprofessional health care team as the day progresses. The report sheet can also be used to document occurrences during the shift. Another suggestion for the novice nurse is to contact a former nursing instructor. Most students have developed a special rapport with one or two instructors. Novice nurses might telephone one of their former instructors to discuss the challenges they face during transition so that the instructor can help with problem solving.

The basic report sheet (Box 24-8) also can be transformed into a unit-specific sheet. For instance if the novice nurse is on a telemetry floor, there might be a section for "rhythms." The orthopedic nurse could include "traction." This form also can be used to establish and set priorities. Once the care has been prioritized, the nurse can begin those critical interventions. However, it also may be possible to delegate tasks to ancillary staff if the tasks are within their scope of practice. This requires the novice nurse to become familiar with the job descriptions of other nursing personnel, such as licensed professional nurses, nursing assistants, or unlicensed personnel, so delegation will be within their defined roles. Remember that the RN cannot do everything.

Clinical Skills

According to Benner's model (1984), the graduate nurse must be allowed to develop clinical skills based on experiences. The novice nurse can develop competence with clinical skills during the orientation phase by asking to observe an experienced nurse perform those skills with which the novice nurse is less familiar. The novice nurse also can provide the nurse manager and mentor with a list of skills that need further practice. The unit's policy and procedure book is a valuable asset. It should describe in detail the steps to follow when performing a procedure. Spend time reviewing the manual before observing the procedure being performed and then ask questions. Take into consideration that there is more than one correct way to perform a skill; remember though, it is not acceptable to take shortcuts that jeopardize the safety of the patient.

Interpersonal Skills

Developing interpersonal skills may be achieved by attending unit meetings, volunteering to serve on committees on the unit or within the agency, and taking an active interest in the nursing unit. These activities aid in socialization into the unit and profession. It is important for all nurses, regardless of their experience, to take part in professional organizations at the local,

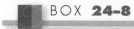

BOX **24-8**

Worksheet

Patient's Name _____	**Patient's Name** _____
Room # _____	Room # _____
Diagnosis _____	Diagnosis _____
Diet _____	Diet _____
Activity status _____	Activity status _____
Lab ordered/time _____	Lab ordered/time _____
IV fluids _____	IV fluids _____

INTAKE/OUTPUT

Urine _____ Stools _____	Urine _____ Stools _____
Other _____	Other _____
IV primary _____	IV primary _____
IV secondary _____	IV secondary _____
Other _____	Other _____

Patient's Name _____	**Patient's Name** _____
Room # _____	Room # _____
Diagnosis _____	Diagnosis _____
Diet _____	Diet _____
Activity status _____	Activity status _____
Lab ordered/time _____	Lab ordered/time _____
IV fluids _____	IV fluids _____

INTAKE/OUTPUT

Urine _____ Stools _____	Urine _____ Stools _____
Other _____	Other _____
IV primary _____	IV primary _____
IV secondary _____	IV secondary _____
Other _____	Other _____

regional, state, or national level. Specialty organizations often provide valuable information and continuing education pertinent to the nurse's area of practice.

As the nurse becomes more confident in his or her nursing abilities and is less stressed by performing tasks, positive relationships with physicians and other members of the intraprofessional team can be developed. Various methods that may be used to develop professional relationships should be emphasized during the orientation period. Nurses in staff development positions can be key players in assisting the novice nurse in developing professional communication skills. Making rounds with physicians and assisting them with procedures open the door for communication. Asking pertinent and relevant questions ensures that the door remains open.

Delegation Skills

Another important skill that novice nurses need to learn is delegating. First, nurses should consider how others have delegated to them. Body language is important when delegating. Look at the person, be pleasant, and leave room for suggestions from the delegatee; however, do not allow the delegatee to resist or intimidate you so that you end up completing the task yourself. After communicating face to face, give a list of tasks in writing or post it at the nurses' station. This leaves little room for misunderstanding. Be willing to change the assignment if there are changes in a patient's condition, new patients are admitted, or you realize that the time needed to perform a task was underestimated. If time allows, it is always good to help those to whom you have delegated tasks. For example, if a nurse passes by a door and the attendant is trying to turn a very large patient, she should enter the room and ask, "How can I best help you turn the patient?" Always take time to give sincere positive reinforcement and say thank you.

Priority-Setting Skills

Now consider the best way to prioritize. How did you prioritize in nursing school? What worked then will probably work now with a few modifications. Remember: if it is not written down, it probably will be forgotten. Keep a notepad and pen in your pocket. Jot down reminders of things to be done and place a number indicating their importance. For example, assume that you have already written the following list:

_____ Start the IV for Mr. B. in room 211.
_____ Check the IV site for Mrs. C. in room 300.
_____ Call the laboratory and check on blood sugar for Mrs. M. in room 215.

Now a call is received from the licensed practical nurse that Mr. T.'s IV line is not dripping in room 212. Next the dietary worker calls to say that when she took the food tray to the patient in room 217, the patient vomited. Then the emergency light goes off in the bathroom of an older, confused patient. Now prioritize. What needs to be done first? First, answer the emergency light; do not even take time to write down this one. Now it is time to reprioritize. The new tasks have been added to the bottom of your previous list. Look over your list below. How would you prioritize these tasks?

_____ Start the IV for Mr. B. in room 211.
_____ Check the IV site for Mrs. C. in room 300.
_____ Call the laboratory and check the blood sugar for Mrs. M. in room 215.
_____ Check Mr. T.'s IV line that is not dripping.
_____ Assist the patient in room 217 who is vomiting.

Now try out your delegating skills. Place a D next to any tasks that can be delegated in the list below.

_____ Start the IV for Mr. B. in room 211.
_____ Check the IV site for Mrs. C. in room 300.
_____ Call the laboratory and check on blood sugar for Mrs. M. in room 215.
_____ Check Mr. T.'s IV in room 212 that is not dripping.
_____ Assist the patient in room 217 who is vomiting.

What had to be considered when you prioritized the tasks? First you needed to consider how much time was required for each task. It usually takes longer to start a new IV line than to check an existing IV site. It also requires less time to determine why an IV is not dripping. However, this is insignificant if the patient needing the IV line started is critical and needs the medication to reduce his or her blood pressure. Delegation may be needed. What tasks can other members perform? The unit secretary can call the lab to check on lab results, and a licensed practical nurse or nursing assistant can assist the patient who is vomiting, provided that you follow up very soon to assess the patient's condition. A nurse must know how to prioritize. Think through each situation. Change the priority as needed or as situations change throughout the shift.

Now that you know ways to develop organizational skills, refine clinical and interpersonal skills, delegate, and set priorities, take time to remember other important areas of your life. Remember the people you may have neglected during school and make it a priority to reestablish special relationships with friends, family, and loved ones.

The following activities show appreciation for yourself and your significant others for all they have endured during your education:

- ◆ Reintroduce yourself to your spouse and close friends. You might even treat them to a special dinner at their favorite restaurant.
- ◆ Participate in your children's activities at school.
- ◆ Read a romance, mystery, or war novel, depending on your taste or mood at the time.
- ◆ Clean your house or apartment. There really is furniture under all those papers.
- ◆ Get a cookbook and try those recipes you have not had time to prepare.
- ◆ Call old friends whom you knew before nursing school.
- ◆ Participate in a health club, learn aerobic exercise, or just walk to improve your health.
- ◆ Enjoy the nursing profession—it really is the best.

Experienced RNs should consider the following to help ease the transition of the novice nurse to the profession of nursing: The novice nurse should not be expected to enter the work environment and be as productive as experienced staff members. It is important for experienced nurses serving on agency committees to serve as advocates for novice nurses by reminding nurse managers and administrators that it is not possible for nursing students to learn everything necessary for professional practice during school. Also remind other members of the nursing unit about this fact. If a novice nurse develops initiative, autonomy, and a desire to become a team member, he or she will succeed.

SUMMARY

The period of transition from novice to competent practitioner is critical. New skills must be learned and refined, professional relationships established, and autonomy gained in nursing practice. Knowledge and skills must be refined over time. The transition from student to RN can be compared with that of butterflies as they emerge from the cocoon. It is unfair to judge them while still nymphs, therefore the nursing profession must withhold scrutiny until novice nurses fly with their beautiful wings spread.

 Additional resources are available online at: http://evolve.elsevier.com/Cherry/

REFERENCES

Adler P: Professional issues. Are we still eating our young? Myth or reality, *Medsurg Nurs* 18(1):62, 2009.

Baltimore JJ: Nurse collegiality: fact or fiction? *Nurs Manage* 37(5):28–36, 2006.

Benner P: *From novice to expert*, Menlo Park, CA, 1984, Addison-Wesley.

Blakeney B: The importance of mentoring, *NSNA Imprint*, November/December, 2005.

Bowles C, Candela L: First job experiences of recent RN graduates, *Nev RNform* 14(2):16–19, 2005.

Center for American Nurses and AzNA: A collaborative approach, *Arizona Nurse*, 2009. Retrieved August 2009, from: CINAHL Plus with full text database www.aznurse.org.

Chapman R, et al: Predicting patient aggression against nurses in all hospital areas, *Br J Nurs* 18(8):476–483, 2009.

Chesnutt BM, Everhart B: Meeting the needs of graduate nurses in critical care orientation, *Crit Care Nurse* 27(3):36–51, 2007.

Childers L: Big brothers, *Future Nurse* Fall:37–40, 2003.

Cybernurse: *Reality shock*. 2000. Retrieved December 2006 from: www.cybernurse.com/wwwboard/messages/1173.html.

DeRung B: Fresh eyes are opened quickly, *Minn Nurs Accent*. 2004, March-April. Retrieved August 2009 from www.mnnurses.org.

Domrose C: The "in" crowd, *Future Nurse* Fall:42–45, 2003.

Domrose C: *Staying power: keeping nurses isn't about showing them the money*. 2000. Available at: www.nurseweek.com/news/Feature/00–07/retain.htm.

Duhart DT: *National crime victimization survey: violence in the workplace, 1993-1999*, Washington, DC, 2001, U.S. Department of Justice.

Farrell GA: From tall poppies to squashed weeds: why don't nurses pull together more? *J Adv Nurs* 35(1):26–33, 2001.

Figley CR: *Compassion fatigue: an introduction.* 2001. Retrieved December 2006 from: www.giftfromwithin. org/html/cmpfatig.html.

Flanagan L, editor: *What you need to know about today's workplace: a survival guide for nurses,* Washington, DC, 1997, American Nurses Publishing.

Gallant-Roman MA: Strategies and tools to reduce workplace violence, *AAOHN J* 56(11):449–454, 2008.

Gries M: *Don't leave grads lost at sea.* 2000. Available at: http://community.nursingspectrum.com/Magazine Articles/article.cfm?AID=800.

Groggin M: *Calm within the storm.* 2001. Available at: http:// community.nursingspectrum.com/MagazineArticles/ article.cfm?AID=3822.

Hertel R: Burnout and the med-surg nurse, *Medsurg Matters* 18(3):1, 2009.

Hinchberger PA: Violence against female student nurses in the workplace, *Nurs Forum* 44(1):37–46, 2009.

Huber D: *Leadership and nursing care management,* ed 3, Philadelphia, 2009, Saunders.

Jennings BM: Work stress and burnout among nurses: role of the work environment and working conditions. In Hughes RG, editor: *Patient safety and quality: an evidence-based handbook for nurses,* Rockville, MD, 2008, Agency for Healthcare Research and Quality, pp 136–158.

John TJ: Your first year as a nurse, *NSNA Imprint.* 2006. Available at: www.nsna.org/pubs/imprint/jan06/Jan06 FeatureTeresa.John.pdf.

Klein E, Dickenson-Hazard N: The spirit of mentoring, *Reflect Nurs Leadersh* 26(3):21, 2000.

Kramer M: *Reality shock: why nurses leave nursing,* St Louis, 1974, Mosby.

Larsen C: *Reality shock and preventing burnout in nursing.* 2000. Available at http://www4.allencol.edu/~lmh0/ CindyL/Burnout.html.

Lee V, Harris T: Mentoring new nursing graduates, *Minority Nurse* 38–41, 2007.

Lofmark A, Smide B, Widblad K: Competence of newly-graduated nurses—a comparison of the perceptions of qualified nurses and students, *J Adv Nurs* 53(6):721–728, 2006.

Longo J, Sherman R: Leveling horizontal violence. *Nurs Manag* 38(3):34, 2007. Retrieved from CINAHL Plus with full text database.

Martin W: Is your hospital safe? Disruptive behavior and workplace bullying, *Hosp Top* 86(3):21–28. 2008. Retrieved from CINAHL Plus with full text database.

Mooney M: Professional socialization: the key to survival as a newly qualified nurse, *Int J Nurs Pract* 13(2):75–80, 2007.

NSNA Leadership University: *Welcome to Leadership University.* 2003. Available at: www.nsnaleadershipu.org.

Occupational Safety and Health Administration: *Guidelines for preventing workplace violence for health care and social service workers.* 2004. Retrieved February 15, 2010 from: www.osha.gov/SLTC/etools/hospital/hazards/workplac eviolence/viol.html.

Olszewski K, Parks C, Chikotas NE: Occupational safety and health objectives of *Healthy People 2010:* part II. A systematic approach for occupational health nurses, *AAOHN J* 55(3):115–123, 2007.

Palmer C: The nursing shortage: an update for occupational health nurses, *AAOHN J* 51(12):510–513, 2003.

Paniagua H, Bond P, Thompson A: Providing an alternative to zero tolerance policies, *BJN* 18(10):619, 2009. Retrieved from CINAHL Plus with full text database.

Pine R, Tart K: Return on investment: benefits and challenges of a baccalaureate nurse residency program, *Nurs Econ* 25(1):13–18, 39, 2007.

Positive Way: *Self-esteem questionnaire.* 2000. Available at: www.positive-way.com/self-est1.htm.

Ramos MC: Eliminate destructive behaviors through example and evidence, *Nurs Manag* 37(9):34–41, 2006.

Ricker F: A supportive nursing model: innovative nurse residency program eases new graduate transition, *Colo Nurse* 108(2):6–7, 2008.

Sherman R, Murphy N: The many merits of mentoring: for both mentor and protege, a successful mentorship increases self-awareness and opens new professional avenues, *Am Nurse Today* 4(2):24–25, 2009. Retrieved from CINAHL Plus with full text database.

Sincox AK, Fitzpatrick M: *Lateral violence: calling out the elephant in the room.* May–June 81(3):8–9, 2008. Retrieved August 2009 from: www.minurses.org.

Sofield L, Salmond SW: Workplace violence: a focus on verbal abuse and intent to leave the organization, *Orthop Nurs* 22(4):274–283, 2003.

Stone S: *Mentoring and modeling for the millennium.* 2000. Available at: www.ajj.com/jpi/deannote/backissu/mar 2000/mentor.htm.

Sullivan EJ, Decker PJ: *Effective leadership and management,* ed 7, Menlo Park, CA, 2009, Addison-Wesley.

Tingle CA: *Workplace advocacy as a transition tool.* 2000. Retrieved December 2007 from: www.lsna.org/newpage 12.htm.

Vance C: Discovering the riches in mentor connections, *Reflect Nurs Leadersh* 26(3):24–25, 2000.

Wells J, Bowers L: How prevalent is violence towards nurses working in general hospitals in the UK? *J Adv Nurs* 39(3):230–240. 2002. Retrieved from CINAHL Plus with full text database.

Zerwekh J, Claborn JC: Role transitions. In Zerwekh J, Claborn JC, editors: *Nursing today: transition and trends,* ed 6, St Louis, 2009, Saunders.

Managing Time: The Path to High Self-Performance

Patricia Reid Ponte, DNSc, RN, FAAN, NEA-BC
Genevieve J. Conlin, MS, MBA, MEd, RN, NEA-BC

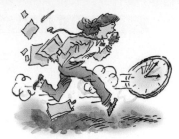

evolve Additional resources are available online at: http://evolve.elsevier.com/Cherry/

Our lives revolve around time: use it as a way to ensure high performance, positive energy, and focus in all aspects of your life.

VIGNETTE

Approximately 4 months ago, Susan Kenny transferred to a position as a staff registered nurse (RN) at an ambulatory cancer treatment center. Today Susan arrived at the chemotherapy infusion room 15 minutes before the start of her shift. She knew it was going to be a busy day, and given her lack of experience in this work setting, she thought she should get a head start on her assignment. She was heading toward the workstation when one of her colleagues stopped her to discuss a holiday party, and they both spoke fervently about how much fun it would be.

Ten minutes later Susan resumed her trek to the workstation. Just as she arrived, the phone rang, and Susan answered it. A patient was seeking information about her appointment time. It took Susan quite a while to open up the computer screen, log in, and find the information, which she communicated to the patient. By now many of her colleagues were on-site, already starting to work on their assignments. Susan looked at her assignment and realized that in addition to her other assigned patients, one of her patients would be receiving the first treatment of a new chemotherapy protocol. She knew that given the time necessary to work with the patient and family, triple-check orders with her physician and pharmacist colleagues, and administer the premedications and chemotherapy, all while monitoring this very ill patient, she would be very busy all day.

While reviewing the new chemotherapy protocol, one of Susan's primary patients came in unexpectedly with a fever and low blood pressure, needing hydration and platelets. The physician gave Susan orders to stabilize the patient and arrange for transfer to the inpatient unit. The hospital was full, so the transfer would take some time. Susan began to get very anxious about being able to complete all of her assigned duties while giving her patients the specialized care and attention they needed. Unfortunately this anxious feeling was becoming a common occurrence in Susan's workday.

Meanwhile Maura Callahan, a staff RN who had been working on the inpatient oncology floor for just less than a year, was passing out 10 AM medications when she received a call from Susan to take report before accepting the patient later in the day when a room became available. Maura was already behind in passing medications because of the new barcoding system *now in use for medication administration. Despite the fact that this system would be safer and more efficient, using the new application took more time in the first few weeks. The training was great, but nonetheless, medication administration took longer. Maura asked the charge nurse if she could take report for her, but the charge nurse said she was in the midst of transferring another patient to the medical intensive care unit.*

Maura took the report from Susan and agreed to accept the patient at 1 PM, when another patient's discharge would be completed and the room cleaned. Maura thought, "How will I ever get finished in time to pick up my daughter from daycare by 4 PM?" Her day was lining up like so many before, not being able to finish her work before the end of the shift. She would have to call her mother to help out again by picking up her daughter.

Both Susan and Maura were working frantically to ensure that patients' needs were met in a timely way, but it seemed impossible to both of them before they decided to call their respective managers and seek assistance.

■ QUESTIONS TO CONSIDER WHILE READING THIS CHAPTER:

1 When Susan arrived on duty, what are some strategies she could have used to be sure she made the most of her early arrival?

2 What factors should Susan and Maura consider when deciding how to prioritize their patient care assignment?

3 What strategies could Maura and Susan consider when deciding how to manage their learning needs and the need to be patient and family focused?

4 What are some strategies that Maura and Susan can use to ensure balance between their work and personal lives?

KEY TERMS

Energy management Ensuring that the right amount of effort matches the right task to optimize an outcome while gauging the amount of personal energy expended or taxed to achieve the desired result.

Goal A tangible, measurable, and attainable act in a specific period of time. It has broad-term results, experiences, or achievements toward which someone is willing to work.

Milieu The physical or social setting in which something occurs or develops.

Novice to expert Five stages of proficiency in the development of skill acquisition and performance within the domain of clinical nursing practice that frames a transition from reliance on abstract principles of the new learner to becoming an involved performer who is engaged in a situation—the expert performer (Benner, 2001).

Objective An identifiable, measurable act that implements one's goal and is typically short termed.

Priority setting The act of deciding what should be done first and what activities should follow sequentially; establishing an ordered list or ranked items based on importance or urgency; method used to determine what actions need to be accomplished ahead of others; represents the execution of ranked items.

Procrastination The act of intentionally and/or habitually putting off doing something that should be done.

Technology management Application of information systems and equipment to enhance work and life activities to maximal benefit.

Time management The development of processes and tools that increase efficiency and productivity within the set standard of time.

LEARNING OUTCOMES

After studying this chapter, the reader will be able to:

1 Understand the unique demands of complex health care environments in today's fast-paced world of high technology and communication transfer and its effects on personal time management.

2 Understand the relationship between personal performance and time management.

3 Understand one's own time management preferences and style.

4 Create an action plan to manage procrastination, distraction, and anxiety.

5 Describe how individual learning and communication styles interact with the ability to manage time effectively.

6 Adopt into daily practice a time management strategy plan unique to one's own style to ensure high-level personal performance in work and home life.

CHAPTER OVERVIEW

The previous scenarios are typical of what happens daily in the lives of busy professionals. Managing multiple priorities during a particular workday and integrating personal and work-related demands is the constant dilemma of so many men and women today. Additionally, performing well in both arenas is a goal of most working professionals. To accomplish the important goals in life, it is necessary to understand your own preferred style of managing priorities, recognize your typical distractions, identify a personal performance approach, and consistently use strategies and tools to make the most of every minute. This chapter is designed to assist students and busy professionals in implementing self-management strategies to better use their time and energy to ensure a highly productive, focused life.

HEALTH CARE TODAY

Health care environments are fraught with incredible complexities: high-acuity patients, vigilant and knowledgeable family members, ever-growing information technology geared toward supporting staff in the care of patients, often tight quarters in which to deliver high-tech care, and little time to interact with patients on an interpersonal therapeutic level. Inter-professional practice models demand collaborative teamwork, when in reality disciplines often function in parallel work processes. The need to move patients quickly from one site of care to another on a constantly growing continuum that reaches into patients' homes is the norm in today's health care environment. Fast-paced clinics, high-tech ambulatory care practice settings, and quaternary care in high-intensity critical care units and operating rooms are typical. The nature of the intimate human element inherent in the delivery of health care makes it like no other work.

As health care continues to evolve and the nation is focused on major healthcare reform to improve access and quality and reduce costs, efficiency has become a critical component when considering the cost and quality of health care delivery (Larkin, 2009). Managing time, organizing care, and maintaining personal health and balance between work and home settings become much more demanding—and essential. Therefore, it becomes critical for each professional working in these dynamic settings to receive education and coaching in managing time, energy, balance, and focus to ensure high performance. Florence Nightingale's words resonate: "Knowing how you manage when you are there [at work]…impacts how your work should be done when you are not there" (1969, p. 35).

PERSPECTIVES ON TIME

Each person has a specific perspective of time, which is based on his or her own experiences, values, education, socioeconomic factors, age, personality, culture, and genetic makeup. To understand an individual's own perspective on time and the resulting behaviors, it is necessary to create opportunities to think introspectively and examine personal preferences, traits, habits, and tendencies. This is the critical first step in achieving an individualized time management strategy and plan.

In her book, *Time Management from the Inside Out,* Julie Morgenstern (2004) presents "10 psychologic obstacles" that influence one's ability to create and sustain focused and productive work habits. As the following 10 obstacles are reviewed, carefully consider how they might affect your own ability to develop productive, energetic work habits.

1. **Unclear Goals and Priorities.** Within a particular work shift or within your life as a whole, if you lack clarity about purpose and expected outcomes, the ability to manage time to meet your desires becomes a futile task.

2. **Conquistador of Chaos.** If you are constantly overburdened with tasks, events, urgent requests, and last-minute cancellations, you are a better crisis manager than manager of time.

3. **Fear of Downtime.** Some individuals fear the possibility of standing still too long. They feel guilty with timeouts or time off. Often this is a result of not wanting to address the larger issues in life. Staying too busy to think keeps long-term planning and personal introspection at bay.

4. **Need to be a Caretaker.** In professions such as nursing the need to be a caretaker is a common devotion and can be very gratifying. However, when this need becomes unbalanced, it can cause you to feel resentful, unappreciated, and overwhelmed.

5. **Fear of Failure.** When you are unable to get to the things that are important to you and are unable to meet your personal goals, it may mean you are afraid of failure. It can be very upsetting to go after your dreams and find out you cannot reach them. Sometimes it is easier to avoid making the effort. Take time to understand what your fears are and to openly address them.

6. **Fear of Success.** You may have been given a message somewhere in your life that you do not deserve to be a success. Therefore, it can be anxiety provoking to garner success and stand apart from others who may distance themselves from you. Take time to think through whether or not this is playing out in your life.

7. **Fear of Disrupting the Status Quo.** Not pursuing your goals for fear of the reactions of those around you is very common. Your family, coworkers, or supervisors may be critical of what you want to pursue. Gradually approaching changes gives you and those around you time to acclimate.

8. **Fear of Completion.** If you are afraid of completing a project that is creative and fun because you are fearful that another similar project will not find its way to you or the project may no longer be important to you, take the time to understand why you are not completing a routine task or a major project that has been with you for some time.

9. **Need for Perfection.** If you are a perfectionist and feel that everything should be completed with the same level of excellence, you are not keeping things in perspective. If you demand extremely high standards for every single task you undertake, you simply will not get everything done.

10. **Fear of Losing Creativity.** Many creative people think that by creating an organized time management structure or approach to life their creative natures or tendencies will

be squelched. However, creating a framework to manage priorities will allow more freedom and time to enhance one's creative juices.

Here are some of the benefits that will result if you take the time to uncover your own tendencies, fears, strengths, and weaknesses (Childre, 2008; Federwisch, 2009; Reid Ponte, 2008):

♦ Improved patient outcomes by implementing a collaborative structure in the work environment

♦ Increased satisfaction with your work accomplishments as a result of applying something new in your setting

♦ Improved interpersonal relations because of your ability to be fully present and engaged to do your best work

♦ Better future direction because there is more attentiveness to proactively managing and engaging in the environment

♦ Improved personal health because of decreased anxiety and a restoration of emotional balance

It is more crucial than ever that you strive to understand what you value, recognize your purpose in life, and determine strategies to ensure that your focus and energy are geared toward your major goals in life. Whether you are trying to organize how to approach a particular workday or trying to balance your personal and work life, the strategies that you will learn and integrate into your daily activities now will play out the rest of your life. Managing energy to ensure high performance is the first step.

ENERGY MANAGEMENT

According to Loehr and Schwartz (2003), "Energy, not time, is the fundamental currency of high performance" (p. 4). Striving to be more efficient and more organized or to manage time and priorities better is all in the interest of becoming a better performer either in one's work or personal life. Loehr and Schwartz also state that only when we are fully engaged do we perform our best. This requires drawing on four separate but related sources of energy: (1) physical, (2) mental, (3) spiritual, and (4) emotional.

Just as we build physical capacity through disciplined exercise and strengthening routines, we can also strengthen our emotional, spiritual, and mental capacities.

Consider Susan from our earlier vignette. Her decision to transfer to the chemotherapy infusion center, her third transfer in 18 months, came only after sheer frustration of not being able to feel in control of her work life and home life. At work Susan felt overwhelmed, underappreciated, and unprepared physically for the daily challenges of 12-hour shifts. She was exhausted every morning, and she fell into bed as soon as she got home. Her energy level was poor. She felt dissatisfied with her inability to spend more time with friends on weekends. Susan could not bear the thought of getting out of bed early another day, even if it was for something fun. Because of this she gained weight over the past 6 months, and the only thing that seemed to make her happy was to visit her sister on Sunday afternoons for shopping and dinner. Getting to work the next day often proved difficult because her motivation was low and her energy level even lower. With this new job Susan was attempting to get back on track. "It's going to be different this time," she said to herself.

Physical Energy

This scenario is not uncommon as novice professionals begin the rigors of full-time work after spending time in college and working part time. Key components of successful transition to a productive, highly energizing experience include paying attention to physical energy through a routine of proper eating, adequate sleep and exercise, frequent breaks during long shifts (about every 90 minutes), drinking plenty of water, and focusing on one activity while collecting thoughts about what to prioritize next. Once the physical capacity of your holistic self is working well, then attention can be paid to your mental, spiritual, and emotional capacities.

Mental Energy

The mental energy that is most potent in ensuring full engagement and high performance is that of realistic optimism. Realistic optimism is seeing the world as it is, but always working toward an optimal solution or goal. Mental energy is the ability to maintain sustained concentration on a task, move flexibly between broad and narrow issues, and be internally and externally focused as needed by the situation. It includes mental preparation, visualization, positive self-talk, effective time management, and creativity. Susan has begun to identify this mental energy in her desire to get back on track. She realizes that change is necessary. To move in this direction Susan needs to spend some time to reflect on the following: (1) What are my major goals in life, and (2) what is my purpose?

Spiritual Energy

Often we do not take the time to reflect about what is important to us. Being in a quiet place helps us identify our vision of life—our purpose and direction in life. Susan has yet to determine her life vision given her frequent job changes and her lack of clarity about how she wants to spend her personal time. Having direction and purpose is the key factor in one's spiritual capacity.

Peter Senge (1999) has identified "personal mastery" as the discipline of continually clarifying and deepening one's personal vision, focusing one's energies, developing patience, and seeing reality objectively. People with a high level of personal mastery live in a continual learning mode, uncovering their personal growth areas.

Emotional Energy

Physical, mental, and spiritual energy provide fuel for building our emotional capacity. Managing emotions skillfully in the service of high positive energy and full engagement is called emotional intelligence. Goleman (1999) suggests that self-confidence, self-control, and interpersonal effectiveness are all key to emotional intelligence. Striving to increase one's emotional capacity—which includes improving one's self-confidence, self-control, self-regulation, social skills, interpersonal effectiveness, empathy, patience, openness, trust, and enjoyment—will result in a more positive, invigorating work experience and personal life.

Understanding how the four energies—physical, mental, spiritual, and emotional—contribute to a fully engaged individual who is productive and happy will help you use the time management skills and strategies described in the following sections of this chapter.

TIME DISTRACTIONS AND ENERGY DISTRACTIONS

We are all subject to distractions in our work and personal lives that may influence our propensity to procrastinate or not reach our goals. It is important to recognize and understand the distractions that inhibit our ability to complete tasks and to meet our objectives and goals. Box 25-1 lists many common internal and external time distractions and energy distractions that each of us may experience in a typical day. It is critical to be aware of those time distractions that affect us. The following section provides specific examples of how to strategically avoid these common time distractions.

BOX **25-1**

Time and Energy Distractions

EXTERNAL TIME AND ENERGY DISTRACTIONS	INTERNAL TIME AND ENERGY DISTRACTIONS
Interruptions	Procrastination
Socializing or visitors	Inadequate planning
Meetings	Ineffective delegation
Excessive paperwork	Failure to set goals and priorities
Understaffing	A cluttered desk or mind
Lack of information	Personal disorganization
Ineffective communication	Inability to say no
Lack of feedback	Lack of self-discipline
Travel	Responding to crises
Inadequate policies and procedures	Haste
Incompetent or uncooperative coworkers	Indecisiveness
Poor filing systems	An "open-door" policy
Looking for misplaced files, etc.	Shifting priorities without sound rationale
Personnel or coworkers with problems	Leaving tasks unfinished
Lack of teamwork	Not setting time limits
Duplicating efforts	Daydreaming
Confusing lines of authority, responsibility, and communication	Attempting too much at once
	Overinvolvement in routine details
Bureaucratic red tape	Making numerous errors
Junk mail	Surfing the Internet
Waiting, meeting delays	Not listening

TIME-MANAGEMENT STRATEGIES

It is easy to apply the perspectives-on-time concept to nurses because many nurses have type A personalities, which means they are oriented toward high achievement. As a result, they are more likely to encounter stress when they mismanage themselves and do not use time appropriately. The reason for this phenomenon becomes clear when some of the common characteristics of high achievers are examined. Nurses tend to go above and beyond for their patients, colleagues, and families, and they set a high bar of achievement for themselves and strive for a positive experience for their patients and families (Lee, 2004).

As high achievers, nurses are often attracted to activities that are challenging, difficult, and even risky. In most cases the activities are complex and time consuming, which forces the person to use self-management to meet the goals and gain internal satisfaction. When these people mismanage themselves in relation to time, it results in frustration and stress. To assist nurses in improving their self-management and time management, many different management strategies have been outlined for review including planning, implementing, and organizing.

Time Management Truisms

Before looking at time management strategies, there are certain truisms to consider:
- ◆ "Nothing changes if nothing changes."
- ◆ "We train people how to treat us."
- ◆ "Everything you own owns you."

These are powerful statements to consider when making decisions about how you manage time.

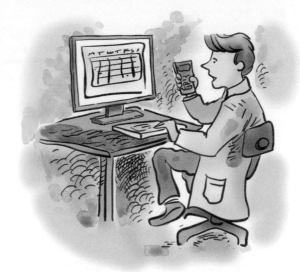

Planning is the most important step in time management.

"Nothing Changes if Nothing Changes." This statement means that a person cannot effect a change on an experience if he or she is not willing to do something differently that could adjust the outcome. This can be meaningful to Susan and Maura in the opening vignette. Each works in an environment where the milieu may and often does change in an instant. Although it is unlikely that either nurse may be able to change her overall work environment, they both own the ability to effect small, gradual changes within themselves that will ultimately affect their work environments. For example, Susan and Maura appreciated the importance of getting Susan's sick patient transferred to Maura's unit, but the priority of that situation was not to give report at that time. There is always an underlying sense of urgency when caring for compromised patients. As Susan and Maura continue to work in their respective settings, each will become more attuned to the true priorities that await them. As they move through the stages of novice to expert nurse, they will be able to build on past experiences to make future ones more successful. The next time Susan has a patient who needs to be transferred to the inpatient unit, she will know that she must first stabilize the patient, then prepare to give report to the inpatient staff nurse.

"We Train People How to Treat Us." A key factor in understanding time management is understanding the behavioral style one possesses. It is helpful to determine your own behavior style and the behavior styles of those who work closely with you. There are four common behavioral types (Skillpath Seminars, 2001):

1. *Self-contained:* Manages self evenly and will express concerns with a situation in a thoughtful, reasonable manner. This person is approachable and fair in decision making.
2. *Open and accepting:* Always willing to help and say yes to requests. This person likely overextends himself or herself and does not share opinions or feedback. This person has the potential to become extremely stressed.
3. *Indirect:* Avoids conflict and will not challenge authority. This person may express concerns to peers, but does not address them with management.
4. *Direct:* Clear and concise about requests; sometimes perceived as curt. This person may be perceived as difficult to approach and/or intimidating.

When you can appreciate the behaviors and personalities of those with whom you work, you are more likely to use this knowledge to your advantage to evoke the responses needed to reach your goals. When you relay a clear message about yourself—how you conduct yourself, manage your time, and interact with others—you set the tone for future interactions, and your colleagues will know what to expect of you. Looking back at the vignette, Susan could have been more direct when talking with her colleague about the upcoming party and asked whether they could talk about the topic more at lunch. This would have allowed her to begin her daily planning sooner. When you are clear and constant in your work, those around you learn to respond to the tone you set.

"Everything You Own Owns You." This statement simply means that those tasks you assume as your responsibility have also assumed your time and energy, thus in turn "owning" you. This implies a deeper meaning than simply "having things to do" (i.e., you cannot assume more tasks until you complete the ones you are already committed to). We need to be cognizant of how the demands we place on ourselves affect our time.

Planning, Organizing, and Implementing to Control the Use of Time

Planning, organizing, and implementing are the key actions a person can use to optimize the use of time. These three actions are sequential and build on each other for successful time management.

Planning for Control

Planning is the most important step in time management. Unfortunately few people expend as much energy planning as they should. Some shy away from planning because they believe it is too time-consuming and never leads to closure. In reality planning allows people to better use their time and can lead to closure in relation to those goals that will produce the most internal satisfaction. For example, 1 minute of planning can transfer to at least 10 minutes of productivity, proving to be a great return on the investment of taking the time to review and plan for the day. If you arrive 10 to 15 minutes early for your scheduled shift and map out the day's priorities, your likelihood of executing those priorities is far greater than had you not taken the time to plan up front.

Having a priority-planning list with you as you work is useful in keeping you on track to accomplish those tasks by the end of the shift or day. Those who plan well also tend to encounter fewer problems when Murphy's law becomes a reality: *If anything can go wrong it will.* Thus it is important to plan before beginning any task, project, or day's activities. Planning involves (1) setting goals and establishing priorities, (2) scheduling activities, and (3) making to-do lists.

Setting Priorities. Prioritizing is about making choices of what to do and what not to do. To prioritize effectively you need to be able to recognize what is important, as well as to see the difference between urgent (must be done immediately) and important (must be done but there may be flexibility as to when the task can be accomplished). A major component of planning is deciding what should be done first and what activities should follow sequentially. The factors that influence how to establish priorities include the following:

- ◆ Urgency of a situation
- ◆ Demands of others
- ◆ Closeness of deadlines
- ◆ Existing timeframe

◆ Degree of familiarity with the task
◆ Ease of the task
◆ Amount of enjoyment involved
◆ Consequences involved
◆ Size of the task
◆ Congruence with personal goals

Unfortunately when considering the use of time, not all of these factors carry the same weight. Factors that are most likely to assist in meeting your goals need to be given more consideration. Setting SMART goals (**s**pecific, **m**easurable, **a**chievable, **r**easonable, and **t**ime-based) may also provide the structure needed to manage these compounding factors we negotiate in our lives (Skillpath Seminars, 2001). Several processes have been proposed to assist people in setting priorities, including the ABC approach, the Pareto principle, and the continuum approach.

The ABC approach is advocated by Lakein (1973) and Mancini (2003). In this approach, a person lists every task that needs to be done. An A is assigned to the high-value items, a B to the medium-value items, and a C to the low-value items. The A items should stand out from the other items because of their worth to the person making the list. Also the A items are likely to require more energy and time, but they should be completed before any of the B or C items. As the A items are completed, you may find that the C items were of such low value that they did not need to be done at all. It is also possible that Monday's C item could become an A item on Friday, reflecting a change in values. Of course this is an arbitrary system that is based on a person's estimation of the value of activities within his or her own life. It allows for reflection and change while maintaining focus.

The Pareto principle is another process that is suggested for setting priorities. This principle is also referred to as the "80-20 rule," suggesting that 80% of the time expended produces 20% of the results, and 20% of the time expended produces 80% of the results (Koch, 2004). The essence is in determining the "vital few" activities that should be done and eliminating the "trivial many." Focusing on one or two tasks at a time supports this concept (Skillpath Seminars, 2001). This principle emphasizes selecting the most productive activities, eliminating trivia, and learning to say no.

The continuum approach to setting priorities encourages a person to select priorities by categorizing or ranking items according to four continuums. As you read about the four continuums, think about Susan's assignment in the opening vignette and consider which of her tasks would have been priorities based on this approach.

◆ **Intrinsic importance**: very important and must be done; important and should be done; not so important and may not be necessary, but may be useful; or unimportant and can be eliminated entirely
◆ **Urgency:** very urgent and must be done now; urgent and should be done soon; not urgent and can wait; time is not a factor
◆ **Delegation:** must be done by me because I am the only one who can do it; can be delegated to A or B; can be dumped because task does not need to be done or delegated
◆ **Visitations and conferences:** people I must see each day; people to see frequently but not daily; people to see regularly but not frequently; people to see only infrequently

Obviously these continuums have varying usefulness, depending on the activity being scrutinized.

Overall it does not matter which method is used to establish priorities as long as priorities are established using a sound rationale. Fortunately, setting priorities becomes easier with practice. If Susan had established her priorities for the day, it is unlikely that talking about the holiday party or calling the inpatient unit to give a report on a patient that would not transfer for several hours would have taken precedence over reviewing the new chemotherapy regimen protocol she would be administering to a patient. Setting priorities would have allowed Susan to better use her time and decreased her anxiety about not managing her assignment appropriately.

Scheduling Activities. Scheduling activities is an important component of planning. It is one way to control Parkinson's law, which states that work will expand to fill the time that is available. By scheduling activities, a person determines how much time is spent on a specific activity. Such time delineations tend to focus attention and activity so that the task gets completed more efficiently and effectively. A schedule of activities can be constructed using a variety of different methods, including hourly time schedules, which are not new to most people because they tend to be used throughout life. Everyone has used an hourly schedule for appointments, classes, or leisure activities. In addition, nurses become adept at using hourly time schedules to administer medications appropriately. Unfortunately, most people, including nurses, do not use time schedules frequently or consistently enough.

The process of scheduling activities is an important part of planning to use your time more efficiently. However, scheduling needs to be done appropriately to ensure adherence. Remember to schedule activities so that they coincide with your internal "prime time," when you concentrate best, and your external "prime time," when you deal best with other people. Typically the first 2½ hours of the workday are the most productive, so plan important tasks according to your most productive time in the day (Skillpath Seminars, 2001). As a general rule, 15 minutes of focused time and energy toward a project equates to 1 hour of productivity. Be sure to include some flexible time just for yourself. In addition, schedules have proven to be most useful when they are written down in ink; a written schedule tends to motivate people, particularly high achievers, because they are averse to deviate from whatever challenges them in black and white.

Establishing a To-Do List. Writing something on paper often is the first step to accomplishing it. A to-do list tends to keep people on track and focused on specific activities. Thus the list should be reflective of your priorities and goals. To-do lists should be made and revised daily to be the most useful in managing your time. Sometimes they require revision more frequently, even hourly, when priorities shift for valid reasons. The list should be legible and easily accessible to review throughout the day. It is helpful to review the list at the end of the shift or day to assess how you achieved or did not achieve your goals. This is an opportunity to reflect on the distractions you experienced so that you can make note of what not to do when the next situation arises. This will also provide you the opportunity to reevaluate your tasks to see what needs to be carried over to the next day. Some people find it useful to construct their lists on notecards, in day-planner calendars, on pocket calendars, in electronic recall devices, on computers, and myriad other ways. There is no right or wrong way to make a to-do list, but it should always be available to you.

Organizing for Control

Organizing yourself and your environment is an important component of time management. Such organization requires that you be able to deal effectively with the following:
- The stacked-desk syndrome
- The art of "no detourism"
- The art of "wastebasketry"
- E-mail and memo mania

The Stacked-Desk Syndrome. This syndrome is exactly what the label implies—a cluttered desk stacked with papers, books, and other things (Penn State, 2009). The syndrome can also apply to the mind when it is cluttered with many thoughts and ideas. Both situations are distractions to accomplishing your goals and will divert your attention sufficiently so that you do not know where to begin. When you lose your concentration, you will again become distracted by the clutter. To deal effectively with this syndrome you must clear both your work area and your mind. To effectively organize or clear a work area, you should:

- Remove everything from the work surface that does not directly relate to the project at hand; only things you need every day should be on your desk.
- Place the phone out of sight, but within reach.
- Remove all personal items, such as calendars, clocks, or photographs, if they are distractors.
- Close the door to the work area when possible, but communicate to colleagues that you may be interrupted in the case of an emergency (Emmett, 2009).

For a nurse this usually means eliminating clutter from a patient's room so that care can be delivered effectively and efficiently. Keep out in the open only things you need to use to carry out the task at hand (e.g., if you are doing a dressing change, you do not need the catheter kit for your next patient in your immediate work space). Another desk management strategy is to assign a work location at the nurses' station for each staff person working on a given shift. This allows the nurse to have a dedicated space to keep schedules and patient charts available, in addition to having computer access, a critical resource for care delivery in today's health care environment.

The Art of "No Detourism." To effectively organize, or clear the mind, you must practice the art of "no detourism." This requires complete concentration on one activity or task until—with no detours—it is completed. It mandates that only one activity at a time be undertaken and that it should be completed before moving to a different task. This method also implies that the task should be completed correctly the first time so that you do not waste time redoing it. Inherent in the concept of "no detourism" is the fact that the tasks undertaken are directly related to personal goals and objectives; thus completing them will result in internal satisfaction. Maura may have benefited from practicing "no detourism." Perhaps she would not have become distracted by the phone call from the infusion unit if she had been focused on passing the medications via the barcoding system.

The Art of "Wastebasketry". Perfecting the art of "wastebasketry" is mandatory for better use of time. The art of physical "wastebasketry" involves "circular filing" (in the trash can or with the delete key on the computer) of any documents, including e-mails or other paperwork that has limited use or needs no response. The goal is to handle a paper (or e-mail) only once, then either act on it (do it), send it along to another appropriate person (delegate it), or throw it away (dump it). Some also refer to this as the TRASH approach: T: throw it away, R: refer it to someone else, A: act on it, S: save it, or H: halt it (e.g., stop junk mail from coming to you) (Skillpath Seminars, 2001). This art involves being sufficiently knowledgeable and skilled to ascertain which documents, e-mails, and paperwork are appropriate candidates for the "circular file" and then daring to follow through. Practicing this art daily will also help in managing the stacked-desk syndrome by reducing much of the clutter.

The art of mental "wastebasketry" also involves organizing your mind to deal with the established priorities. This requires using selective perception to attend only to those tasks at hand.

It also assists in discarding useless information. Mental "wastebasketry" is a valuable skill to perfect in relation to effecting a better use of time.

E-Mail and Memo Mania. Keep electronic mail brief and to the point. Do not procrastinate in responding. Use correct form and proper etiquette and be accurate. Also keep in mind that a phone call may be a sufficient and more efficient means of response and often more appropriate. The consensus regarding e-mails is that too many of them are generated unnecessarily, which may constitute a major time distraction. It is beneficial to allot specified periods throughout the workday to review, filter, and respond to e-mail, as appropriate. Taking 10 minutes every morning to review your e-mail messages will allow you to prioritize those activities that may be time sensitive. Make sure to review your e-mail inbox at least once again around the lunch hour or midday, then again at the day's end to wrap up unfinished business.

E-mail has become the primary method of communication for the majority of individuals in professional, health care, and academic settings. It is an expedient route to contact people, regardless of their location. It is also a useful way to conduct business with a group of people concurrently, when appropriate, because of the ability to share information with many parties at once. Keep in mind, however, that e-mail is a professional channel of communication, and messages should contain a greeting, a clear body of text, specific and clear requests for information, and an acceptable closing to the message. Messages should also be free of grammatical and typographic errors. Chapter 18 provides additional information about how to use e-mail effectively.

Implementing for Control

Implementing for control refers to carrying out those activities that assist people in managing time use. The implementing activities include:

- Attacking the priorities
- Finding "extra" time
- Handling paperwork appropriately
- Avoiding procrastination
- Delegating appropriately
- Controlling interruptions, such as phone calls, meetings, and visitors
- Learning the art of saying no
- Rewarding yourself
- Using technology

Further exploring these activities clarifies how they can be easily implemented in daily life.

Attacking the Priorities. It is important to attack the priorities early to gain control of your time. Delay in beginning tasks will only result in crises when deadlines or personal goals are not met. One of the most cited reasons for delaying this process is fear—a very real symptom of procrastination—usually fear of failure, although it could be a fear of something else. Regardless, it is important to analyze your fears to be able to identify the source and to determine whether the fear is valid or exaggerated in order to manage it to obtain the results you established (Emmett, 2009; Vestal, 2009). If the priority is a big project or large task, it can be successfully approached by examining how the project can be divided up into smaller, more manageable tasks.

Finding "Extra" Time. The concept of finding extra time seems paradoxical because in reality everyone has the same amount of time. The concept actually relates to how people choose to use their time. In some cases a different use of time may result in additional time for accomplishing goals. A few ways to produce extra time are:

◆ Using commuting time and coffee breaks to relax so that designated working hours are more productive
◆ Instituting working lunches periodically, such as twice a week

Certainly there are other ways individuals might choose to alter their use of time. The key is knowing which activities can be altered without being detrimental to overall functioning. For example, perhaps giving up 30 minutes of television watching or reading each evening would work for some, but not if that is the only relaxation time that is available daily. Sacrificing downtime for more work may decrease overall productivity. It may be a case of working longer, but not smarter, so less actually gets accomplished.

Handling E-Mail and Paperwork Appropriately. The rule regarding paperwork is to handle it only once. Decide to act on the paperwork, delegate it, or toss it. Shuffling papers or e-mails, filing, and retrieving are time wasters. Plan to prevent becoming mired in paperwork. Perfecting the art of "wastebasketry" will assist in handling paperwork and e-mails appropriately. Another tip is to set aside a specific time each day for dealing with all e-mail and paperwork.

Avoiding Procrastination. Procrastination is a bad habit that ranks high on the list of time wasters. It has been referred to as an obstacle to success, "the cat burglar of time management" and a "hidden fear of conflict" (Mancini, 2003). It can wear many disguises, including fear, laziness, indifference, overwork, and forgetfulness. Procrastination most frequently is evident when a person is faced with an unpleasant task, a difficult task, or a difficult decision. Usually procrastination is easily recognizable because it involves doing low-priority rather than high-priority tasks, and it always welcomes interruptions. Procrastination is the art of "never doing today what can be put off until tomorrow." The result is less productivity, less internal satisfaction, and more stress.

The first step in avoiding procrastination is being able to recognize when it is occurring. The second step is being able to admit that what is occurring is procrastination. Once those two steps are accomplished, the work of overcoming procrastination can begin. Following are mechanisms for overcoming procrastination:

◆ Identify the tasks that are being put off.
◆ Ask why the task is being avoided.
◆ Determine whether the task could or should be done by someone else.
◆ Identify consequences of the procrastination.
◆ Set priorities in relation to the task.
◆ Establish deadlines and adhere to them.
◆ Focus on one aspect at a time.
◆ Do not strive for perfection if 95% or 98% will be just as effective (Emmett, 2009).

The last item is clearly one in which good clinical discernment must be exercised, because there are clearly instances when providing nursing care that anything less than 100% could cause harm. It also helps if you can eliminate those tasks that make up the procrastination. For example, if rearranging the desk, the furniture, or even the medication cart is part of how a person procrastinates, then eliminate that activity by changing the work location or environment. Most important, emphasize the benefits that are to be gained by completing the task and accomplishing the goals that will provide internal satisfaction.

Delegating Appropriately. Most simplistically, delegation is the art of giving other people tasks to be accomplished. In reality, however, there is nothing simple about delegation. It usually requires considerable time and energy to delegate, but the rewards are greater in the overall context of accomplishing goals. Mancini (2003) and Skillpath Seminars (2001) identify the following important benefits of delegation:

- Extends the results that can be accomplished from what one person can do alone to what he or she can manage through others
- Frees time for more important tasks
- Assists in developing the initiative, skills, knowledge, and competence of others
- Maintains the responsibility and decision level
- Is often more cost-effective

With these potential benefits, it would seem that everyone would want to use delegation. Unfortunately this is not the case. Many barriers, internal and external, can hinder the delegation process.

A brief exploration of those barriers may clarify why delegation is such a problem for some people. The internal barriers to delegating include the following: a personal preference for how tasks get accomplished, demanding that everyone know all the details, believing that no one else can complete the task as well, lack of experience in delegating, insecurity, fear of being disliked, lack of confidence in others, perfectionism resulting in overcontrol, lack of organizational skill, failure to delegate authority commensurate with the responsibility delegated, indecision, poor communication skills, and lack of commitment to the development of others.

The external barriers to delegating are either inherent in the situation or in the person to whom something is being delegated. External barriers within the situation may include stringent policies that mandate who can do what, low tolerance of mistakes, the criticality of the decisions, implementation of a management-by-crisis style, confusion regarding responsibilities and authority, and understaffing. External barriers to delegation that reside within the person to whom tasks are being delegated include lack of experience, lack of competence, avoidance of responsibility, overdependence on others, disorganization, procrastination, work overload, and immersion in trivia and clutter (Mancini, 2003). When the barriers are identified and overcome, the delegation process can proceed. Implementing the following steps will facilitate appropriate delegation (also see Chapter 19 for a complete discussion of delegation in the clinical setting):

- Identify exactly what is to be delegated and why.
- Select the best person for the task; this may be the person most qualified or it may be the person whose development the delegator chooses to contribute to.
- Communicate the assignment in detail, perhaps even including written instructions.
- Involve the delegatee in establishing the objectives and deadlines for the task.
- Have the delegatee repeat the details of the task.
- Give the person the authority for accomplishing the task.
- Provide adequate resources and support as needed.
- Schedule regular meetings for progress reports.
- Establish controls and monitor the results.
- Evaluate the process and progress of the delegatee.
- Let the person do the job.
- Enjoy the results of having the delegated task completed and being able to accomplish other tasks simultaneously (Mindtools, 2006).

It is not prudent to take shortcuts when delegating tasks because the results might be different than what was originally intended. Avoiding delegation shortcuts is an important consideration because the nurse who does the delegating also retains accountability for the task.

Delegation would have been useful to Susan in the opening vignette. It could have helped her meet her patient care goals and decrease her anxiety. Unfortunately Susan was overwhelmed, and she could not identify those things that needed to be done or direct someone else to do them. In addition, she had not established any priorities, so it was difficult for Susan to plan for appropriate delegation. Ignoring the availability and influence of other colleagues can perpetuate a rather self-critical and individualist perspective of time management (Waterworth, 2003). As seen in the vignette, this can lead to a failure to address problems in the organization of work and in the coordination of patient care within the health care team.

Controlling Interruptions. To focus on your priorities it is important to establish uninterrupted blocks of time. Frequent causes of interruptions are telephone calls, meetings, and visitors, particularly the drop-in type. Learning how to control such interruptions will assist in accomplishing more in less time. One of the easiest ways to manage incoming calls is to not answer them during time that is scheduled for other activities. An answering machine, voice mail service, or an assistant can take the message to be responded to later. "Later" should refer to the time that was preestablished for returning telephone calls. A good example of controlling interruptions in the opening vignette would have been for Susan to ask the unit secretary to assist the patient requesting information about an appointment.

Most people schedule callbacks for times when their productivity level is lower or during their downtime. Also telephone calls can be controlled by the tone and verbiage used. If a person chooses to invite conversation and ensure a longer call, using a vague, open-ended greeting will accomplish that purpose. If a person chooses to focus the call specifically on its purpose, a specific, factual, informative greeting will enhance the productivity of the call and shorten its length. For example, "Hi, Bill, how are you? How are things going?" definitely invites the person to reply at length, whereas "Hi, Bill, I have two questions that I need for you to answer" tends to condense the telephoning session. Also being prepared for the conversation with all of the pertinent facts readily available helps to focus the conversation and to shorten the call.

Meetings can become a major time waster if they are poorly managed and nonproductive. The first step in controlling this interruption is deciding whether to attend. Such a decision should be based on an evaluation of the potential productivity of the meeting. For example, is the meeting absolutely necessary? Does the agenda contain items that you should be informed about? Is it necessary for you to contribute to the discussion? Will decisions be made that will affect you and your functioning? Are you conducting the meeting? These questions should guide the decision (Mancini, 2003). Once a person is committed to attending a meeting, he or she is responsible for helping to ensure that the meeting remains focused and productive. The person conducting the meeting not only shares those same responsibilities but also has a more direct role in effecting the outcome. Steps for conducting a productive meeting are presented in Box 25-2.

Visitors, particularly unplanned visitors, also create interruptions. One way to decrease the number of visitors is to seclude yourself during specific times by closing the door to others, physically and mentally. Managing visitors in today's health care environment can be difficult, given the fact that family members are able and welcome to accompany their ill members for extended periods and in a variety of settings. Educating family members can be a time-consuming task in a nurse's day. It is important to ensure that this time is factored into

BOX **25-2**

Managing Effective Meetings

PREMEETING WORK

Step 1—Determine the specific purpose(s) for the meeting (What do you want to accomplish in the meeting?).

Step 2—Create a list of meeting topics, such as "revisions to nursing handbook" or "new admission policy." Create a fact sheet related to each topic (if appropriate) to distribute with the agenda.

Step 3 Determine the meeting attendees. The meeting attendees are individuals, groups, or department representatives with valuable insight or who are affected by decisions made during the meeting.

Step 4—Determine the date, time, and location for the meeting, and invite attendees. To maximize meeting attendance, ask attendees what date and time would work with their schedules.

Step 5—Create the meeting agenda. It should contain the following components:
- Title of the group meeting
- Date, time, and location of the meeting
- The purpose(s) for the meeting in sentence form
- Agenda items, time allotted for each item, and person responsible for reporting on each item. Agenda items titled "Next meeting agenda items," "Rate the meeting," and "Assign roles for next meeting" should be listed as the last three items and allotted 3 to 5 minutes each.

Step 6—Send the meeting agenda out at least 1 week before the meeting so that attendees come prepared. Send a meeting reminder 2 days before the meeting.

DURING THE MEETING

Step 1—Ensure that the participants' comfort needs are met by arranging the seating in an oval or circular shape and preferably around a table.

Step 2—Ask for volunteers to fulfill the following roles:
- *Leader:* The leader is usually the person calling the meeting. This person is responsible for completing all six of the meeting prework steps.
- *Timekeeper:* The timekeeper monitors and intervenes as necessary the time allocations for each agenda item and announces the time remaining until the end of the meeting.
- *Recorder:* This person records the major points of the meeting on paper, flipchart, or board. The person records at the level of detail requested by the group and then captures major summary points, decisions, action steps, and assignments in the meeting minutes, which should be distributed with the agenda before the next meeting.

Step 3—The leader guides the meeting by:
- Processing one agenda item at a time.
- Allowing the timekeeper to do his or her job to keep the meeting on track.
- Debriefing the end of the meeting by asking these questions: "What went well with the meeting?" and "What can we improve upon for the next meeting?" These questions should be used at the end of each meeting to improve subsequent meetings.

one's schedule because communicating with family members is an inevitable and important occurrence.

Learning the Art of Saying No. "No" is such a small word, but it is sometimes more difficult to say than any 14-syllable word. The first step in learning the art of saying no is determining when to say it. The cost-benefit ratio of each opportunity must be evaluated in relation to the overall goals. If the activity will be a benefit overall, obviously it must be given careful consideration. If it will not be a significant benefit, decline gracefully but emphatically. There isn't a need to provide an elaborate qualifier to your "no" response; a clear, succinct reply is acceptable (Patterson et al, 2002). For example, when asked to review a clinical guideline, do not refuse based on the fact that you are overworked and do not have a free minute for 3 weeks. The person requesting the review is likely to agree that the later timeframe will be fine, in which case, you find yourself committed to doing something that has low benefit unless you create another excuse. Instead be polite and gracious in the refusal but do not allow leeway to be manipulated into saying yes. Always consider the opportunity that "no" offers in terms of your overall goals.

Rewarding Yourself. All people function more productively when they are motivated. The sources of motivation vary from person to person. A person needs to identify his or her motivators and use them as rewards for accomplishing goals. It is important to identify long- and short-term rewards so that they can be implemented appropriately. Most people are familiar with rewarding themselves in exchange for doing something, and they do it frequently. For some it is a way of life. It usually amounts to bargaining with yourself to facilitate the completion of a task. For example, "If I finish reading these two work-related articles, then I can read my novel for 30 minutes," or "If I complete this paper, I will treat myself to ice cream." You should know which rewards work best and use them appropriately to accomplish long-term goals.

Using Technology. Many of today's technologic advances can be used to improve time management. Most health care settings have adopted more uses of technologic resources to better improve the use of time and enhance patient care. Many health care organizations use electronic health records (EHRs), which allows for multiple users to access a patient's record at the same time to document and to review information. There are also electronic order entry systems now in place, in which clinicians enter orders and activate orders that are then transmitted to the pharmacy to fill the medication request. Patient acuity rating systems are now completed online and used by admitting departments to send patients to the appropriate units for care.

Just about every workplace has a professional office system that supports e-mail and scheduling activities. The scheduling features available can be very useful for staff in the planning phase of time management. However, there are advantages and disadvantages to most of the new technologic devices. If it takes longer to look up a telephone number in a computer system than using a traditional phonebook, for example, it makes sense to review that process for efficiency before determining which system would provide a best practice.

Many people today use personal digital assistants (PDAs) or smart phones to synchronize their personal and professional calendars. The PDA also becomes a valuable resource in the clinical setting when programmed with drug information and lab value databases, which allow a nurse to have a wealth of information at her or his fingertips without having to carry or look for resource manuals. However, when considering the many technologic devices available, keep in mind the tools and devices should improve workflow and processes, not hinder them or create cumbersome ones (Brafman and Beckstrom, 2006). Also remember that taking time to learn to use new technology correctly will pay off in the long run by increasing effective use of time. Once the strategies have been implemented, it is important to continue to use them to achieve your goals and gain internal satisfaction.

CONTINUING TO SUCCEED

Improving time management to enhance self-performance and accomplish goals is a lifelong process. The process becomes easier the longer you engage in it, but time management still requires continual attention and energy. Obviously, time management does not just happen—it requires a strong personal commitment. Lakein (1973) suggests that it is important to continue doing the following to succeed:

- ◆ When feeling overwhelmed, always stop and plan activities.
- ◆ Keep focused on priorities and act accordingly.
- ◆ Avoid favorite forms of procrastination.
- ◆ Maintain a positive attitude about the established goals, or revise them so that they coincide with your value system.
- ◆ Do something for yourself every day.
- ◆ Continue to work on overcoming your fears.
- ◆ Resist doing the easy but unimportant tasks.

In addition, delete the words "if only" from your vocabulary. Regret is a luxury and a great time waster. Significant time is expended rehashing mistakes or determining how to make something perfect when it was a one-time occurrence that is now over. Such time usually is not productive unless you will encounter similar situations in the future. It is more productive to admit mistakes, accept responsibility for them, and move on. Thus the words "if only" should be replaced with "next time," and the incident itself should be filed in the mental circular file to leverage for the future (Skillpath Seminars, 2001). The reader is encouraged to review the tips for continuing success in managing time presented in Box 25-3.

BOX **25-3**

Tips for Successful Time Management

1. Clarify objectives, put them in writing, and establish a priority list to work from.
2. Focus on objectives, not on activities.
3. Set at least one major objective for each day and achieve it.
4. Record a time log periodically to analyze how time is used and to document bad habits.
5. Analyze everything in terms of objectives.
6. Make a to-do list every day that includes daily objectives and priorities and time estimates to accomplish them.
7. Schedule time every day to ensure that the most important things are accomplished first.
8. Make sure the first hour of every workday is productive.
9. Set time limits for every task undertaken.
10. Take the time to do the task right the first time so that time will not be wasted doing it over.
11. Institute a quiet hour of uninterrupted time each day to work on the most important tasks.
12. Develop the habit of finishing whatever task is started.
13. Conquer procrastination and learn to do tasks now.
14. Make better time management a daily habit.
15. Never spend time on less important things when it could be spent on more important things.
16. Take time for yourself—time to relax, time to live, time to just be.
17. Develop a personal philosophy of time that is consistent with your values.
18. Know how you currently spend your time.
19. Identify your "prime productive time."
20. Do tomorrow's planning tonight.
21. Ask yourself often, "Why am I doing what I am doing right now?"
22. Handle each piece of paper only once.
23. Delegate whenever possible and delegate wisely.
24. Identify your high payoff items (80-20 principle).

From www.time-management-guide.com. Retrieved May 2009; Skillpath Seminars: *Managing multiple projects, objective and deadlines*, Mission, KS, 2001.

SUMMARY

This chapter has focused on how to better manage your energy to control one of our most precious and seemingly scarce resources—time. Time management is important to achieving any personal or professional goals, and it helps decrease frustration and anxiety in high achievers. Without time management most professionals could never achieve their established goals, and for nurses, many patient care activities would never get completed, perhaps resulting in poor outcomes for the patient. Susan's and Maura's experiences in the opening vignette are an example of what your life could be like in nursing, unless strategies for better self-management are implemented. Thus it is important in your professional career to initiate habits related to time management that will continue throughout the years. Start asking Lakein's question frequently throughout the day: "What is the best use of my time right now?" (Lakein, 1973). You may be surprised to learn that the answer does not coincide with your current activity. When that occurs, stop and implement the strategies for self-management to better control your time. You will become more productive and gain internal satisfaction as a result.

evolve   Additional resources are available online at: http://evolve.elsevier.com/Cherry/

REFERENCES

Benner P: *From novice to expert: excellence and power in clinical nursing practice*, Upper Saddle River, NJ, 2001, Prentice-Hall.

Brafman O, Beckstrom RA: *The starfish and the spider*, New York, 2006, Penguin Group.

Childre D: *De-stress kit for the changing times*, Boulder Creek, CA, 2008, Institute of Hearthmath.

Emmett R: *Manage your time and reduce your stress: a handbook for the overworked, overscheduled, and overwhelmed*, New York, 2009, Walker Publishing Company, Inc.

Federwisch A: On the hour: collaboration helps hospitals fine-tune hourly rounding, *Manage Leadersh*:48–49, 2009.

Goleman D: *Emotional intelligence*, New York, 1999, Bantam Books.

Koch R: *Living the 80/20 way: work less, worry less, succeed more, enjoy more*, Boston, 2004, Nicholas Brealey Publishing.

Lakein A: *How to get control of your time and your life*, New York, 1973, Signet.

Larkin H: Will we make history? *Hosp Health Netw* 83(2):20–25, 2009.

Lee F: *If Disney ran your hospital: 9½ things you would do differently*, Bozeman, MT, 2004, Second River Healthcare Press.

Loehr J, Schwartz T: *The power of full engagement*, New York, 2003, Free Press.

Mancini M: *Time management*, New York, 2003, McGraw-Hill.

Mindtools: *How to: delegating work to other people*. 2006. Available at: www.mindtools.com.

Morgenstern J: *Time management from the inside out*, New York, 2004, Henry Holt and Co.

Nightingale F: *Notes on nursing: what it is and what it is not*, New York, 1969, Dover Publications.

Patterson K, et al: *Crucial conversations: tools for talking when the stakes are high*, New York, 2002, McGraw-Hill.

Penn State College of Agricultural Sciences: *Cooperative Extension Orientation Learning Modules*. 2009. Retrieved May 2009 from: http://cas.psu.edu/docs/casadmin/NSO/StackedDesk.html.

Reid Ponte P: Nurse executive: the four principles of management. In Adams LT, O'Neil EH, editors: *Nurse executive: the purpose, process, and personnel of management*, New York, 2008, Springer.

Senge P: *The fifth discipline*, New York, 1999, Doubleday.

Skillpath Seminars: *Managing multiple projects, objective and deadlines*, Mission, KS, 2001. Retrieved May 2009 from: http://Time-Management-Guide.com.

Vestal K: Procrastination: frustrating or fatal? *Nurse Leadersh* 7(2):8–9, 2009.

Waterworth S: Time management strategies in nursing practice, *J Adv Nurs* 43(5):432–440, 2003.

Contemporary Nursing Roles and Career Opportunities

Robert W. Koch, DNS, RN

evolve   Additional resources are available online at: http://evolve.elsevier.com/Cherry/

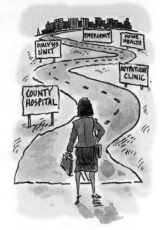

*The career path for nurses
is long and wide.*

VIGNETTE

When Eric Sanders graduated 15 years ago, he thought he would work in the hospital his entire career. However, with so many changes in the economic forces affecting health care and the resulting shift of clients outside acute care, more opportunities exist for him. Eric can take his skills and seek new ones to have a choice of practice roles and settings. Being a registered nurse now gives him more options for practice than he ever thought possible.

■ QUESTIONS TO CONSIDER WHILE READING THIS CHAPTER:

1 What community-based opportunities exist for graduate nurses?

2 How can a new nurse gain knowledge about the role of the parish nurse, forensic nurse, or other unique nursing roles?

3 What unique skills do nurses working in community settings need?

KEY TERMS

Advanced practice nursing Based on knowledge and skills acquired through basic nursing education, with licensure as a registered nurse (RN) and graduate education and experience that includes advanced nursing theory, physical assessment, and psychosocial assessment and treatment of illness. Includes nurse practitioners (NPs), certified nurse-midwives (CNMs), certified registered nurse anesthetists (CRNAs), and clinical nurse specialists (CNSs).

Clinical nurse leader (CNL) The CNL is a master's degree–prepared generalist who oversees the care coordination of a distinct group of patients in any setting. The CNL actively provides direct patient care in complex situations, evaluates patient outcomes, and has the decision-making authority to change care plans when necessary. This clinician puts evidence-based practice into action to ensure that patients benefit from the latest innovations in care delivery and is envisioned as a leader in the health care delivery system.

Doctor of nursing practice (DNP) The DNP is an expert in advanced nursing practice who has an earned clinically focused doctorate degree in nursing.

Interprofessional team Health care team composed of professionals from different disciplines including chaplains, nurses, dietitians, pharmacists, physical therapists, physicians, respiratory therapists, social workers, and speech language pathologists who cooperate, collaborate, communicate, and integrate care to ensure that care is continuous and reliable.

Nursing roles (1) Traditional duties and responsibilities of the professional nurse, regardless of practice area or setting, such as the roles of care provider, educator, counselor, client advocate, change agent, leader and manager, researcher, and coordinator of the interprofessional health care team. (2) Duties and responsibilities of the professional nurse that are guided by specific professional standards of practice and usually are carried out in a distinct practice area (e.g., flight nurse, forensic nurse, and occupational nurse).

LEARNING OUTCOMES

After studying this chapter, the reader will be able to:

1 Evaluate the effect of the current health care environment on the future role of nurses.

2 Analyze the influence of current demographic characteristics of RNs in the United States on contemporary nursing roles.

3 Differentiate among various innovative nursing practice roles today.

4 Differentiate between the roles of advanced practice nurses and other RNs in various settings.

5 Describe the role of the CNL.

CHAPTER OVERVIEW

The health care system continues to change as social and economic factors create a state of constant evolution. Professional nurses respond by creating innovative alternatives to traditional nursing practice to meet these new challenges. As nurses proactively define solutions to today's health care dilemmas, multiple career opportunities emerge.

In the past, most nurses considered acute care hospitals the main practice setting available on graduation. Few other career choices were available. Public health nursing was one of few exceptions providing variety in the nursing job market. As health care moves from inpatient treatment to outpatient and home care, and acute care shifts to health promotion and disease prevention, the U.S. culture seeks alternative settings to meet this growing need. This shift in health care settings creates a variety of choices for nurses exploring career opportunities.

Nurses today have more liberty to explore and even create job opportunities. Nurses may continue to select the hospital acute care setting or venture into less traditional nursing roles. Nurses must claim ownership of nontraditional roles as they emerge in the health care job market. As professionals, they should exercise their influence to develop and support new nursing roles.

This chapter presents an overview of some key opportunities available for RNs today in the United States. Included are demographics of today's nurses, in addition to implications for the future. This chapter examines the traditional and less traditional options available and the current and future issues for roles in professional practice.

NURSING—MUCH THE SAME, BUT BIGGER AND BETTER

In the past, describing the role of RNs was simple because there were few opportunities for variation. Today exploring job opportunities for RNs is more complicated because nurses can practice in literally hundreds of diverse settings with a broad variety of clients. The proliferation of career opportunities for nurses is growing. Although nursing roles have expanded, the traditional functions of the nurse remain intact. Box 26-1 summarizes the roles nurses assume in any employment role or setting.

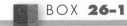
BOX **26-1**

> ## Professional Nursing Roles
>
> | | |
> |---|---|
> | Care provider | Leader and manager |
> | Educator and counselor | Researcher |
> | Client advocate | Coordinator of the interprofessional health |
> | Change agent | care team |

Care Provider

The role of care provider is basic to the nursing profession. As the provider of care the nurse assesses client resources, strengths and weaknesses, coping behaviors, and the environment to optimize the problem-solving and self-care abilities of the client and family. The nurse plans therapeutic interventions in collaboration with the client, physician, and other health care providers. In addition, the nurse takes responsibility for coordination of care that involves other health professionals or resources, providing continuity and helping the client deal effectively with the health care system. As part of this role, caring is always central to nursing interventions and is an essential attribute of the expert nurse.

Educator and Counselor

Multiple factors increase the need for nurses to serve as educators. Today the emphasis is on health promotion and health maintenance, in addition to management of disease conditions. The role of nurse counselor has been elevated to new heights. More than ever, nurses encourage clients to look at alternatives, recognize their choices, and develop a sense of control in a rapidly changing health care environment.

Client Advocate

Professional nurses find that the role of client advocate is essential in various situations with a multitude of client populations. Promoting what is best for the client, ensuring that the client's needs are met, and protecting the client's rights remain important responsibilities of the professional nurse.

Change Agent

When nurses first adopted the role of "change agent," few individuals anticipated to what extent nurses would fulfill this role. However, nurses have expanded their role as change agents in many ways. The profession continues to identify client, patient safety, and health care delivery problems; to assess individual and organizational motivation and capacity for change; to determine alternatives; to explore possible outcomes of the alternatives; and to assess cost-effective resources in infinite health-related situations.

Leader and Manager

The leadership role of the professional nurse is paramount to the health care system. Nursing leadership varies according to the level of application and includes:

- ◆ Improving the health status and potential of individuals or families
- ◆ Ensuring that safe, high-quality care is provided across all health care settings
- ◆ Increasing the effectiveness and level of satisfaction among professional colleagues providing care

◆ Managing multiple resources in a health care facility
◆ Raising citizens' and legislators' attitudes toward and expectations of the nursing profession and the health care system

There is little doubt that the management role of the nurse has become more important. Nursing management includes planning, giving direction, and monitoring and evaluating nursing care of individuals, groups, families, and communities.

Researcher

During the past decades, nursing has taken its place among other disciplines in the production and use of research specific to its profession. Although the majority of researchers in nursing are prepared at the doctoral and postdoctoral levels, an increasing number of clinicians with master's degrees are participating in research as part of their advanced practice role. Nurses prepared at the baccalaureate and associate degree levels are also participating in research. These nurses may be assisting with data collection, critiquing research findings, and using these findings in practice. More nursing interventions are based on nursing research than in the past.

Coordinator of the Interprofessional Health Care Team

Interprofessional teams consist of collaborative practice relationships among several disciplines of health care professionals. These disciplines may include nursing, medicine, pharmacy, nutrition, social work, case management, and other allied health professionals, such as physical therapists, respiratory therapists, occupational therapists, and speech therapists. Chaplains or pastoral care representatives also serve a valuable role on the interprofessional health care team. These teams are found in all health care delivery settings and function most effectively when their focus revolves around the needs of the client.

Interprofessional teams are valuable because professional members bring in-depth and specialized knowledge and skills to the interaction process. In an age of exploding information, the roles of interprofessional team members complement one another. Through the formal and informal communication of ideas and opinions of team members, health care plans are determined. A plan of care developed by the interprofessional team is considered a valuable health management tool.

Interprofessional teams refer to coordination between and among disciplines involved in providing client care. The collaborative process involved in interprofessional health care transcends a single health profession to create comprehensive work outcomes. This team process can improve the quality of care, increase client satisfaction, increase nursing satisfaction, and reduce hospital cost by decreasing hospital length of stay and increasing nurse retention.

Successful health care team models that use concepts related to interprofessional health care include pain management, nutritional support, skin care, rehabilitation, mental health, and hospice. Discharge planning, which emerged as a major focus of health care delivery in the 1980s and involves developing a plan of treatment that ultimately results in the discharge of the client from the health care facility, is built on the concept of interprofessional care, with each discipline involved in providing care for the client included in developing the discharge plan.

Client education is another area in which collaboration of disciplines is absolutely essential. Health care professionals must understand one another's contributions to client education and ensure that the information clients and families receive is consistent and complete. This will produce the best possible health outcomes for clients and families.

In Box 26-2 some of the more common roles of interprofessional health care team members are addressed, and the website of their associated professional organization is listed. These team members are involved in client care to varying degrees, depending on client needs for the specific talents and knowledge of each team member. This list contains selected professional roles contributing to the interprofessional health care team approach, but there may be more in a given team.

The following case study provides an excellent example of the role of various members of the interprofessional health care team. Multiple professional caregivers provide health care within the limits of each provider's expertise. The joint efforts of all professionals provide the opportunity for a better overall outcome.

CASE STUDY

John was discussing a problem with a coworker over his cell phone as he approached the intersection. He did not notice the truck approaching on his left side so he did not see the STOP sign. After evaluation in the emergency department, John was diagnosed as post motor vehicle accident with multiple trauma, closed head injury, several rib and leg fractures, lacerations, and internal injuries. His physician ordered multiple diagnostic tests, laboratory tests, medications, and treatments. His nurse monitored his physical status and carried out the orders written by the physician. The nurse organized the tests and procedures and managed his pain. The pharmacist reviewed and supplied the medications ordered and analyzed potential interaction effects of the multiple pharmaceutical agents. A respiratory therapist was consulted to perform breathing treatments to facilitate lung expansion and prevent respiratory complications. After surgical repair of his fractured leg, physical therapy was consulted to assess John's condition and his need for physical reconditioning. A plan of care was determined to enhance his mobility. His long recuperation led to mild depression and spiritual distress. The nurse who assessed these symptoms made arrangements for the chaplain to visit John and discussed the possibility of pharmacotherapy for depression with the physician and pharmacist. Throughout John's period of care, all involved practitioners communicated their assessments and worked together to provide collaborative interventions for holistic care. In addition, all interprofessional team members collaborated in medical rounds and discharge planning meetings to plan and coordinate John's care.

NURSES TODAY: WHO ARE THEY, AND WHAT ARE THEY DOING?

The phrase "a typical nurse" became a misnomer as the profession entered the twenty-first century. Nursing roles are so diverse that no typical role or practice setting exists. Nurses are the largest occupation in health care with a total of more than 2.5 million, with 59% working in a hospital setting. Projections state that nursing will create the largest number of new jobs of all occupations in the future as more specialties and diverse work options emerge. Overall jobs for nurses are projected to expand 23% between 2006 and 2016, with some specialties such as home care services and physician offices growing up to 39%. Nurses can specialize in basically four ways: work or treatment setting, disease category or condition, organ or body system, or population. Some nurses specialize in more than one of these (U.S. Department of Labor, 2008.).

Examples of specialization in work or treatment settings include ambulatory care nurses, critical care nurses, trauma or emergency nurses, home-care nurses, holistic care nurses, medical-surgical nurses, hospice nurses, perioperative nurses, transplant nurses, psychiatric nurses, or rehabilitation nurses. Examples of nurses who specialize in disease category or condition are oncology nurses, addictions nurses, ostomy and wound care nurses, developmental disabilities nurses, diabetes management nurses, HIV-AIDS nurses, and genetics nurses. Organ or body systems can differentiate nurses as cardiovascular nurses, dermatology nurses, urology nurses, orthopedic nurses, nephrology nurses, gastroenterology nurses, gynecology nurses,

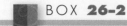

BOX **26-2**

Interprofessional Health Care Team Members

Nurse (RN): Often the coordinator of the team. RNs take licensure examinations after completing associate degree, diploma, or baccalaureate degree preparation from an accredited school of nursing. RNs are able to obtain specialty certification for advanced skills and/or advanced degrees. RNs use the nursing process in client care in any health care setting.
American Nursing Association
www.nursingworld.org

Physician (MD or DO): Often the leader of the team, the physician diagnoses and prescribes treatment interventions for clients. Medical doctors (MDs) or doctors of osteopathy (DOs) complete 4 years of medical school and board examinations. Physicians can complete postgraduate training, including internship, residency, and fellowship training in a specialty area. Physicians also complete state licensing examinations and function in all health care arenas.
American Medical Association
www.ama-assn.org

Pharmacist (RPh or PharmD): Responsible for providing drug therapy for positive client outcomes; activities include drug information services, client and health care staff education, dispensing medications and client monitoring, adverse drug reaction reporting, research, concurrent drug use evaluation, and consultative services in areas such as pain management and nutritional support. Pharmacists complete baccalaureate preparation, an internship period, and licensing board examinations. Pharmacists can complete additional specialized training, certifications, and/or advanced degrees. In some states, the PharmD, or doctor of pharmacy degree, is now the educational requirement for entering practice.
American Pharmaceutical Association
www.aphanet.org

Physician assistant (PA): Works under the supervision of the MD or DO and performs assessments, procedures, or protocols approved by the physician. PAs complete a baccalaureate degree with specialized PA training (usually 2 years) and state licensure.
American Academy of Physician Assistants
www.aapa.org

Dietitian (RD or LD): Provides nutritional therapy and support to ensure that the nutritional needs of the client are met. Activities include involving both client and family in dietary assessment and teaching, identifying resources for food purchase and preparation, and identifying areas of food-drug interactions. Dietitians complete a baccalaureate degree from an accredited nutrition or food service administration program and national board examinations and may also complete state licensure and advanced educational preparation.
American Dietetic Association
www.eatright.org/public

Physical therapist (PT): Attends to the client's needs for movement. Activities include assessing physical strength and mobility needs and developing a plan of strengthening exercises for the client with movement dysfunction, maintaining range of motion and muscle tone, and identifying assistive devices that may be needed. A physical therapist may also be expert in the area of wound care. The basic educational requirement is a baccalaureate degree in a physical therapy program and completion of a national certifying examination. Advanced degrees are available.
American Physical Therapy Association
www.apta.org

Speech language pathologist (SLP): Assists clients who are communicatively impaired by intervening in speech, language, and/or swallowing disorders related to receptive language, expressive language, speech intelligibility, voice disorders, alaryngeal speech, or prosody and cognitive impairments; plays an important role in evaluation and treatment of swallowing disorders. Therapists complete a master's degree from an accredited school, a 1-year fellowship, and a national certifying examination.
American Speech-Language-Hearing Association
www.asha.org

Continued

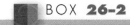

BOX **26-2**

Interprofessional Health Care Team Members—cont'd

Occupational therapist (OT): Plans activities that assist and teach clients with physical disabilities to become independent in activities of daily living, such as dressing, grooming, bathing, and eating. Once self-care goals have been met, the OT can help the client perform daily responsibilities of caring for a home and/or returning to work. Educational requirements include completion of an occupational therapy program of study at the baccalaureate, graduate certification, or master's degree level. Graduates must complete a period of supervised clinical experience and state licensure examinations.
  American Occupational Therapy Association
  www.aota.org
Respiratory therapist (RT): Responsible for assessment and maintenance of the client's airway and respiratory equipment used for diagnosis and therapy of respiratory disorders. Activities include client assessment, aerosolized medication administration, sputum sampling, arterial and mixed venous blood sampling, pulmonary function testing, cardiopulmonary stress testing, and sleep studies; may also be involved in conducting pulmonary rehabilitation programs. RTs complete a program of study and take a national certifying examination. If the program of study is completed in an associate or bachelor's degree program, the level of credentialing examination is different.
  American Association for Respiratory Care
  www.aarc.org
Social worker: Uses skills to help clients, families, and communities address psychosocial needs. Activities include educating clients, families, and staff about community resources, discharge planning, financial counseling and identifying financial resources, crisis intervention, referring to community resources, abuse and neglect reporting, completing advanced directives, assisting with resolving ethical dilemmas, evaluating behavior and mental disorders, and conducting support groups. Social workers complete a minimum of baccalaureate preparation in the field and may pursue advanced degrees.
  National Association of Social Workers
  www.naswdc.org
Chaplain or pastoral representative: Attends to the spiritual and emotional needs of the client and family. Activities include providing pastoral counseling and support and sacramental ministry and liturgical celebrations; not all pastoral representatives share the same religion as the client or family members but must be able to acknowledge the differences among religions and help assist the person with spiritual needs. Basic education requirements vary based on the setting and religious affiliation. The Association for Clinical Pastoral Education is a multicultural, multifaith organization devoted to improving the quality of ministry and pastoral care offered by spiritual caregivers of all faiths.
  Association for Clinical Pastoral Education
  www.acpe.edu

ophthalmic nurses, or respiratory nurses. Nurses can be recognized by the population they serve, such as neonatology nurses, pediatric nurses, or gerontology nurses. Nurses such as CNSs, nurse anesthetists, nurse-midwives, and NPs have more direct patient contact, whereas case management nurses, infection control nurses, forensic nurses, legal nurses, nurse educators, nurse administrators, or nurse informaticists have little or no contact with patients. Truly these diverse opportunities are increasing in the world of health care (U.S. Department of Labor, 2008).

Demographics for Registered Nurses

Preliminary findings indicated that there were an estimated 2,909,467 RNs in the United States as of March 2004, representing a 7.9% increase above survey results in 2000. Of this total nursing population, 83.2% were employed in nursing, whereas 16.8% were not, an increase of 10% more than 2000 data. Approximately 58.3% of this group was employed full time in the profession, with 25% of nurses working part time. In 2004 the average age of the RN population was 46.8 years, compared with 45.2 in the 2000 survey report. In 2004 the largest group was ages 45 to 49.

Although the nursing profession continues to be preponderantly female, the number of men working as RNs significantly increased in the past decade. The 2004 report indicates that the number of male RNs increased to 5.7%, up from 5.4% in 2000 (Bureau of Health Professions, 2004).

Changes in racial or ethnic backgrounds were reported as well. The March 2004 survey reports that 81.8% of RNs were white or non-Hispanic, whereas 10.6% reported being from one or more racial and/or ethnic backgrounds. Some did not specify this information on the survey (http://bhpr.hrsa.gov/healthworkforce/rnsurvey04/2.htm).

Changes also are occurring in the educational preparation of RNs. There has been a substantial increase in the number of nurses graduating from associate degree nursing programs over the past decade. Although not as dramatic an increase, baccalaureate-prepared nurses also are increasing in number. In 2004 nurses reported their highest degree as 17% diploma, 33.7% associate degree, 34.2% baccalaureate degree, and 13.0% master's or doctoral degree (Bureau of Health Professions, 2004).

Advanced practice nurses now comprise 8.6% of the RN population, up from 7.3% in 2000. NPs lead this group in numbers, followed by CNSs, nurse anesthetists, and nurse-midwives. Nurse practitioners and CNSs make up 81% of the advanced practice group (Bureau of Health Professions, 2004). Acute care hospitals remain the common worksite for RNs, although there has been a trend toward outpatient settings. In 2005 56% of RNs reported working in hospitals, down from 59.1% in 2000.

The next largest area of employment was in community and public health settings—a total of 14.9%, down from 18.3% in 2000. About 11.5% work in physician-based practices, nurse-based practices, or health maintenance organizations (HMOs), up from 10% in 2000. Other worksites include educational settings, occupational health settings, nursing management, prisons and jails, and insurance companies (Bureau of Health Professions, 2004).

The Health Resources and Services Administration (HRSA) is part of the U.S. Department of Health and Human Services. The Bureau of Health Professions, a division of HRSA, provides national information on the health professions workforce in this country. You can explore demographic changes in nursing online at ftp://ftp.hrsa.gov/bhpr/nursing/sixth.pdf.

Hospital Opportunities

Despite enormous changes in hospital care, jobs in the hospital environment will be available for a long time. In the hospital, a nurse provides direct care for people who are ill and unable to care for themselves. Another function of the direct-care role is to help the client and family in managing the illness event. Hospital positions can range from staff nurse to administrator and may entail any of the clinical specialties and most of the target populations identified in Table 26-1. Determining the area of clinical interest depends mainly on personal preferences.

Depending on the region of the United States, the new graduate's degree of choice in the clinical setting is highly variable. However, if the desired arena for work in hospital-based acute care is not available, it may be wise to accept an alternate position, watchful of an opportunity to transfer when a position becomes available in an area of clinical preference. Such an approach is perceived as a willingness to be flexible and to learn. Accepting assignments in an open, cooperative spirit provides more opportunities for the beginning nurse to learn about the organization and gain important experiences. Furthermore, working as a staff nurse offers many learning opportunities in addition to the immediate client-centered ones.

TABLE **26-1**

Trends in Health Care Delivery Systems

FROM	TO
Acute inpatient care	Life span care
Focus on the individual	Focus on aggregates or populations
Product of care orientation	Value of care orientation
Number of hospital admissions	Number of lives covered (capitation)
Managing organizations	Managing networks
Managing departments	Managing markets
Coordinating services	Documenting quality and outcomes

If the choice of the clinical setting has been based on experiences as a student, the new graduate needs to be prepared to have different perceptions in a new role. At a minimum, experiences that are highly enjoyable on the limited-time basis of a student schedule may feel different when the new graduate functions in that role full time. It also is good to have a mix of experiences and learning opportunities before making a definitive decision.

Misleading perceptions about functioning in various clinical arenas are not limited to new graduates. Often a person perceives or believes that one clinical area is the ideal choice, only to find that it is not what he or she wanted. For example, Jane Patrick, RN, wanted to work with sick children and successfully landed a position on the pediatric unit after a couple of years' experience as a staff nurse on an adult surgical wing. Despite her eagerness for the position, Jane found it difficult to adjust to the unit. The distress of the children in the unit was painful to her, and she found herself depressed and unhappy. She began to dream about the children for whom she was caring and was increasingly unable to provide nursing intervention that entailed discomfort for the child. Jane was not in the right place.

It is critical that nurses stay attuned to their reactions and respond in a constructive manner to self-discovery, such as Jane's. Internal transfers in large hospitals and health care organizations that offer a continuum of care are common; the probability is high that Jane will find a position that is deeply satisfying in another area.

In addition to clinical emphasis, nursing within hospitals offers almost endless opportunities for diversity. Staff level positions in a hospital can be on many different units, and working different shifts on those units presents different work environments, approaches to work, and priorities for client care. Some examples follow.

Infection Control. The infection control nurse assesses the total incidence of infections within the hospital. Clients who suffer an infection while in the hospital are comprehensively reviewed to ensure prompt and accurate treatment and timely containment of the client's infection so that it is not passed to other clients or staff. The infection control nurse must also conduct a thorough analysis to determine the source of the infection and its onset. If the infection is determined to have been contracted during hospitalization, an investigation is initiated to assess the sequence of events leading up to the infection, and an action plan is developed to prevent future occurrences. A position such as this enables the nurse to have hospital-wide interactions and functioning. Knowledge of epidemiology and outstanding interpersonal skills foster full participation in the infection assessment process. Infection control nurses may work in community settings and hospitals.

Quality Management. Although the parameters of a position in quality management may vary from setting to setting, the basic premise is to ensure that outcomes in client care services are consistent with established standards. Benchmarking activities to establish such standards have been under way on a national level for the past few decades. Quality management nurses assess the compliance of the agency or institution with established standards and explore variations from these established standards. Chart reviews and ongoing interaction with the staff of the agency are integral components of a quality management position. Chapter 20 provides a more in-depth overview of the quality management process.

Specific Client Services. An almost endless list of specific client services can be found in hospitals, depending on the hospital's size and function within the community. Some nursing positions might be self-evident, such as the intravenous team on which the nurse provides support and interventions with the insertion and maintenance of intravenous therapies. Other services might relate to ostomy care, counseling, support groups, or health education related to a specialty area.

Coordinator Positions. Some hospitals have various coordinator positions, such as trauma nurse coordinator. The nurse in this position is responsible for the coordination and integration of the clinical and administrative requirements of the trauma victim. Consisting of equal parts of program and case management, the trauma nurse coordinator role involves overseeing the care of the client from the point of injury through acute care to rehabilitation and back to society. Maintenance of a comprehensive database on the management of trauma victims is an important part of this position. Another example of a coordinator position for a highly specialized area is the organ donor coordinator, who procures organs and oversees the transplantation program. Coordinators require considerable experience in the specialty in which they practice.

Variations on Traditional Roles in Nursing

As clients shift from hospital to ambulatory and home care, the role of the community nurse has evolved beyond the traditional public health nurse concept. Although still based in the framework of the traditional public health nurse concept, nurses today take their critical care skills once used only in an acute care setting into the home, where clients recover from illness and surgery. Pharmacologic and technologic advances make the care of chronic and critically ill clients in their homes a cost-effective option. For example, therapies such as dobutamine administration or chemotherapy were once considered too risky for home administration. Today adequate teaching of the client and family members and careful monitoring make these therapies a daily occurrence in clients' homes.

Clients can be monitored through home visits by RNs, expanded technology, radiographs, or telemetry at home. Uterine monitoring for high-risk obstetric clients is common as vital signs of the mother and baby are observed by telephone modem. All these changes increase the need for home-care nurses who are expert clinicians and client educators.

Hospice Nurse. As more clients with terminal illness choose to stop aggressive treatment, hospice nursing has flourished. More than 4100 hospice programs exist in the United States. The growth of hospice was seen by the 1.45 million clients receiving these services in 2008. According to the National Hospice and Palliative Care Organization (NHPCO), 38.5% of all Americans who died in 2008 with cancer received hospice care.

BOX **26-3**

Helpful Websites and Online Resources

Air and Surface Transport Nurses Association
www.astna.org
Airline nursing (flight nursing)
www.flyingnurse.com
All nurses
http://allnurses.com
American Academy of Nurse Practitioners
www.aanp.org
American College of Nurse-Midwives
www.midwife.org
American College of Nurse Practitioners
www.acnpweb.org
American Forensic Nurses
www.amfn.com
American Nurses Informatics Association
www.ania.org
CareeRxel for Nurses
www.careerxel.com
Bureau of Health Professions—Division
of Nursing
www.bhpr.hrsa.gov/nursing
International Association of Forensic Nurses
www.forensicnursing.com/html/about.html
International Parish Nurse Resource Center
http://ipnrc.parishnurses.org
Johnson & Johnson
www.discovernursing.com
National Association for Healthcare Quality
www.nahq.org

National Association of Clinical Nurse
Specialists
www.nacns.org
National Association of School Nurses
www.nasn.org/Default.aspx?tabid=279
National Committee for Quality Assurance
www.ncqa.org
National Hospice and Palliative Care
Organization
www.nhpco.org
Preliminary findings: 2004 National Sample
Survey of Registered Nurses
*http://bhpr.hrsa.gov/healthworkforce/-reports/
rnpopulation/preliminaryfindings.htm*
Nelson, Valerie: "Shattering the myths about
forensic nursing," 1998
*www.nurseweek.com/features/98-7/
forensic.html*
Nursing specialties
www.allnurses.com/Nursing_Specialties
Quality management
www.ncqa.org and www.nahq.org
"So, you wanna be a flight nurse?"
www.seaox.com/wannabe.html
Travel nursing
*www.healthcaretraveler.com/healthcaretraveler/
static/staticHtml.jsp?id=40099*
Trauma nursing
http://trauma.org

Hospice and palliative care nurses treat the symptoms of those with progressive terminal disease. These nurses work holistically with clients and families to maximize quality of life rather than focus on the quantity of life remaining. To learn more about the hospice concept, visit the NHPCO website at: www.nhpco.org/templates/1/homepage.cfm (Box 26-3).

Informatics Nurse Specialist. As health care systems face the inevitable need for data management for decision making, another nursing role has emerged—the informatics nurse specialist. Nursing informatics (NI) focuses on management and processing of health care information. The Joint Commission (TJC) recognized the increased need for information management in the clinical client care settings. The 1994 Joint Commission standards define information management as critical to organizational success. Nurses are well positioned to assume these roles because they best understand client care processes. The American Nurses Credentialing Center (ANCC) has developed a certification examination for nurses who demonstrate beginning levels of competency to become certified as informatics nurses. The ANA *Scope and Standards of Nursing Informatics Practice* states, "Nursing informatics is a specialty that integrates nursing science, computer science, and information science to manage and communicate data, information, and knowledge in nursing practice. Nursing informatics facilitates the integration of data, information, and knowledge to support patients, nurses, and other providers in their decision-making in all roles and settings. This support is accomplished through the use of information structures, information processes, and information technology" (2000, p. 17). More information is available on the ANA Informatics Association website (see Box 26-3).

Occupational Health Opportunities. Nursing within the framework of specific occupational groups (e.g., automobile manufacturing, textile plants, etc.) has long been a career option for nurses. Within these settings the nurse designs and implements a program of health promotion and disease prevention for employees and assists with immediate health needs as necessary. In this primary care milieu, the nurse assesses the need for programs about specific topics of importance to the health of the employees. Some examples of these might be breast-screening programs for female employees and information on early identification of prostate cancer for male employees. Other programs might revolve around the management of developmental events, such as empty nest syndrome, menopause, care for aging parents, or retirement.

In addition to services related to maintaining the health of employees, the occupational nurse is responsible for the assessment of the work environment to ensure the safety of the employees. Examples of significant environmental improvements in the health of U.S. workers are clean air programs, antismoking-on-the-job campaigns, and eliminating the use of asbestos in heating or insulation of buildings. All these activities pose special challenges to the occupational health nurse. The nurse in this setting develops procedures to be followed in the event of illness at work, including the management of health care emergencies.

Opportunities also exist in specific industries. For example, within the airline industry the nurse is responsible for airline safety through maintaining the health of employees. Protection of the employee's health is a component of the role, as is the effect of the health of the employee on the safety of the airline and its passengers. The nurse must be vigilant in the assessment of employee health problems that could affect overall airline safety. An obvious function is alcohol and drug screening. Protocols for the maintenance of employee health programs in the airline industry must be strictly followed and enforced, as required by government regulation.

Nonetheless, the heart of this nursing position still lies with providing care to people, which sometimes can place the nurse in a difficult position. In the ongoing monitoring of the health of the employees, the nurse often is the first to spot a deviation from health that could affect the career and livelihood of an employee. Such an example is hypertension. If an employee is developing high blood pressure, which will affect his or her employment status, that employee may encourage the nurse to "hear" the blood pressure in the qualifying range.

Occupational health and employment screening activities are entwined with urgent care and travel assistance for passengers. Although occasionally an emergency situation develops with a passenger or an employee, most of the client problems are travel related. For example, international travel to some countries requires comprehensive precautions regarding immunizations and inoculations. Airport nurses were critical in screening passengers on international flights during such times as with the severe acute respiratory syndrome (SARS) crisis in 2003. Also passengers may forget prescribed medications, or medications may be lost in baggage. Short-term problems, such as fear of flying, are also managed.

Another form of transportation provides a career opportunity: cruise ship nurse. Generally when people think of taking a cruise, they do not plan on getting sick—nor do nurses usually consider career possibilities in the industry. However, many cruise ships are as large as small cities. The role of the nurse in this setting is similar to that of the airline nurse with respect to the health of the employees and the safety of the passengers. The unique elements of the ship relate to special sanitation requirements, such as testing and culturing the water supply, and managing the total health needs of the passengers. The nurse is responsible for instructing the staff on the basic elements of emergency care and transport. Primary patient care needs are similar to those found in an emergency department. Additional career information can be found at: www.carnival.com/CMS/Fun_Jobs/Shipboard-Medical_Recruiting.aspx.

Quality Manager. Another role that is attractive to nurses is that of quality manager. This reflects the need for health care providers to assess opportunities for process improvement, implement changes, measure outcomes, and then start the improvement process over again. Quality management nurses research and describe findings and look for opportunities to improve care. The result of quality assessment studies may produce critical pathways or algorithms defining care and expected client outcomes. Basic and advanced knowledge of quality management tools is essential, although practice may vary from setting to setting. For instance in the inpatient setting, the quality management nurse needs strong clinical skills, such as those that might be acquired in medical-surgical practice, intensive care units, or the operating room. Experience in home care would be an advantage for a quality management nurse if employed in that setting. Interpersonal skills are important because to be successful in this role, the nurse must build relationships and rapport with people and groups across the organization. The role of quality manager is one that promotes improved care for health care recipients in a variety of settings. For more information, visit the quality management websites listed in Box 26-3 and see Chapter 20.

Case Manager. This role has had a rich tradition in community and public health nursing and now has gained more prominence in acute care. Case managers coordinate resources to achieve health care outcomes based on quality, access, and cost. The complexity of case management practice is obvious in the era of chaotic systems caused by recent changes in the health care market, in which providers, services, and coverage details are constantly changing. Case managers identify the best resources at the lowest cost to achieve the optimal health outcome for the client. Case managers are often nurses, but can also be other professionals, such as medical social workers.

Flight Nurse. Flight nursing is a specialty for nurses who desire autonomous practice and the opportunity to use advanced clinical skills. Practice is diverse because clients are all ages and from all backgrounds with different health problems. Critical care experience, with certification in advanced cardiac life support, is necessary. Most programs prefer experienced nurses in critical care and/or emergency department nursing. The two types of flight practice available are military, such as in the Air Force Reserves or active duty, and civilian flight nursing. To learn more, visit the website "So, you wanna be a flight nurse?" (see Box 26-3). Nurses who enjoy a fast-paced diverse practice in an unstructured setting may find this role a good fit. For more information, call the Air and Surface Transport Nurses Association, formerly known as the National Flight Nurse Association, at 1-800-897-NFNA (6362) or visit their website (see Box 26-3).

Telephone Triage Nurse. Another career option is that of telephone triage nurse. In this practice, nurses interact with clients on the telephone to assess needs, intervene, and evaluate. This position requires excellent communication and assessment skills, in addition to problem-solving skills. Telephone triage is used in a variety of settings, including emergency departments and physician practices.

Forensic Nurse. Forensic nursing may well be one of the fastest-growing nursing specialties in the twenty-first century. This is likely due to the epidemic increase in violence and resulting trauma in this country. The ANA's *Scope and Standards of Forensic Nursing Practice*, published by American Nurses Publishing, serves as a professional guide for nurses working in or entering this evolving specialty. Forensic nursing applies nursing science to public or legal proceedings in the scientific investigation and treatment of trauma and/or death of victims of violence, abuse, criminal activity, and traumatic accidents. The forensic nurse may provide direct services to individual clients and consult with and/or be an expert witness for medical and law enforcement. To learn more about this exciting practice, visit the International Association of Forensic Nurses (IAFN) website (see Box 26-3). The American Forensic Nurses' Organization offers distance-learning programs through the Internet (see Box 26-3).

School Nurse. Most registered professional nurses employed in school health are generalists prepared at the baccalaureate level who function as consultants or coordinators. The newer role for school nurses is school health manager or coordinator and includes functions, such as policymaking, case management and program management activities, and health promotion and protection activities. The National Association of School Nurses defines the role as "a specialized practice of professional nursing that advances the well-being, academic success, and life-long achievement of students. To that end, school nurses facilitate positive student responses to normal development; promote health and safety; intervene with actual and potential health problems; provide case management services; and actively collaborate with others to build student and family capacity for adaptation, self-management, self-advocacy, and learning" (NASN, 2009; see Box 26-3).

Travel Nurse. For the person who wants to travel and still work as a nurse, travel nursing may be an answer. This role is expanding as the demand for nurses grows nationwide. Benefits and company programs vary, but many include travel reimbursement allowance for assignments, in addition to free housing, free insurance, travel money, free phone card use, and other benefits. Sign-on bonuses may also be offered. If these benefits are not important to the nurse, higher wages may be available. Some companies allow nurses' pets to travel with them. Assignments are usually for a minimum time, such as 12 weeks, but others may last as long as a year. For more information, visit the travel nurse website (see Box 26-3).

Parish Nurse. The role of parish nurse has become a recognized specialty in a growing professional practice. In 1998 the ANA, in collaboration with the Health Ministries Association, established the scope and standards of this professional practice. This role focuses on health promotion within the beliefs, values, and practices of various faith communities. In these contexts, health is seen as a sense of physical, psychologic, social, and spiritual well-being. Health is further viewed as being in harmony with self, others, the environment, and God. The parish nurse functions as counselor, teacher, referral agent, volunteer coordinator, and integrator of spiritual care and health. Although all communities do not have a hospital or clinic, most have a faith community, providing an exciting setting in which to teach disease prevention and health promotion.

The late Granger Westberg (1988), founder of this role in the mid-1980s, proposed that clergy can and already do more in the field of preventive medicine than traditional physicians. Westberg's efforts focused on getting the medical establishment to recognize faith communities as partners in keeping people well. He stated that churches, even though they may not realize it, are in the health business. In this role, parish nurses participate in joint ministry with other staff members, helping to integrate faith and health for healing and wholeness. For more information on this practice, visit the website of the International Parish Nurse Association (see Box 26-3).

Nursing Educator. Preparation for nurse educators occurs at the graduate level. Nursing educators should be competent in clinical practice either at the advanced generalist or specialist level (Southern Region Education Board, 2002). They should be prepared in the specialty area in which they teach and match the needs of the institution that hires them. Nursing educators assume leadership in curriculum development, instruction, and evaluation. Knowledge of the learning process and classroom and clinical teaching methods that include engagement and "virtual teaching" is essential. The role of faculty or nursing educator can be very rewarding for those nurses who enjoy lifelong learning and mentoring. Individuals who assume these roles usually are expected to have not only teaching responsibilities, but evidence of scholarship and service to the community.

Clinical Nurse Leader (CNL). The CNL is a master's degree–prepared generalist who oversees the care coordination of a distinct group of patients in any setting. The CNL actively provides direct patient care in complex situations, evaluates patient outcomes, and has the decision-making authority to change care plans when necessary. This clinician puts evidence-based practice into action to ensure that patients benefit from the latest innovations in care delivery and is envisioned as a frontline leader in the health care delivery system.

Doctor of Nursing Practice (DNP). The DNP is an expert in advanced nursing practice who has an earned clinically focused doctorate degree in nursing. DNPs include advanced practice nurses, such as CRNAs, NPs, CNSs, and CNMs, in addition to nurse administrators whose expertise is in advanced systems of care. This is a professional doctorate as opposed to the academic doctorate, which is the doctor of philosophy (PhD) that prepares individuals for a research career. Other professions that receive a professional doctorate are pharmacists who receive a PharmD, physicians who receive the MD, and lawyers who receive the JD. In 2004 The American Association of Colleges of Nursing (AACN) published a DNP position statement that called for a transformational change in the education for advanced practice nurses. They recommended that nurses practicing at the highest level should receive doctoral degrees.

Other Unique Roles

Career opportunities described in this chapter should not be considered an exhaustive list of possibilities. Nurses now have selections for practice areas never before considered. Nurses should adopt an attitude of openness, an attitude of creativity, and a willingness to take a chance to explore these different possibilities. Nurses can let their imaginations take them to unknown settings or explore uncharted waters. To do this, they must develop confidence in their abilities and talents and be willing to venture outside the norm. Many websites have been developed to portray nursing as an attractive career with endless opportunities—one lists more than 50 categories of roles for nurses with links and discussions areas (see Nursing Specialties, Box 26-3). In addition to exploring pertinent websites, examine the Pfizer publication, *Opportunities to Care: The Pfizer Guide to Careers in Nursing (2002)*, a "must have" guide that profiles the life and work of nurses in the field.

There are those detractors in the nursing profession who would limit the possibilities for the profession, claiming that many of the aforementioned alternatives are not really "nursing." However, this mindset severely limits the expansion of professional nursing in a changing health care environment. For nursing to thrive, new roles need to be defined and refined for future success of the discipline.

One way to settle this dispute within the nursing profession is to evaluate new nursing roles through the definition established by the ANA in nursing's social policy statement (2003):

> "Nursing is the protection, promotion, and optimization of health and abilities, prevention of illness and injury, alleviation of suffering through the diagnosis and treatment of human response, and advocacy in the care of individuals, families, communities and population" (p. 6).

Therefore, evolving nursing roles should be evaluated based on the ability of the new role to fit this accepted definition. Does the newly created role require assessment, diagnosis, planning, implementation, or evaluation to human responses? Does the newly created role require the knowledge and expertise of a professional nurse? By answering these questions, nurses can see that nursing is now more encompassing than "traditional" nursing.

ADVANCED PRACTICE NURSING

Much is written in the professional and lay literature about advanced practice nursing. Although new roles in advanced nursing may be forthcoming, the term "advanced practice nurse" (APN) includes nurse practitioners (NPs), certified nurse-midwives (CNMs), certified registered nurse anesthetists (CRNAs), and clinical nurse specialists (CNSs).

Each specialty of APN has unique differences although they share key elements. All APNs make independent and collaborative health care decisions and engage in active practice as expert clinicians. APNs are educationally prepared through master's level education to assume responsibility and accountability for the health promotion, assessment, diagnosis, and management of client problems, including the prescription of medication (AACN, 2002).

Nurse Practitioner (NP)

NPs engage in advanced practice in a variety of specialty areas, such as family, adult, pediatric, geriatric, women's health, school health, occupational health, mental health, emergency, and acute care. Typically, NPs assess, diagnose, and manage medical and nursing problems. Health promotion and maintenance, in addition to disease prevention, are the emphases of their practice. Some NPs diagnose and manage acute and chronic diseases of their selected population.

Job responsibilities of NPs include taking client histories; conducting physical examinations; ordering, performing, and interpreting diagnostic tests; and prescribing pharmacologic agents, treatments, and therapies for the management of client conditions. Frequently the NP serves as a primary care provider and consultant for individuals, families, or communities.

NPs have advanced education, with specific emphasis on pathophysiology and pharmacology. Certification is achieved via written examination after the completion of a master's level program. Several professional organizations offer certification for NPs. For example, the National Certification Board of Pediatric Nurse Practitioners certifies pediatric NPs; adult NPs or family NPs may be certified by the American Academy of Nurse Practitioners. For more information, visit their websites (see Box 24-3).

NPs achieve registration and licensure by state boards of nursing or other designated agencies. The state boards of nursing regulate NP practice and prescriptive authority and can vary from state to state.

The National Advisory Council on Nurse Education and Practice (NACNEP), established by Title VIII of the U.S. Public Health Service, provides a nurse practitioner workforce report (see Box 26-3). The American College of Nurse Practitioners' website offers further professional information (see Box 26-3).

Clinical Nurse Specialist (CNS)

CNSs are APNs who possess clinical expertise in a defined area of nursing practice for a selected client population or clinical setting, such as oncology, pediatrics, geriatrics, psychiatric-mental health, adult health, acute-critical care, and community health. This practice specialty emphasizes the diagnosis and management of human responses to actual or potential health problems.

The CNS functions as an expert clinician, educator, consultant, researcher, and administrator. The CNS monitors the care of clients and collaborates with physicians, nurses, and other members of the interprofessional health care team. The emphasis of this advanced nursing practice is to provide clinical support that improves client care and client outcomes.

CNSs are educated in graduate nursing programs. Their expertise is acquired from combining graduate study with clinical experience. The educational program for CNSs features an intense study of nursing theories and knowledge from other disciplines. Programs emphasize advanced scientific concepts, research methodologies, and supervised clinical practice.

CNSs practice within a systems model paradigm, which means that in performing their role CNSs evaluate each client in the context of his or her social environment. These APNs view clients as individuals who are part of a larger society entering a complex health care delivery system. This practice philosophy prompts the CNS to use a comprehensive approach to client care.

As consultants CNSs are called on for expert clinical advice within and outside the clinical setting. Their consultation function frequently consists of problem solving with a client who may be a colleague, an individual, family, group, agency, or community. Problems may be related to provider competence, equipment, facilities, or health care delivery systems.

CNSs contribute to research in their area of specialization, generating and refining research questions, interpreting research findings, applying them to clinical practice, and educating other nurses about research findings. As teachers CNSs educate clients, families, and communities. The CNS functions as a role model or preceptor for nurse generalists and students in a variety of clinical settings (ANA, 2004).

With the advent of the CNL (described previously), there has been some confusion with the role of the CNS. However, the AACN (2006) supports both the CNL and the CNS as distinct and complementary roles with their differences summarized as follows:
- CNLs are educated as generalists, whereas CNSs are prepared for specialty practice.
- CNLs operate primarily on the clinical level involving small, frontline nursing units; CNSs are engaged at the clinical frontline level and organizational systems levels.
- CNLs coordinate and implement client care; CNSs design and evaluate patient-specific and population-based programs.
- CNLs evaluate and implement evidence-based practice; CNSs have the added responsibility of generating new evidence.

The NACNEP, established by Title VIII of the U.S. Public Health Service, provides a CNS report (see Box 26-3).

Certified Registered Nurse Anesthetist (CRNA)

Established in the late 1800s, nurse anesthesia is recognized as the first clinical nursing specialty. Nurse anesthesia practice developed in response to requests from surgeons seeking a solution to the high morbidity and mortality attributed to anesthesia at that time. The most famous nurse anesthetist of the nineteenth century, Alice Magaw, called the "mother of anesthesia," worked at St. Mary's Hospital in Rochester, Minnesota. Magaw was instrumental in establishing a showcase of professional excellence in anesthesia and surgery. In 1909 the first formal educational programs preparing nurse anesthetists were established.

Since World War I nurse anesthetists have been the principal anesthesia providers in combat areas of every war in which the United States has been engaged. Although nurse anesthesia educational programs existed before World War I, the war sharply increased the demand for nurse anesthetists and, consequently, the need for more educational programs.

Founded in 1931, the American Association of Nurse Anesthetists (AANA) is the professional association representing more than 27,000 nurse anesthetists nationwide. The AANA promotes education, practice standards, and guidelines and affords consultation to private and governmental entities regarding nurse anesthetists and their practice.

The AANA developed and implemented a certification program in 1945 and instituted mandatory recertification in 1978. The association established a mechanism for accreditation of nurse anesthesia educational programs in 1952. Additional information is available at the AANA website (see Box 24-3).

The educational preparation of CRNAs occurs at the graduate level or in association with traditional institutions of higher education, most commonly in schools of nursing or health sciences. The educational curriculum in the anesthesia specialty ranges from 24 to 36 months in an integrated program of academic and clinical study. The academic curriculum consists of a minimum of 30 credit-hours of formalized graduate study in courses such as advanced anatomy, physiology, pathophysiology, advanced pharmacology, principles of anesthesia practice, and research methodology and statistical analysis. All programs require approximately 1000 hours of hands-on clinical experience. Students gain experience with clients of all ages who require medical, obstetric, dental, and pediatric interventions.

Admission requirements to a nurse anesthesia educational program include a bachelor of science degree in nursing, licensure as an RN, and a minimum of 1 year of acute care nursing experience. Nurse anesthetists are required to successfully complete a written examination for certification as a CRNA.

Recertification, which includes practice and continuing education requirements, must be met every 2 years. CRNAs are qualified to make independent judgments relative to all aspects of anesthesia care based on their education, licensure, and certification. CRNAs provide anesthesia and anesthesia-related care on request, assignment, or referral by a client's physician, most often to facilitate diagnostic, therapeutic, or surgical procedures. In other instances, CRNAs perform consultation or assistance for management of pain associated with obstetric labor and delivery, management of acute or chronic ventilatory problems, or management of acute or chronic pain through the performance of selected diagnostic or therapeutic blocks.

The laws of every state permit CRNAs to work directly with a physician or other authorized health care professional, such as a dentist, without being supervised by an anesthesiologist. TJC does not require anesthesiologist supervision of CRNAs, nor does Medicare. In some cases a provider, payer, or medical staff bylaws may require anesthesiologist supervision. However, these decisions are not based on legal requirements (AANA, 2009).

Certified Nurse-Midwife (CNM)

According to the American College of Nurse-Midwives (ACNM, 2004), certified nurse-midwives are primary care providers of women's health care, focusing particularly on pregnancy, childbirth, the postpartum period, care of the newborn, and the family planning and gynecologic needs of women. This practice occurs within a health care system that provides consultation, collaborative management, or referral, as indicated by the health status of the client.

A CNM is educated in the two disciplines of nursing and midwifery and possesses evidence of certification according to the requirements of the ACNM. A CNM has successfully completed prescribed studies in midwifery and has met the requisite qualifications to be certified. A CNM is legally qualified to practice in one or more of the 50 states. The ACNM supports educational programs for CNMs at the certificate and the degree level, but opposes mandatory degree requirements for state licensure.

The ACNM claims that mandatory degree requirements would limit access to maternity and gynecologic services for women. Several national reports specifically recommend placing greater reliance on CNMs to increase access to prenatal care for underserved populations. These reports also recommend that state laws be supportive of nurse-midwifery practice.

The entry-level nurse-midwife is a primary health care professional who independently provides care during pregnancy, birth, and the postpartum period for women and newborns within their communities. Therefore, the CNM is an individual who has successfully completed an ACNM-accredited educational program in nurse-midwifery and passed the national certification examination administered by the ACNM Certification Council. Additional information is available at the ACNM website (see Box 24-3).

Midwifery care occurs within a variety of settings, including homes, birthing centers, clinics, and hospitals. The nurse-midwife works with each woman and her family to identify their unique physical, social, and emotional needs. Services provided by the CNM include education and health promotion. With additional education and experience, the nurse-midwife may provide well-woman gynecologic care, including family planning services. When the care required extends beyond the CNM's abilities, the midwife should have a mechanism for consultation and referral.

CNMs are an expanding group of professionals. In March 2004, midwives in the United States numbered 13,684 as compared with 9232 in 2000 (Bureau of Health Professionals, 2004). In 2004 there were 45 accredited nurse-midwifery education programs in the United States. Approximately 56.5% of CNMs have a master's degree, and 4.8% have a post-master's certificate. Nurse-midwifery practice is legal in all 50 states and the District of Columbia and is reimbursed by Medicaid in all 50 states. They can prescribe medications in 48 states. Areas of practice include care to women from puberty through menopause, including gynecologic and wellness services, family planning and contraception care, preconception counseling, prenatal care, labor through childbirth and afterbirth care, and menopause counseling and care (ACNM, 2004).

Nurse Administrator or Nurse Executive

Although not formally considered an APN, the nurse administrator or nurse executive has an important advanced role within nursing. It is vital that individuals be knowledgeable about the business of the health care system and the profession of nursing. Nursing administration unites the leadership perspective of professional nursing with the various aspects of business and health administration. The practice of nursing administration focuses on the administration of health care systems for the purpose of delivering services to groups of clients.

Individuals who assume a nurse executive role typically hold a master's degree. Master's and doctoral level programs that offer degrees in nursing administration are available, although some nursing executives are educated in additional disciplines, such as business.

Nursing administration research focuses on organizational factors and management practices and their effect on nurses, health care delivery systems, and client outcomes. Nursing administration is concerned with establishing the costs of nursing care and examining relationships between nursing services and quality client care. Nurse executives are called on to view problems of nursing service delivery within a broader context of policy analysis and delivery of health care services.

Nursing administration is an integral part of any organization that provides health care. Nurse administrators lead and direct large groups of nurses and ancillary personnel. They manage large budgets and are responsible for provision of quality care at reasonable cost. They serve at all management levels in health care organizations and in the community.

WHAT ABOUT THE FUTURE?

The future of nursing is brighter than ever. Because of never-ending changes in the health care environment, many new jobs will result. Growth of the nursing profession also will be prompted by technologic advances in client care, which allow an increased number of health problems to be detected early and managed quickly. A greater number of sophisticated health-related procedures are already performed not only in hospitals but also a variety of settings, such as clinics and physicians' offices. Health maintenance organizations, ambulatory surgicenters, and church health centers are only a few of the places where the public will receive their health care. Nursing can be a vital component of the "alternative setting" movement that is on the forefront of health care reform.

As the focus of health care shifts to disease prevention and modification of lifestyles, the opportunities for nurses will follow. Nursing also can benefit from the increased emphasis on primary care because prevention is the only true mechanism to reduce health care expenditures. Professional nursing services should be viewed as a cost-effective way to provide disease prevention and health promotion activities in multiple areas of the community, including industry, business, and commerce. Wellness and disease prevention, historically fundamental to the nursing profession, are becoming more meaningful and revitalized concepts within the larger health care system.

The need for the traditional role of the hospital nurse will always exist. In fact with a shift to more community services, the intensity of hospital nursing care is likely to increase because only those in most need are treated there. Increases in client acuity will expand the need for professional nursing within the hospital setting. However, the most rapid growth for nursing employment is expected in outpatient facilities, such as same-day surgery, rehabilitation, and chemotherapy infusion centers.

Nurses also will see job opportunities continue to develop in home health care. Many factors contribute to this phenomenon. The increasing numbers of older persons with disabilities require nursing care to minimize their functional loss and optimize their quality of life. Another factor that promotes home care is the consumer's preference for care in his or her own home. Home care is a feasible option with recent technologic advances. Complex health care treatment that was once thought only possible in the hospital setting is now a reality in the home. Professional nurses who are able to perform complex procedures and comprehensive client assessments will be invaluable to the home-care industry.

Financial pressures on hospitals to discharge clients as soon as possible are producing increased admissions to nursing homes, skilled nursing facilities, and long-term rehabilitation units. In addition, because more individuals are living into their ninth and tenth decades, the number of people entering nursing homes or assisted-living facilities will increase. The opportunity for nursing is tremendous in the long-term care arena because no other discipline can offer the multiple skills that nursing has to offer to the aging population.

Despite this bright outlook, the nursing profession must heed the old cliché that "opportunity only knocks once." If nurses fail to seize their opportunities, other less-qualified health care providers will attempt to move into this advantageous position. Nursing professionals must demonstrate their contribution to health care and publicly market their potential. The nursing profession historically has requested a chance to prove its worth in producing cost-effective, quality health care—now is the time.

SUMMARY

This chapter has explored the various roles available to professional nurses today. Social and economic trends influencing the development of new nursing roles in innovative practice settings have been discussed. Nurses who are interested in developing new roles should be encouraged by the examples provided by nurses who first envisioned and created new roles. Traditional, nontraditional, and advanced practice nursing roles offer many exciting opportunities for professional growth and satisfaction. The diversity and challenge available to professional nurses today are unparalleled.

 evolve   Additional resources are available online at: http://evolve.elsevier.com/Cherry/

REFERENCES

American Association of Colleges of Nursing: *Nurse practitioner primary care competencies in specialty areas: adult, family, gerontological, pediatric, and women's health*, Washington, DC, 2002. Available at: www.nonpf.com/finalaug2002.pdf.

American Association of Colleges of Nursing: *Doctor of nursing practice (DNP) position statement*, Washington, DC, 2004. Available at:www.aacn.nche.edu/DNP/DNPPositionStatement.htm.

American Association of Colleges of Nursing: *AACN statement of support for clinical nurse specialists*, Washington, DC, 2006. Retrieved May 2009 from: www.aacn.nche.edu/publications/pdf/CNS.pdf.

American Association of Nurse Anesthetists: *Qualifications and capabilities of the certified registered nurse anesthetist*, 2009, www.aana.com.

American College of Nurse Midwives: What is a midwife? 2004. www.midwife.org.

American Nurses Association: *Scope and standards of nursing informatics practice*, Washington, DC, 2001, American Nurses Publishing.

American Nurses Association: *Nursing's social policy statement*, ed 2, p. 6, Washington, DC, 2003, American Nurses Publishing.

American Nurses Association. *Nursing: scope and standards of practice*, Washington, DC, 2004, American Nurses Association.

Bureau of Health Professions, Division of Nursing, Health Resources Service Administration: *The Registered Nurse Population: Findings from the 2004 National Sample Survey of Registered Nurses*, Washington, DC, March 2004. http://bhpr.hrsa.gov/healthworkforce/rnsurvey04/preface.htm.

National Advisory Council on Nurse Education and Practice: *Meeting the challenges of the new millennium: challenges facing the nurse workforce in a changing health care environment*, Wasington, DC, January 2008, U.S Department of Health and Human Services.

National Association of School Nurses. 2009. Retrieved May 2009 from: www.nasn.org/Default.aspx?tabid=279.

Nelson, Valerie: "Shattering the myths about forensic nursing," 1998. Available at: www.nurseweek.com/features/98-7/forensic.html

Pfizer Pharmaceuticals Group (Friedman R): *Opportunities to care: the Pfizer guide to careers in nursing*, New York, 2002, Pfizer Pharmaceuticals Group.

Southern Region Education Board, Council on Collegiate Education for Nursing: *Nurse educator competencies*, pp. 6–7, 2002. Available at: http://publications.sreb.org/2002/02N04_Nurse_Competencies.pdf.

US Department of Labor, Bureau of Labor Statistics: *Occupational outlook handbook*, 2008-2009 edition, Washington, DC. Retrieved May 2009 from: www.bls.gov/oco/ocos083.htm.

Westberg GE: Parishes, nurses, and health care, *Lutheran Part* 6:26–29, 1988.

ADDITIONAL RESOURCES

Abendroth DA: *How expert hospice nurses find meaning in their work*, Ann Arbor, MI, 2006, ProQuest.

American Association of Colleges of Nursing: *White paper on the role of the clinical nurse leader*, Washington, DC, 2007, AACN Publications.

Bemis PA: *Nurse entrepreneurs: tales of nurses in business*, ed 3, Rockledge, FL, 2004, National Nurses in Business Association.

Buppert C: *Nurse practitioners business practice and legal guide*, ed 3, Sudbury, MA, 2007, Jones and Bartlett.

Frederickson K: *Opportunities in nursing*, New York, 2003, McGraw-Hill.

Hebda TL, Czar P: *Handbook of informatics for nurses and healthcare professionals*, ed 4, Boston, 2008, Prentice-Hall.

Holleran RS: *Flight nursing: principles and practice*, ed 2, Cincinnati, OH, 1996, Mosby.

Mezey M, et al: *Nurse practitioners: evolution of advanced practice (advanced practice nursing)*, New York, 2003, Springer.

Solari-Twaddel P, McDerrmot MA: *Parish nursing: development, education, and administration*, Philadelphia, 2006, Mosby.

Stevens S: *Forensic nurse: the new role of the nurse in law enforcement*, New York, 2006, Thomas Dunne Books/St Martins Press.

Wallace C: *Kaplan legal nurse certification*, New York, 2008, Kaplan Publishing.

Job Search: Finding Your Match

Susan R. Jacob, PhD, MSN, RN

evolve Additional resources are available online at: http://evolve.elsevier.com/Cherry/

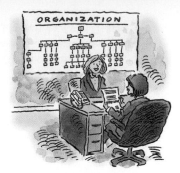

Finding the right match can be exciting.

VIGNETTE

"For 2 years I've struggled to meet deadlines for term papers, nursing care plans, and examinations," sighed Leslie. *"Now that graduation is almost here, I'm scared that I don't know enough to be a 'real nurse.' And I'm confused about where to begin and what kind of nursing position I should seek. This first job seems so important."*

■ QUESTIONS TO CONSIDER WHILE READING THIS CHAPTER:

1 How should the new graduate in the scenario decide where to apply for that first position?

2 What kinds of questions should the applicant ask about a prospective position?

3 How can the applicant demonstrate knowledge, skills, and experience to the recruiter?

KEY TERMS

Orientation Activities that enhance adaptation to a new environment.
Portfolio A collection of evidence demonstrating acquisition of skills, knowledge, and achievements related to a professional career.
Professional objective Occupational position for which one aims.
Résumé Summary of a job applicant's previous work experience and education.

LEARNING OUTCOMES

After studying this chapter, the reader will be able to:

1 Use the interview process to evaluate potential employment opportunities.

2 Prepare an effective résumé and nursing portfolio.

3 Compare and contrast various professional nursing employment opportunities.

4 Summarize the employment process.

We thank Kathryn S. Skinner, MS, RN, CS, and Laura H. Day, BSN, MS, RN for their contributions to this chapter in the 4th edition.

CHAPTER OVERVIEW

This chapter helps student nurses prepare to successfully negotiate their first employment as professional nurses. They learn the importance of networking, researching available opportunities, and examining their personal aptitudes, interests, lifestyle priorities, and long-term goals to find the best job fit.

Readers are shown how to create and use cover letters and résumés to market themselves in written introductions and how to prepare for and actively participate in a recruitment interview. The chapter describes what can be expected from a recruiter and how to obtain the information needed to make thoughtful and rewarding job choices. Putting these recommendations into practice will ensure the new graduate of the best chance for finding a good job match as an entry-level nurse practicing in a suitable work environment.

EXPLORING OPTIONS

The job market for graduate nurses is extensive. There are many opportunities in urban as well as rural areas. Health care economics ride a roller coaster from robust to lean times, but the high demand for the skills of professional registered nurses (RNs) remains constant, and the potential for finding suitable employment is good. Trends in health care delivery direct today's health care providers to change their orientation from disease to health and from inpatient to outpatient services, which leads to a growing need for professional nurses in nonacute community-based care settings, such as primary care clinics, ambulatory surgery centers, and home, school, and work environments. However, although rapid changes in health care delivery systems continue to create new and varied opportunities outside the acute care settings where nurses have traditionally practiced, hospitals remain the most likely starting place for new graduates to acquire general experience helpful in opening career path doors. In fact with a nursing shortage there is an increased demand for nurses to work in acute care settings.

Numerous marketing strategies have been tried in an effort to aggressively attract bright, energetic new graduates in times of demand and short supply. For some institutions in selected areas of the country, cost seems irrelevant. Sign-on bonuses, expense-paid weekends to visit institutions in other parts of the United States, promises of tuition reimbursement for continued education, student loan repayment, and low-interest loans for new cars, just to name a few, have been offered as enticements. However, in other areas of the country, for the first time in several years, it is taking graduates longer to find employment than in the past when it was common for new graduates to have promises of employment prior to graduation. Ultimately, being aware of one's own qualities and taking advantage of networking opportunities are more important keys to finding just the right match in today's job market.

Knowing Oneself

The choice of a first nursing position deserves careful study. For some the opportunities seem to be a smorgasbord of possibilities, all of them attractive. The neophyte nurse should carefully explore any job under consideration and its responsibilities in light of his or her own personal qualities. Some students find it helpful to consult an instructor, job counselor, or a trusted nursing mentor for objective input and perspective. An experienced nurse can see the pros and cons that may not be visible to a new nurse. A thoughtful review of general interests, abilities, and strengths, especially those pointed out by clinical instructors, in addition to attention paid to the types of patients who have provided the greatest emotional reward is essential.

Other important considerations are one's physical and emotional stamina, energy level, and responsibilities to others—spouse, children, and other family members; volunteer commitments; and social activities—all of which make legitimate demands on one's schedule. Long-term goals must be factored into the first job choice as well. Is the first job a stepping stone to an advanced degree, to a narrowly specialized area of nursing, to a traveling nurse position, or to a management role? Selection of a position that fits the nurse's abilities, lifestyle, and career aspirations will affect job satisfaction, career advancement, and overall sense of success and happiness.

Finding the right practice environment is essential to long-term success and job satisfaction. The American Association of Colleges of Nursing (AACN) developed a white paper titled *Hallmarks of the Professional Practice Environment*, which can be accessed at: www.aacn.nche.edu/Publications/positions/hallmarks.htm. Based on this paper, a brochure for graduates of nursing schools was developed, titled "What Every Nursing School Graduate Should Consider When Seeking Employment." This brochure identifies eight key characteristics or hallmarks of the professional practice setting and suggests that applicants ask the following questions about the employer they are considering—Does the potential employer:

- Manifest a philosophy of clinical care emphasizing quality, safety, interdisciplinary collaboration, continuity of care, and professional accountability?
- Recognize the value of nurses' expertise on clinical care quality and patient outcomes?
- Promote executive-level nursing leadership?
- Empower nurses' participation in clinical decision making and organization of clinical care systems?
- Demonstrate professional development support for nurses?
- Maintain clinical advancement programs based on education, certification, and advanced preparation?
- Create collaborative relationships among members of the health care team?
- Use technologic advances in clinical care and information systems?

Box 27-1 provides other statistics and information to request from a potential employer.

BOX **27-1**

Statistics and Information That Applicants May Request from a Potential Employer

- RN vacancy rate and RN turnover rate
- Patient satisfaction scores (preferably a percentile ranking)
- Employee satisfaction scores
- Average tenure of nursing staff
- Education mix of nursing staff
- Percentage of registry or travelers used
- Key human resource policies (e.g., reduction in workforce; tenure vs. performance criteria)
- Copy of the most recent TJC report and the number of contingencies cited
- Information about whether the nurses are unionized
- Copy of contract

From American Association of Colleges of Nursing (AACN): *What every nursing school graduate should consider when seeking employment,* Washington, DC, 2002, AACN.

The numbers of hospitals seeking and receiving Magnet hospital credentialing are growing, and where these work environments are available, the nurse may wish to consider these organizations. Generally, hospitals with Magnet status have demonstrated excellence in areas such as low RN turnover rates, adherence to standards of nursing care as defined by the American Nurses Association (ANA), and mechanisms in place for staff participation in decision making (Nursing 2009CareerDirectory, 2009). The American Nurses Credentialing Center (ANCC) lists all Magnet hospitals on its website at www.nursingworld.org/ancc/magnet/getall.cfm.

Many graduate nurses have discovered that working in an environment that did not match well with their personal attributes and long-term goals not only made them miserable but also damaged their future employment options. Poor job fits lead to frequent job changes, which could lead to poor references and the attachment of the label "job hopper."

Appropriate job choice is critically important and can be costly to the new graduate. Accordingly, an ineffective hiring decision can also be expensive for the employer. Some estimate the cost of recruiting, placing, and orienting a new nurse to be from two to two and one half times the average RN salary—but the costs are more than financial (Donna Herrin, personal communication, 2009). Critical to effective selection is high-level nurse leader competency in resource management processes and attention to creation of an effective healthful practice environment. A great decision on the part of the new graduate and the nurse leader will have better outcomes for the individual nurse in areas of job satisfaction and retention and overall organizational outcomes, employee engagement and retention, and patient outcomes.

Networking

The investigative process of researching potential employers begins with networking at school, in the community, and within student nurse organizations. One may question other nurses, employees, and former employees, especially alumni of one's own school, who have worked in various settings. Faculty will have pertinent observations based on their experiences with clinical sites in the community. It is also valuable to listen to neighbors, friends, and family members who have been patients.

Employment sections of newspapers, particularly Sunday editions, contain advertisements for job openings and provide names to contact for further information. Some employers now offer "phone-a-thons" inviting nurses to speak directly with recruiters or nursing department supervisors. Websites, open houses, health care job fairs and virtual online career events are great places to pick up information about institutions. Recruitment materials and brochures often contain interesting facts about the organization, such as the mission, vision, and values statements and goals, available services, and information about associate benefits.

The Internet offers links to actual jobs and information on career planning. Most hospital and large health care systems maintain websites to post their employment needs and invite applications online. The Internet is a cost-effective recruiting method, and larger health care systems expect early communications to take place by fax and e-mail. Applicants who use this method to follow-up on a job posting should pay particular attention to the application and résumé that is sent electronically, making sure there are no errors before submitting materials online. If there is no response to Internet inquiries within a week, applicants should follow up with a phone call. Examples of Internet sites that are helpful in exploring job opportunities, writing résumés, and preparing for employment interviews are included in Box 27-2.

If a new graduate is seeking a position in a large community with multiple job choices available, this informal research will help to narrow the list to the best place to begin the job

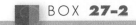

BOX **27-2**

Helpful Websites and Online Resources

www.aacn.nche.edu/Publications/positions/
  hallmarks.htm
www.careerxel.com
www.discovernursing.com
www.nsna.org/career
www.medsearch.com
www.monster.com
www.nursecredentialing.org/magnet.html

www.nursingspectrum.com
www.nursing-jobs.com
www.nursingworld.org
www.nurse.com
www.nursingcenter.com
www.nursezone.com
www.rnwanted.com
www.careerbuilder.com

application process. Later in the interview, the applicant may wish to describe to the recruiter how his or her search resulted in this employer being the number-one choice over others for the graduate's first job. This process of researching potential employers will continue through the interview process. Assessing the climate of the work environment is a valuable tool in "finding a match" and is discussed more thoroughly later in this chapter.

WRITTEN INTRODUCTIONS

Three of the most important steps in a job search are writing a cover letter, preparing a professional résumé, and assembling a professional portfolio. These tools introduce the applicant to a prospective employer. The first impression should be persuasive; there may not be a second chance. Presenting oneself on paper can make a difference, perhaps the difference between getting a desired interview and being passed over in favor of someone else. These written introductions should present a conscientious, mature, competent, committed professional who would be an asset to an agency that prides itself on its nursing services

How to Write a Cover Letter

The cover letter (Box 27-3) is a chance to sell oneself and make the recruiter look forward to meeting an attractive candidate. A convincing cover letter will show how this candidate is different and convey to the recruiter why he or she is the best fit for the position. The letter should also address why this institution is the applicant's first choice.

A cover letter should reflect the nurse's own style of writing, should never appear to have been copied from a book, and should be tailored to the particular job. Like any business document it should be clean, direct, and letter perfect. It should be attractive and effortless to read. There must be no obvious erasures, no typing errors, no evidence of correction fluid, and no grammar or spelling mistakes. Everything should fit on a single page of 8½ by 11–inch white, heavyweight bond paper with ample margins on the top, bottom, and sides.

The letter should be addressed to a specific person. If the person's name or title is unknown, refer to a marketing brochure or call the recruitment office to ask for correct title and spelling of the appropriate person's first and last names.

If spelling is not your strength, use the spell-check tool on the computer, but do not depend on its accuracy. Using a dictionary and asking a competent friend to proofread the final copy is also a good idea. Poor typists would be well served to pay someone to type for them. A sloppy letter will cast doubt on one's abilities to practice as a professional.

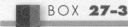 BOX **27-3**

Cover Letter

April 8, 2010

Ms. Donna Henderson, RN, MS
Director of Nurse Recruitment
Charleston Memorial Hospital
1600 Beckley Avenue
Memphis, TN 38104

Dear Ms. Henderson:

I would like to apply for a new graduate position on a cardiology nursing unit at Charleston Memorial Hospital. After graduating from Smith College with a BSN on June 6, I will be ready to start work immediately. I plan to take the RN licensing examination in early July.

Through reading about your hospital and my own personal experience in a recent clinical rotation at Charleston Memorial, I have learned that your institution is a modern, professional one with an emphasis on quality patient care. For this and many other reasons, I am convinced that Charleston Memorial is where I want to work as a nurse.

I will be in Memphis on April 20-25 and will call to schedule an appointment to see you then. My phone number at home is 555-912-3120; my cell phone number is 555-200-9999.

I look forward to meeting you and discussing how I can contribute to Charleston Memorial Hospital.

Sincerely,
(Sign your name here in pen)
Bonnie McCray Pino

Enclosure

The body of the letter should be single-spaced, three or four block paragraphs long, with a blank line between paragraphs, and organized as follows:

- Paragraph 1 should be a statement of purpose that tells the recruiter what kind of position is being sought, the writer's expected date of graduation, state licensing status, and the date the writer will be ready to begin work.
- Paragraph 2 should emphasize the writer's suitability. The implied message should be "I'm just the person for the job" without going into all the details that will be included in the résumé. A sentence should describe past work or educational experiences that relate to the agency's particular needs and philosophy. The more homework the nurse has done in learning about the institution, the more convinced the recruiter will be. Finally, refer to the enclosed résumé.
- Paragraph 3 should request an interview appointment and give a range of dates of availability. It is a good idea for the writer to promise a telephone call "next week" or "soon" to schedule a meeting time and provide a telephone number where the writer can be reached, if the number is different from the permanent telephone number listed on the résumé.
- The letter can end with a "written handshake," such as, "I look forward to meeting with you to discuss available nursing positions in your institution"—a cautiously optimistic note.
- The letter closes with "Sincerely," and after four lines of space for a signature, the writer's name is typed. A line is skipped, and "Enclosure" is typed on the left margin to indicate that a résumé is enclosed.

The letter should be proofread carefully, signed, and copied; and the copy filed. If the nurse has chosen to use different approaches with different institutions, it would be wise to review the cover letter before the interview.

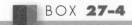

BOX **27-4**

Résumé

Bonnie McCray Pino
416 Melody Avenue
Bristol, TN 37620
555-912-3120 (Home)
555-200-9999 (cell)
E-mail: bpino@xyz.com

Professional objective:	Staff nurse position (cardiology)
Licensure:	Eligible to take NCLEX after June 6, 2010
	Anticipated date of NCLEX: July 2010

Education:
2006-2010	Smith College School of Nursing
	Bristol, TN
	BSN, June 6, 2010
2003-2006	Oakview High School
	Nashville, TN
	Diploma, June 2006

Experience:
May 2009-August 2009, St. Mary's Hospital, Knoxville, TN
Patient Care Assistant: Assisted RNs in providing basic nursing care including feeding, bathing, ADL, and patient teaching in a pediatric setting
June 2008-August 2008, Drs. Smith and Jones OB/GYN office, Bristol, TN
Office Assistant: Accompanied patients to treatment area, weighed, and recorded vital signs

Honors:	Sigma Theta Tau International, 2006
	Who's Who Among American High School Students

Professional Organizations: Tennessee Student Nurses Association, 2007-2010
References: Provided on request

One week later the writer should follow up by telephone to be sure the letter was received. This attention to detail and follow-through will impress the recruiter or personnel office and improve chances of getting an interview soon. These telephone calls usually become mini-interviews, and the applicant should be extra courteous, aware that it usually is the secretary who controls the interview schedule. By keeping a written list of all contacts made, the new graduate will be able to add the flattering personal touch of acknowledging previous telephone contacts when meeting them for the first time during the interview process.

The cover letter serves as the foundation on which all other follow-up is built: résumé, call for appointment, and interview. What is presented in the letter should prompt the person responsible for hiring to take a close look at the enclosed résumé.

How to Prepare a Résumé

A résumé is a short account of one's career or professional life (Box 27-4). The résumé is different than a curriculum vitae (CV), which is a chronologic account of one's entire educational and professional work experience, usually required by academic institutions for educator positions. The résumé is the most appropriate format for the new graduate and will complement the cover letter by filling in important details about educational and work experiences. An effective résumé should compress education and employment history into an attractive, easy-to-read one-page summary. A wealth of valuable information can be communicated simply and straightforwardly by saying more with less. The key is writing concisely. For example, "BSN with high honors" speaks for itself. Citing exact grade point average or "dean's list" standing adds little. Succinct ways to convey a message will be found by experimenting with phrases and word choices. Avoid pompous language and use of the passive voice. Instead use active verbs, such as *improved, established, trained, administered, prepared, wrote,* and *evaluated.* Pepper the résumé with such words, and it will read easily.

A basic résumé contains three essential sections: (1) identifying information; (2) education; and (3) work experience. In addition, optional information may include professional objectives, honors, achievements, and memberships in professional organizations. A well-designed résumé will mark the writer as a career-minded professional, just what recruiters are seeking. A succinct well-organized résumé indicates that the applicant is focused and organized in other areas as well.

The first section of the résumé, the identifying information, contains the applicant's name, address, and home and work telephone numbers, followed by licensure information. The states of licensure and license numbers are listed. Graduating students should indicate when and where the National Council of Licensing Examination (NCLEX®) was taken or will be taken.

If the résumé writer opts to include a professional objective, it should come next. Some interviewers like to see this because it shows that the nurse has put some thought into career planning. Keep in mind, though, that it is limiting to put forth a singular objective that ties the nurse to only one particular clinical area. If there is no such opening available in that department, the recruiter will consider the applicant an unlikely candidate to pursue. It is better to have an objective statement that is broad and general.

The second section should include details about education, including degrees and diplomas awarded, names and locations of schools, and graduation dates, starting with the most recent graduation and degree in reverse chronologic order.

The third section will present the information apt to be the greatest help in obtaining a job: work experience and employment history. Many recruiters are nurses themselves, so a detailed description of what a routine job entails is not needed. Instead efforts should be directed toward illustrating any special knowledge or contributions. The new graduate's résumé might reflect student accomplishments or elaborate on jobs in which he or she has demonstrated skills also applicable to nursing responsibilities, such as organization of tasks, time management, delegation to subordinates, and ability to work well with others. Start with current or most recent position and work backward, including place of employment, job title, dates worked, and responsibilities. List accomplishments while employed, including number and type of patients cared for, any special techniques used, or any participation in the development of programs, policies, or forms pertinent to the position.

This section closes with optional information, such as seminars attended, honors received, and memberships in professional organizations. It is not advisable to list community activities or activities from more than 5 years ago unless it can be clearly shown that they are pertinent to a nursing career. Similarly, exclude personal information, such as marital and health status, age, number of children, and hobbies. This information is not job related and should not be used by the employer to screen applicants.

References do not need to be included in the résumé, but should be ready for presentation in a neatly typed, photocopied list when requested from any future employer. Simply state, "references provided on request" or "references available." When someone agrees to be listed as a reference, take time to discuss what prospective employers may want to know. Former instructors or former employers may require written permission before releasing information. As the job search continues, keep references informed of the names of employers who may be inquiring.

Produce the résumé neatly and inexpensively, preferably on a computer or word processor, because a good résumé will be used repeatedly with revisions, and the nurse will want to be able to produce an up-to-date version without completely rewriting it. Production methods should be kept as simple as possible. It is not necessary to go to the added trouble and expense of having the résumé professionally typeset and printed. Having it neatly typed and reproduced using good-quality photocopying services suffices. To make the text easy to read, use one style of serif font throughout, in 11- or 12-point size. Again have someone review the final copy for typing errors, then use a photocopying service for "quick copying" onto good-quality white or ivory paper. It is important to remember that when it comes to résumés, appearances do count. A well-formatted résumé that is properly organized and neatly typed makes a great first impression.

How to Prepare a Portfolio

The nursing portfolio contains more information than a résumé and provides documentation to support the résumé. The portfolio introduces the professional nurse to recruiters, employers, admissions committees, and potential supervisors in a visual and tangible way. It includes traditional documents, such as a résumé, license to practice and certifications, educational documents (diplomas, transcripts, etc.), and examples of significant professional, community, and student activities (Box 27-5).

The simplest way to build a portfolio is to start with an attractive three-ring binder. A table of contents gives interviewers a map to guide their review of the information. Dividers can separate sections, each with its own cover page, and plastic sleeves or pocketed pages work well to hold loose items. Appropriate documents are assigned to each section. Make copies

BOX **27-5**

Documents for Professional Portfolio

PROFESSIONAL CREDENTIALS
Résumé
Licenses
Certifications
Specialty practice certifications
Basic cardiac life support (BCLS)
Advanced cardiac life support (ACLS)

EDUCATIONAL CREDENTIALS
Diplomas
Transcripts
Continuing education certificates
Honors and awards (including program from
    awards ceremony, letters regarding awards,
    newspaper articles)

RESEARCH AND SCHOLARLY ACTIVITY
Publications
Teaching materials for patients, staff, handouts
Case studies
Photo of poster sessions, classroom presentations
PowerPoint outline of presentation
Student papers and projects

PROFESSIONAL ACTIVITIES
Membership cards
Evidence of service as an officer or leader
    in student organizations
Community involvement and volunteer activities
Performance evaluations
Letters of recommendation

Adapted from Sherrod D: The professional portfolio: a snapshot of your career, *Nurs Manag* 36(9):74-75, 2005.

of important originals, such as diplomas, certifications, and licenses that would be difficult to replace. Include samples of letters from grateful patients, congratulations from peers, and complimentary notes from supervisors. Highlight sentences in longer letters or performance appraisals that address the information considered to be most important for the reader to note. The graduate nurse may want to include supervisor evaluations from non-nursing positions to demonstrate leadership qualities, dependability, and attention to detail, characteristics also relevant to the nursing work setting.

Graduation is the perfect time to create a career portfolio, one that will be easy to build on and update as the nursing career evolves. If documents are created on the computer, updates and revisions will be easy when the nurse pursues new and different professional roles and responsibilities. Many baccalaureate educational programs require students to create such a portfolio as part of their preparation for graduation and entry into the first job—and increasingly boards of nursing are making portfolios (or other methods for documenting evidence of competency) mandatory for relicensure (Sherrod, 2005).

Nurses who present portfolios to the recruiter may have a competitive edge over nurses who do not.

HOW TO INTERVIEW EFFECTIVELY

No matter how qualified and self-confident a person may feel, sitting across the desk from an interviewer can be intimidating. One's conduct in the recruiter's office may determine whether a job offer is made. Being a little anxious is normal, but panic is not. When the applicant has made a good first impression in the cover letter and résumé, he or she can expect to be called for an interview. The graduate's task then becomes to enter the interview prepared to answer and ask questions that will help determine whether this organization, with its available job opportunities, is a good match.

Every agency has its own hiring and interviewing policies. Generally the smaller the organization and the more decentralized the nursing department, the more involved the lower-level manager is in the recruitment and hiring process. The same person who interviews nurse applicants also may be the manager, staff development instructor, quality assurance director, employee health nurse, or chair of the product standards committee. A large organization with many employees may have a separate human resources department with a nurse recruiter on staff. Within such large organizations, the hiring process becomes more complicated and more formal; applicants are more tightly screened, and the hiring decisions are further removed from the actual work position.

Not all "nurse recruiters" are nurses themselves, which may make a difference in the kind of information exchanged in the interview. A non-nurse is not likely to be able to fully discuss questions that pertain directly to a nurse's job description, patient care workload, and nursing responsibilities. The applicant does not have to answer questions that are not job related. In fact some questions are not legally allowed to be asked (Box 27-6). After a job offer is made, certain non–job-related questions may be asked, but not before. They should not be a part of deciding whether the applicant is offered a position.

How to Prepare: Planning Ahead

It is recommended that interview appointments be made as early as possible and that senior students not wait until graduation day. Ideally interviews should be scheduled at least 2 months prior to graduation. Job hunting takes time, and appointments are not easily scheduled near nursing school graduation dates because these tend to be busy weeks for recruiters.

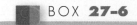

BOX **27-6**

Legal and Illegal Areas of Questioning

Some questions are inappropriate to be asked of an applicant before a job offer is made.

LEGAL	ILLEGAL
Educational preparation	Race
Licensure status	Creed
Work experience	Color
Reasons for leaving previous jobs	Age
Reasons for applying to this institution	Nationality
Qualifications for this job	Marital status
Strengths and weaknesses	Sexual preference
Criminal convictions	Religious beliefs
	Number of children or dependents
	Financial or credit status

How to Prepare: Self-Talk

As the day approached, Mary obsessed about the interview, thinking to herself, "What if they ask me something I cannot answer, and I go blank like I used to do in clinicals when the instructor quizzed me about my patient's medicines? I will look like an idiot, and maybe even start to cry." The night before the appointment, Mary could not sleep.

Your thoughts dictate your reality. Nurses, especially new nurses, should be aware of what they are saying to themselves. The applicant who thinks, "Why would anyone want to hire a graduate nurse with no practical experience like me?" will project a lack of self-trust that may be interpreted by the recruiter as lack of enthusiasm or even incompetence. If instead the graduate thinks, "I have successfully completed a difficult nursing course of study. I am now ready to take on the responsibilities of a professional. With orientation, on-the-job training, and the support of experienced nurses, I can succeed as an RN. I have everything I need to begin practice." This reality-based self-talk is an important internal dialogue for establishing feelings of confidence before the job interview.

The reality is that all graduates have met the criteria for graduation from a nursing education program and have been deemed ready by that credentialing body for an entry-level position as an RN. The final test of competence to practice, the NCLEX® examination, will provide further proof. Graduate nurses who fear failure of this final test must remind themselves of those now successfully practicing who preceded them from the same educational program with the same preparation.

How to Prepare: Rehearse

A simple visualization of how the graduate wants to appear to the recruiter can bring about the self-assurance needed to create an attractive candidate. It is helpful to mentally review and be prepared to describe pride in any past work experiences, especially the parts of any job that relate to what is required of a nurse. Even baby-sitting jobs can validate a worker as a responsible adult if that person worked consistently for the same family and showed stability and good judgment as a trusted caretaker for children. Applicants tend to discount minimum-wage, part-time, adolescent, or summer employment, but these experiences often reveal a great deal about the applicant: Would attendance records attest to the worker's dependability? Was the worker given greater responsibility over time? Was the worker allowed to open or close the business? Handle the cash receipts? Consider the following scenario.

CASE STUDY

The only job Sam had before nursing school had been working at the customer service desk at a large children's toy store, where he scheduled and supervised the cashiers. His title was "designated key carrier," which he listed on his résumé. The interviewer reasonably interpreted this to be a position that demonstrated the employer's trust in Sam.

Remember that it is not only the graduate's academic standing or honors and awards that measure success as a student. Perhaps the student was not in the top 10% of the class, but was active in student affairs. Perhaps the student was chair of a student government committee or a contributor to the campus newspaper. The graduate should be prepared to describe other areas of student accomplishments.

Unfortunately many nurses are not accustomed to selling themselves and are uncomfortable in situations in which they need to be able to discuss their best attributes and market their qualifications. Therefore, after rehearsing in your own mind how to present these qualifications to interviewers, it would be wise to rehearse with another person, role-playing the expected interview dialogue. Role-play with another student or an experienced nurse (even better), rehearsing answers to questions the interviewer is expected to ask. Practice descriptions of the key points of past employment. A few minutes spent in rehearsing with another will contribute to composure and self-confidence in the actual situation.

Finally, it is important for the graduate to remember that the job interview is not an examination to pass or fail, nor is it an interrogation. It is an exchange of information—the recruiter hoping to find a potential employee to fill a staff vacancy and the applicant hoping to find employment as a nurse in this organization. Each has responsibilities for informing the other, and each has rights to obtain information from the other (Box 27-7).

How to Prepare: The Interview Itself

Dress Appropriately. Business-appropriate clothing, such as a neat dress, suit, or pantsuit, projects a professional attitude. Casual attire projects a casual attitude. Jeans are not acceptable, nor are shorts or any clothes that are too short, too tight, too revealing, or too trendy. Conservative and simple are always best. "Dressing for success" influences not only the impressions others have, but also the wearer's own behavior. When people are dressed to look their best, attitudes improve and levels of self-confidence increase. Facial makeup should be light, and the use of perfume or cologne should be avoided. Many institutions are fragrance free because of patients' and employees' allergic reactions to perfumes. Large, distracting jewelry should be avoided.

Arrive on Time. Arriving late for a job interview creates a poor first impression. Be considerate of the interviewer's time and agenda. If delayed call to reschedule. To arrive too early can make the interviewer feel rushed or the applicant appear overanxious; however, 10 to 15 minutes early is a reasonable target.

Bring a Résumé. Even if a résumé has already been submitted, the applicant should bring extra copies. The recruiter may have routed the mailed copy to a manager for review. Applicants probably will be asked to complete an employment application, and the résumé is a ready

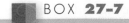

BOX **27-7**

Applicant's Rights

Applicants have the right to:
- Be informed of available positions at an institution and the minimal qualifications required.
- Apply for any available position for which they are qualified.
- Be seriously and fairly considered for any available position for which they are qualified.
- Be interviewed, be shown a job description, and be made aware of the requirements and expectations of the job.
- Have the work schedule discussed.
- Be informed of the benefits package.
- See the nursing unit and meet the manager if they are being seriously considered.
- Be made aware of the orientation program.
- Be given an expected time by which a decision will be made.

reference for past employers and dates of employment. Social security card, driver's license, and the nursing license, if available, also will be requested as necessary parts of the identification process. Some agencies request that a current cardiopulmonary resuscitation card be made available to photocopy. These documents will be easy to produce if the applicant has also brought a professional portfolio folder.

The Interview

The interview is the most time-consuming and subjective part of the employment process. For professionals it is appropriate for interviews to be unstructured, using open-ended questions; both recruiter and applicant will have questions. The initial interview can be expected to last 30 minutes to 1 hour. Being prepared is the key, and planning answers to the questions most likely to be asked is the best way to prepare. Eight of the most frequently asked questions follow.

1. What Positions Interest You? The interviewer needs to know whether there are positions available in the applicant's area of interest and whether the applicant has the required qualifications to fit the vacant positions. If there is no fit in interest or qualifications with jobs available, neither applicant nor recruiter need waste much more time in the interview.

Because titles and position names vary from organization to organization, it is better to answer the question with favorite clinical experiences. Applicants might share short- and long-term goals and how they visualize laying the groundwork today for tomorrow's professional roles. A good response might be, "I'm interested in a position that will help me grow as a professional and give me opportunities to develop greater competency as a nurse. Ultimately, I would like to work as a critical care clinical nurse specialist." If interest, qualifications, and the available positions match, the interviewer will want to start planning secondary interviews and tours.

2. Tell Me About Your Work History. Even if previous jobs were not nursing related, the applicant can highlight the responsibilities carried out, the skills acquired, and how those skills can transfer to the professional nursing role. This is the point at which the interviewer will get an idea of motivation, drive, energy level, and reliability. No new graduate will be expected to have all the knowledge and skills of an experienced RN; however, when answering, the graduate may stress other aptitudes, such as verbal skills or interpersonal skills. It is best to start with the current or most recent job and proceed backward. A new graduate might discuss student clinical experiences, which clinical areas were favored, and why.

3. How Did You Choose to Apply for a Job Here? Any previous investigative homework done on the institution is useful and helps to form honest responses. For example, an applicant might say, "This hospital has a reputation for its quality care, and I like that," or "I am interested in research and have heard you have a nursing research committee for staff nurses."

4. Do You Want a Full-Time or Part-Time Position, and Which Shift Do You Prefer? If there is a need or desire for a particular schedule, the nurse should be honest and ask for that schedule. If the recruiter does not have that schedule available, ask what is available so that a decision can be made. Can the nurse be flexible to accept an undesirable shift until a preferred one becomes available? Part of one's investigation of an institution should include looking at a current list of posted positions. Particularly with smaller agencies, if what the nurse desires is not posted, it may be beneficial to ask for a particular schedule but, if willing, express an interest in working a schedule that is posted. For example, "I'm willing to work the evening shift posted for the medical-surgical unit; however, I'm most interested in moving into a day position in labor and delivery."

5. What Are Your Strengths and Weaknesses? Sometimes this question may be asked in less direct ways, such as, "What are some of the areas you know you need to improve?" or "How have your skills developed in your advanced nursing courses?" Honesty always is best. By asking this question the interviewer may only be trying to pinpoint the special skills and preferences of the nurse. For example, with what kind of patients has the nurse been most effective, and which ones proved most difficult? The clearer the applicant can be in articulating specific talents and deficiencies, the more closely the recruiter will be able to match the candidate to a position suited to his or her abilities. The closer this match, the more likely the employee will flourish and be able to use special talents.

6. It Is Not Advisable to Avoid the Issue of Weaknesses. Everyone has them. It is better to admit them, but to present them in a positive way. In addition, it may be helpful to tell the interviewer what is being done to correct weaknesses. For example, "Sometimes I tend to see the big picture and have to remind myself to pay more attention to the details. I've started keeping lists, and they seem helpful." Another suggestion might be, "I have limited bedside nursing experience, but I am excited about building on the clinical skills I have learned in school."

7. What Would You Do If...? The recruiter probably will ask some situational questions related to decision making and critical thinking skills. The nurse will be asked to explain how to assess a particular situation, set priorities, decide what should be implemented first for a patient, and what can be delegated. Rather than fabricate an answer about unfamiliar circumstances, one can honestly say, "I've never been in that situation, but I think I would..." or "I was in a similar situation in which...occurred, and this is what I did in those circumstances."

8. Why Should We Hire You? This is an opportunity to share the special assets that the applicant would bring to the employer's institution. Without embellishment or selling oneself short, it is important to convey pride in being a nurse and conviction that one has something special to offer.

9. What Questions Do You Have? Usually the interview ends with the interviewer asking whether there are any questions. This is an opportunity for the applicant to demonstrate initiative, and one should take advantage of it, although not to excess. In an effective interview with an experienced interviewer, most questions regarding salary, benefits, and human resource policies will have been addressed (Box 27-8). If not this is the time to ask. Should a tour of the nursing unit and a meeting with the supervisor be arranged, many concerns will be answered then. Box 27-9 presents a list of suggested questions.

Mentally reviewing practiced responses to these questions will give the applicant confidence. The more information gathered, the easier it will be to make a decision, and the more likely it is that the nurse will be happy in the long term.

BOX **27-8**

What to Expect a Recruiter to Communicate

Recruiters should inform applicants of basic human resource policies regarding job descriptions, compensation, benefits, and staff development, including:

- Conditional period
- Job descriptions
- Shift rotation
- Weekend rotation
- Salary
- Staff development
- Parking
- Security
- Health insurance and other insurance benefits
- Preemployment physical examinations
- Credit union
- Overtime
- Scheduled paydays
- Paid time off
- Leaves of absence
- Employee discounts
- Transfer and promotion policies
- Resignation policies
- Preemployment policies
- Pay increases

BOX **27-9**

Appropriate Questions for the Applicant to Ask

1. May I see the job description for the position we are discussing?
2. What is the nurse-to-patient ratio?
3. What support staff are available on the unit to assist nurses?
4. What about clerical help and support services? What nursing care delivery systems or models are practiced here (team nursing, primary nursing, centralized, decentralized)?
5. How available are physicians? Admitting physicians and house staff?
6. How often are nursing care conferences held on this unit?
7. What type of nursing documentation is used?
8. How long is the orientation program? What does the program include? What continuing education programs are available after my initial orientation?
9. How will my performance be evaluated? How often, and by whom?
10. What exact schedule or shift will I be working in this position?
11. What will my salary be? Is there a shift differential?
12. Are there differentiated practice levels or roles and differentiated pay scales for nursing congruent with differences in educational preparation, certification, and other advanced nursing preparation?
13. How are pay increases decided?
14. What other benefits are there (health, life insurance, vacation time, tuition reimbursement, retirement plan)?
15. What input do staff nurses have in decision making about nursing practice?

THE APPLICANT'S TASKS
Assess the Climate of the Work Environment

As mentioned in the discussion of researching potential employers, there are ways other than direct questioning to learn a lot about the institution. Every organization has its own personality and atmosphere. The first impression probably came from the secretary who answered the phone when the applicant called for an appointment with the recruiter, followed by the greeting on arrival at the recruiter's office. A tone of respect and pride in being associated with the organization may have been communicated in the first encounter. Every subsequent encounter builds on the first.

In the hallways of the agency, how do people acknowledge each other? A visit to the employee cafeteria to buy a cup of coffee or a sandwich at mealtime can be enlightening. Are nurses eating there? Does it seem that the staff members are enjoying themselves? Pick up for later reading any available in-house publications, such as employee newsletters or bulletins.

Ask for a Tour

If the interviewer does not automatically offer a tour of the unit, the applicant can request to see it and will certainly want to meet with the person who would be the immediate supervisor. Some employers will arrange for the recruit to actually shadow a staff nurse for part of a shift. To get an accurate feel for the unit, the applicant should pay close attention to the pace, the tone of the staff interaction, and the morale. Is this a group the prospective employee would like to join? Are the manager's philosophy and management style similar to the applicant's own?

The astute applicant can get an accurate feel for the nursing unit's culture and personality if the manager's interactions with staff are observed. Is the manager accessible to the staff and supportive in response to them? How are telephone calls and other interruptions handled? How well do people seem to be getting along? Pay attention to the way people on the unit relate to each other—nurses to physicians, nurses to families, nurses to nurses. How are the patients responded to on the intercommunication system? Notice the efficiency with which staff work. How rushed are they? Also note bulletin boards and any public displays of staff recognition (e.g., "employee of the month" plaques or brag boards). Even a second visit to the unit might be requested before a final decision is made. The more information gathered, the easier it will be to make a decision (Sirgo and Coeling, 2005).

Some managers offer opportunities for the applicant to meet with staff, and formal interviews with staff nurses may be scheduled as a routine part of the hiring process. This gives the applicant a closer view of the actual work organization and gives representative staff members a chance to have a voice in selecting new coworkers. Staff nurses provide bedside care to patients and best understand the qualities appreciated in a good team member. Whether the introduction to staff is a formal interview or a casual conference room encounter, the applicant can be made to feel welcome and wanted while learning about the real work and the real workers of the agency. Now that firsthand knowledge has been obtained, if the applicant confers again with these employees and former employees are consulted before applying, he or she can ask more informed questions.

Follow-up

Thank-You Letter. A follow-up letter thanking the recruiter is a courtesy and a reminder of the nurse's interest in receiving a timely response (Box 27-10). If the nurse does not hear from the employer within a reasonable length of time (1 to 2 weeks) after the interview, it is appropriate to inquire by telephone about the status of a hiring decision.

BOX **27-10**

Interview Follow-up Letter

April 24, 2010

Ms. Donna Henderson, RN, MS
Director, Nurse Recruitment
Charleston Memorial Hospital
1265 Beckley Avenue
Memphis, TN 38104

Dear Ms. Henderson:
It was a pleasure meeting with you on Monday. I now have a clear picture of what I might expect as a new graduate nurse in your hospital. Everyone on the units I visited was very friendly.

I look forward to hearing from you with good news about a position at Charleston Memorial. I can be reached in the afternoons at 555-912-3120 or on my cell, 555-200-9999.

Thank you again for your time and interest.

Sincerely,
Bonnie McCray Pino

Avoid Impulse Decisions. If offered a position and time is needed to make a decision, the applicant should postpone a decision and should not feel pressured into acceptance while still unsure. An offer to telephone the recruiter with an answer within an agreed-on time is appropriate.

If there are other job opportunities, certainly comparisons need to be made by weighing the pros and cons of each position and each organization. How do benefits compare? What are the possibilities for movement within the systems laterally and vertically? How available are continuing education opportunities to staff nurses? How do observations of the work culture fit with the nurse's ideas of what is needed to support professional success? Does the schedule that is offered fit the applicant's lifestyle? When a decision has been reached, a telephone call should be made promptly to the recruiter, whether the answer is yes or no.

Weighing Options. What questions might be asked of oneself while weighing the merits of one position against others? Remembering that no job is perfect, the following four questions should be considered.

Does the Position Match the Nurse's Qualifications? Although it is flattering to receive a job offer for a position for which a nurse has little or no preparation, one should not be influenced by such a compliment. When there is a nursing shortage, a position that is beyond an applicant's present skills and experience may sound wonderfully challenging, when in actuality it may be overwhelming and a disastrous beginning for a new graduate. Being overzealous, overconfident, and overanxious to please can only lead to feelings of guilt and inadequacy if the job is not appropriate. It is wiser to accept a position in which adequate orientation and clinical support exist, which would allow the graduate to gain the experience and preparation necessary to accept a position requiring more skills at a later time.

What Are the Actual Responsibilities of the Job? The newly hired nurse has the right to completely understand what will be expected in the position offered, including the overall and daily responsibilities and the length and nature of on-the-job training that will be provided.

What will the supervisory responsibilities be? How many and what skill level employees will be under the RN's leadership? What orientation is planned to prepare the RN for practicing independently? Are there arrangements for a preceptor to guide the graduate through the difficult transition of entering a first nursing job? Reality shock can be anticipated, and the more assistance a new graduate receives in adjusting to the new role of the nurse, the more likely the beginner is to be successful and satisfied.

Does This Position Lead the Nurse in the Direction of Projected Career Goals? Is the offered job a step toward meeting long-term career objectives? For example, a graduate who wants to be a nurse-midwife someday would be wiser to accept a position in postpartum, if labor and delivery is not available, rather than accepting a position in neurosurgery just because it offers a slightly higher salary or a few more weekends. No position or job change should be accidental or the result of a snap decision. Wise career moves result from deliberate planning and purposeful preparation.

How Will the Work Be Compensated? Experienced nurses often advise novices that money, although important, is not the only reward associated with a job. However, money does matter, especially to a new graduate who may have subsisted on a limited income while in school. It is common for loans to have accumulated, along with unpaid bills. Inadequate salary can be a real source of job dissatisfaction, of course, but with 24-hour responsibilities, nurses traditionally have basic salaries that include other income-contributing factors, such as shift differentials, weekend differentials, holiday pay, paid vacation days, and expected salary increases over time. Compensation comes in other packages besides paychecks. There are policies that allow for maternity leaves, medical leaves, tuition reimbursement, sick days, discounts on prescriptions and health insurance, retirement benefits, and malpractice insurance coverage, all of which affect income in indirect but important ways. As is true in other areas of consideration, the better the total compensation package fits one's needs, the greater the likelihood that one will remain satisfied with the job.

Well-prepared job applicants will have listed those benefits they consider essential, and these vary with individual circumstances. For example, the essentials for someone who is the sole family breadwinner probably include health insurance, paid time off, and an employer-provided retirement plan. Available child care would be especially important for parents of preschool children. Box 27-11 further helps applicants evaluate potential employment opportunities.

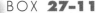

BOX **27-11**

Assessment Tool for Decision Making

When weighing options for employment, consider those measures of a professional work climate evident in written documentation and visible in the patient care areas. The following observations should guide the new graduate in making an informed decision.
- Standards of nursing practice are evident and are an integral part of patient care.
- Nurse-to-patient ratio is adequate and adjusted for patient acuity.
- Orientation is structured, individualized, and adequate for new graduates.
- Opportunities for horizontal transfer and advancement exist within the system.
- The salary is competitive and reasonable.
- Benefits are competitive.
- Continuing education is available, and staff members are encouraged to attend.
- A nurse administrator is responsible for delivery of nursing services.

THE EMPLOYER'S TASKS

In any agency providing nursing services, its nurses are the indispensable employees. The selection of new nurse employees is a critically important responsibility, and it is the recruiter's duty to make sure the best selection is made.

First, the nurse must meet the minimal requirements for the position desired. For example, 1 year of experience might be required for a nurse to work a weekender program or in a critical care area. Operating room (OR) experience may be required for OR nursing positions, and perinatal nursing experience may be required for labor and delivery positions. A secondary consideration is the nurse's suitability for contributing to the mission of the health care delivery system. The recruiter is selling the organization to the applicant and measuring the skills and aptitudes the applicant would bring to the organization.

The bottom line for any employer who provides health care services to the public is to ensure that its nursing staff practices safely. Recruiters are looking to uncover anything that would impair a nurse applicant's ability to provide safe nursing care, such as incompetence, unprofessional conduct, unreliability in attendance, chemical dependency, or record of criminal activity. For screening, recruiters have four primary sources of information: the application, interview impressions, test results, and references.

Applications are validated. Work history and references are checked to ensure accuracy. Previous supervisors are asked about attendance, dependability, performance, attitude, ability to get along with others, integrity, and eligibility for rehire. The applicant's stated reason for termination is compared with information obtained from work references. The employer has a right to obtain reasonable information about the people who are hired. Most employment applications ask whether the applicant has ever been convicted of a crime other than a minor traffic violation. The question is about convictions, not arrests, and the response is verified by a background or criminal record check. Response to this or any other question in the application process must be honest and truthful. Each institution has its own policies regarding convictions, but most are vitally concerned about their responsibilities regarding negligent hiring. If an applicant committed a crime that, if repeated while in the employ of the institution, would cause harm to patients, families, other employees or the institution, the applicant is rejected.

A physical examination is often required. This usually is done on-site and at the employer's expense. It may involve obtaining the applicant's full medical history and vital signs, routine blood tests, a urine drug screen, and sometimes a chest radiograph. The purpose of the examination is to ensure protection for patients and to ensure that the caregiver can carry out the necessary physical responsibilities of the job. For example, are illegal mood-altering substances evident that would impair the nurse's abilities and judgment? Are there physical limitations the institution should know about to determine whether any special accommodations are necessary to allow the candidate to perform the usual duties associated with the position?

Even with a job offer made and a date for employment set, actual start dates are contingent on receipt of documentation of these final screenings, plus a reference check to verify the résumé; these items establish the practitioner's safety and reliability. Other parts of screening for safety might include paper-and-pencil testing, such as skills tests, pharmacology tests, and in some cases, psychologic testing for specialty areas.

Although a preemployment pharmacology test is becoming less common than in past years, many institutions still give such a quiz to determine basic knowledge of routinely administered medications, their purposes, and side effects. Simple dosage questions and calculation methods may be asked. Some questions may be situational ones, such as, "What would you do in this case?" or "The first nursing action in this scenario should be... ."

A few larger institutions also may administer a clinical skills test. This might be conducted in a simulated laboratory setting, where frequently used patient care equipment is set up. Usually a staff development instructor accompanies the nurse through a series of stations where the nurse would be asked to plan and perform the appropriate nursing actions. Examples might be starting cardiopulmonary resuscitation on a simulated patient, demonstrating the proper procedure for starting an intravenous line, or talking through an assessment of a patient.

It is far better to be prepared and even better to be proactive and offer to produce some of the documentation required. For instance the nurse may be able to get a written reference from a former employer or a statement from a physician sooner than the institution can. The employment start date depends on the receipt of all the necessary information, so it would expedite the process if the hopeful employee volunteered to initiate some of the documentation gathering or even have references in hand with other documentation at the time of interview.

Once an applicant is selected, the agency has committed itself to costly training, orientation, and additional benefits that may cost as much as 30% to 40% of the employee's salary. A major element of control, which any organization possesses, is its ability to choose its employees. When the selection process is thorough, it is a sign to the committed professional that this is a reputable employer.

SUMMARY

If not offered a position, the new graduate should still feel good about himself or herself. There may have been several candidates for that same position. Perhaps it was not the best match for one's skills or preferences. There is victory in having had an opportunity to practice interview skills. Preparation, practice, and perseverance will reward the nurse with a job that is better suited to his or her personality, values, qualifications, and skills. New graduates have internalized standards of practice from their nursing education experience. On graduation they must decide where to begin to put those standards to work in real-life terms handling real responsibilities with real patients. The question becomes, "Can school and work values be reconciled in this nursing environment?" When adequate groundwork in pursuit of a job has been laid, the answer should come easy.

 Additional resources are available online at: http://evolve.elsevier.com/Cherry/

REFERENCES

Herrin D, American Association of Nurse Executives (AONE): *Personal communication*, September 1, 2009.

Nursing2009CareerDirectory. What's the attraction of Magnet hospitals? Nursing2009CareerDirectory Magnet section, p. 26, January 2009.

Sherrod D: The professional portfolio: a snapshot of your career, *Nurs Manag* 36(9):74–75, 2005.

Sirgo C, Coeling H: Work group culture and the new graduate, *AJN* 105(2):85–87, 2005.

ADDITIONAL RESOURCES

American Journal of Nursing, January 2010, 2010 Career Guide, Vol 40, No. 1(Suppl), Philadelphia, 2010, Lippincott, Williams, and Wilkins.

Dennison RD: What goes into your professional portfolio and what you will get out of it, *Am Nurse Today* 42–43, (January) 2007.

Ulrich BT, et al: Magnet status and registered nurse views of the work environment and nursing as a career, *J Nurs Adm* 39(Suppl 7-8):554–562, 2009.

Williams M, Jordan K: The nursing professional portfolio: a pathway to career development, *J Nurs Staff Dev* 23(3):125–131, 2007.

NCLEX-RN® Examination

Tommie L. Norris, DNS, RN

⊜volve   Additional resources are available online at: http://evolve.elsevier.com/Cherry/

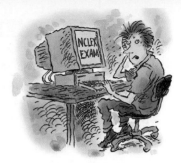

Adequate preparation for the NCLEX-RN® examination can reduce panic and ensure success.

VIGNETTE

Consider for a moment how nursing and licensure examinations have changed as society has changed. Nursing is a reflection of society's values, knowledge, and needs. Test items or questions found on the NCLEX-RN examination today have little resemblance to questions asked on state board examinations administered during the early part of the century. The examination of that era dealt with practical issues and consisted mainly of knowledge-based questions that had little to do with assessment, application, evaluation, or need. Consider, for instance, the following questions taken from the 1919 state board questions and answers for nurses (Foote, 1919):

- *What are the advantages of fireplaces?*
- *How would you sterilize silkworm-gut and silk sutures?*
- *What care regarding nourishment would you give a gynecological patient to prevent a common discomfort?*
- *Give some general rules for preparing meats.*
- *Give three common complaints that the public makes about graduate nurses.*

■ QUESTIONS TO CONSIDER WHILE READING THIS CHAPTER:

1 What is the purpose of the NCLEX-RN examination?

2 What type of questions can I expect on today's NCLEX-RN examination?

3 What is the best way to prepare for the examination?

KEY TERMS

Compulsory licensure Requirement that must be met to legally practice or work as a registered nurse (RN). Licensure is a prerequisite to practice in each state and U.S. territory.

Computer adaptive testing (CAT) A type of testing taken on a computer, in which a person is given a test question to answer, followed by a subsequent question that is leveled based on the whether the candidate correctly answered the first question. For example, a person missing a question dealing with assessment might be given another assessment question to determine the person's competency with assessment, or a person answering a knowledge-level question correctly could receive a question at the application level of Bloom's taxonomy.

NCLEX-RN examination NCLEX stands for National Council Licensure Examination, an examination taken by qualified graduates of approved schools of nursing. Graduates successfully taking the NCLEX-RN examination are granted a license to practice as RNs.

After studying this chapter, the reader will be able to:

1 Explain the purpose of the NCLEX-RN examination.

2 Evaluate various methods of preparation for the NCLEX-RN examination.

3 Create a personal plan for preparing for the NCLEX-RN examination.

4 Analyze the relationship between the nursing process and client needs as they relate to NCLEX-RN test items.

5 Compare various review courses designed to aid in review for the NCLEX-RN examination.

CHAPTER OVERVIEW

This chapter helps student nurses prepare to successfully pass the NCLEX-RN examination. The purpose of the NCLEX-RN is discussed and an overview of the format and content is given. Various strategies for preparing for the exam are given, and students are encouraged to develop a personal plan of study.

ARE YOU PREPARED FOR THE NCLEX-RN EXAMINATION?

You are pursuing a degree in nursing and plan to take the NCLEX-RN licensure examination on graduation. Do you know what to expect on the exam itself? Do you feel you have the knowledge necessary for NCLEX-RN examination success? If not you should be interested in this chapter, which offers an overview of the format and content you can expect on the test and strategies for success.

THE NCLEX-RN EXAMINATION

The NCLEX-RN examination and licensure to practice nursing go hand in hand. To receive a license to practice as an RN in the United States and its territories, candidates must furnish evidence of competency to provide safe and effective nursing care by successfully completing the NCLEX-RN examination (National Council of State Boards of Nursing [NCSBN], 2009).

There are three types of RN programs: (1) 2-year associate degree programs usually found in community or junior colleges, (2) hospital-based diploma programs, and (3) baccalaureate degree or higher programs found in 4-year colleges and universities or academic health centers. Graduates from all programs take the same NCLEX-RN examination. The examination tests content common to all these programs is job related and reflects current entry level nursing practice (NCSBN, 2009). Individuals taking the examination must have graduated from approved schools of nursing.

Purpose of the NCLEX-RN Examination

The purpose of the NCLEX-RN examination is to:

1. Safeguard the public from unsafe practitioners.
2. Assist state boards of nursing in determining candidates' capabilities for performing entry-level RN positions.

To keep the NCLEX-RN examination current, the National Council of State Boards of Nursing (NCSBN) conducts a practice analysis on a 3-year cycle by investigating current practice that entry-level nurses are performing in various health care settings in the United States. Six thousand newly licensed nurses are asked to prioritize 150 nursing care activities and state how often they perform them. These activities are then evaluated based on the context, frequency, and effect on client safety (NCSBN, 2009). The most recent RN practice analysis was completed in 2008. Based on the results of this practice analysis, NCSBN revised and implemented the current test plan in April, 2010. To view the latest practice analysis visit: www.ncsbn.org/1235.htm.

Characteristics of the NCLEX-RN Examination

The NCLEX-RN examination is a pass-fail exam and has been computerized since 1994. Before that time it was a paper-and-pencil exam requiring 2 days to complete. Today the NCLEX-RN examination is offered at more than 3400 Pearson Professional Centers throughout the country, can be taken at the candidate's convenience, and can be completed in 6 hours or less, which includes examination instructions and breaks. The results of the examination are sent to candidates within a month after they have taken the examination. In some states, candidates may receive unofficial results by telephone or e-mail, or they may check the state board website for licensure verification.

Computer Adaptive Testing. The NCLEX-RN examination uses CAT, which is a test-administering technique that uses computer technology and measurement theory. As a candidate answers questions on the examination, CAT adapts to the level of the candidate's knowledge, skills, and ability. All examinations are consistent with the NCLEX-RN examination test plan, which controls inclusion of nursing content. Candidates have ample opportunity to demonstrate their competence because the examination does not end until stability of the pass or fail result is certain or time runs out (NCSBN, 2009).

A tutorial is administered before the examination actually begins, providing candidates with experience in using the computer in CAT situations. Candidates should carefully read an entire question and all possible answer options before selecting an answer. Candidates may request assistance regarding the use of the computer at any point, even during the NCLEX-RN examination. In addition, they may find it helpful to view the PowerPoint candidate tutorial before going to the testing center. This tutorial, provided by NCSBN, may be accessed at the following website: www.ncsbn.org.

Skipping Questions and Changing Answers. Candidates taking the NCLEX-RN examination are not allowed to skip questions and return to them at a later time or to change answers to questions once an answer has been selected and entered into the computer. These actions would defeat the purpose of adaptive testing because CAT selects questions based on the examination taker's knowledge, skills, and abilities. Candidates are not disadvantaged using this method of testing because CAT has a built-in self-correcting mechanism (www.ncsbn.org).

Question Format

All of the information needed to answer a particular question appears on one computer screen, so candidates do not need to see the previous or next screen for answer determination. Questions are presented in traditional top-down format, in which the question is presented, followed by the potential answers to it. Questions appearing on the computer screen will be either traditional multiple-choice or alternate item format.

Traditional Format: Multiple-Choice, One Option. With this type of format, the candidate is presented a question, followed by four possible responses. The candidate is asked to select the one option that best answers the question. Multiple-choice, one option format is the style most commonly used on the examination. See the following example.

*The nurse has received the following information about assigned clients. The nurse should **first** assess:*

a. *A 64-year-old client who had a total knee replacement 3 hours ago and has 15 mL of serosanguineous drainage in the collection device.*

b. *A 32-year-old client who had closed reduction of a fractured right malleolus 5 hours ago and has swelling of the right toes.*

c. *A 9-month-old client admitted 6 hours ago with vomiting, whose vital signs are temperature, 37.6° C (99.7° F); pulse, 124; respirations, 26.*

d. *A 6-week-old client who was admitted 2 hours ago with nasal flaring and has a pulse oximetry reading of 90%.*
(Answer: d)

Alternate Item Format

Because of the nature of CAT, the type of item presented to the candidate will depend on the content area.

Consequently, candidates may or may not receive alternate item format questions on their exams. Possible alternate item formats include:

◆ **Hot spot (questions based on illustrations and charts).** With this type of item the candidate is asked to identify one or more area(s) on a picture or graphic. See the following example:

Identify the point of maximal impulse (PMI):

1. *A*
2. *B*
3. *C*
4. *D*

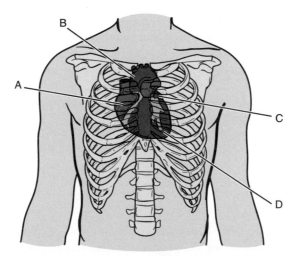

(Answer: D)

◆ **Multiple-response, multiple-choice questions.** The candidate is presented with a question, followed by five or more responses. The candidate is asked to check all responses that are correct; partial credit is not given. See the following example:

A nurse is caring for a 47-year-old female client who has been diagnosed with hypothyroidism. Which of the following manifestations might the nurse expect the client to report? (Select all that apply.)

a. Intolerance to heat
b. Periorbital edema
c. Weight loss
d. Menorrhagia
e. Constipation
f. Fatigue
(Answer: b, d, e, and f)

♦ **Fill-in-the-blank.** The candidate is presented with a question to which the answer must be typed, instead of selecting from among a set of four options. In some cases candidates may be asked to calculate values, such as dosages. A drop-down calculator is available for the candidate to use. See the following example:
A nurse is completing the intake and output record for a client who had a left total knee replacement 1 day ago. The client has had the following intake and output during the shift:
Intake: 3 oz apple juice
½ serving oatmeal
8 ounces water
1 cup fruit-flavored gelatin
½ cup beef broth
800 mL of 0.45 sodium chloride (half-strength saline), IV
Output: 1200 mL of urine
50 mL from the drainage tube
How many milliliters should the nurse document as the client's intake?
(Answer: 1490 mL)

♦ **Graphic option identification.** The candidate is presented with a picture or a graphic image rather than text and asked to identify a particular area.
♦ **Drag and drop (prioritize).** The candidate is presented with a set of responses to a question and asked to place them in order or to prioritize. See the following example:
A nurse is preparing to perform a sterile dressing change. In what order would the following steps be performed?
1. Gather supplies.
2. Set up the sterile field.
3. Assess the wound.
4. Explain the procedure to the patient.
5. Remove the soiled dressing.
6. Document the dressing change.
Type your answer in the box below (Note: Do not use spaces or commas between the numbers in the answer.) Candidates may also be asked to click on the steps and drag item in the correct order.
(Answer: 1, 4, 5, 3, 2, 6)

♦ **Chart exhibit.** The candidate is asked to seek additional information in a patient's chart to answer the question. See the following example in which the candidate must look in the chart to find pertinent information to report:
A patient is ordered Lanoxin 0.25 mg daily. The nurse assesses the patient's heart rate as 48 beats per minute. Prior to calling the physician what additional information is needed?
a. Potassium 2.8 mEq/L

> b. *Arterial blood gases (Pa_{O_2}), 95*
> c. *History of kidney stones*
> d. *Diet: 1800 calorie*
> *(Answer: a)*

◆ **Audio.** Each candidate is furnished with earphones and listens to an audio clip. The candidate is asked to identify specific assessment findings. See the following example: *Candidate listens to an adventitious breath sound such as crackles. Candidate will be asked to identify abnormal finding.*

Candidates should note that any of the item formats, including standard multiple-choice items, may include tables, graphic images, or charts. Candidates can find additional information on alternate item formats on Pearson Vue's website at: www.pearsonvue.com/nclex/#tutorial.

Cognitive Domains and the NCLEX-RN Examination

NCLEX-RN examination questions use Bloom's original cognitive levels of knowledge, comprehension, application, and analysis and the revised taxonomy of remember, understand, apply, analyze, evaluate, and create (Anderson and Krathwohl, 2001; Bloom, Englehart, and Furst, 1956). These levels may be viewed as four consecutive steps, with knowledge being the lowest, most fundamental step and analysis being the highest, most highly evolved of the steps. Because nursing requires application of knowledge, skills, and abilities, the majority of NCLEX-RN exam questions are written at the application or higher cognitive level and critical thinking skills (NCSBN, 2009). Following is a description of the four cognitive levels of Bloom's taxonomy used on the NCLEX-RN exam.

Knowledge Questions

As the lowest and simplest level of learning within the cognitive domain, knowledge is remembering or recalling information. This may include knowing selected facts, such as normal range of serum potassium or common terminology, such as dyspnea. Giving definitions and examples are common skills at this cognitive level because this level requires no understanding or judgment.

Comprehension Questions

Comprehension, the second level of Bloom's cognitive domain, is the fundamental level of understanding or the ability to grasp or summarize information or material or restate in one's own words. The following is an example of a comprehension level question:

> *A patient is ordered a clear liquid diet. The nurse can offer the patient which of the following on the food tray?*
> a. *Orange juice*
> b. *Lime Jell-O*
> c. *Skim milk*
> d. *Tomato soup*
> *(Answer: b)*

Application Questions

The third cognitive level, application, refers to the ability to use learned information in new situations. This level involves applying abstract theories and principles in new concrete or practical situations, solving mathematical problems, constructing charts and graphs, and making inferences. Information learned is applied to deliver safe and effective nursing care. The following is an example of an application level question:

> An adult patient with a history of alcoholism, 24 hours after gastric resection surgery, is complaining of pain rated as 9 on a scale of 1 to 10, with 10 being most severe. The nurse reviews the orders and prepares to administer morphine 2 mg intramuscularly. Before administration of pain medication, which assessment is a **priority** that must be completed by the RN?
> a. Bowel sounds and degree of nausea
> b. Respiratory rate and level of consciousness
> c. Heart rate and ambulatory status
> d. History of addiction to narcotics and potassium level
> (Answer: b)

Analysis Questions

The highest cognitive level used on the NCLEX-RN examination, analysis, requires complex thought processes and includes the ability to reduce material into its fundamental parts so that relationships may be understood. Included in this level are questions of drawing conclusions, setting priorities, forming hypotheses, and creating something new. The majority of items are written at the application level or higher because the practice of nursing necessitates that nurses apply knowledge, skills, and abilities to problem solve. The following is an example of a question written at the analysis level:

> A patient exhibits tetany and a positive Trousseau sign. The following lab values were reported: Sodium 140 mg/dL, potassium 5 mEq/mL, calcium 8 mg/dL, and magnesium 3 mg/dL. These clinical manifestations and laboratory findings are consistent with which electrolyte disorder?
> a. Hyponatremia
> b. Hypomagnesemia
> c. Hypocalcemia
> d. Hypokalemia
> (Answer: c)

Candidates taking the examination answer a minimum of 75 questions to a maximum of 265 questions. The NCSBN (2009) advises that the length of an NCLEX-RN examination be based on the performance of the candidate on the examination and has established a goal to be 95% sure of pass-fail decisions. After a minimum number of questions have been answered, the computer stops when there is 95% certainty that the candidate is above the passing standard and the candidate passes or 95% certainty that the candidate is below the standard and the candidate fails. Candidates whose ability is extremely close to the passing standard receive a maximum number of items and a decision is based on whether the candidate's performance has been consistently above or below the passing standard.

COMPONENTS OF THE NCLEX-RN EXAMINATION TEST PLAN

The test plan for the NCLEX-RN examination is based on the current nursing practice of entry-level RNs. According to NCSBN (2009): "The NCLEX examination assesses the knowledge, skills and abilities that are essential for the nurse to use in order to meet the needs of clients requiring the promotion, maintenance or restoration of health" (p. 1). The NCLEX-RN examination test plan is framed by four major categories of client needs, which are further subdivided into a total of six subcategories (NCSBN, 2009):

(1) Safe, effective care environment

   ◆ Management of care
   ◆ Safety and infection control
(2) Health promotion and maintenance
(3) Psychosocial integrity
(4) Physiologic integrity
   ◆ Basic care and comfort
   ◆ Pharmacologic and parenteral therapies
   ◆ Reduction of risk potential
   ◆ Physiologic adaptation

Each of these will be examined individually, followed by a discussion of several processes that are fundamental to nursing and integrated throughout the client needs categories and subcategories.

Client Needs

The goal of nursing for client care in any setting is preventing illnesses; alleviating suffering; protecting, promoting, and restoring health; and promoting dignity in dying (NCSBN, 2009). The organizing framework of the NCLEX-RN examination is client needs. This is a broad component that "provides a universal structure for defining nursing actions and competencies across all settings for all clients" (NCLEX, 2009, p. 3).

Safe and Effective Care Environment. This category pertains to the provision and direction of nursing care delivery to safeguard clients, their families or significant others, in addition to health care providers. This category is further subdivided into two categories: management of care, from which 16% to 22% of the test plan is constructed, and safety and infection control, from which 8% to 14% of the test plan is constructed (NCSBN, 2009). Within this section the nurse should have the knowledge, skills, and ability to meet the client's needs for a safe and effective environment.

Health Promotion and Maintenance. This category relating to client needs pertains to the provision and direction of nursing care that takes into consideration the projected growth and development principles, early detection and prevention of health problems, and plans to realize best possible health. Six to 12% of NCLEX-RN examination questions are related to this category.

Psychosocial Integrity. In this category, "The nurse provides and directs nursing care that promotes and supports the emotional, mental, and social well-being of the client and family/significant others experiencing stressful events, as well as clients with acute or chronic mental illness" (NCSBN, 2009, p. 5). Psychosocial integrity is addressed in 6% to 12% of NCLEX-RN examination questions.

Physiologic Integrity. This category entails the provision and direction of nursing care delivery to protect the client and family or significant others, in addition to health care providers. This category is further subdivided into four subcategories: (1) Basic care and comfort, accounting for 6% to 12% of the test plan, is directed at the provision of comfort and assistance while performing activities of daily living; (2) pharmacologic and parenteral therapies, accounting for 13% to 19% of the test plan, is concerned with medication and parenteral therapies administration; (3) reduction of risk potential, accounting for 10% to 16% of the test plan, correlates with reducing the risk of clients developing complications related to their current conditions or treatments; and (4) physiologic adaptation, accounting for 11% to 17% of the test plan, is the management or coordination of care for clients with acute or chronic and life-threatening disease processes (NCSBN, 2009).

Integrated Processes

Processes that are fundamental to nursing are integrated throughout the previously noted client needs categories and subcategories (NCSBN, 2009):

- Nursing process
- Caring
- Communication and documentation
- Teaching and learning

For example, a question may be a health promotion and maintenance question that has to do with assessment or a psychosocial integrity question that also addresses implementation. All questions relate to some activity in which an entry-level nurse may engage when caring for or managing a patient. A more complete overview of these integrated processes follows.

Nursing Process. Success on the NCLEX-RN examination relies on a sound working knowledge of the nursing process. The NCSBN (2009) defines nursing process as "a scientific problem-solving approach to client care that includes assessment, analysis, planning, implementation, and evaluation" (p. 3). The nursing process is applicable to all situations in which the nurse and patient interact and may be used with any theoretic framework. Cox and associates (2007) expand the definition to incorporate the cognitive (mental), psychomotor (motor and mental), and affective (feelings or emotions) processes used to design care.

Assessment. Assessment is the first step of the nursing process and establishes a database for the client. Just as the nursing process provides a foundation for nursing practice, assessment provides the foundation for the nursing process. Assessment includes gathering information or data about an identified client. Depending on the nurse's focus, the client may be a person, a family, a group of people, or a community.

Information about a client comes from a variety of sources, including the client, the family and significant others, laboratory or radiographic reports, physician records, hospital or clinic records, and other caregivers. Client data are typically classified as subjective and objective. Simply put subjective data are the client's perception or understanding of a specific event or phenomenon. It is his or her opinion, such as the degree of pain experienced during an episode of angina. Objective data are observable and measurable by the nurse and come from various patient records. Blood pressure, heart rate, and the presence or absence of edema are examples of objective data.

Cox and associates (2007) suggest two additional classifications of client data—historical and current. Historical data relate to health events occurring before the current health problem or admission to the health care system. Current data include information specific to the current health problem or admission. Historical and current data may occur as subjective or objective information.

Assessment also includes verification and communication of data. Seeking additional client-related information, such as laboratory work or talking with the family, may confirm data. Communication of data may be accomplished by verbal report to other health care workers or by written or computerized record.

Analysis. Analysis is the second step or phase of the nursing process. Client-related data gathered during assessment provide the basis for analysis. During this phase the nurse classifies or groups assessment data and identifies actual or potential client problems. During classification data also are validated and interpreted, and additional data may be required. Numerous frameworks exist for categorizing data. Included in the frameworks are Gordon's functional health patterns, Maslow's hierarchy of needs, and the NANDA International (NANDA-I) human response patterns (Cox et al, 2007). Nursing diagnoses are determined based on classification of data. A working definition of nursing diagnosis is provided by NANDA-I:

> A nursing diagnosis is a clinical judgment about individual, family, or community responses to actual or potential health problems/life processes. Nursing diagnoses provide the basis for selection of nursing interventions to achieve outcomes for which the nurse is accountable (American Nurses Association, 1999).

As with assessment, nursing diagnoses must be communicated in a reliable format. It is important to remember that there must be congruency between the client's needs or problems and the nurse's ability to realistically meet those needs.

Planning. Planning is the third phase of the nursing process and includes setting realistic and measurable mutual goals, developing interventions to meet or resolve identified patient needs or problems, and modifying goals as necessary. Included in planning of care are ranking nursing diagnoses, documenting expected outcomes for each goal, and setting realistic target dates for the accomplishment of each goal. Goal setting should include the collaboration of members of the interdisciplinary health care team, the client, his or her family, and significant others as indicated. As with the previous phases of the nursing process, the plan must be communicated to other members of the health care team to ensure continuity of care.

Implementation. The fourth phase of the nursing process is implementation. This stage includes initiating and carrying out nursing interventions or nursing actions to achieve the goals set in the planning phase of the nursing process. In discussing nursing actions, Cox and associates (2007) wrote:

> Nursing action is defined as nursing behavior that serves to help the client achieve the expected outcome. Nursing actions include both independent and collaborative activities. Independent actions are those activities the nurse performs using his or her own discretionary judgment and that require no validation or guidelines from any other health care practitioner (e.g., deciding which noninvasive technique to use for pain control or deciding when to teach the patient self-care measures). Collaborative actions are those activities that involve mutual decision making between two or more health care practitioners (e.g., a physician and nurse deciding which narcotic to use when meperidine is ineffective in controlling the patient's pain) (Cox et al, 2007, p. 6).

Each nursing action should be geared toward achieving a particular goal of care. Included in the implementation phase are (1) organizing and managing care; (2) actually performing patient care; (3) overseeing and coordinating the delivery of care; (4) delegating nursing actions to other health care workers; (5) teaching or counseling the client, his or her family, significant others, and other caregivers; and (6) communicating and exchanging patient-related information with other health care workers (Cox et al, 2007).

Evaluation. To evaluate, data must be collected to document the progress the patient has made, or not made, in relation to the stated goal. Once data have been collected and analyzed, the nurse must decide what action to take or what modification to make regarding the goal. In all instances, the nurse will make one of three choices:
1. Resolve the plan because the patient has achieved the goal.

2. Continue the plan because the patient is still making satisfactory progress toward the goal, but did not achieve the goal during the original timeframe.
3. Revise the plan because the patient is not making satisfactory progress toward the goal (Cox et al, 2007).

As with the other phases of the nursing process, evaluation involves documenting and illustrating the patient's responses to the care provided.

Caring. NCSBN defines caring as "the interaction of the nurse and client in an atmosphere of mutual respect and trust. In this collaborative environment, the nurse provides encouragement, hope, support and compassion to help achieve desired outcomes" (NCSBN, 2009, p. 3).

Communication and Documentation. NCSBN defines communication and documentation as "the verbal and nonverbal interactions between the nurse and the client, the client's significant others and the other members of the health care team. Events and activities associated with client care are validated in written and/or electronic records that reflect standards of practice and accountability in the provision of care" (NCSBN, 2009, p. 3).

Teaching and Learning. NCSBN defines teaching and learning as "facilitation of the acquisition of knowledge, skills and attitudes promoting a change in behavior" (NCSBN, 2009, p. 3).

PREPARING FOR THE NCLEX-RN EXAMINATION

There is no one best method for preparing to take the NCLEX-RN examination. Success depends on a candidate's nursing knowledge and ability to use that knowledge, test-taking skills, and confidence level. The best preparation any candidate can have is what the candidate brings from his or her nursing program.

Some measure of preparation for the NCLEX-RN examination after graduation from nursing school is a must for all candidates seeking success on the examination. Candidates should NOT convince themselves that they do not need to review because average or above-average grades were made in their academic and nursing coursework, nor should they decide that review will serve no purpose because average or below-average grades were made in their coursework.

In preparing for the NCLEX-RN examination it is important to remember that review is a personal undertaking. What works for one candidate may not work for another and vice versa. Use study and review methods that have proven successful in the past.

Consider the following when preparing for the NCLEX-RN examination:

◆ *Perform a needs assessment.* Determine content areas of strengths and weaknesses. Look at previous academic and nursing coursework, class notes and handouts, examination grades, and grades made on nursing care plans or process papers. If your school uses nationally normed assessment examinations, use the report to determine areas of strengths and weaknesses. The rationale provided when reviewing these exams provides a wealth of information and validates the correct answers. Talk with faculty in courses in which weakness or difficulty existed. Determine where the greatest amount of review is needed. Be honest in performing the needs assessment. The foundation for success or failure on the NCLEX-RN examination may be determined here.

◆ *Determine the number of days or weeks necessary for review.* Candidates with a strong nursing knowledge base may need less time than candidates with weaknesses. As with the needs assessment, candidates should be realistic in planning the amount of review time needed.

◆ *Decide what method of review will be used.* Individual and group study have strong and weak points. Strong points of individual study include having total control over content and time spent in review. Weak points include having no immediate resources to explain or assist with understanding difficult concepts. Candidates with weakness in disciplining themselves may have problems sticking to review schedules and focusing on specific content with individual study. Strong points of group study include the support that members can give each other and learning from others in the group. Also many minds working together are stronger than one working alone. Weak points of group study include a lack of preparation of some group members, weaker members of the group holding the rest back, and a tendency of the group to focus on topics that have more to do with socialization than review. Candidates using study groups should insist on members coming to sessions prepared to work.

◆ *Decide what materials or resources will be used during review.* Textbooks and class notes from nursing or nursing-related courses, such as anatomy and physiology, psychology, or nutrition, are helpful. Computer-assisted instructions used during the nursing program may be available. Numerous NCLEX-RN exam review books are available (prices range from around $20 to $50). Many review books include a computer disk or CD to be used during review. Make sure that these computer aids are compatible with the type of computer you will be using during review.

◆ *Structure review time.* Schedule review during times of peak performance. Learning is enhanced when reviewing for short blocks of time, around 50 minutes, instead of reviewing for several unbroken hours at a time. Candidates should remember that they are reviewing for an examination, not cramming for one.

◆ *Control the review environment.* Keep noise and distraction at a minimum. Have adequate space and lighting for review. Control the room temperature when possible; if not possible, dress for the environment. Have all materials needed for review, including soft drinks and snacks, close at hand so that time is not wasted gathering these items during review time. Make sure that friends and family know not to interrupt during review time.

◆ *Have a game plan for each review session.* Develop a review schedule complete with subject matter to be considered and specific tasks to be completed during each session. Stick to the schedule.

◆ *Learn concepts and principles, not isolated facts.* The NCLEX-RN examination tests a candidate's ability to apply, analyze, and evaluate nursing knowledge and does not focus on isolated events. Candidates whose past test-taking success has been based on memorization rather than actual learning have an increased risk for failure on the NCLEX-RN examination.

◆ *Use learning techniques that have proven successful in the past.* Students have different learning styles and therefore benefit from different learning techniques. Students might choose to use flash cards or note cards, underscore key points, take notes or outline material, or capture pertinent information on a tape recorder for later playback. Students should quiz themselves or ask others to pose questions.

◆ *Seek qualified help when reviewing information that is particularly difficult.* Faculty members are an excellent resource. Be cautious when asking peers for assistance because they may not understand the material as well as they think they do.

◆ *Practice taking NCLEX-type examinations, paying particular attention to the rationales or reasons provided for correct and incorrect answers.* Successful test takers know why a specific option is correct or incorrect. Even though candidates may spend as much time as they

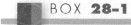

BOX **28-1**

Helpful Websites for the NCLEX-RN Examination

National Council of State Boards of Nursing
  www.ncsbn.org
NCLEX-RN 2010 Test Plan
  www.ncsbn.org/2010_NCLEX_RN_TestPlan.pdf

NCLEX-RN Course Review
  www.nclexinfo.com

want on a question when actually taking the examination, they should get into the habit of taking about 1 minute for each question. Poor time management may cause a candidate to not have enough time to complete the test and therefore be unsuccessful on the NCLEX-RN examination. Practice also will help reduce test anxiety. NCLEX-type examinations are commonly found in NCLEX-RN exam review books.

◆ *Use the Internet.* It provides numerous sources that may aid in preparation for the NCLEX-RN examination. Box 28-1 provides a partial listing of available sites that might be helpful.

◆ *Avoid excessive stimulants (e.g., caffeine) to increase review time.* The best learning takes place when heads are clear.

◆ *Maintain a healthy, positive attitude toward reviewing and taking the NCLEX-RN examination.* Have confidence in your abilities to be successful on the examination. Remember that even practicing nurses with years of experience do not know everything there is to know about every aspect of nursing and that the goal on the NCLEX-RN examination is to demonstrate minimal competency for an entry-level RN position, not competency for an advanced RN position.

FOOD FOR THOUGHT WHEN SELECTING AN NCLEX-RN REVIEW COURSE

Just as there is no one best method for preparing to take the NCLEX-RN examination, there is no one best review course for a candidate to take in preparation for the NCLEX-RN examination. The most important thing to remember is that a review course is exactly what it says it is—a review course. Such courses are designed to reconsider or reexamine content common to the three types of nursing programs.

The purpose of a review course is to enhance or polish what candidates already know from their nursing programs. Review courses are not intended to teach totally new concepts. If candidates have an extreme weakness in one or more content areas, the review course may not provide enough content to bring the candidate up to speed on the topic.

Numerous companies and people offer review courses. Each review offering has strong and weak points, and what appeals to one candidate may not appeal to another. Some offer financial discounts or other incentives if more than one candidate from a school of nursing registers for their course.

Review courses usually are expensive and last from 1 or 2 days to a complete workweek. Some courses provide books, CDs, or other written materials. Others may offer additional materials for a fee. Some courses will refund a part or all of the cost of the review if a candidate takes their review course and is unsuccessful in taking the NCLEX-RN examination.

Review courses may or may not be taught by competent people. Nurse educators who are teaching faculty at schools of nursing teach many review courses. However, people with no substantial background in nursing may teach some courses. A review course is no better than the person or people teaching it.

The decision to take a review course in preparation for taking the NCLEX-RN examination is a personal one. Some candidates find the structure and schedule of a review course helpful in preparation. Other candidates may find the structure and schedule restrictive and overly time-consuming.

Candidates seriously interested in taking an NCLEX-RN exam review course should look to the faculty at their school of nursing for guidance. Many faculty have had experience with review courses or may teach review courses. Candidates should also talk to peers who have recently graduated about recommendations for review courses. Serious candidates also should obtain written information from several different review course offerings and compare and contrast among the offerings. Selection of a review course should be based on more than the cost of the review program—it should meet the candidate's unique needs.

SUMMARY

Success on the NCLEX-RN examination is needed to obtain a license and practice as an RN. Most candidates taking the NCLEX-RN examination are successful. Of the 66,531 first-time, U.S.-educated candidates taking the examination during the first two quarters of 2009, approximately 89.52% were successful (NCLEX-RN results, 2009). The key to success on the NCLEX-RN examination is sound preparation from the nursing program, adequate preparation for the examination, and confidence in oneself.

 ⓔvolve Additional resources are available online at: http://evolve.elsevier.com/Cherry/

REFERENCES

American Nurses Association (ANA): *Nursing classification ii. Definition and criteria for classification*, 1999. Retrieved October 2009 from: www.nursingworld.org/mods/archive/mod30/cec25.htm.

Anderson LW, Krathwohl DR, editors: *A taxonomy for learning, teaching, and assessing: A revision of Bloom's taxonomy of educational objectives*, New York, 2001, Addison-Wesley Longman.

Bloom BS, Englehart MD, Furst EJ: *Taxonomy of educational objectives: the classification of educational goals. Handbook I. Cognitive domain*, New York, 1956, David McKay.

Cox HC, et al: *Clinical applications of nursing diagnosis: adult, child, women's, psychiatric, gerontic, and home health considerations*, ed 5, Philadelphia, 2007, FA Davis.

Foote J: *State board questions and answers for nurses*, Philadelphia, 1919, JB Lippincott.

National Council of State Boards of Nursing (NCSBN): *NCLEX-RN® examination test plan for the National Council Licensure Examination for Registered Nurses*. Retrieved October 2009 from: www.ncsbn.org/2010_NCLEX_RN_TestPlan.pdf.

Index

Page numbers followed by f, t, or b indicate figures, tables, or boxes, respectively.